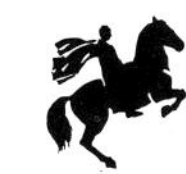

Nikolai N. Korpan (ed.)

Basics of Cryosurgery

SpringerWienNewYork

Nikolai N. Korpan, MD, PhD
Professor of Surgery,
Vienna International Institute
for Cryosurgery
Department of Surgery, Evangelical
Hospital Vienna-Waehring
Vienna, Austria

Active Membership in national, European and international societies: Austrian Society of Surgery, Ukrainian Society of Surgery, Swiss Society of Surgery, European Society for Clinical Investigation, Co-founder and Board Member of the European Society of Cryosurgery, Alumni Gold Club, European School of Oncology, Arbeitsgruppe 'Kryochirurgie-Deutschland', International Society of Cryosurgery, International College of Surgeons, International Society of Surgery, International College of Angiology, The New York Academy of Sciences, The American Association for the Advancement of Science, Founder and Head of the Vienna International Institute for Cryosurgery, Founder and President of the International Association of Inventors 'Perpetuus', Vice President of the European Society of Cryosurgery.

Printed in Slovenia

Typesetting: Scientific Publishing Services (P) Ltd., Madras
Printing: Gorenjski Tisk, Kranj

Printed on acid-free and chlorine-free bleached paper

SPIN: 10760709

With mostly color figures and illustrations

CIP data applied for

ISBN 3-211-83701-9 Springer-Verlag Wien York

Dedication

'Fiat lux!'
'Dum spiro, spero'

This unique basic publication in the field of modern cryosurgery at the begin of the third millennium is dedicated to surgeons and indeed to all doctors and specialists throughout the world, especially to those in oncology, cryosurgery and cryotechnology, who in their devotion to the service of medical science are helping patients in the fight against malignant tumors.

I would like also more specifically to dedicate this book to those in Austria, my second home, who, on my second start as a doctor and surgeon, had confidence in my professional and scientific abilities and who have over the years continued to give me their friendship and support.

Further, I would like to express my deep appreciation to all of my colleagues, the nurses, secretaries, administration, and patients in the Vienna hospitals, especially the Evangelical Hospital in Waehring, who have in one way or the other contributed to this book.

Nikolai N. Korpan

Foreword by Jose Carlos d'Almeida Gonçalves

Cryosurgery is an elegant method that has become an important branch of surgery in many medical specialities as a result of the progress made in understanding its pathophysiology and in improving its practical applications. In fact, the cryosurgical approach has been used empirically for millennia but only in the second half of the last century was it investigated on a scientific basis. Since then it has attained a high level of precision and fine adjustment to the meticulous procedures required by modern surgery. Over the last four decades, it has become an important, widespread and indispensable method of treatment that gives excellent results, equivalent to and often better than, other surgical modalities.

In the past, there was a definite distinction between medical and surgical specialities and many of these, such as pneumology, hepatology and dermatology, were exclusively medical. In recent times, the boundaries between the two have been fading away. The dynamic evolution in the knowledge and practice of medical specialties forced their practitioners to broaden their activities to most surgical aspects of their patients' diseases. Modern cryosurgery provided one of the answers to this need. For certain areas of treatment, it is a method that, when correctly learned, can be properly performed even by physicians who are not especially inclined to surgical activity.

Over the last few decades technical advances have led to the appearance of new and frequently expensive apparatuses in other therapeutic modalities, some of which excited the enthusiasm of young physicians. Despite such competition, supported by strong lobbies, cryosurgery remains an indispensable method in many specialities. When indicated, it can replace other surgical treatments for many pathological conditions, with at least equivalent results but, in most cases, with considerable advantages. Some notoriously intractable conditions that were insoluble, like multiple metastases of the liver, inoperable bronchial carcinoma and external advanced cancers, can now be treated cryosurgically, always with great palliative relief, and even leading, in a considerable number of cases, to actual cure. Among the important advantages of cryosurgery that should be stressed are that it has fewer complications than other surgical techniques and permits the treatment of frail and elderly patients for whom conventional surgery is not indicated or presents risks. Physicians not acquainted with cryosurgery may fear frequent infections resulting from cryogenic necrosis. However, these are extremely rare, even for internal tumors or bulky external cancers.

In dermatology, one of the fields in which cryosurgery is more frequently used, this form of treatment has many advantages: its results are at least as good, and many times better, than those of other modalities; generally, it is less time consuming and less expensive than other treatments; most treatments can be performed in an outpatient clinic. Unfortunately, some young physicians - especially dermatologists - are misled by the apparent simplicity of the cryosurgical technique in treating small lesions and have a tendency to slight the rigor of the surgical protocol. They are surprised when their results are worse than those reported internationally, and attribute their failure to the method, instead of recognizing the limits of their skills or technical knowledge. It must be stressed that, even for small skin or mucosal lesions, the cryosurgical protocol must be as carefully observed as that of any other surgical method. No one would risk performing conventional surgery without adequate study and training. The same applies to cryosurgery.

Modern cryosurgery had its beginnings in the 1960s, expanded and progressed thereafter, having become, in the meanwhile, a precise therapeutic tool. The neurosurgeon Irving S. Cooper was the pioneer researcher who, in the '60's, devised a sophisticated apparatus to freeze part of the basal ganglia in order to improve symptoms of some neurological diseases. His work awakened the interest of physicians in other specialities who, in the years following, adapted cryosurgery to their own fields of activity and created adequate instrumentation. The late dermatologist Setrag A. Zacarian was one of the first to understand the value of cryosurgery and became an enthusiastic practitioner and researcher. He had a wonderful, open personality and contributed to spreading interest in cryosurgery both in his own specialty and in others. He studied its application to skin lesions (benign and malignant) and published his first book on the subject in 1969. Later, he edited several books (1973, 1977, 1985) with the collaboration of other physicians, many of whom were not dermatologists. Because of his competence, enthusiasm and the ease with which he related to other people, his books and excellent papers had a considerable impact in the medical community and contributed strongly to promoting interest in the advantages and possibilities of the method. Over the following years the practice of cryosurgery developed, first in the USA and Italy and, then, world-wide. I believe that, at present, it is extensively used in China and Eastern Europe, but my information on cryosurgical activity in these countries is sparse, due to difficulties in communication.

William G. Cahan was the first surgeon to understand the possibilities and advantages of cryosurgery in the treatment of advanced cancer of the skin and breast, and did invaluable pioneering work in this field, also in the 1960s. This was developed further in subsequent years, particularly in Argentina, Portugal and Japan. In the latter country, Shigeo Tanaka performed over 50 cryomastectomies on advanced inoperable breast cancer, the largest number ever that had such excellent results. It has been demonstrated that, in addition to being an excellent palliative treatment, cryosurgery can cure many advanced malignancies that are beyond the limits of other therapeutic modalities.

The first International Congress of Cryosurgery was held in Vienna, Austria, in 1971. Three years later the International Society of Cryosurgery was founded during the Second International Congress, in Torino, Italy. Dr. Giovanni Sesia – whose contribution to the cryosurgical treatment of prostatic cancer constituted a remarkable advance in this area – was the first elected president. Since then, international congresses have taken place every three years, which has contributed greatly to maintaining interest in and enthusiasm for cryosurgery and to disseminating the knowledge of its ongoing advances. In the meantime, cryosurgery has successfully spread to other specialties.

Coinciding with the rise of cryosurgery, a new field of science was born, cryobiology, which studies the effects of subzero temperatures on biological systems. Cryobiology has undergone spectacular progress and has developed in two practical directions: one, to improve the understanding of the pathophysiology of cryodestruction of cells and tissues, and the other, to create techniques of cryopreservation of living cells, tissues and organs. Its importance is increasing continuously and it has become an important section of science in general and of medicine in particular, as well as an indispensable basis for bio-industry. To achieve efficient cryosurgical treatment it is indispensable to have a good grasp of cryobiology as a basis for a clear understanding of the pathophysiology of cryonecrosis. This is why it constitutes an important part of this book.

The discovery of immunogenic effects, with cure or regression of metastases of prostate cancer after cryosurgery, led to a hope of similar results in other fields of oncology, which, until now, has been only partially fulfilled. Experimental work in rodents with tumors induced by viral and chemical agents proved the existence of cryoimmunology in these animals. Similarly, the positive effects of cryosurgery in the treatment of cutaneous melanoma were clinically known, but Breitbart, and Weyer and collaborators succeeded in proving their existence in the laboratory.

Cryosurgery is an alternative choice for the treatment of selected patients with internal tumors. I. S. Cooper, as long ago as 1963, suggested the use of cryosurgery for the destruction of primary and metastatic tumors of the liver, because cryosurgery has several well-known advantages over classic surgery: 1) it is effective in inducing tumor cell necrosis; 2) it spares more normal tissue than resection, with less risk of hemorrhage and dissemination of cancer cells; 3) it makes the treatment of unresectable tumors possible, particularly those involving large vessels; 4) it allows retreatment; 5) it may induce an immunostimulating effect against residual cancer.

In a further important development, J.-P. Homasson and M. O. Maiwand devised adequate cryosurgical techniques to treat bronchial carcinoma. The cryosurgical treatment of prostatic cancer is currently a commonly used technique world-wide. The efficacy of hepatic cryosurgery was supported by animal experiments and clinical evidence in a limited number of patients. Xin-Da Zhou reported in 1988 the cryosurgical treatment of 60 patients with primary liver cancer. He asserted that cryosurgery was the treatment of choice for unresectable primary liver cancer when the whole tumor mass can be frozen in patients without hepatic failure. This assertion was confirmed by Nikolai N. Korpan in a long-term, prospective randomized clinical trial between 1985 and 1997. He concluded that hepatic cryosurgery is a safe and effective modality for the treatment of liver metastases, with results at least comparable to those of conventional surgery.

To my knowledge, no important books have been published on cryosurgery in the English language over the last decade. The last ones were published in 1990: one by E. G. Kuflik and A. A. Gage and the other edited by E. W. Breitbart and Elzbièta Dachów-Siwiéc, both on the cryosurgery of skin lesions. Therefore, an updated and comprehensive textbook was greatly needed.

We should be grateful to Professor Dr. Nikolai N. Korpan, the Editor of this book, for filling this lacuna. When he invited me to collaborate on this book we had never met. We became acquainted during a General Meeting of the Board of Directors of the European Society of Cryosurgery; I was very impressed with his intelligence, energy and determination. He is an innovative researcher, a scientist and a therapist, with a good sense of leadership. Professor Korpan has dedicated himself especially to the study of the surgical treatment of the liver, bile ducts and pancreas, has published many papers and is the author of three books. Co-founder in 1997 and vice president of the European Society of Cryosurgery, he is also founder and president of the Vienna International Institute for Cryosurgery. Also an inventor, he has devised 31 patents, some of which are for cryoprobes that guarantee an even and persistent temperature, something current cryoprobes fail to do. I think that Professor Korpan is the right person to edit this book.

This book is designed to be of practical use, being aimed at those already trained in cryosurgery who want to improve their knowledge and skills. Other goals are to stimulate the interest of and offer a scientific basis to those who are not yet familiar with this important mode of therapy. The Editor was therefore committed to producing a clear, comprehensive and lavishly illustrated textbook.

Considerable attention was devoted in this book to the biology of cryodestruction and to practical procedures in the various modalities of cryosurgical treatment, which are meticulously described, as well as to their advantages, disadvantages, limitations and complications. This book received contributions from outstanding international specialists. Contributors resisted the temptation to write long reviews and strove to write clear and practical essays. The reader will find some overlap in texts written by different authors, but this has the advantage of offering distinct views on certain topics, which tends to be highly enlightening.

A comprehensive compendium of theoretical, experimental and clinical data reflecting the dynamic evolution of cryosurgery, this book constitutes a challenge to those who want either to improve their skills or to acquire an important new technique for improved treatment of their patients.

Jose Carlos d'Almeida Gonçalves JS, MD
President of the International Society of Cryosurgery
Head, Department of Dermatology
District Hospital of Santarem, Portuguese Institute of Oncology
Portugal

Editor's Preface

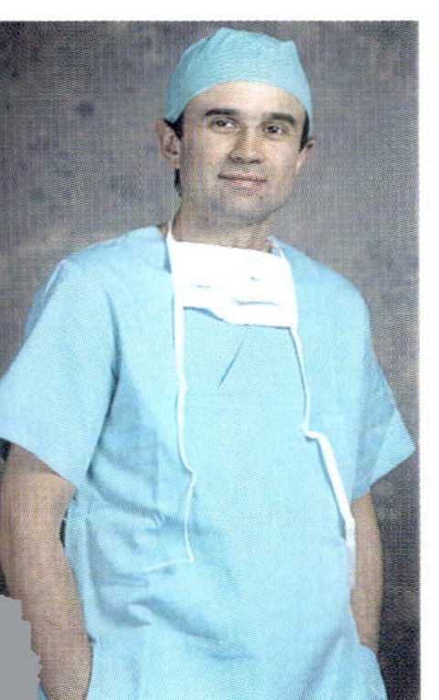

Ars longa, vita brevis est,
Hippocrates (ca. 460-377BC)

This book on the basic aspects of modern cryosurgery is the first on the subject to appear at the start of the third millennium. It aims to be an important contribution to the further development of this branch of medicine and to its future indispensability.

"Basics of Cryosurgery" is a unique contribution in that no book previously has concentrated in one source the available scientific data on the numerous theoretical, experimental and clinical investigations that have been performed in the field of cryosurgery. The chapters are written by well-known authorities in the field of cryosurgery who have not only seen the triumphs but have learned to avoid the pitfalls of their endeavours and have helped many patients escape what was thought to be an unavoidable fate. I admire their wisdom and skill and thank them for their willingness to share their experiences.

This work is offered as a basis for the further development of the cryosurgical approach. The book is also directed to practising surgeons, oncologists, dermatologists, urologists, thoracic and orthopedic surgeons, proctologists, gynecologists, pulmonologists, plastic surgeons, otorhinolaryngologists, as well as to medical residents. Further, the book is recommended to engineers, scientists and all who are interested in modern surgical oncology, especially oncological cryosurgery, as well as in the development of twenty-first century cryotechnology.

The intent of this book is to cover the entire field of cryosurgery. Included are chapters on such special topics as cryochemotherapy and experimental cryoimmunology on animals, including histopathological studies and assays of organ function, in addition to clinical evidence. The book is organized into a general section pertinent to all of cryosurgery followed by chapters dealing with specific operative areas of modern cryosurgery.

A special feature of this book is its emphasis on indications and contraindications for cryosurgery, advantages, side-effects and disadvantages, pre- and post-operative imaging of cryosurgery, and different kinds of radical and palliative cryosurgical treatment of benign and malignant tumors.

I am greatly indebted to all those who have contributed to this work, whether with advice, color illustrations or design. My thanks to each of them for a job well done!

Prof. Dr. Nikolai N. Korpan
Vienna, Austria

List of Contributors

Boris I. Alperovich, M.D., Dr.Med.Sc.

Professor of Surgery
Siberia Medical University
Department of General Surgery
Tomsk
Russia

Joao A. Amaro, M.D.

Department of Dermatology
District Hospital of Santarem
Lisbon
Portugal

M. Angebault, M.D.

Centre Hospitalier Specialise en Pneumologie
Chevilly-Larue Cedex
France

Duke K. Bahn, M.D.

Chairman, Department of Radiology
Hospital in Rochester, Prostate Center
Michigan
USA

Franz Beer, M.D.

Pathologisch-Bakteriologisch-Humangenetisches Institut
SMZO-Donauspital
Vienna
Austria

Jacob Bickels, M.D.

Department of Orthopaedic Oncology
Tel-Aviv Sourasky Medical Center
Tel-Aviv
Israel

Douglas O. Chinn, M.D.

Urology and Cryosurgery
Chinn Urology Medical Group, Inc.
Arcadia
USA

Rodney P. R. Dawber, M.A., M.B., Ch.B., F.R.C.P.

Consultant Dermatologist
Oxford Hospitals and
Clinical Lecturer in Dermatology
University of Oxford
U.K.

M. Gipponi, M.D.

National Institute for Cancer Research
Division of Surgical Oncology
Genoa
Italy

Jose Carlos d'Almeida Gonçalves, M.D.

President of the International Society of Cryosurgery
Head, Department of Dermatology
District Hospital of Santarem
Portuguese Institute of Oncology
Lisbon
Portugal

Gerhard Hochwarter, M.D.

Consultant General Surgery
Department of Surgery
SMZ-Ost Donauspital
Vienna
Austria

Jean-Paul Homasson, M.D.

Past-President of the International and European Society of Cryosurgery
Medical Chief, Centre Hospitalier Specialise en Pneumologie
Chevilly-Larue Cedex
France

Yoshiaki Hosaka, M.D.

Professor and Chairman
Department of Plastic and Reconstructive Surgery
Showa University Medical School
Tokyo
Japan

Shigeo Ikeda, M.D.

Department of Dermatology
Saitama Medical School
Saitama
Japan

Shuichi Ikekawa, M.D.

Department of Dermatology
National Cancer Center Hospital
Tokyo
Japan

Kazuyuki Ishihara, M.D.

Department of Dermatology
National Cancer Center Hospital
Tokyo
Japan

Thomas B. Julian, M.D.

Division of Surgical Oncology
Allegheny General Hospital
Pittsburg
USA

Irina R. Khramova, M.D.

Department of Dermatology with Cosmetology
Orenburg State Hospital
Orenburg
Russia

Tatjana B. Komkova, M.D., Dr.Med.Sc.

Professor of Surgery
Siberia Medical University
Department of General Surgery
Tomsk
Russia

Nikolai N. Korpan, M.D., Ph.D., F.I.S.S., F.I.C.S.

Professor of Surgery
Head, Vienna International Institute for Cryosurgery
Department of Surgery
Evangelical Hospital Vienna-Waehring
Vienna
Austria

Calvin H.L. Law, M.D., F.R.C.S.C.

McMaster University
Department of Surgery
St. Joseph's Hospital
Surgical Oncology
Hepatobiliary and Pancreatic Surgery
Minimally Invasive Surgery
Hamilton, Ontario
Canada

Omar Maiwand, M.D.

President of the European Society of Cryosurgery
Vice President and Co Chairman of the International Society of Cryosurgery
Consultant Thoracic Surgeon
Royal Brompton & Harefield NHS Trust
Harefield Hospital, Hill End Road
Harefield
Middlesex
U.K.

G. Margarino, M.D.

National Institute for Cancer Research
Division of Surgical Oncology
Genoa
Italy

P. Mereu, M.D.

National Institute for Cancer Research
Division of Surgical Oncology
Genoa
Italy

Cecília Moura, M.D.

Department of Dermatology
District Hospital of Santarem
Lisbon
Portugal

Peter Nordin, M.D.

Läkarhuset Göteborg
Göteborg
Sweden

Peter Olson, M.D.

Department of Pathology and Laboratory Medicine

Allegheny General Hospital
Pittsburg
USA

Yoed Rabin, D.Sc.

Associate Professor
Department of Mechanical Engineering
Carnegie Mellon University
Pittsburg
USA

Daniel Luna Sabate, M.D.

Vice President of the European Society of Cryosurgery
Thoracic Medicine
Hospital N.S.Aranzazu
San-Sebastian
Spain

Marco Scala, M.D.

National Institute for Cancer Research
Division of Surgical Oncology
Genoa
Italy

H.W. Bart Schreuder, M.D., Ph.D.

Orthopaedic Surgeon
Department of Orthopaedics
University Medical Center St. Radboud
Nijmegen
The Netherlands

Franz Sellner, M.D.

Associate Professor of Surgery
Department of Surgery
Kaiser-Franz-Josef-Spital
Vienna
Austria

Shigeo Tanaka, M.D.

Tanaka Clinic
Obusemachi, Nagano
Japan

Ved R. Tandan, M.D., M.Sc., F.R.C.S.C., F.A.C.S.

Assistant Professor
McMaster University
Department of Surgery
St. Joseph's Hospital
Surgical Oncology
Hepatobiliary and Pancreatic Surgery
Minimally Invasive Surgery
Hamilton, Ontario
Canada

Iwan S. Tchekman, M.D., Dr.Med.Sc.

Professor of Pharmacology
Head, Chair of General and Clinical Pharmacology
National Medical University of Kyiv
Kyiv
Ukraine

Wilson S. Wong, M.D.

Cryosurgical Center of Southern California
Alhambra Hospital
USA

Jaroslav V. Zharkov, Dipl. Eng., Designer

Director
Cryosurgical Industrial Research Institute 'Pulse'
Kyiv
Ukraine

Christos C. Zouboulis, M.D.

Professor of Dermatology
Department of Dermatology
University Medical Center Benjamin Franklin
The Free University of Berlin
Germany

Contents

Part I

Basic Principles of Cryosurgery

1. Cryosurgery in the 21st Century

Nikolai N. Korpan

1.1 Introduction

If the cautery was for hundreds of years an indispensible tool for the physician – and is today used only for hemostasis or the removal of the smallest skin tumors, and in veterinary medicine – so today cryosurgery provides results as effective but at far lower risk.

"Cold surgery" is at the start of a path that promises to lead a very long way.

Disease statistics of recent decades reveal the increasing frequency of cancer 'and cancer deaths, and this in spite of exorbitantly risen expenditures for diagnostics and therapy (major equipment, intensive care, etc.). The situation has by no means improved in recent years and the treatment modes are still of limited effectiveness.

A new way of thinking must determine the future of cancer research and treatment. We need new approaches to new discoveries and new therapies.

Modern cryosurgery, which is a particularly sparing surgical technique, is today internationally respected and gaining ground. Long years of practical experience and numerous internationally published papers have provided evidence of the good results obtained with this method. At the same time it has become clear that the best use of this method has only become possible through the development of efficient medico-technical devices.

The theoretical, experimental and clinical knowledge that has been gathered throughout the world is making it possible to successfully treat various kinds of benign and malignant tumors in different specialties. In Austria, modern cryosurgery has been in use since 1996. The "cold stream" ("white surgery") method has successfully been integrated into the field of surgery. Many patients who faced a seemingly inevitable fate have been helped with this method. Since then more than 2000 patients have received cryosurgical treatment, either in targeted tissue or an entire organ, both on an in-patient and an out-patient basis (Fig. 1.1.A–1.1.H).

Patients who have undergone cryosurgery with excellent results are often happy to talk about their experiences (Fig. 1.2.A–1.2.B).

The most extraordinary successes have been achieved with "cold surgery". For many cancer patients it borders on the miraculous. Not only did they regain their previous quality of life and thus also their will to live, most important of all they were also pain free. They did not require general anesthesia and were either outpatients or very briefly inpatients. This new surgical technique offers the patient a number of advantages. With the use of a high tech system, the pathological tissue that is embedded in healthy tissue is destroyed with a precisely targeted ray of cold in a temperature range of −170°C to −196°C. The treated tissue is turned to ice, so to speak. In consequence, and in contrast to traditional methods, there is no bleeding or blood loss. Every cancer cell – the entire tumor mass – is deep frozen and destroyed, which prevents the further growth of the cancer and – most importantly – the development of metastases. The use of the cryomethod usually does not require general anesthesia, the duration of surgery is short, there is no or only minimal scar formation and thus the cosmetic results are excellent. As simple as the technique seems, it is just as important to have the necessary specialized know-how. The proper regulation of the freezing process (formation of the cryozone – aseptic necroses), the extent and depth of the freeze, the correct dose of cold, the appropriate number of treatment cycles and the correct duration of application – all require clinical and experimental knowledge.

The essense of cold surgery is the destruction and removal of only pathological changes, both on the surface as well as within tissue (skin, mucosa). In surgery on inner organs (liver, pancreas, etc.), cryosurgery is combined with conventional surgical techniques.

The reliable destruction of tumors requires the use of high-tech medical devices. Among these state-of-the-art devices are the new generation of cryoinstruments produced by the industrial company 'Pulse' (Kiev, Ukraine).

1.2 What is Cryosurgery?

Cryo-, freeze- or cold-surgery is the operative cutting of tissue or the targeted destruction of pathological tissue by induced cold necrosis at temperatures down to −196°C. Tumors are usually not excised but shock-frozen. In these cases vacuum-isolated cryoinstruments (cryoprobes, cryoscalpels, cryoclamps) are used. These instruments are cooled to −170°C to −196°C by the evaporation of liquid nitrogen.

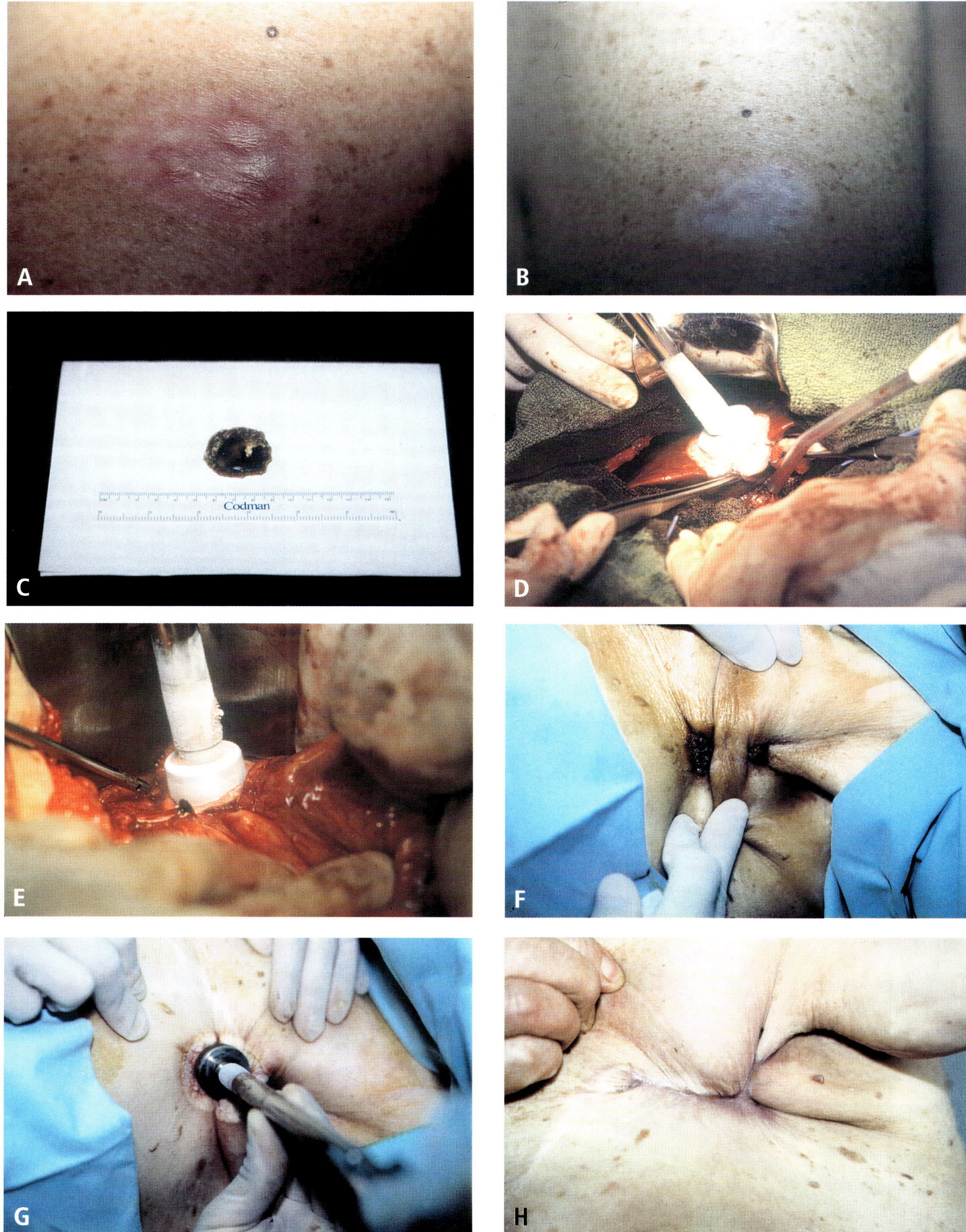
A
B
C
Codman
D
E
F
G
H

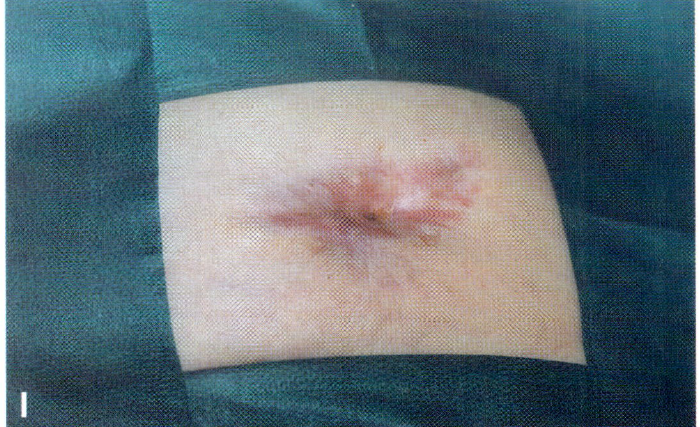

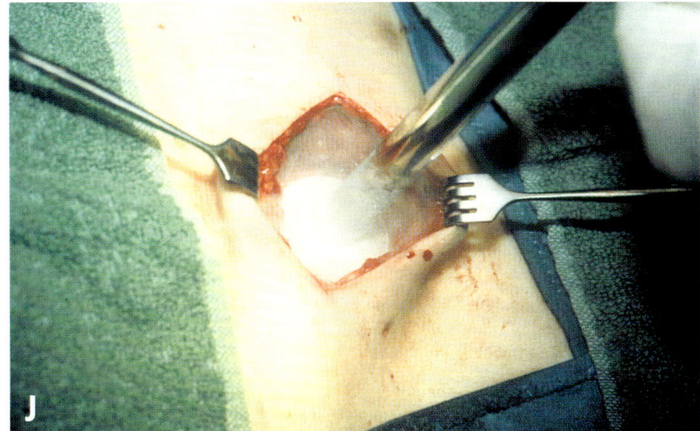

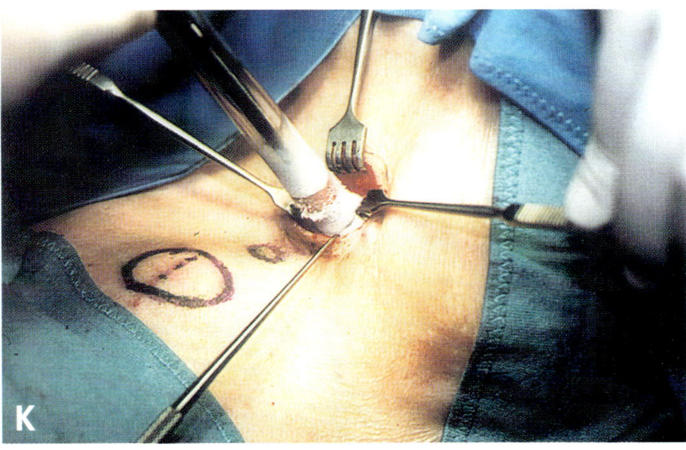

Fig. 1.1.I–K. Patient with ulcerated cancer on the right breast: 1 year after cryosurgical operation with local anesthesia; no recurrence (**I**). Patient with primary breast cancer: view of the subcutaneous cryosurgical operation (**J**). Patient with lymph node metastases: subcutaneous double freeze-thaw cycle at a temperature of −180°C for 3 min each freeze (**K**).

The prerequisites for the art of cryosurgery include not only long experience in the use of the instruments but also experimental and clinical knowledge. In the last 15 years, Dr. Nikolai N. Korpan and his colleages in co-operation with engineer Jaroslav V. Zharkov have developed and refined new cryosurgical techniques for operative procedures in patients with liver and pancreas tumors, breast cancer, lymph node metastases, and recurrent skin cancer (Korpan et al. 1985, 1987, 1996, 1997, 2000).

Cryosurgery is established in medical practice both as a single technique as well as supplementary to other oncological treatments. The development of the cryocautery (on the Cooper principle), which makes the destruction of large areas of tissue by extreme hypothermia possible, was the technical prerequisite for a cryosurgical method applicable in general surgery. However, the reliable destruction of tumors requires the use of high-performance devices. The new generation of high-technology cryodevices produced, for example, by 'Pulse' make the use of modern cryosurgery in different areas of medicine possible.

1.3 Main Mechanisms of Action

Numerous theoretical and experimental studies *in vitro* and *in vivo* have been carried out to understand the action of low temperatures on tissue (1–5). It has been determined that the processes of ice crystallization are here of primary importance (6). Current opinion holds that one of the most important elements contributing to the action of subzero cold is intracellular ice formation, which damages the delicate cell structures (7). Also important in cryoactivity is the formation of extracellular ice, which is followed by cell and tissue

Fig. 1.1.A–H. Patient with recurrent basal cell carcinoma (BCC) on the right upper arm. Excellent results one (**A**) and two (**B**) years after cryosurgical operation. Crust has fall off 5 weeks after cryosurgical procedure (**C**). Patients with liver and pancreas tumor: intraoperative view of the liver metastasis (**D**) and pancreas head carcinoma (**E**) during the double cryosurgical session. Patient with local recurrence after breast ablation of left side: pre- (**F**) and intraoperative (**G**) view of the percutaneous cryosurgical operation with local anesthesia. The patient has been disease-free for 4 years (**E**).

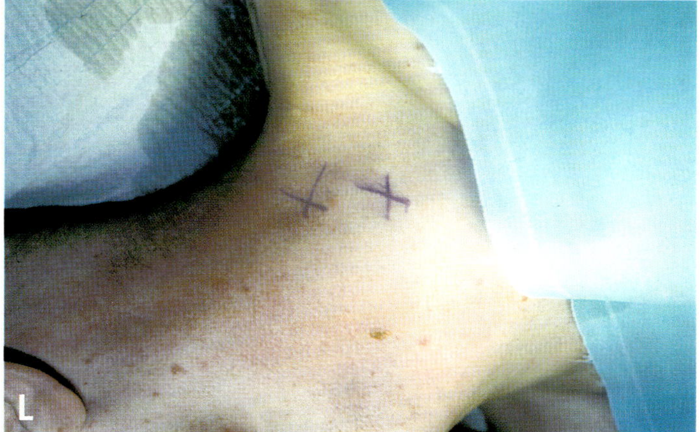

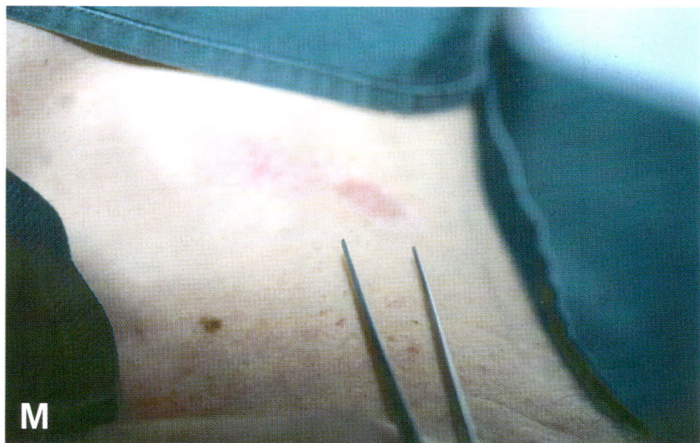

Fig. 1.1.L–M. Patient with lymph node metastases: location of the lymph node metastases marked preoperatively (**L**). The same patient: view of the wound healing process 4 weeks after percutaneous cryosurgical operation (**M**).

dehydration as well as protein denaturation and rupture of the cell membranes. But the major effect on cell damage and cell destruction in cryoactivity is exerted by the speed of freezing and of thawing of the tissue (8).

The macroscopic picture resulting from the influence of cold on different organs is almost always identical (8,9). At first one notices a mild hyperemia. This is followed by a hint of a change in color of the tissue to livid, after which a snow-white area of solid ice builds around the cryoprobe, which expands as the temperature sinks and the effect of the action of cold increases. Then the ice formation decelerates and finally ceases at –196°C. After thawing, the tissue has regained its original color and consistency. In the hours immediately following, the area of focus swells up with edema, and after 3–4 days a completely necrosed focus with a discolored gray surface has formed.

Several days later the process of regeneration begins with the sloughing off of the necrotic tissue. After about 4 weeks the deep necrotic crater is entirely replaced by course granulation tissue.

Microscopically the picture is similar. Total cell dissociation with interstitial bleeding can be seen – a hemorrhagic infarction immediately followed by the formation of an unstructured, homogeneous mass, i.e., a coagulation necrosis. With the sloughing off of the necrotic mass, a seam of fibroblasts appears in the border foci that intitiates regeneration absent of leucocytic infiltration (aseptic necroses). Finally a hypocellular stoma rich in connective tissue fibers forms.

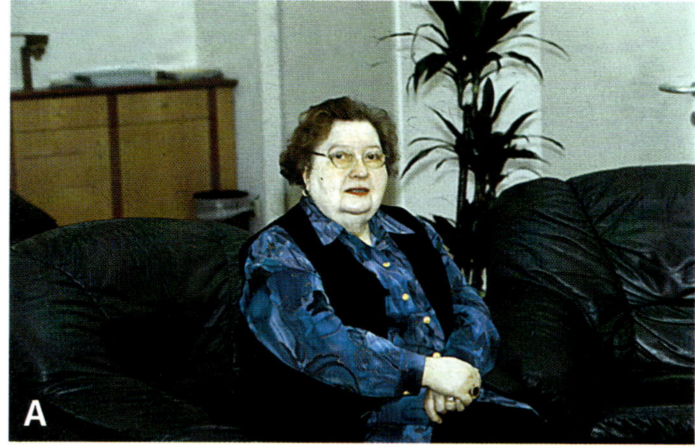

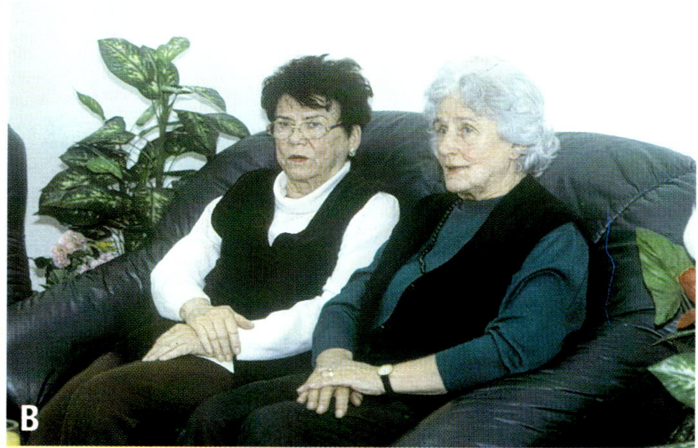

Fig. 1.2.A–B. Patient with breast cancer in advanced stage: about 1 year after cryosurgical operation there is no evidence of recurrence of disease in the breast; the patient is in good health (**A**). Excellent curative and cosmetic results after cryosurgical operation about 2 years after cryosurgery in patient with recurrent basal cell carcinoma (BCC) on the femur (**B**, patient left) and about 3 years after cryosurgery in patient with recurrent BCC on the lower lip (**B**, patient right).

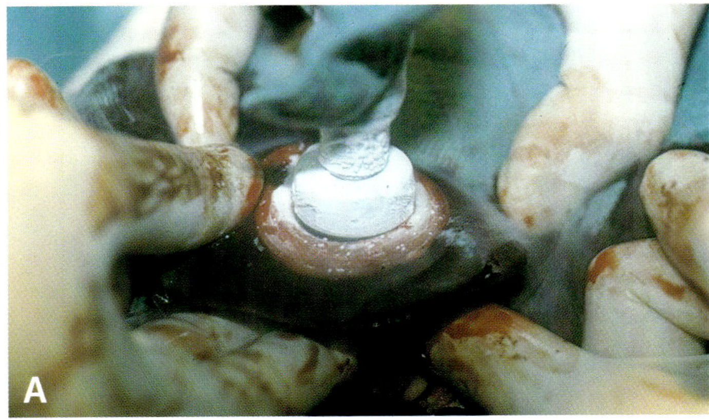

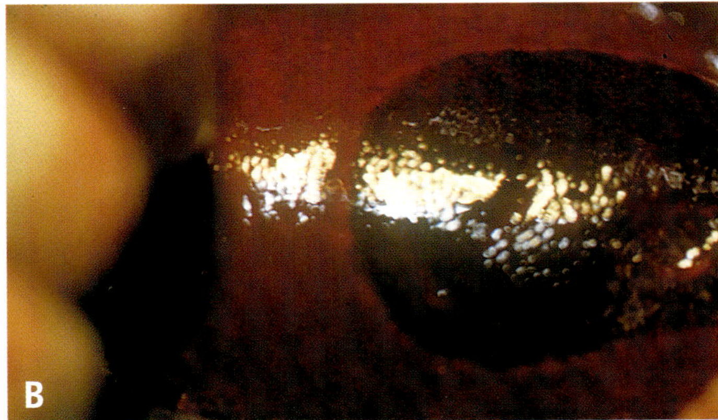

Fig. 1.3.A–B. An animal experiment. View of cryosurgical operation on the liver with the sharp demarcation line during cryosurgery (**A**) and thawed post-cryosurgical lesion (**B**)

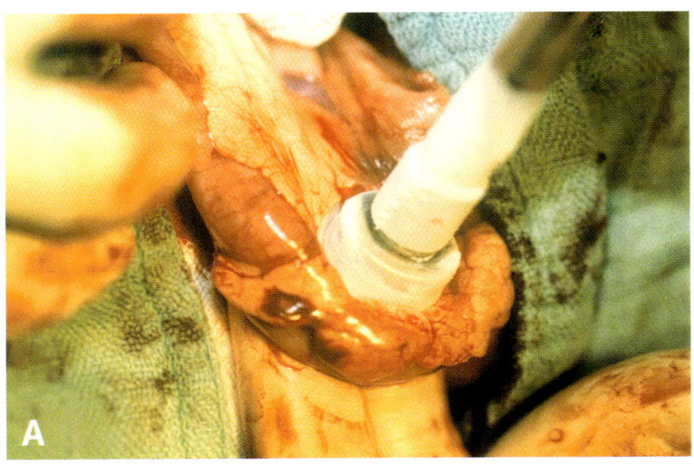

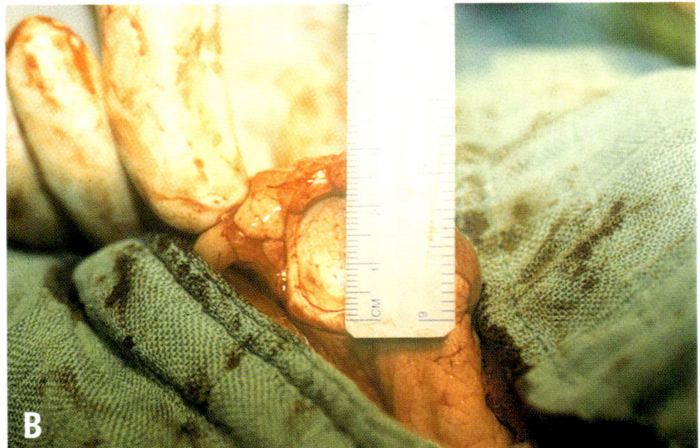

Fig. 1.4.A–B. An animal experiment. View of cryosurgical operation on the pancreas with sharp demarcation line during single freeze-thaw cycle (**A**). The post-cryosurgical zone is clearly defined by a demarcation line (**B**)

Under the electron microscope, swelling of the mitochondria, fragmentation of the plasma membranes, and thickening of the nuclei can be seen.

Our own experimental studies in the animal model on dog livers showed that the cryodestruction zone of the liver parenchyma had a sharp, well defined line of demarcation with clearly discernible contours (Fig. 1.3. A–B, Fig. 1.4. A–B). On the fifth postoperative day the liver parenchyma that had been frozen was now a pronounced necrosis of homogeneous substance. In the following weeks, granulation tissue formed. Four weeks later loose connective tissue with numerous blood vessels formed in the cryozone, after 9–10 weeks there was tight connective tissue and after 12 weeks the transformation of the cryozone of the liver parenchyma to connective tissue was complete.

1.4 General Surgical Indications

On the basis of long-term medico-technical experience, the indications for cryosurgery especially in the treatment of cancer have been further defined.

These indications are:

- Benign and malignant skin cancers (papillomas, moles, warts, basaliomas, melanomas, hemangiomas)
- Skin metastases
- Primary and secondary liver, pancreas, and colon cancer
- Operable and inoperable liver metastases, rectal and anal carcinomas
- Primary as well as secondary breast cancer (local recurrence, skin mestastases)

- Lymph node metastases (but not every type)
- Scar and keloid formation including painful and tight scar and keloid formations
- Hemorrhoidal nodules
- Rectal and perianal fistulas
- Varicose ulcers
- Patients at high risk of hemorrhage (patients on Marcoumar or other blood-thinning medications)

The most important areas of medicine in which cryosurgical methods are applied:

- General surgery
- Oncology, including surgery of the breast
- Dermatology
- Urology
- Gynecology
- Ear-nose-throat (ENT)
- Orthopedics
- Neurosurgery
- Plastic (including cosmetic) surgery
- Thorax surgery

Contraindications for cryosurgical interventions are not known at present.

1.5 What are the Latest Developments in Cryosurgery?

- The development of unique state-of-the-art high-performance medico-technical cryoinstruments and devices.
  a) 21 national patents (Austria)
  b) 5 world-wide patents
- The development of new operations
- Innovative cryotechnology with healing cold

1.6 The Advantages to the Patient of Modern Cryosurgery in Comparison to Conventional Surgical Methods

- Short duration of surgery
- Minimal operative and anesthesia trauma
- Surgery without bleeding
- Surgery without the scalpel
- Surgery without scar formation. In external treatment (e.g., facial tumors) scars are largely avoided
- Prevention of metastasis at time of excision of tumor – there is no "cutting"
- Good cosmetic result: no scars
- Surgically uncomplicated results, the high rate of curative success, short hospital stays, lower hospital costs, as well as increased quality of life for the patient
- Anesthesia is usually unnecessary, as the cold itself functions as an anesthetic
- The period of convalescence is a fraction of that usual for stationary hospital admissions
- The resorption of tissue so frozen appears to have a sort of "vaccination" effect, although this effect cannot be scientifically explained to date
- The stationary hospital stay of the patient is significantly shorter than with conventional surgery
- No local complications stemming from the area of surgery
- Quick and technically simple method of tumor removal
- Both benign and malignant tumors are easily extirpated
- Improved subjective state of the patient through palliative cryosurgical methods, lessening of pain (freedom from pain or pain reduction) and fetor, as well as improvement in the general condition of the patient by containment of tumor growth.

1.7 Optimal Cryoparameters

- Optimal freeze speed 300°C/min
- Freeze temperature of −170°C to −196°C
- Spontaneous thawing
- Duration of application

Crash treatment:	10 sec
Short treatment:	1 min
Medium-length treatment:	3 min
Long treatment:	5–7 min, in special cases longer

- Number of sessions: 1–5
- Volume of the cryozone: 1–180 cm^3
- Constancy of temperature at the tip of the probe
- The freeze process should proceed automatically in line with the previously established values

1.8 Cryosurgery Today

The enormous efficiency (performance), the surgically uncomplicated results, the high rate of treatment success, as well as the enhanced quality of life of the patients will doubtless contribute to an upsurge in the use of this method in the near future.

2. Cryosurgery and Cryotechnology – Future Safety in Medicine

Nikolai N. Korpan and Jaroslav V. Zharkov

2.1 Concept of Technical Requirements for Cryosurgical Equipment

One of the crucial factors which have influenced the development of cryosurgery is the standard and the technical competency of cryosurgical devices; i.e., the efficiency of cryosurgery in curative practice first of all depends on the technical proficiency of the cryosurgical devices used to perform cryooperations.

On the basis of our own theoretical, experimental and practical experience, and after examining the work of cryosurgery schools the world over, but also on the basis of our own know-how (21 national patents, including 5 world-wide patents), we have elaborated a concept of modern cryosurgical technology which can be used universally. It is produced by an automated system known as 'Universal Cryosurgical Complex' (UCC). It will make it possible to apply the main advantages of the cryosurgical method in all fields of medicine. The UCC is illustrated below and consists of the following three cryosurgical systems:

- 'Cryosurgical System, Mobile' – CSM
- 'Cryosurgical System, Stationary' – CSS
- 'Cryosurgical System, Ambulatory' – CSA

The mobile cryosurgical unit (Fig. 2.1) is produced as a compact installation with a cryogenic system, and an automatic steering block which activates the cryogenic process. Storage of the cryoagent (10 l) provides uninterrupted cryoactivity for 3-4 hours and makes it possible to perform cryooperations in surgery, gynecology, urology, proctology, dermatology, etc., at out-patient clinics.

The stationary cryogenic unit is new and an absolute must in any modern operating theatre. The unit, with a complete set of cryosurgical instruments, is situated above the operating table and fixed at the required angle so as to fully relieve the surgeon's hand during operations which can last several hours.

The ambulatory (portable) cryosurgical unit is provided in a case and consists of a steering block and a small cryoblock (weighing 1.5 kg, plus 400 ml of liquid nitrogen), a set of cryodevices and applicators. It is easy to transport and can be used for performing a single cryodestruction of not more than 40 cm^3 of tissue volume. The set can be powered during transport of the patient, or on site, from the electric network of an automobile, as it can run on a car battery.

The way the cryosurgical complex is constructed has made it possible to increase the number of the various cryodevices and applicators for the three cryosystems and thus it has become possible to involve all branches of medicine. All the above-mentioned units have a block in the center to which the various cryodevices and applicators for use in different fields of medicine can be attached. All these cryosystems contain the unique cryoelements (heat-exchangers, cryodevices and applicators, electromagnetic valves, heaters, cryopipelines, etc.), which satisfy all the above-mentioned requirements. Mechanized cryosystems allow the realization of different parameters of cryoactivity and make it possible to conduct cryobiological investigations with the very best technology and under optimal conditions.

All the cryosystems mentioned above are based on the latest achievements in the field of cryo-heat-exchange, cryomaterial-science and mechanization of the cryo-processes.

The new cryosurgical automated systems 'Universal Cryosurgical Complex' (UCC) has been constructed on our basic know-how, which includes the design and manufacture process of porous heat-exchangers, the technology of electron-vacuum welding for thin-wall components, the design of electromagnetic valves for cryogenic liquids, and the results of clinical investigations of the new system in different fields of medicine.

The technical data are as follows:

– volume of the cryodestruction zone	1–180 cm^3
– liquid nitrogen capacity	10 litres
– freezing temperature range	20–196°C
– time needed to reach working temperature	a max. of 5 min.
– thawing time	2–3 min.
– power consumed	a max. of 600 W
– voltage	220 V. 50 Hz
– weight	10 kg

The main advantages of the UCC system are:

- high cooling capacity
- quarantining the cryodestruction of the specified volume

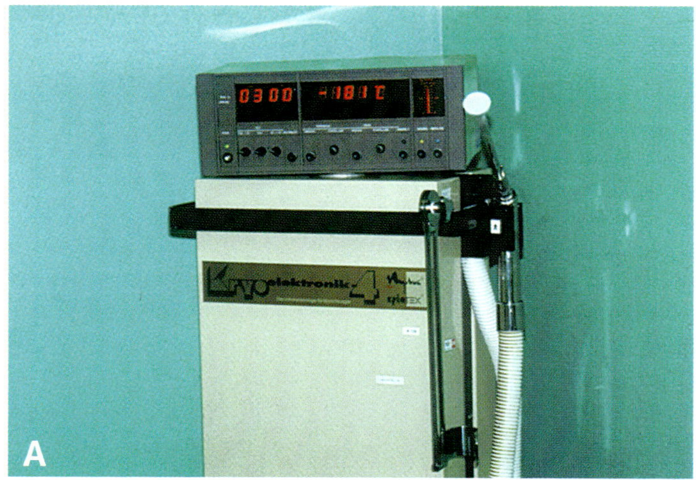

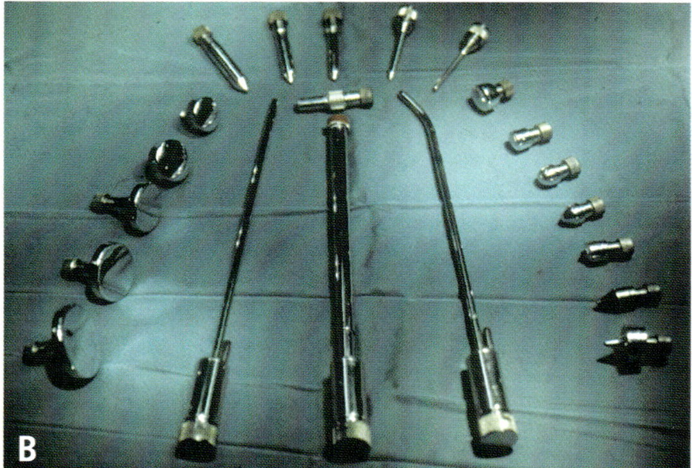

Fig. 2.1. Cryosurgical System, Mobile. General view (**A**) and set of the new universal needles and probes for cryosurgery (**B**)

- enabling a choice for different oncological operations
- high accuracy of measurement
- stabilization of the temperature required for cryosurgery, and the provision of a specially developed mathematical formula for very precise estimation of the cryodestruction zone, which is symmetrical around the axis of the probe
- the availability of three kinds of cryosystems, different cryoinstruments and probes make it possible to realize various cryosurgical procedures (application, penetration, spraying, clamp) which can be used in almost all fields of medicine
- the high reliability of vacuum and cryogenic equipment provided by the use of the advanced technologies of the electronic beam and of laser welding

When one analyzes the technical facilities of the cryosurgical systems in the suggested complex and compares them to those on the market today, it is possible to conclude that, as far as their technical standard is concerned, our cryosystems are three to five years ahead of their potential competitors.

In this study we have analyzed one of the most essential factors influencing the development of cryosurgery, namely the condition and standard of the cryosurgical appliances and their influence on the development of the method in general, and we have put forward our own conception of cryosurgical techniques.

Finally, the findings in cryobiological investigations, which have described the mechanisms of cryodestroying biological cells, have made it possible to formulate the main technical requirements for cryosurgical devices. Our recommendations for the further development of cryosurgical techniques are based on various experimental and clinical results of the application of the cryomethod in different branches of medicine. We have deliberately used our own prodigious experimental and clinical material.

2.2 Requirements for Modern Cryosurgical Technology

Findings in cryobiological investigations which describe cryodestructive mechanisms make it possible to formulate the main technical requirements of cryosurgical devices. The elaboration and improvement of any medical technique begins by trying to satisfy the main technical requirements so that the appliance will prove efficient in medical practice.

Having studied the construction of many cryosurgical instruments made in different countries and based on various ways of attaining very low temperatures, one can now say that cryosurgical techniques have been going in the wrong direction. The first simple appliances appeared long before the main mechanisms for cryodestruction of biological cells was known. Technical requirements which could perhaps have been realised had not yet been established. Thus, for a long time, many scientists, who had applied the simple techniques without effect, no longer believed that cryosurgery had a future and stopped promoting it.

The main technical parameter for effective cryodestruction is the provision of a low enough, sub-zero temperature in the biological tissue, followed by deliberate thawing. This very low temperature, in turn, is defined by the temperature of the working surface of the cryoinstrument which is in contact with the bulk tissue to be frozen. The results of experimental studies show that if the cryosurgical device provides temperatures of −170°C to −196°C on the working surface of the cryoinstrument which is in contact with the bulk of the tissue to be frozen, then in this case most of the cells die. If the temperature is not lowered quickly enough in the course of the cryosurgical procedure, there is an increasing probability that cells will be preserved in the bulk of the tissue which is to be frozen, and recurrences of malignant malformations become possible. Thus, during cryoactivity the temperature of the working surface of the cryodevice which is in contact with the tissue should not be higher than −170°C.

Another condition which must be fulfilled is the provision of great accuracy in measuring and stabilizing the correct temperature at which cryoactivity is carried out.

Our new cryosurgical technology is able to create sub-zero temperatures of down to −196°C where they are required, that is, where the cryosurgical instrument makes contact with the tissue, and this accurate freezing procedure can, moreover, be repeated again and again. Although essential for cryosurgery to be effective, repeated lowering of the temperature to such a degree has up to now not been possible.

Simplicity, reliability, efficiency and safety are, of course, also essential qualities of this new technology.

Stability and the possibility of repeating several freeze-thaw cycles accurately, as well as the other above-mentioned requirements are provided by the construction of the cryosurgical unit and the all-important peculiarities of its functional structure, especially the accuracy of the steering.

In recent decades cryosurgical devices invented by different firms have appeared on the market. Although they are reasonably complicated automatic systems, they do not satisfy the main requirement, namely the very low temperatures required for cryoactivity. Because of their construction, devices currently on the market cannot produce a temperature of less than −120°C on the working surface of the cryodevice which is in contact with the human organ and cannot, therefore, guarantee cryodestruction. This is why the cryosurgical method has not spread more extensively and why its possibilities have been neglected.

Part II

Experimental Aspects of Modern Cryosurgery

3. Experimental Cryosurgery

Temperature Measuring and Evaluation of Tumor Cell Viability in Different Zones of an Ice Ball. Practical Application of *in vitro* Experimental Results

A.M. Granov with contributions by D.G. Prokhorov, A.P. Andreev, G.P. Pinaev, G.G. Prokhorov, and A.V. Vlasova

3.1 Introduction

The cryogenic treatment method has found wide application in many branches of surgery, including surgical oncology, for the treatment of tumors of various locations. The advantages of this method over traditional techniques are based on experimental and clinical experience. They are absence of tumor resistance to cryosurgical application, limited area of exposure, and monitoring of injurious effects of low temperatures on biological structures, presence of hemostatic and anesthetic effects, favorable course of a wound process following tissue cryolysis, and almost complete absence of general negative reactions of the organism.

The practical value of the cryosurgical method is determined also by the possibility of treating neoplasms resistant to radiation and chemotherapy, to use it as a sparing treatment in elderly patients with concomitant diseases, and when tumors are located in surgically non-accessible areas.

The goal of radical cryosurgical interventions for malignant tumors is the complete destruction of tumor cells. The damage to cells is achieved by cooling them to subzero temperatures (−186°C) with the help of metal cryoprobes directly in contact with tumor tissue. An ice ball forms around the cryoprobe, involving the tumor. It is obvious that normal tissues surrounding a tumor should be minimally damaged. It is especially important that normal tissue in the immediate proximity of a tumor be protected, in order to avoid cold damage, which can lead to postoperative complications.

Cryosurgical treatment is widely applied in various branches of medicine as an alternative to existing classic techniques or in addition to them. Cryoequipment with different technical characteristics, most frequently employing liquid nitrogen or argon as a cooling agent, is used.

In spite of the fact that the cryogenic treatment method has been known for quite a long time, comprehensive answers to many questions associated with cryoablation processes are still not available. At present much research is being carried out to increase the efficiency and safety of cryosurgical operations. Analyzing the scientific data obtained and comparing them with the results of more recent experiments and clinical data, many authors anticipate that cryosurgical treatment will become one of the leading treatment options for malignant tumors in the near future (Korpan 2000, Onik and Lugnani 1999).

"Science progresses, destroying itself every 25 years", Pasteur wrote. Some data considered to be indisputable in the past is of only historical interest today. It is possible that many of the existing methods of treatment of malignant tumors will be abandoned in the future.

At present the accuracy of various monitoring techniques for the cryoablation process is well investigated. Tacke et al. (1998) performed cryoablation of rabbit livers under MRI guidance. Histological examination 7 days after cryotherapy confirmed that the liver lesions were of the same size as had been predicted by the images of the ice ball (35). Stephenson et al. (1996) studied histological changes after cryoablation for the treatment of selected renal tumors in a canine model. Histological studies in animals killed up to 1 week after cryoablation revealed complete coagulative necrosis within the cryolesion (34). Nakada et al. (1998) performed laparoscopic renal cryotherapy in swine. Under external ultrasound guidance, two 3-mm cryoprobes were positioned in the lower pole of the kidney, and the double-freeze technique was performed using puncture or contact application. Kidneys treated with both methods demonstrated cell death and subsequent necrosis within the ice ball (23). Edmunds et al. (2000) studied the tissue changes following cryoablation in human renal tumors. A 3-mm argon-gas-based cryoprobe was placed directly into each tumor. A single 15-minute freeze preceded an active thaw (helium gas) for each lesion. Ice ball dimensions were monitored by intraoperative ultrasonography. Histologically, freezing of renal tissue resulted in coagulative necrosis and hemorrhages within the boundaries of the cryolesions. There was a zone of demarcation between the viable and nonviable tissue (12).

However in a series of works (15,17,29,30, 35,37) the discrepancy between sizes of actual ice balls and sizes seen under the instrumental guidance has been emphasized. Depending on the method of monitoring (Ultrasound, CT or MRI) the error is from 4 to 8 mm (36). Grampsas et al. (1995) have found that the necrotic area resulting from cryodestruction appeared much smaller than predicted by intraoperative ultrasound (17).

Steed et al. (1997) studied a correlation between thermosensor findings and transrectal ultrasonography findings during prostate cryoablation. Two cryosurgeons, working together and blinded to the actual temperature, used sonographic observations to estimate the temperature until they believed that the gland was adequately frozen. The operators were not able to accurately predict subzero temperatures by transrectal ultrasonography evaluation. Moreover, the bias and magnitude of the error were significant and might lead to inadequate freezing of the prostate during attempted cryoablation (33).

Intraoperative ultrasound guidance still remains the main method of control of the cryoprobe position and of ice ball formation during prostate or liver cryosurgery.

Ultrasound control gives precise evidence of the external borders of an ice ball because approximately 100% of the signal is reflected from the ice ball (Saliken et al. 1995; Onik et al. 1995; Bischof et al. 1997). However, the use of ultrasound guidance alone is frequently not sufficient for the monitoring of the freezing process. The adequate control of the ice ball formation in many respects determines the success of the operation and the appearance of complications associated with inadequate freezing during cryoablation (Steed et al. 1997).

On the one hand, it can be explained both by the presence of a "critical angle shadowing effect" (Onik et al. 1995) and by the fact that tumor cells can remain unaffected and keep their ability to divide on the periphery of an ice ball. Therefore the method of continuous thermomonitoring of tumor freezing was introduced into cryosurgery (Watson 1995; Chinn et al. 1996).

Thermomonitoring is especially important for normal tissues in the immediate proximity of a tumor, cold damage to which can lead to postoperative complications (for example, radical cryoablation of a prostate for a cancer). In that case the thermocouples, located on the periphery of the prostate, will provide the signal to stop freezing.

The ultrasound control and thermocouples, placed on the periphery of the prostate, give a rather precise picture of the peripheral part of an ice ball, but the location of the isotherms and the condition of cells inside various zones of an ice ball remains unclear. A number of scientific studies in cryosurgery are devoted to investigating the location of critical isotherms inside an ice ball and mechanisms of cell destruction during freezing (15,20,24,26,35–38).

In accordance with new experimental evidence, the accumulation of clinical experience and the development of new cryounits, allowing freeze and thaw rates to vary, the initial protocols of cryosurgery have changed considerably. All future experiments will differ from previous ones, in that materials and methods, as well as parameters of the performed experiments and cryosurgical equipment, will be updated. The goal of all studies is the same – increase in the efficacy and safety of cryosurgical operations.

The analysis of the literature shows that all authors are interested in the following:

1. Radical cryoablation of malignant tumors or metastases
2. Cryodestruction of a tumor or metastases before organ resection or removal
3. Cryosurgery for non-malignant tumors and precancerous diseases
4. Palliative cryodestruction of malignant tumors or metastases
5. Combination of cryosurgical treatment with other treatment methods

3.2 Objective

1. Determination of the temperature parameters inside an ice ball.
2. Assessment of viability of cells after cooling in various zones of an ice ball.
3. Development of practical recommendations on the basis of experimental results.

3.3 Material and Methods

1. The temperature in an ice ball around cryoprobes 3.8 mm in diameter (cryoequipment: liquid nitrogen based Candela Cryotech LCS 3000) was measured with ten thermocouples of 150 microns diameter.
2. Determination of the number of affected cells (line A-131 epidermoid carcinoma) at temperature regimens corresponding to various zones of an ice ball.
3. The study of viability of unaffected frozen tumor cells.
4. The use of the obtained results in cryosurgery for prostate cancer.

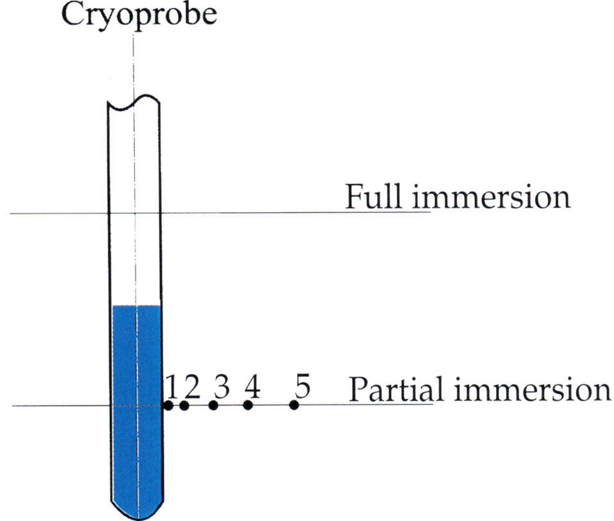

Fig. 3.1. Location of thermocouples respective to the cryoprobe

Standard cryoprobes were used for prostate cryoablation in our experiments. The diameter of each cryoprobe is 3.8 mm, and the length is 170 mm. The active (cooled) tip (length – 25 mm) was placed in a 5-liter container, filled with different liquids or colloidal media. The temperature parameters of the formed ice ball were investigated both at complete immersion of the active part of a cryoprobe and at its superficial location (Fig. 3.1).

In the experiments, the temperature around the cryoprobe was measured by ten thermocouples with a diameter of 150 microns. Small dimensions and low thermoinertia of the measuring elements made it possible to reduce measuring errors to a minimum. The first thermocouple was close to a cryoprobe surface, subsequent ones were located 5, 10, 16, and 26 mm from the longitudinal axis of a cryoprobe. The data from the thermocouples were registered discretely at 10-sec intervals.

In an isotonic solution (0.9% NaCl) where temperature was maintained at a constant level of +38°C, the definitive size of an ice ellipse was 22 × 37 mm. Temperature at the center of an ice ball reached its maximum of −186°C within two minutes from the moment of switching on the cryoequipment, and on the periphery of the ice ball the temperature was lowered in 10 min to −6°C. The −40°C isotherm was 8 mm from the surface of the cryoprobe.

Direct physical measurement of an ice ball was accompanied by ultrasound guidance. The Aloka SSD-630 (Japan) and Sono Diagnost 360 Philips (Germany) ultrasound units with convex and linear ultrasound probes were used. The average error of ultrasound estimation was up to 10% of the actual size of an ice ball increasing with the size of the ice ball.

In a gelatinous medium (+38°C) in which there is no convection, the process of ice formation was more intense.

The shape of the frozen area represented an ellipse of 35 × 47 mm in case of complete immersion of an active tip, and a hemisphere of 53 mm diameter in case of its partial immersion. The critical isotherm (−40°C) reached 10 and 16 mm from the cryoprobe surface after an ice ball diameter became stable (Table 3.1).

In the clinical study the control measurements were made during cryoablation for prostate cancer and metastases of colorectal cancer to the liver with the help of standard cryosurgical thermocouples.

During the experiments, the essential differences between parameters of ice balls after the first and second freeze without any change of cryoprobe position were revealed. The differences are presented in Fig. 3.2.

The diameter of an ice ball at the first freezing was 35 mm, at the second 42 mm; the temperature pattern showed a decrease inside and at the periphery of an ice ball. The temperature at the center of an ice ball reached the maximum (−186°C) within two minutes of switching on the cryoequipment, and on the periphery of the ice ball it fell to −6°C in 10 min.

It is necessary to note that the cooling rate of tested cryoequipment depends on the level of the

Table 3.1. Characteristics of ice balls during first freezing

	Radius of the critical isotherm (−40°C)	Diameter of an ice ball
Full immersion	10 mm	35 mm
Partial immersion	16 mm	53 mm

AFTER FIRST FREEZING AFTER SECOND FREEZING

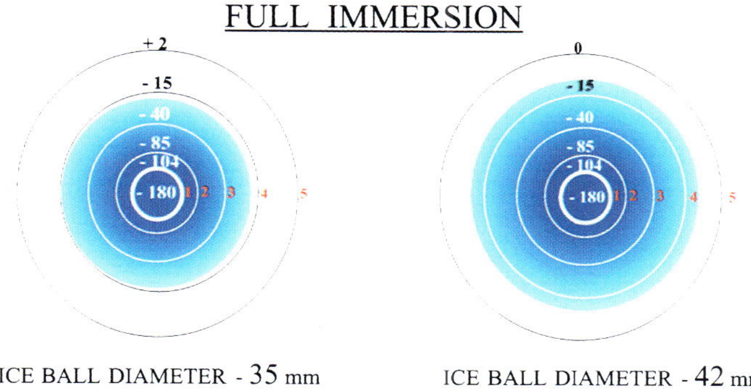

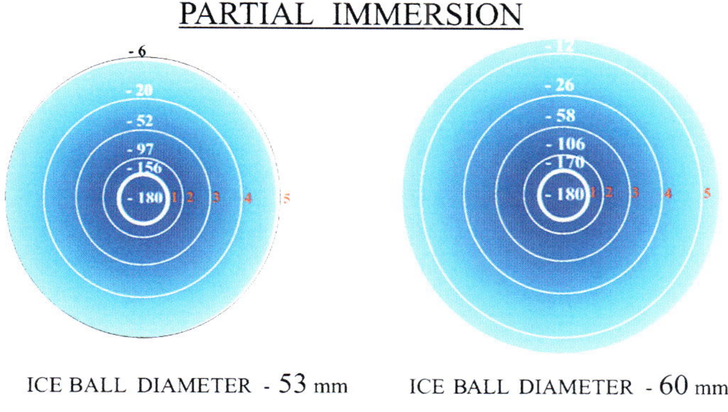

1,2,3,4,5 - THERMOCOUPLES

Fig. 3.2. The differences in ice balls after single and double freezing in gelatinous medium

coolant in the Dewar flask and the number of cryoprobes cooled simultaneously (27). The maximum cooling rate in the medial zone of an ice ball that can be achieved with recommended parameters for this cryounit is no more than 15°C per min. Liquid nitrogen based cryoequipment has some inertia in the freeze-thaw processes. When discontinuing freezing and in the transition to the thawing process, there is no immediate change in the size of an ice ball and its temperature. In some cases a small increase in the diameter of an ice ball in the first minute after an active thawing process began was noted.

In experiments with cell cultures, temperature regimens corresponding to various zones of an ice ball were simulated. The viability of cells after freezing and thawing was estimated by adhesive properties and the ability to divide. All experiments were carried out *in vitro*. It is worth noting that *in vivo* cells are more resistant to unfavorable environmental factors such as cold or ischemia. In our experiments we tried to take this into account.

The cell cultures A-431 (epidermoid carcinoma) and HeLa (carcinoma of cervix uteri) were cooled in the cryocamera ICE-CUBIE 1810 (SY-LAB, Austria).

Cell suspension or cell deposit after centrifugation of a suspension at 1000 g for 3 minutes were exposed to liquid nitrogen vapors. Freezing of cells was carried out at different rates of cooling, end temperatures and exposure time.

After freezing, cells were thawed up to +37°C and transferred to a Petri dish for culture (medium DMEM with addition of 10% embryonal serum at a temperature of +37°C in a CO_2 incubator).

In the first experiments it was found that cells in the suspension are very sensitive to low temperatures and died quickly. In contrast, the cells in the centrifuged suspension appeared to be much more resistant to cooling.

Following the first series of experiments comparing the resistance of cells lines HeLa and A-431 to cold it was determined that A-431 cells are more resistant to freezing. Therefore, all further experiments were carried out only with the centrifuged suspension line A-431. The cell culture (line A-431 epidermoid carcinoma) was cooled at temperature regimens corresponding to various zones of an ice ball.

At first, the cell culture was cooled at a rate of 1°C and 10°C per minute down to final temperatures of −5°C to −60°C without any additional exposure to end temperature (see Diagram 3.1).

At a low cooling rate (1°C/min) a gradual decrease in the number of unaffected cells with a decrease in the end temperature was noted (from 95% at −5°C to 33% at −50°C). When cooled down to −60°C, 46% of cells were not affected. At higher cooling rates (10°C/min), the viability of

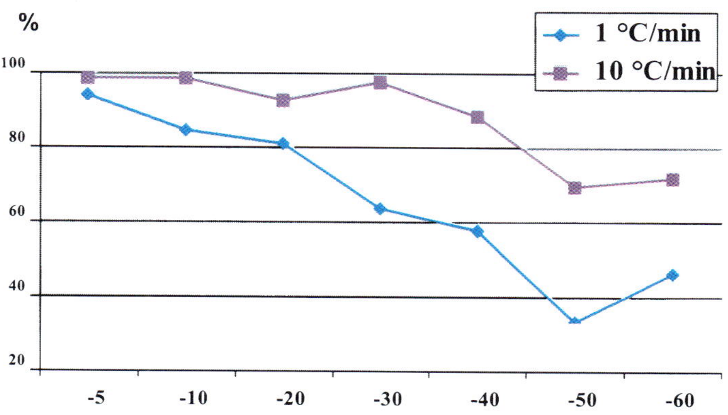

Diagram 3.1. Percentage of unaffected cells after freezing without exposure to end temperature

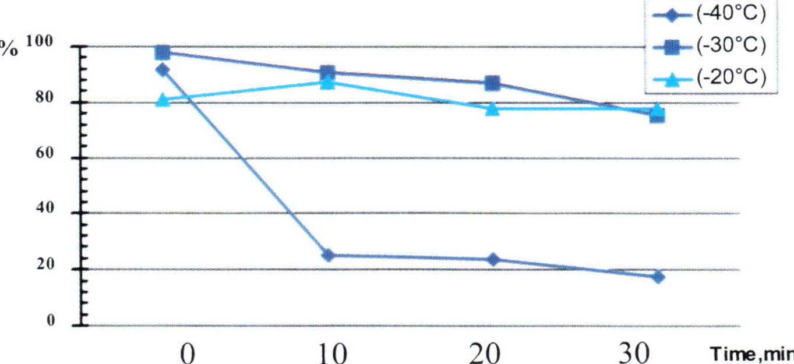

Diagram 3.2. Percentage of unaffected cells after freezing with further exposure to end temperature

cells increased. When cooled from −10°C down to −40°C, cell deposits did not show a significant decrease in number of affected cells. Only after cooling down to −50° and −60°C, the proportion of unaffected cells was reduced to 70%.

This protocol of tumor cryolysis (single freezing without additional exposure to end temperature) is rarely used in radical cryosurgical operations. Therefore all parameters of further experiments have been changed in order to meet as much as possible the requirements of actual cryosurgical protocols for prostate and liver cryoablation.

When frozen cells were exposed to the same end temperatures for 10–30 minutes, the proportion of undamaged cells essentially decreased. The results are presented in Diagram 3.2. The exposure of cells at temperatures of −20°C and −30°C did not essentially influence the number of unaffected cells. At a temperature of −30°C, a decrease in the number of unaffected cells following the 10-min exposure was observed. Further exposure of cells to this temperature did not essentially influence cell damage.

A considerable destruction of cells was achieved, if cells were exposed to a temperature of −40°C for even 10 min. The number of unaffected cells was reduced by approximately 60% during this period (from 92% to 25%). The prolongation of the exposure time to 20 and 30 min did not significantly reduce the amount of unaffected cells, reaching 18% in 30 min. Thus, the best results were obtained at an end temperature of −40°C at an exposure not less than 20 min (more than 80% of cells were completely destroyed).

In spite of the fact that after the exposure to low temperatures an appreciable number of cells appear not to be destroyed, it does not mean, however, that they remain viable. Actually, further experiments show that among undamaged cells only an insignificant part retain the ability to divide.

The experiments estimating the viability were carried out according to the protocols of the previous experiments.

In Table 3.2 the viability of cells after cooling without exposure to end temperatures are presented. Cells cooled at temperatures from −5°C down to −30°C retained their ability to attach, plate and divide. At end temperatures from −40°C to −60°C the ability of cells to attach to the substrate was reduced. Part of them attached to the substrate only in 24 hours, but without dividing further and died within 5 days.

When cells are exposed to temperatures of −20°C to −40°C the viability of cells differs (see Table 3.3). Cells frozen down to −40°C, irrespec-

Table 3.2. Viability of cells after freezing without exposure to end temperatures

T °C	V = 1°C/min				V = 10°C/min			
	% of unaffected cells	Viability			% of unaffected cells	Viability		
		2 hrs.	24 hrs.	5 days		2 hrs.	24 hrs.	5 days
−5	94.5	++	+++	+++	98	++	+++	+++
−10	85	++	+++	+++	99	++	+++	+++
−20	81.3	+	+++	+++	93	++	+++	+++
−30	64	—	+	++	98	++	+++	+++
−40	58	—	+	—	89	—	+	+_
−50	33.5	—	+	—	70	—	+	—
−60	46.5	—	+	—	72	—	+	—

"—" - complete cell destruction
"+" - attaching to the substrate
"+" - attaching + plating
"++" - attaching + plating + dividing
V - velocity of temperature change

Table 3.3. Viability of cells after freezing with further exposure to end temperatures

T °C	Time, min	V=1°C/min				V=10°C/min			
		% of unaffected cells	Viability			% of unaffected cells	Viability		
			2 hrs.	24 hrs.	5 days		2 hrs.	24 hrs.	5 days
−20	0	81.3	+	+++	+++	93.0	++	+++	+++
	10	87.5	—	++	+++	85.0	++	+++	+++
	20	78.0	—	+	++	79.0	—	++	+++
	30	78.0	—	—	++	68.0	—	—	++
−30	0	64.0	—	+	+	98.0	++	+++	+++
	10	21.0	—	+	—	91.0	—	+	++
	20	19.0	—	+	—	87.0	—	+	++
	30	18.5	—	+	—	75.6	—	+	+
−40	0	58.0	—	+	—	83.9	+	++	++
	10	20.0	—	+	—	25.5	—	+	—
	20	18.0	—	+	—	24.0	—	—	+_ _
	30	16.2	—	+	—	17.5	—	—	+_ _

"—" - complete cell destruction
"+" - attaching to the substrate
"++" - attaching + plating
"+++" - attaching + plating + dividing
V - velocity of temperature change

tive of the exposure rate, underwent direct destruction, or died during the hours following thawing, forming *"a zone of direct cell destruction"*. Changes in the temperature range from −40°C to −6°C, which corresponded to the temperature on the periphery of an ice ball, exerted damaging action on the cell culture. After thawing, however, more than 75% of tumor cells retained their ability to divide. We defined this area as a "zone of partial cell damage".

Thus, the picture presented earlier (Fig. 3.2) of the isotherm arrangement in an ice ball will appear as follows (Fig. 3.3).

"A zone of direct cell destruction" corresponds to the inner area of an ice ball forming around the cryoprobe within a temperature range of −180°C to −40°C, while a so-called *"zone of partial cell damage"* corresponds to the peripheral part of an ice ball. The distance between the outer border of an ice ball, seen under ultrasound guidance, and the −40°C isotherm ranged from 10 mm to 17 mm.

The comparison of the results obtained in the experiments with the conditions of cryosurgical operations is of special interest.

The posterior surface of the prostate is known to lie in immediate proximity to the rectal wall. Normally this distance is less than 10 mm (Fig. 3.4). When performing radical cryosurgical operations on a prostate, the external border of an ice ball (visible under ultrasound guidance) corresponds to the external borders of the prostate, following its shape (Fig. 3.5). The −40°C isotherm, however, which is the border of a destructive zone, encircles the inner area of an ice ball 10–12 mm from the outer surface of an ice ball seen under ultrasound guidance, the peripheral parts of a prostate remaining outside the critical isotherm (Fig. 3.6).

Judging from the ultrasound image during cryosurgery, surgeons are led to suppose that the ice ball extends over the entire prostate, whereas, in fact, the peripheral part of the prostate, corresponding to a "zone of partial cell damage" still contains viable cells.

The cryoablation of the prostate for cancer will be radical should the entire prostate be involved in a "zone of direct cell destruction". Under these conditions, the external borders of an ice ball will be displaced outside the prostate, which leads to cooling normal adjacent tissues (Fig. 3.7).

The zone of partial cell damage does not exert a sufficient damaging effect to destroy a tumor, but is dangerous to the rectal wall. Overcooling of a rectal wall during cryoablation of a prostate inevitably leads to its damage. Clinically, it means the appearance of severe post-operative complications.

It is necessary to emphasize that various models of cryoequipment create different physical characteristics of the formed ice balls, various rates of cooling and thawing as well as various opportunities for temperature monitoring in cryosurgical interventions (30,31–34). Nevertheless, with each model the fact that the border of an ice ball ob-

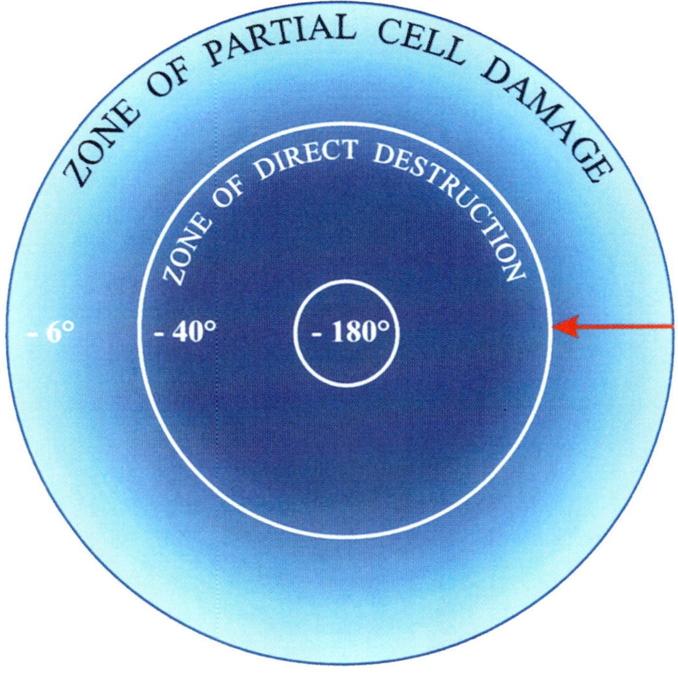

- length from 10 to 17 mm

Fig. 3.3. Scheme of division of an ice ball into zones of cell viability

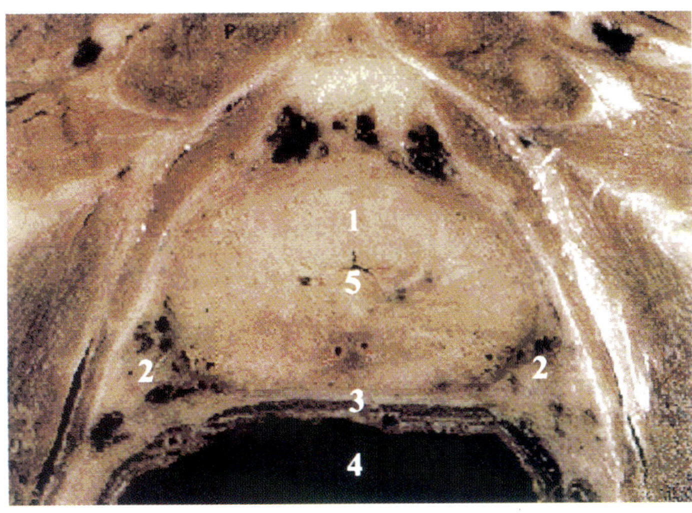

Fig. 3.4. Cross-section of a normal human prostate. **1** prostate, **2** neurovascular bundles, **3** rectal wall, **4** rectum, **5** urethra

served under ultrasound guidance does not correspond to the border of the cryosurgical zone, remains valid from the practical point of view.

We would like to draw the attention of the reader to the fact that we tested a specific liquid

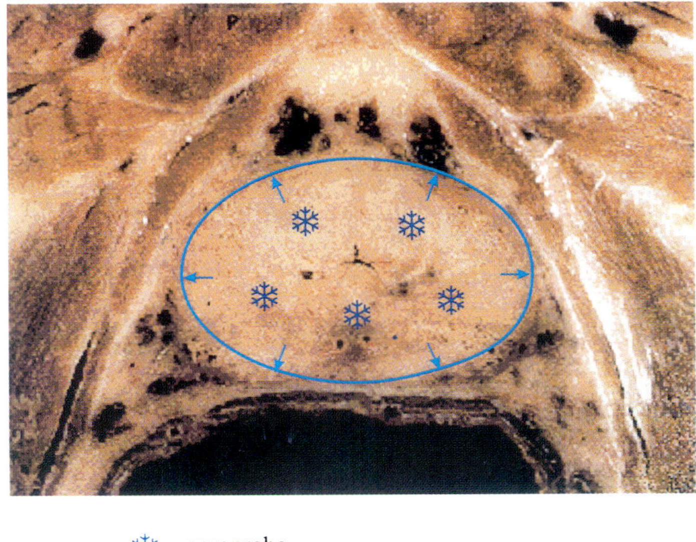

- cryoprobe

- ice front

Fig. 3.5. External borders of an ice ball visible under ultrasound guidance

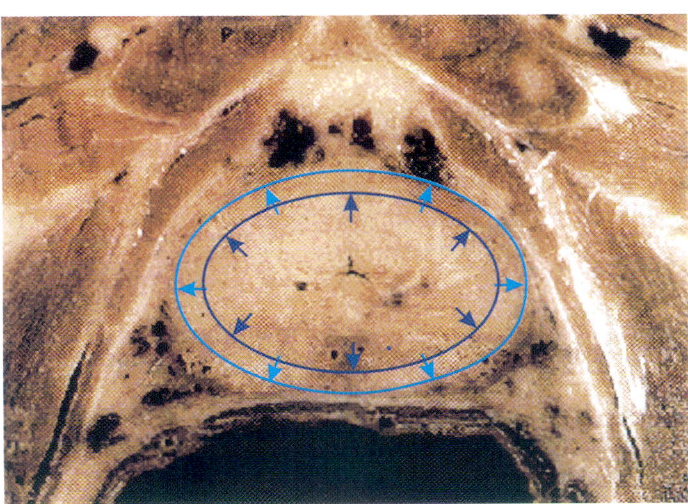

- zone of direct cell destruction (- 40 °C)

- zone of partial cell damage (- 6 °C)

Fig. 3.6 Approximate isotherm arrangement during prostate cryoablation

nitrogen based cryounit. The temperature parameters inside ice balls produced by other cryounits, using other types of cooling agents, may differ from our data. In our opinion the most important parameter of any ice ball is the distance from its external border to the critical isotherm (−40°C), which surrounds the "zone of direct cell destruction".

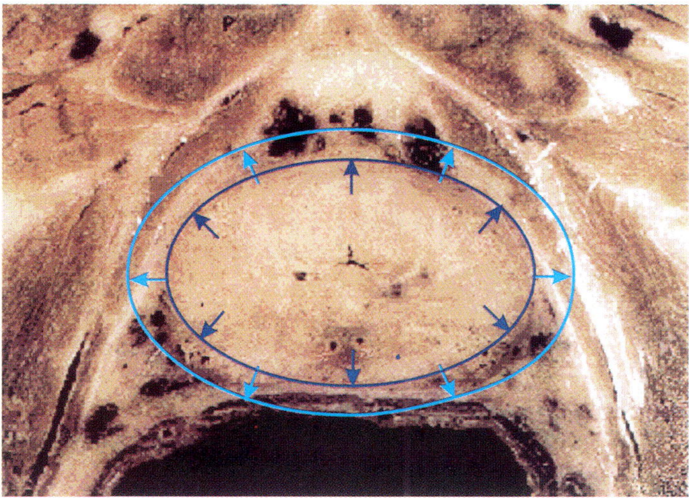

← - zone of direct cell destruction (- 40 °C)

← - ice front = zone of partial cell damage (- 6 °C)

Fig. 3.7. Approximate isotherms arrangement during prostate cryoablation with the reference to the "zone of partial cell damage"

3.4 Conclusion

The presence of a "zone of partial cell damage" inside the ice ball limits to some extent the indications for radical cryosurgery on the prostate for a malignant tumor located in the parts of the posterior prostate closest to the rectal wall, and requires development of protective measures for adjacent normal tissues.

References

1. Arnott J. On the treatment of cancer by the regulated application of an anaesthetic temperature. Churchill, London, 1851.
2. Berger WK, Schuder G Feifel G. Temperature distribution pattern in liver tissue in freezing procedures with new cryoprobes. Chirurg 1996; 67 (8): 833–838.
3. Bischof J, Christov K, Rubinsky B. A morphological study of cooling rate response in normal and neoplastic human liver tissue: cryosurgical implications. Cryobiology 1993; 30 (5): 482–492.
4. Bischof JC, Smith D, Pazhayannur PV, Manivel C, Hulbert J, Roberts KP. Cryosurgery of dunning AT-1 rat prostate tumor: thermal, biophysical, and viability response at the cellular and tissue level. Cryobiology 1997; 34 (1): 42–69.
5. Chosy SG, Nakada SY, Lee FT, Warner TF. Monitoring renal cryosurgery: predictors of tissue necrosis in swine. J Urol 1998; 159 (4): 1370–1374.
6. Cooper JS. Cryogenic Surgery. New Engl J Med 1963; 268 (14): 748–749.
7. Cooper JS. Cryogenic surgery of the basal ganglion. J Am Med Ass 1962; 81: 600–604.
8. Cozzi PJ, Lawson JA, Lynch WJ, Morris DL. Critical temperature for in vivo cryoablation of human prostate cancer in a xenograft model. Br J Urol 1996; 77 (1): 89–92.
9. Cozzi PJ, Lynch WJ, Collins S, Vonthethoff L, Morris DL. Renal cryotherapy in a sheep model, a feasibility study. J Urol 1997; 157 (2): 710–712.
10. Demichev NP. The development of cryogenic method in osseous oncology. Vestn Khir 1986; 136 (5): 139–144.
11. Dilley AV, Dy DY, Warlters A, Copeland S, Gillies AE, Morris RW, Gibb DB, Cook TA, Morris DL. Laboratory and animal model evaluation of the Cryotech LCS 2000 in hepatic cryotherapy. Cryobiology 1993; 30 (1): 74–85.
12. Edmunds TB Jr, Schulsinger DA, Durand DB, Waltzer WC. Acute histologic changes in human renal tumors after cryoablation. J Endourol 2000; 14 (2): 139–143.
13. El-Shakhs SA, Shimi SA, Cuschieri A. Effective hepatic cryoablation: does it enhance tumor dissemination? World J Surg 1999; 23 (3): 306–310.
14. Fay T. Early experience with local and generalized refrigeration of the human brain. J Neurosurg 1959; (16): 239–260.
15. Ferris DG, Ho JJ. Cryosurgical equipment: a critical review. J Fam Pract 1992; 35 (2): 185–193.
16. Gage AA, Baust J. Mechanisms of tissue injury in cryosurgery. Cryobiology 1998; 37 (3): 171–186.
17. Grampsas SA, Miller GJ, Crawford ED. Salvage radical prostatectomy after failed transperineal cryotherapy: histologic findings from prostate whole-mount specimens correlated with intraoperative transrectal ultrasound images. Urology 1995; 45 (6): 936–941.
18. Kaplan SA, Greenberg R, Baust JG. A comparative assessment of cryosurgical devices: application to prostatic disease. Urology 1995; 45 (4): 692–699.
19. Keijser LC, Schreuder HW, Buma P, Weinans H, Veth RP. Cryosurgery in long bones: an experimental study of necrosis and revitalization in rabbits. Arch Orthop Trauma Surg 1995; 119 (7–8): 440–444.
20. Larrey DJ. Surgical Memoirs of Campaigns of Russia, Germany and France. Carey and Leo. Philadelphia, 1932.
21. Marcoue RS, Miller TR. Treatment of primary and metastatic bone tumors by cryosurgery. J Amer Med Ass 1969; 207: 1890–1894.
22. Marcoue RS, Sadrich J, Huvos AG, Grabstald H. Cryosurgery in the treatment of solitary and multiple bone metastases from renal cell carcinoma. J Urology 1972; 108 (4): 540–547.
23. Nakada SY, Lee FT Jr, Warner T, Chosy SG, Moon TD. Laparoscopic cryosurgery of the kidney in the porcine model: an acute histological study. Urology 1998; 51 (5A): 161–166.
24. Neel UB, Ketcham AS, Hammond WG. Cryonecrosis of normal and tumor bearing rat liver patientiated by inflow occlusion. Cancer 1971; (28): 1211–1218.
25. Pirogov NI. Beginnings of general field surgery taken from observations in the military-hospital practice and memoirs of the Crimean war and the Caucasian expedition. Dresden, 1866.
26. Pogrel MA, Yen CK, Taylor R. A study of infrared thermographic assessment of liquid nitrogen cryotherapy. Oral Surg Oral Med Oral Pathol Oral Radiol Endod 1996; 81 (4): 396–401.
27. Rewcastle JC, Hahn LJ, Saliken JC, McKinnon JG. Use of a moratorium to achieve consistent liquid nitrogen cryoprobe performance. J Surg Oncol 1997; 66 (2): 110–113.
28. Rewcastle JC, Sandison GA, Hahn LJ, Saliken JC, McKinnon JG, Donnelly BJ. A model for the time-dependent thermal distribution within an iceball surrounding a cryoprobe. Phys Med Biol 1998; 43 (12): 3519–3534.
29. Rewcastle JC, Sandison GA, Saliken JC, Donnelly BJ, McKinnon JG. Considerations during clinical operation of two commercially available cryomachines. J Surg Oncol 1999; 71 (2): 106–111.
30. Schuder G, Pistorius G, Fehringer M, Feifel G, Menger MD, Vollmar B. Complete shutdown of microvascular perfusion upon hepatic cryothermia is critically dependent on local tissue temperature. Br J Cancer 2000; 82 (4): 794–799.
31. Shakhov VYu, Kochenov VI, Ovsyanikov VYa, Rylkin AI, Konev VYe, Aranzhereev AYu. Concerning improved cryodestruction procedures in management of neoplasms. Vopr Oncol 1983; 29 (9): 33–37.
32. Smith DJ, Fahssi WM, Swanlund DJ, Bischof JC. A parametric study of freezing injury in AT-1 rat prostate tumor cells. Cryobiology 1999; 39 (1): 13–28.
33. Steed J, Saliken JC, Donnelly BJ, Ali-Ridha NH. Correlation between thermosensor temperature and transrectal ultrasonography during prostate cryoablation. Can Assoc Radiol J 1997; 48, N 3: 186–190.

34. Stephenson RA, King DK, Rohr LR. Renal cryoablation in a canine model. Urology 1996; 47 (5): 772–776.
35. Tacke J, Adam G, Speetzen R. MR-guided interstitial cryotherapy of the liver with a novel, nitrogen-cooled cryoprobe. Magn Reson Med 1998; 39 (3): 354–360.
36. Tacke J, Speetzen R, Heschel I, Hunter DW, Rau G, Gunther RW. Imaging of interstitial cryotherapy – an in vitro comparison of ultrasound, computed tomography, and magnetic resonance imaging. Cryobiology 1998; 38 (3): 250–259.
37. Weber SM, Lee FT Jr, Chinn DO, Warner T, Chosy SG, Mahvi DM. Perivascular and intralesional tissue necrosis after hepatic cryoablation: results in a porcine model. Surgery 1997; 122 (4): 742–747.
38. Yudin SS. Notes on field surgery. Moscow, Russia, 1943.

4. Cryoimmunology and Cryoimmunotherapy

Cryochemotherapy. An Animal Experiment and Clinical Evidence

Shunichi Ikekawa with contributions by Kazuyuki Ishihara, Shigeo Tanaka, and *Shigeo Ikeda*

4.1 Introduction

Disturbance of the microcirculation occurs in the frozen tissue after cryosurgery. Immediately after the thawing phase, the vessels of the frozen tissue are constricted for a moment followed by vasodilatation, hyperemia, and vascular stasis. Accordingly thrombosis and complete circulation arrest develop (8,19) leading to tissue death (cryonecrosis). In an experiment using Syrian hamster cheek pouch, Zacarian et al. (19) found that injected Evans blue leaked around the vessels during the thawing phase, while the circulation had been completely arrested. We empirically knew of a synergistic effect of a combination of cryosurgery and an anticancer drug, as Benson (4,5) reported the effectiveness of treating squamous cell carcinoma of the head and neck by a combination of cryosurgery and regional intraarterial continuous infusion chemotherapy for 48 hours. The patients with primary and advanced carcinoma or recurrent carcinoma who received 5-fluorouracil (5-FU) had a good prognosis. We also have had a substantial experience of a striking effect of local administration of anticancer drugs combined with cryosurgery, particularly with oil-bleo (30 mg of bleomycin sulfate suspended in 2 ml of sesame oil), which does not easily disperse and is trapped for an unusually long time in the tumor, thus multiplying the anticancer activity.

To elucidate this phenomenon, changes in the vascular volume and vascular permeability after cryosurgery were analyzed quantitatively by means of radioactivity assay technique. And, different responses of the vessels of normal tissue and cancer tissue to freezing intervention were investigated. Our results in this experiment gave evidence that the tumor vessels dilate and increase in permeability sharply and quickly after cryosurgery, hence the anticancer drug would be concentrated in the tumor. It was noted that there is a characteristic difference between tumor vessels and normal vessels after cryoinjury. Many authors (2,3,9–11,14,15,18) have reported on the functional features of tumor vessels, the pharmacological reactions of tumor vessels to such agents as vasoactive drugs (2,3,9–11,18) and angiotensin II (15). Lack of significant response of tumor vessels to heating has also been reported. (14) Further, the vascular bed of a tumor is known to be different from vessels of normal tissue and lacking autoregulation of blood flow (15). The second problem is the timing of administration of anticancer drugs in combination with cryosurgery, and the third, the kinds of agents applicable. As far as we know, peplomycin (16) (a novel analog of bleomycin that exhibits less pulmonary toxicity than bleomycin), 5-FU, and DTIC (17) (dimethyl-triazenoimidazloecarboximide) are trapped in the tumor, but adriamycin is not. Peplomycin was trapped in the tumor 5 min, 1 or 3 hr after cryosurgery. Essential is the timing of administration of anticancer agents when the vascular volume and vascular permeability reach their peaks after cryosurgery, and selection of the proper agents. Many efforts to increase concentration of anticancer drugs in the tumor, e.g., regional selective or even super selective intraarterial infusion chemotherapy and selected enhancement of tumor blood flow by angiotensin II, (15) etc., have been reported. Cryochemotherapy, however, provides trapping of the anticancer agents in the tumor or periphery of the tumor. Hence it is not only a combination therapy but a new mode of cancer therapy, as we stress in this study. It deserves much attention as an anticancer strategy.

4.2 Experiment

I. *Tumor-host system:* B16 melanoma/BDF_1 mice. BDF_1 mice, 6–7 weeks old, mean body weight of 16.5 g, supplied by Charles River Japan Co., and B16 melanoma maintained by subcutaneous inoculation into C57BL/6 mice at 2-week intervals at the National Cancer Center Japan, were used. B16 melanoma, 5×10^5 cells/mouse, was inoculated intradermally into the back of the mice on both left and right sides, and approximately 10 days after the inoculation the one grown to 8 mm in diameter underwent cryosurgery, and the other was left untreated as a control.

II. *Instrumentation:* Cryosurgical instruments used for this experiment was liquid nitrogen (LN_2)-driven portable type CS-76 (Frigitronics of Connecticut Inc., USA), equipped with a 6 mm in diameter cylindrical probe-tip adaptor, the same as clinically used. Cryosurgery was performed by the contact method, 2-cycle freezing for 40 sec each cycle at −196 °C for the tumor and 20 sec each cycle for the normal skin, so as to freeze the normal skin to the same extent as the tumor.

III. *Determination of anticancer agents:* (1) Peplomycin (16) by a paper disk method showing antimicrobial activity against *Bacillus subtilis* PCI219 (1); (2) Adriamycin by a fluorescence method associated with the anthracyclin moiety (12).

IV. *Changes in vascular function:* Vascular volume and vascular permeability were measured according to the method of Song and Levitt (13). Blood withdrawn from an untreated healthy mouse was transferred into a heparinized tube and incubated with sodium chromate ^{51}Cr (300 CrCi/ml of blood, New England Nuclear) for 45 min at 37 °C in a water bath under gentle shaking. Then red blood cells were washed with physiological saline and centrifuged 3 times to remove unbound ^{51}Cr. ^{125}I-labeled human serum albumin (30 I-Ci/ml Amersham Japan Co., Tokyo) was added to the ^{51}Cr-labeled red blood cells, and the volume was adjusted to the original blood volume with physiological saline. Quantities of the mixture, 0.1 ml was injected into the mice through the tail vein. One hour after the injection, 0.3 ml of blood was withdrawn by cardiac puncture, and the tumor or normal skin was extirpated. The radioactivity of ^{51}Cr and ^{125}I in the blood and tissue was counted with a gamma-counter (ARC-300, Aloka Co., Japan). The dry weight of the tissue was determined after drying overnight at 110 °C, and the vascular volume and vascular permeability were calculated by the following formulae:

Vascular volume:

$$\text{ml of blood/g of tissue} = \frac{^{51}\text{Cr activity/g of tissue}}{^{51}\text{Cr activity/g of blood}}$$

Vascular permeability:

$$\text{ml of plasma extravasated in 1 hr/g of tissue} = \text{total plasma in g of tissue} - \text{intravascular plasma in g of tissue}$$

$$\text{where total plasma} = \frac{^{125}\text{I activity/g of tissue}}{^{125}\text{I activity/ml of plasma}}$$

and intravascular plasma =

$$\text{vascular volume} \times \left(1 - \frac{\text{hematocrit}}{100}\right)$$

V. *Trapping of anticancer agents into the tumor*, tissue distribution in blood, liver, and kidney: (1) Peplomycin, 40 mg/kg was administered intraperitoneally 1 hr before and 5 min, 1 and 3 hr after cryosurgery. The mice were sacrificed 1, 2, 4, and 8 hr after the administration. Samples were collected and examined for the determination of the drug concentration. Each group consisted of five or six mice. Figure 4.1 is the time course of the peplomycin level in blood, liver, and kidney. All showed a rapid decrease in the peplomycin level, and no difference was observed between peplomycin alone and peplomycin combined with cryosurgery. However, as shown in Fig. 4.2, when peplomycin was administered 5 min after cryosurgery, the peplomycin concentration in the tumor was significantly higher than in the control tumor. When peplomycin was administered 1 and

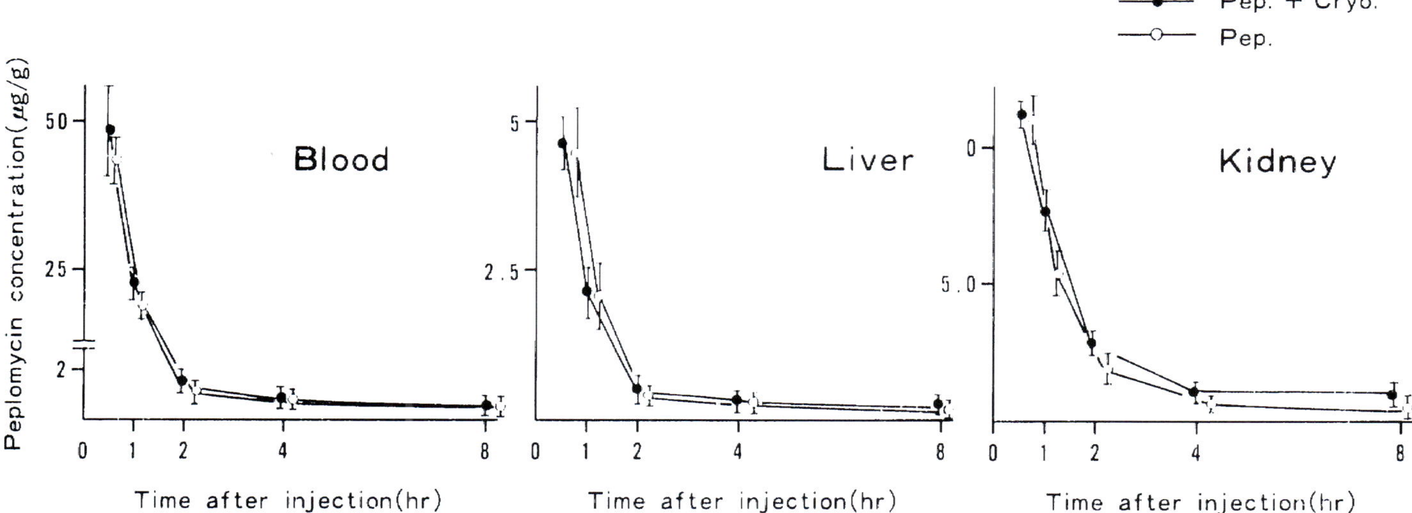

Fig. 4.1. Concentration of peplomycin in organs after cryosurgery (blood, liver, kidney)

3 hr after cryosurgery, we observed that the drug was still concentrated in the frozen tumor. But when the drug was administered an hour before cryosurgery, this concentration was not seen.

(2) Adriamycin, 8 mg/kg was administered intraperitoneally. Figure 4.3, which depicts the adriamycin level in blood, liver, and kidney, also shows a rapid decrease in tissue level with no difference between adriamycin alone and adriamycin combined with cryosurgery, identical to the course of peplomycin. Figure 4.4 shows the time course of the adriamycin level, given 5 min after cryosurgery. The adriamycin level in the cryosurgically treated tumor was rather lower than that of the untreated tumor. Therefore, in contrast with peplomycin, adriamycin was not trapped in the frozen tumor.

As reported in the early experiments in animals, the blood level of adriamycin decreases rapidly. Adriamycin has a certain tissue affinity and is strongly adsorbed by the tumor or normal tissue (12,18). Hence adsorption by the frozen tumor or frozen normal tissue may be lower than adsorption by non-frozen tissues.

VI. *Vascular volume and vascular permeability in the tumor and normal skin after cryosurgery:* As for the difference in functional characteristics in response to cryoinjury between the normal vessels and the tumor vessels, the results revealed that the vascular volume of the frozen tumor was approximately seven times that of the untreated tumor 30 min after cryosurgery and then fell to the control level within 1 hr (Fig. 4.5). Also, the vascular permeability of the frozen tumor was approximately eight times that of the untreated tumor 1 hr after cryosurgery (Fig. 4.5). However, in regard to the changes in vascular volume and

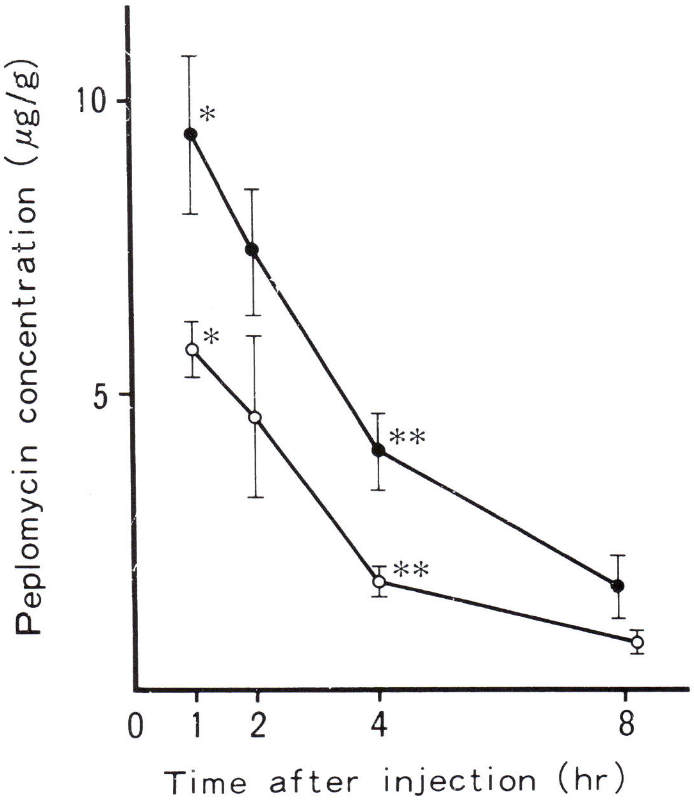

Fig. 4.2. Peplomycin concentration in the tumor after cryosurgery. Combined cryosurgery and peplomycin (●), peplomycin alone (○). Mean ± SE. Significant by student's t test, $P<0.05$ (*), $P<0.02$ (**)

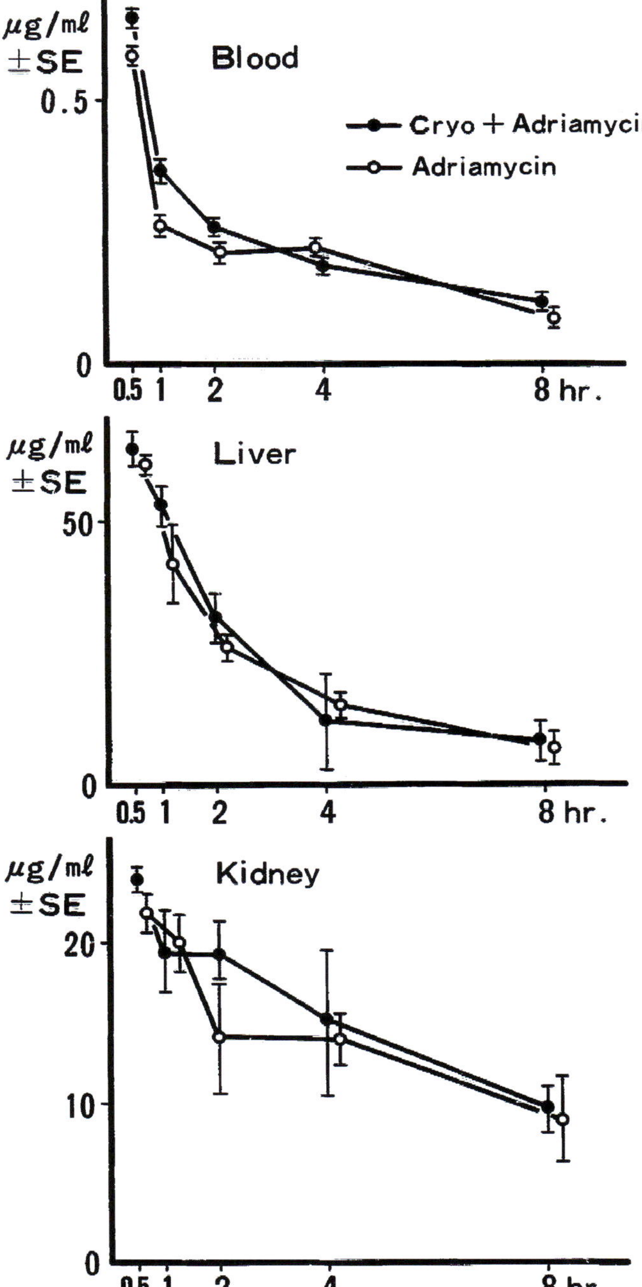

Fig. 4.3. Concentration of adriamycin in organs after cryosurgery (blood, liver, kidney) Mean ± SE

vascular permeability of the normal skin after cryosurgery, the vascular volume of the frozen normal skin was approximately 12 times that of the normal untreated skin 1 hr after cryosurgery and decreased gradually (Fig. 4.6), and the vascular permeability of the frozen normal skin was approximately 17 times that of the normal untreated skin 2 hr after cryosurgery (Fig. 4.6).

VII. *Low recurrence rate and increased survival* in an animal experiment with B16 melanoma treated by cryochemotherapy: B16 melanoma was inoculated to BDF_1 mice, and when the tumor grew to 10 mm in diameter, the size not completely destroyed by cryosurgery, the tumor was frozen at −196 °C for 40 sec in each of 2 cycles. DTIC, 300 mg/kg was administered intraperitoneally immediately after cryosurgery, and the recurrence rate was recorded. The rate of recurrence in the group treated with cryosurgery and DTIC was 75.0%, whereas it was 86.7% in the control group, treated by cryosurgery alone (Fig. 4.7). The time to recurrence in the group treated with DTIC was shorter than in the control group. The difference between the two groups was statistically significant as determined by the Wilcoxon test. The growth of the tumor remnants after cryosurgery was inhibited by the anticancer drug, which had been trapped during cryosurgery.

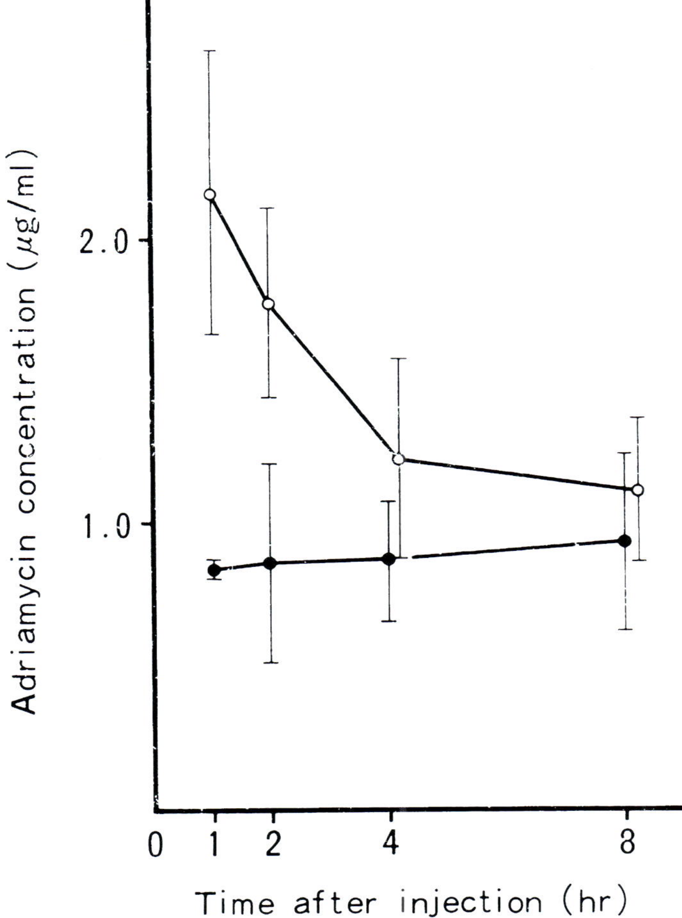

Fig. 4.4. Adriamycin concentration in the tumor after cryosurgery. Combined cryosurgery and adriamycin (●), adriamycin alone (○). Mean ± SE

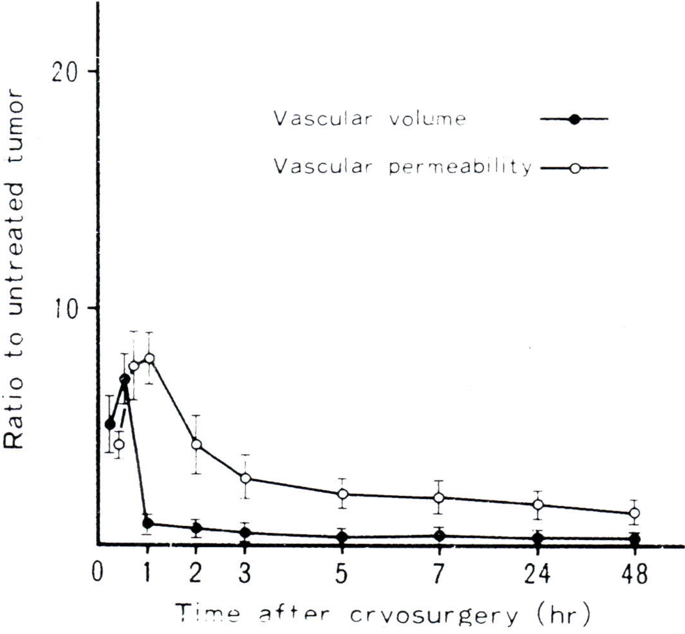

Fig. 4.5. Vascular volume and permeability after cryosurgery of the tumor. Vascular volume (●), vascular permeability (○). Mean ± SE

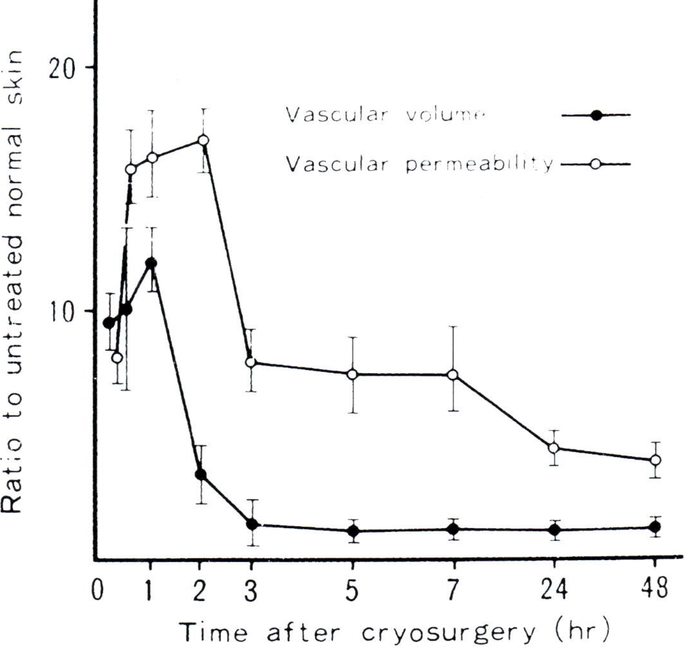

Fig. 4.6. Vascular volume and permeability after cryosurgery of the normal skin. Vascular volume (●), vascular permeability (○). Mean ± SE

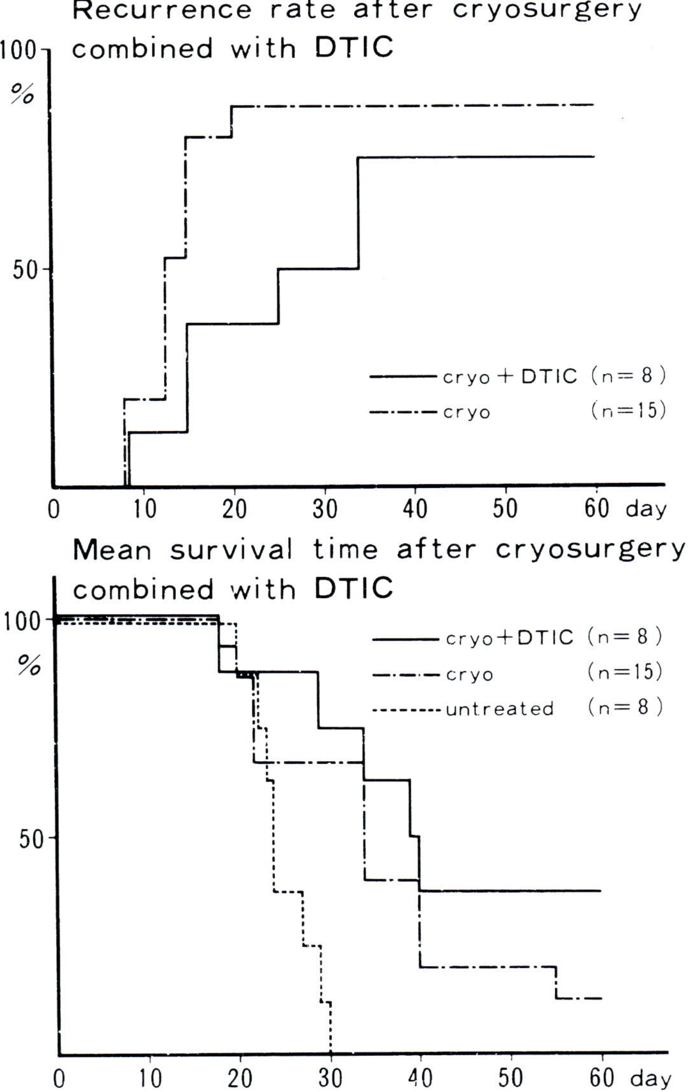

Fig. 4.7. Recurrence rate after treatment by cryosurgery alone or in combination with DTIC. Combined cryosurgery and DTIC (—), n = 8. Cryosurgery alone (— • —), n = 15

4.3 Clinical Evidence

As described earlier, the local injection of an oil-type anticancer agent, e.g., oil-bleo had a striking effect against squamous cell carcinoma in conjunction with cryosurgery. Two representative cases are demonstrated as follows:

Case 1. Tongue cancer, recurrent, a 46-year-old male. A recurrent tumor on the left side, found November 1986 (Fig. 4.8A). Oil-bleo, 30 mg, was injected intratumorally and on the periphery of the tumor, and was immediately followed by cryosurgery. The result was complete cryoablation of the tumor and no recurrence since then, more than 14 years later, leaving a tissue defect but no tongue dysfunction (Fig. 4.8B). Total extirpation of the tongue was avoided.

Case 2. Tongue cancer, recurrent, in an 85-year-old female. The tumor invaded mandibular bone

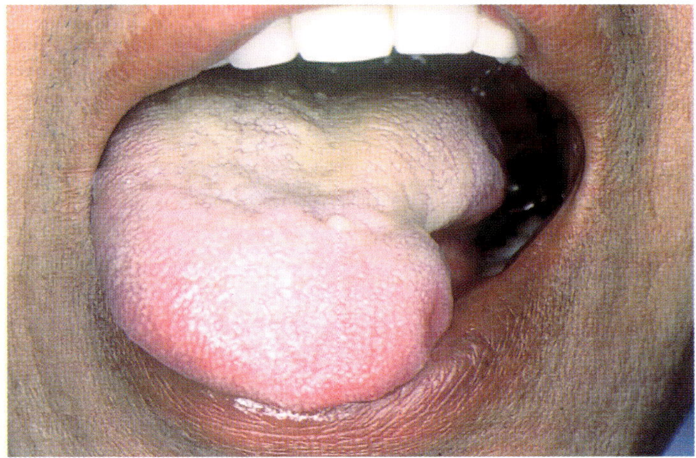

Fig. 4.8B. Appearance 10 years later. Shows tissue defect and a scar, but no recurrence since cryochemotherapy

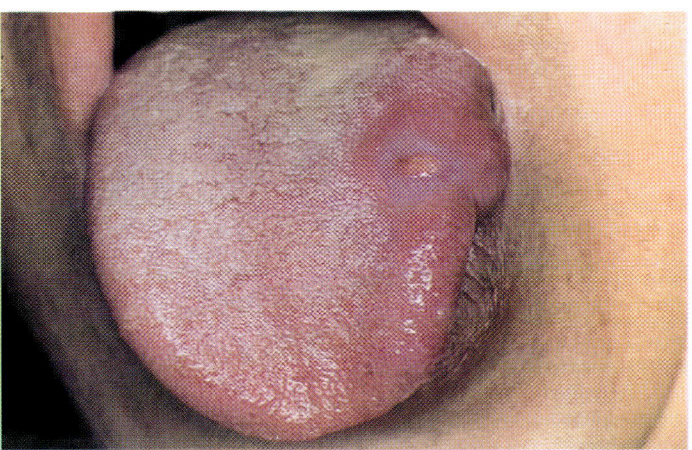

Fig. 4.8A. A tongue cancer male, 46 y. A recurrent tumor on the left margin before cryosurgery

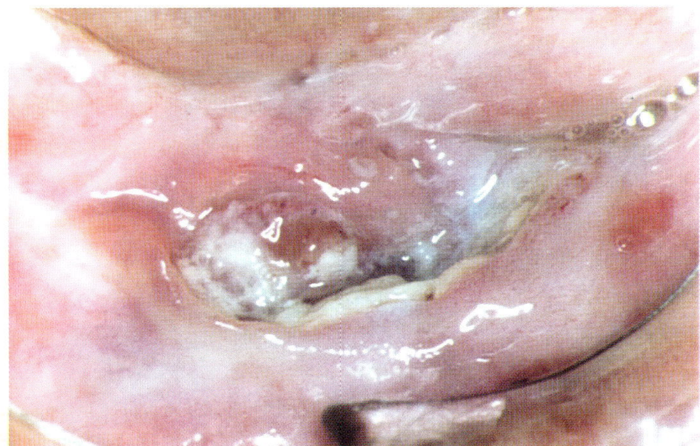

Fig. 4.9A. A tongue cancer, recurrent, female, 85 y. The tumor invaded mandibular bone

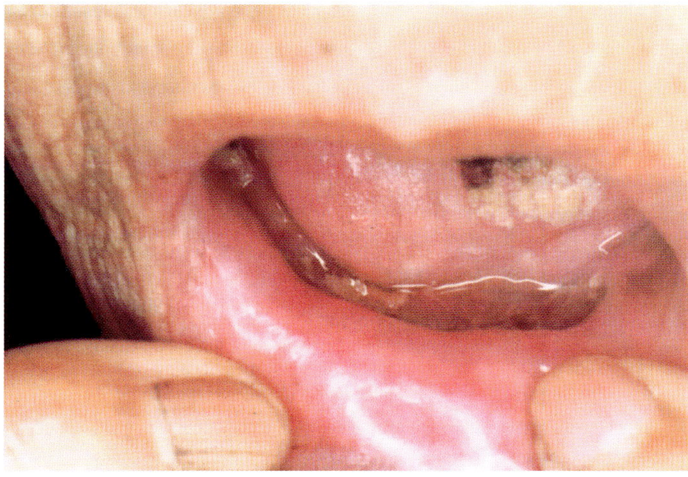

Fig. 4.9B. Six months after cryochemotherapy. Tongue functions are maintained, and no tumor cells detected afterwards

(Fig. 4.9A). Cryosurgery, immediately after injection of oil-bleo, 30 mg intratumorally and in the adjacent area, resulted in unexpected eradication of the tumor, and no recurrence thereafter (Fig. 4.9B).

4.4 Comments

With cryochemotherapy certain anticancer drugs accumulate in a high concentration within or at the periphery of the tumor, thus multiplying the effect of the treatment. Fujimura (6) in an animal experiment reported on the combination of cryosurgery and 5-FU for treatment of an Ehrlich tumor, in which the uptake of 5-FU was significantly increased in the tumor margin, but not in the center, when administered from 3 to 24 hrs after cryosurgery. Therefore, it is essential that anticancer agents should be administered while the vascular permeability is highest, one hour after cryosurgery, but vascular volume decreases abruptly and markedly after cryosurgery. In this respect, locally long-lived oil-based anticancer agents are of preference for use in conjunction with cryosurgery as the strategy against head-and-neck cancer.

References

1. Abe F, Yoshioka O, Ebihara K, Koyu A, Suzuki H, Inoue H, Kodama A, Matsuda A (1978) Studies on organ distribution, adsorption and excretion of peplomycin sulfate. Jpn J Antibiot (Tokyo) 31: 886–894.
2. Abrams HL (1964) Altered drug response of tumor vessels in man. Nature (London) 201: 167–170.
3. Ackerman NB, Hechmer PA (1977) Effects of pharmacological agents on the microcirculation of tumors implanted in the liver. Bibl Anat 15: 301–303.
4. Benson JW (1972) Regional chemotherapy and local cryotherapy for cancer. Oncology 26: 134–151.
5. Benson JW (1975) Combined chemotherapy and cryosurgery for oral cancer. Amer J Surg 130: 596–600.
6. Fujimura K (1982) Experimental studies on cryochemotherapy. Acta Obstet Gynecol Jpn 34: 21–29 (in Japanese).
7. Kimura K, Fujita H, Sakai Y (1971) Blood levels, tissue distribution and clinical effects of adriamycin. In: Proceedings, 1st International Symposium on Adriamycin, Milan, Italy. Springer, Wien New York, pp. 124–134.
8. Lenz, H (1972) Cryosurgery of the cheek pouch of the golden Syrian hamster. Int Surg 57: 223–228.
9. Matton J, Appelgren L, Karlsson L, Peterson HI (1978) Influence of vasoactive drugs and ischemia on intratumor blood flow distribution. Eur J Cancer 14: 761–764.
10. Papadimitrou JM, Woods AE (1974) Structural and functional characteristics of the microcirculation in neoplasma. J Pathol 116: 65–72.
11. Rankin JG, Jirtle R, Phernetton TM (1977) Anomalous response of tumor vasculature to norepinephrine and prostaglandin E_2 in the rabbit. Cir Res 41: 496–502.
12. Rosso R, Ravazzoni C, Esposito M, Sala R, Santi L (1972) Plasma and urinary levels of adriamycin in man. Eur J Cancer 8: 455–459.
13. Song CW, Levitt SH (1970) Effect of X irradiation on vascularity of normal tissue and experimental tumor. Radiology 94: 445–447.
14. Song CW (1978) Effect of hyperthermia on vascular functions of normal tissues and experimental tumors. J Natl Cancer Inst 60: 711–713.
15. Suzuki M, Hori K, Abe I, Saito S, Sato H (1981) A new approach to cancer therapy: selective enhancement of tumor blood flow with angiotensin II. J Natl Cancer Inst 67: 663–669.
16. Takahashi K, Ekimoto H, Aoyagi S, Koyu R, Kuramoshi H, Yoshioka O, Matsuda A, Fujii A, Umezawa H (1979) Biological studies on the degradation products of 3-[(S)-1′-phenylethyl-amino] prophylamin-obleomycin: a novel analog (peplomycin). J Antibiot (Tokyo) 32: 36–42.
17. Venditti JM (1976) Antitumor activity of DTIC in animals. Cancer Treat Rep 60: 135–140.
18. Yong SW, Hollenberg NK, Kazam E, Berkowitz DM, Hainen R, Sandor T, Abrams HL (1979) Resting host and tumor perfusion as determinants of tumor vasculature response to norepinephrines. Cancer Res 39: 1898–1903.
19. Zacarian SA, Stone D, Clater M (1970) Effect of cryogenic temperatures of microcirculation in the golden hamster cheek pouch. Cryobiology 7: 27–39.

5. Experimental Cryoimmunology

Shigeo Tanaka, Tetsuo Ohkuma, and Zenichiro Ishii

5.1 Introduction

Cryosurgery *per se* aims at a local effect, namely, destruction *in situ* of neoplasms resistant to conventional treatments, but it also elicits an immunologic reaction (cryoimmunologic reaction). In animal experiments, production of antibodies in consequence of freezing treatment was first reported by Yantorno et al. (14) and Shulman et al. (9) in rabbit normal accessory glands, and these antibodies were proved to be tissue- or organ-specific and species-specific. Antibodies in serum in syngeneic mice tumor systems were demonstrated by Blackwood et al. (3). And Ablin et al. (2) elicited antibodies reactive with prostatic tissue in man, as demonstrated by the immunofluorescence technique. Further, Mochizuki (6) reported transfer of tumor-specific immunity by infusion of the cryoimmune lymphocytes to other rats, showing establishment of passive antitumor immunization.

A number of clinical reports suggesting induction or stimulation of tumor-specific immune reaction in consequence of cryosurgery in man were published in the 1970s (1,5,11,13). The mechanism of action is still unknown, but apparently involves both humoral and cell-mediated immunity, the latter playing an important role in the tumor-specific immune reaction.

Histologically, this is represented by the lymphoid infiltration into the target area, as a manifestation of the immunologic reaction of the host. Most of the infiltrating lymphocyte subsets into the tumor tissue are comprised of T cells, later defined as the "tumor infiltrating lymphocytes (TIL)". This was first verified in our animal experiments and the characteristics of cryoimmunologic reaction, organ-specific and tumor-specific, were determined. Growth arrest of the tumor cells owing to a cryoimmunologic reaction was demonstrated in man in our recent clinical study (12) by means of the immunohistochemical technique.

In the following the design of our experiments on cryoimmunology is described.

5.2 Augmentation of Cryoimmunologic Reaction

I. 1. Histopathologic verification of cryoimmunologic reaction in animals: appearance of TIL in Vx2 carcinoma of rabbits.
   2. Cross reactivity of cryoimmunologic reaction in allogeneic tumor systems in mice.
   3. Strict tumor-specificity in a syngeneic tumor system in mice.

II. 1. Intensification of cryoimmunologic reaction with adjuvant immunopotentiators in mice.
   2. Intensification of cryoimmune reaction by certain immunopotentiators in man, evaluated by blastoid transformation of lymphocytes by PHA (phytohemagglutinin), a preliminary study.

III. Demonstration of possible cryoimmunointensification therapy. Growth arrest of tumor cells indicated by immunohistochemical staining: immunostain of the encoded proteins of oncogenes.

(1) *Histological verification of cryoimmunologic reaction in Vx2 carcinoma-bearing rabbits:* Rabbits (Japan White) were implanted with Vx2 carcinoma subcutaneously on both sides of their back, 5×10^6 cells to the right back and 1×10^6 cells to the left back. Eight days later, tumors on both sides were established. Then, the tumor on the right side was destroyed by cryosurgery, at −120°C for 3+2+1.5 min, 3-cycle freezing, while the tumor on the left side was left untreated. Histopathologic examinations were made on the 17th day after cryosurgery. Figure 5.1 is a photomicrograph of the left tumor of the control rabbit, showing infiltrative proliferation into the dermis. Figure 5.2 is a photomicrograph of the tumor on the right side, which underwent cryosurgery. Necrosis of subcutaneous fatty tissue ensued, and no tumor cells are observed. However, the tumor on the left side of the same rabbit shows central necrosis and liquefaction of the tumor (Fig. 5.3), and the tumor residue is circumscribed by reactive granulation, rich in cells and newly grown capillaries. Cell components of this area consist mainly of TIL, as defined later, plasma cells, monocytes, and macrophages (Fig. 5.4). This granulation tissue results from the interstitial reaction against cancer, and this phenomena can be interpreted as a manifestation of the antitumor immunity.

(2) *Specificity of antitumor activity evaluated by challenge test*

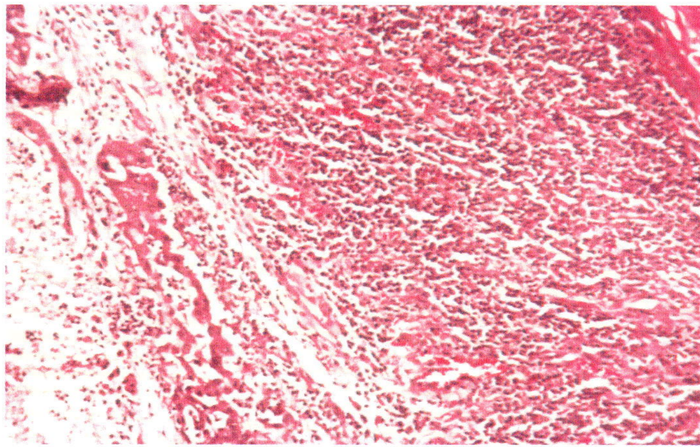

Fig. 5.1. Vx2 carcinoma in a control rabbit (H.E.×50). The tumor shows infiltrative proliferation into dermis

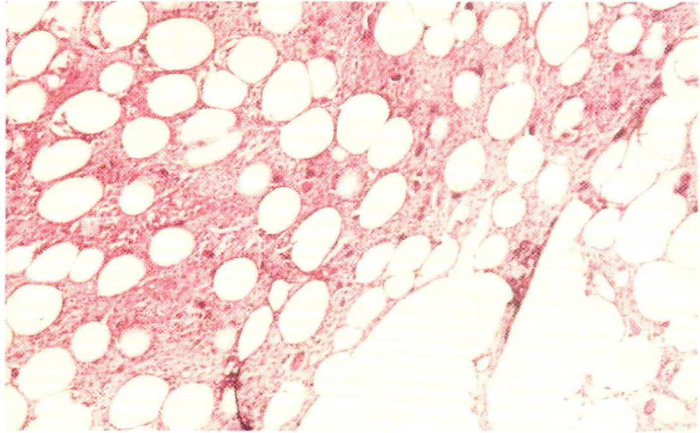

Fig. 5.2. Cryonecrosis of Vx2 carcinoma of the right side, the 17th postoperative day (H.E.×50). No tumor cells are recognized. −120°C, 3-cycle freezing, 3+2+1.5 min, contact method, LN_2

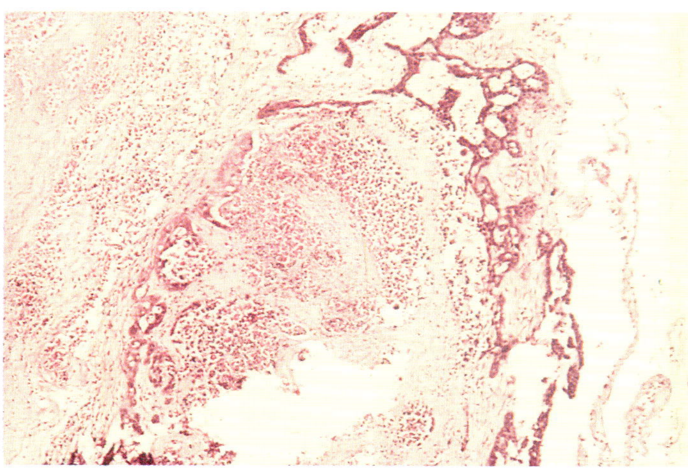

Fig. 5.3. Encapsulated, regressing tumor of the nontreated left side, 17 days after cryosurgery of the right side tumor (H.E. ×50). Central necrosis and liquefaction are obvious, and the tumor residue is circumscribed by reactive granulation tissue rich in cells and newly grown capillaries

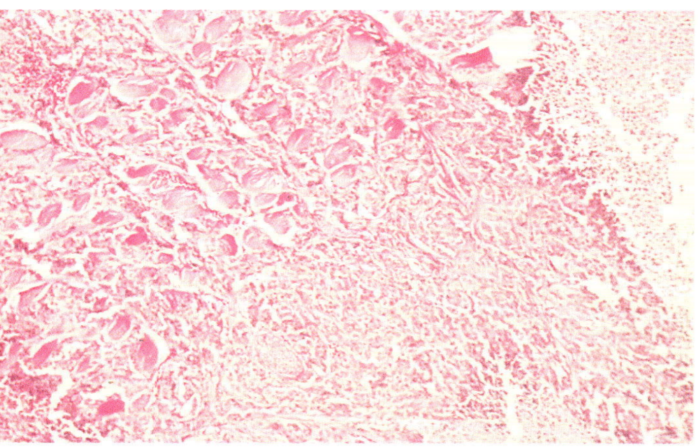

Fig. 5.4. Marked lymphoid infiltration observed in the reactive granulation tissue, in the juxtatumor regions (H.E.×50)

(a) *Cross-reactivity of cryoimmunologic reaction in allogeneic tumor systems in animals.* In some allogeneic systems, cross-reactivity was observed. Vx2 carcinoma-immune rabbits rejected Vx7 carcinoma under certain conditions. Incidentally, both Vx2 and Vx7 carcinomas are originated from the same Shope Papilloma. Histologically, Vx7 retains characteristics of squamous cell carcinoma, suggesting its epithelial origin, whereas Vx2 exhibits anaplastic type carcinoma. And, in the sarcoma 180/ICR mice tumor system, cryosurgery-treated mice resisted the intraabdominal challenge of Ehrlich ascites carcinoma, although not the challenge of the same sarcoma 180 (Table 5.1).

(b) *Strict tumor-specificity in syngeneic tumor system in mice.* In the syngeneic MethA/BALB/c tumor system, cryosurgically acquired MethA immune mice did not reject BAMC1, a fibrosarcoma induced by the same methylcholanthrene originated by the same host, as seen in Table 5.2. This indicates the strict specificity of antitumor activity or the tumor-specificity of cryoimmunity acquired by the cryotreatment in syngeneic tumor systems, in accordance with the report of Faraci et al. (4).

(c) *Time course of antitumor activity estimated by challenge test.* Antitumor activity induced by cryosurgery was tested in allogeneic and syngeneic murine tumor systems. In the sarcoma 180/ICR mice tumor system, rechallenge was performed on the 4th, 7th, and 21st day after cryosurgery and increase in life span (ILS) was observed. Maximum antitumor activity (ILS of 56.4%) was noted in the group which received rechallenge of the tumor on the 7th day (Table 5.3). The same trial was performed in the syngeneic MethA/BALB/c system, indicating maximum activity in the early period –

Table 5.1. Mean survival time of cryosurgery-treated sarcoma 180/ICR mice when challenged by Ehrlich ascites carcinoma

S180 (sc)	Cryo	5×10^4 cells ip challenge		MST (days) (mean ± SD)	60 days survivors/ total
		S180	Ehrlich		
+	+		+	59.5 ± 1.1	5/6
+	–		+	37.8 ± 18.2	1/5
+	+	+		22.2 ± 4.7	0/5
–		+		18.8 ± 2.2	0/5

Note: MST, mean survival time: SD, standard deviation.

Table 5.2. Tumor size of BAMC1 challenged to cryosurgically acquired MethA-Resistant BALB/c mice

Mice	No. of BAMC1 challenged	Days after BAMC1 challenge		
		11	20	36
MethA immune	1×10^6 cells	3.8 ± 1.6*	9.5 ± 2.8	19.2 ± 0.6
MethA immune	5×10^5	2.0 ± 0.8	5.7 ± 1.4	13.3 ± 1.3
Control	1×10^6	3.0 ± 0.4	6.8 ± 0.6	17.3 ± 2.8

* Mean ± SD, mm.

Table 5.3. Time course of antitumor immunity estimated by challenge test. (1) sarcoma 180/ICR mice (Allogeneic)

Challenge days after cryosurgery[a]	MST (days) (mean ± SE)	ILS (%)	60 days survivors/ total
4	20.3 ± 0.8	8.0	0/8
7	29.4 ± 6.3	56.4	2/8
14	17.9 ± 2.0	–4.8	0/8
21	18.8 ± 0.6	0.0	0/8
Control	18.8 ± 0.6	0.0	0/8

[a] 5×10^4 cells of sarcoma 180 ip challenge. ILS, increase in life span.

Table 5.4. Time course of antitumor immunity estimated by challenge test. (2) MethA/BALB/c Mice (Syngeneic)

Challenge days after cryosurgery[a]	MST (days) (mean ± SE)	ILS (%)	60 days survivors/ total
4	50.6 ± 5.8	97.7	6/8
7	48.8 ± 4.7	90.6	4/8
14	37.8 ± 5.3	47.7	2/8
21	40.4 ± 8.6	58.7	4/7
Control	25.6 ± 1.7	0.0	0/8

[a] 1×10^5 cells of MethA ip challenge.

on the 4th day (ILS of 97.7% after cryosurgery) – and minimum activity on the 14th day (Table 5.4).

(d) *Beneficial and adverse effects.* Dose-dependent effects of some biological response modifiers (BRM), levamisole and BCG, upon combined treatment with cryosurgery in a syngeneic B16 melanoma/BDF_1 mice tumor system were investigated (7). Levamisole, 1 mg/kg/day or 5 mg/kg/day was administered intraperitoneally every other day eight times pre- and postcryosurgery or surgical amputation of the original tumor. Eight days after cryosurgery, B16 melanoma was challenged, and growth of the tumor was measured. Combined treatment with 1 mg/kg/day of levamisole showed a suppression of the tumor growth with cryosurgery. But administration of 5 mg/kg/day had no effect. Likewise, BCG, 0.5, 1, and 2 mg/mouse/day was injected into the foot pad every 3 days six times. Results indicated that no effect was observed with 0.5 mg, significant tumor suppression ($P<0.05$) with 1 mg/mouse/day (cryosurgery predominant), whereas tumor progression was noticed with 2 mg/mouse/day. These facts indicate existence of an optimum dose in immunomodulators when combined with cryosurgery. An overdose holds the danger of resulting in tumor progression (or rather, immunologically induced aggravation), hence extreme caution must be exercised when using these materials (BRMs) as adjunct to cryosurgery.

5.3 Intensification of Cryoimmunologic Reaction

(1) *Augmentation of cryoimmunologic reaction and intensification of the tumor-specific immunity (cryoimmunointensification):* In an experimental tumor system in ICR mice, sarcoma 180 was implanted subcutaneously, and 7 days later, the established tumors were destroyed by cryosurgery. Certain boosters, EA, EA_3, EA_5, or EA_6 (8) were administered 10 mg/kg/day intraperitoneally prior to and after cryosurgery for 10 days (Fig. 5.5). EA is the acetone precipitate of a hot water extract of an edible mushroom, *Flammulina velutipes* (Curt. ex Fr.) Sing.; EA_3: β-1,3-glucan; EA_5: heteropolysaccharide; and EA_6 is a protein-bound polysaccharide fraction derived from EA and the component characteristic to the *Flammulina velutipes*. Seven days after cryosurgery, sarcoma 180 again was implanted intraperitoneally, and increase in life span of the animals was observed. As depicted in Fig. 5.5, the administration of EA_6 resulted in a marked increase in life span of the animals when used in conjunction with cryosurgery. In view of

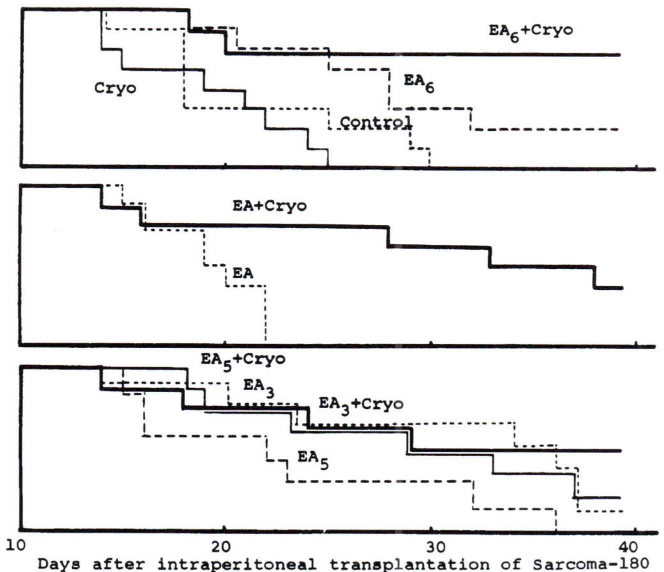

Fig. 5.5. Effect of cryosurgery on sarcoma 180 solid tumor and combined administration i.p. of EA, EA_3, EA_5, and EA_6 on the increase in life span of ICR mice, challenged by the same tumor intraperitoneally

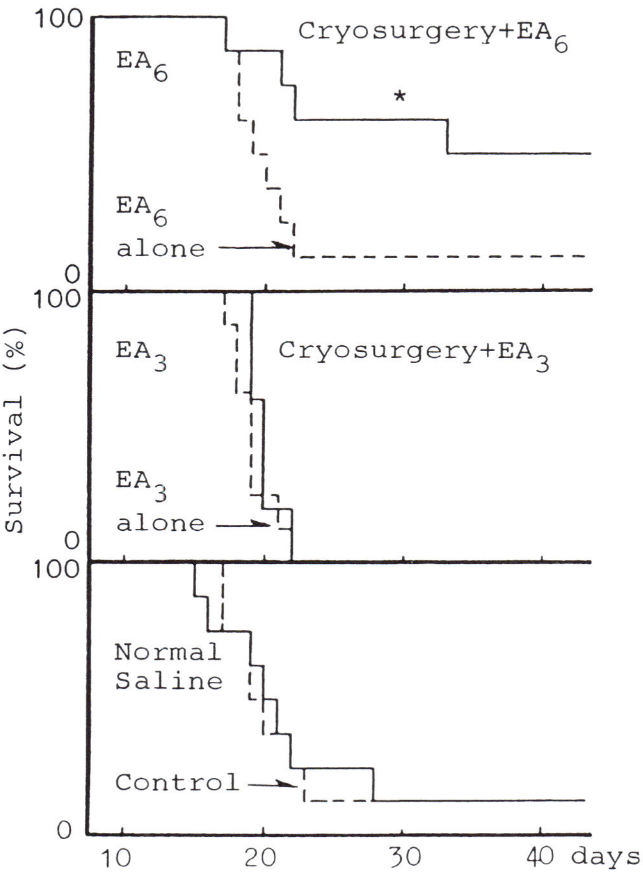

Fig. 5.6. Increase in life span of ICR mice, treated by combined cryosurgery and EA_3 or EA_6 p.o., challenged by sarcoma 180 intraperitoneally. 1) EA_3 or EA_6 was orally administered to ICR mice 50 mg/kg daily for 10 days. Cryodestruction of established tumor (sarcoma 180) was performed on day −7. Mice were challenged with ascites tumor of sarcoma 180 i.p. (5×10^4 cells) on day 0. $^*P < 0.05$ as compared with the control group

the results in this tumor system thus far, cryosurgery alone hardly induces immunity sufficient to reject the same tumor when challenged intraperitoneally. However, adjunctive use of an effective booster such as EA_6 will exert synergistic action and intensify latent cryoimmunity to a valuable degree.

(2) When one of those boosters, EA_3 was administered orally in conjunction with cryosurgery (Fig. 5.6), EA_3 gave no beneficial effect, i.e., it probably was not absorbed by the intestine or it underwent degradation, but EA_6 showed significant effect in increase in life span of the animals when administered either i.p. or p.o.

(3) Assays on immune parameters in animals: Parameters as described below are old by now, but to assess the host's immune function when cryo-

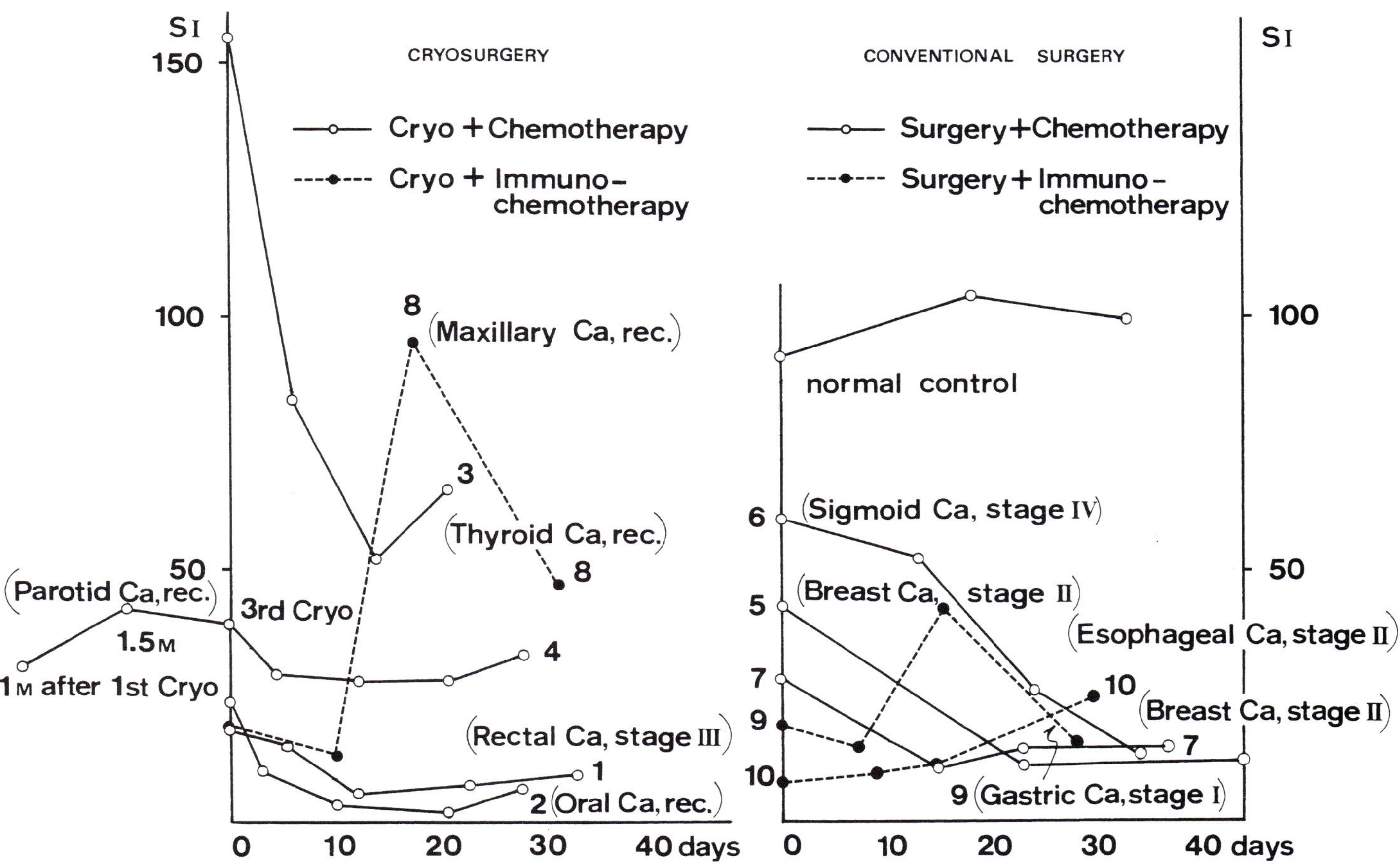

Fig. 5.7. Blastoid transformation of lymphocytes by PHA before and after surgery in man (supermicromethod using whole blood culture, July–August 1980, February-March 1981) SI: stimulation index. *TNM classification revised according to UICC 1997

surgery was combined with oral administration 100 mg/kg/day of EA_6, the following tests were carried out (7).

(a) Delayed hypersensitivity reaction (DHR) by sheep red blood cells (SRBC), representing T lymphocyte function, i.e., cellular immunity; (b) an increase in number of splenic antibody-forming cells (plaque-forming cells: PFC), representing IgM production, i.e., humoral immunity; (c) carbon clearance test, representing function of the reticuloendothelial system. The results of the DHR and PFC tests denoted the most increase in activity when cryosurgery was combined with EA_6, suggesting that this material activates both cellular and humoral immunity after cryosurgery. As for the carbon clearance test, practically no difference was observed between the experimental groups, indicating no possible participation of the reticuloendothelial system (7).

(4) Blastoid transformation of lymphocytes by PHA as a marker of cryoimmunointensification before and after cryosurgery in man, a preliminary study: Figure 5.7 depicts a follow-up of five examples each of PHA-blastoid transformation of lymphocytes in the cryosurgery group and the conventional surgery group, expressed by a stimulation index (SI) pre- and postcryosurgery, by means of the supermicromethod utilizing whole blood cell culture. (10) The general immunity in man decreases for a short while postsurgically. We generally combine chemotherapy as an adjunct to surgery, but as a rule, commencing 2 weeks after the operation. Cases No. 5 and 7 of stage II breast cancer and Case No. 6 of stage IV sigmoid cancers are good examples of those who received conventional surgery with chemotherapy, indicating the low immune response lasted more than 1 month even in the stage II cancer. Cryosurgery-treated patients never showed postcryosurgical immune stimulation, but apparently they had a tendency to recover 4 weeks after cryosurgery. In all, the postoperative course was uneventful and the general condition of the patients was well maintained. Case No. 3 is a patient with recurrent thyroid cancer, showing a high SI before cryosurgery. This patient was treated by cryosurgery only, but SI marked the lowest level on the 14th postoperative day, and recovery on the 21st day after

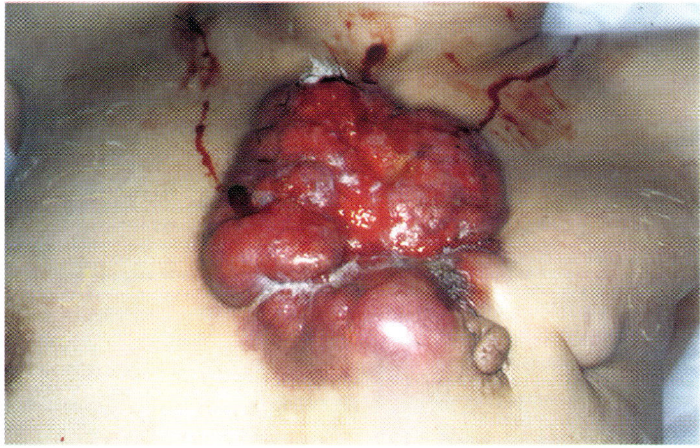

Fig. 5.8. An advanced bilateral breast cancer, female, 67 y. The left main tumor was ulcerating and bleeding

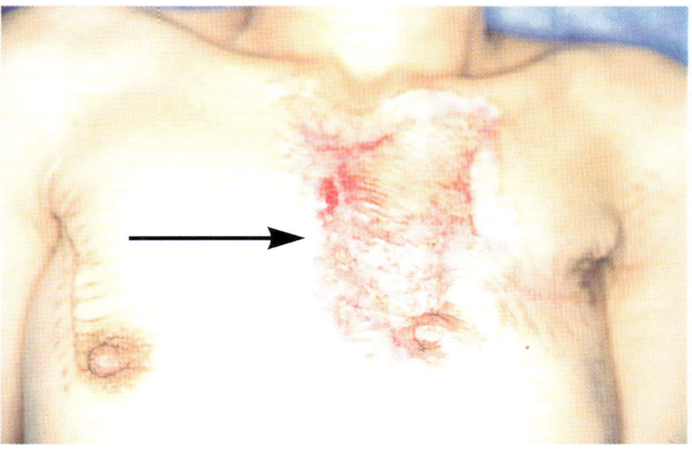

Fig. 5.9. After sequential cryosurgery, necrotomy followed by a mesh skin graft. A persistent small local recurrence is seen at the right margin of the skin graft (arrow)

cryosurgery. These facts indicate the necessity of the combined use of adjuvant immunopotentiators with cryosurgery (cryoimmuno-intensification therapy). Indeed, cases No. 8 and 9, which were given such a booster (FEH-1: a crude hot water extract of *Flammulina velutipes* Sing.), exhibited peaks in SI on the 14th postoperative day.

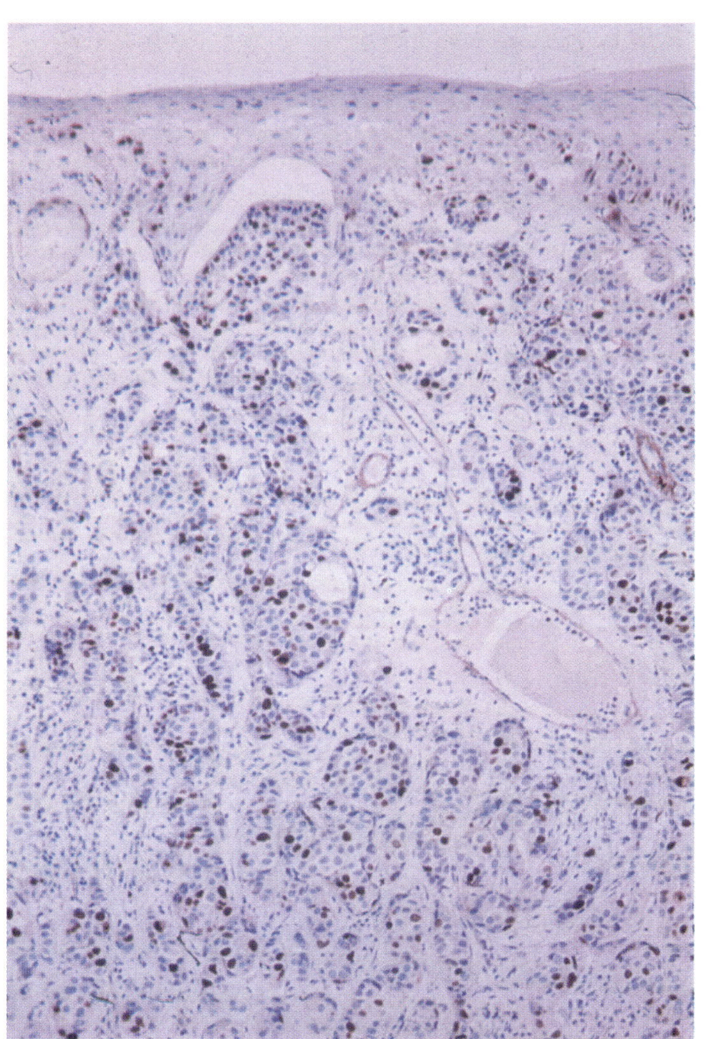

Fig. 5.10. Ki-67 stain before treatment: positive. ×10

5.4 Demonstration of Possible Cryoimmuno-intensification Therapy

Growth arrest of the tumor cells verified by immunohistochemical staining for the encoded proteins of oncogenes and oncosuppressor genes: A case report. A 67-year-old female, with an advanced bilateral breast cancer (12), continuously bleeding from the ulcerating tumor (Fig. 5.8), was treated by extensive cryosurgery. TNM classification was impossible, but biopsy revealed ductal adenocarcinoma with scirrhous pattern. In consideration of the patient's extremely poor general condition, only single cryosurgery was attempted to stop bleeding as palliation, and chemotherapy or radiotherapy was ruled out of the treatment regimen. But in effect, it almost eradicated the main tumor and the patient's general condition was improved. Thus additional surgery followed: lumpectomy of the bilateral breast with axillary lymph node dissection. The lymph nodes in the left supraclavicular region and neck disappeared spontaneously. One year later, after 2-month immunotherapy with FEH-G (a granule preparation made of FEH-1, a hot water extract of *Flammulina velutipes* Sing.), a small persistent skin tumor, a local recurrence which had not enlarged, along the right margin of the skin graft (Fig. 5.9) was resected for immunohistochemical examination: p53, Ki-67,

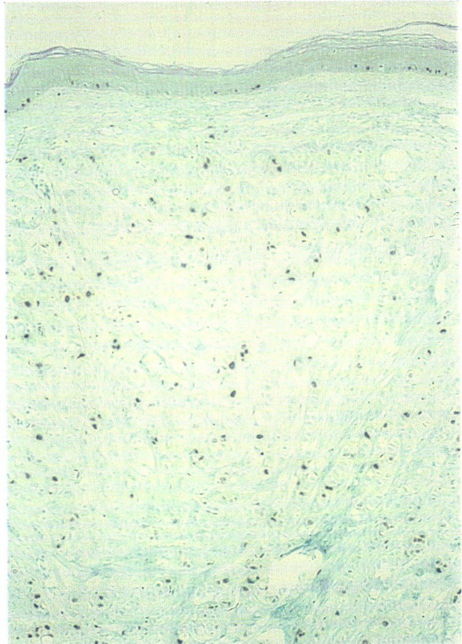

Fig. 5.11. Ki-67 stain after immunotherapy: negative. ×10

BCL-2, estrogen receptor, and progesterone receptor. Results of immunostain before and after the immunotherapy revealed negative stain of Ki-67 after the treatment (Figs. 5.10, 5.11), indicating no actively proliferating cells in the tumor after the immunotherapy. Expression of p53 and of BCL-2 was negative, the estrogen receptor had turned negative at the termination of immunotherapy, and the progesterone receptor was negative throughout the course of treatment. This evidence demonstrates the growth arrest of the tumor after the immunotherapy, at least locally, in spite of apoptosis being practically absent at the termination of immunotherapy. Both hormone receptors were negative, and indicated endocrine therapy is no longer effective; hence cryoimmunointensification was strongly suggested.

References

1. Ablin RJ, Soanes WA, Gonder MJ (1971) Prospects of cryoimmunotherapy in cases of metastasizing carcinoma of the prostate. Cryobiology 8: 271–279.
2. Ablin RJ, Gonder MJ, Soanes WA (1974) Elution of cell-bound antiprostatic epithelial antibodies after multiple cryotherapy of carcinoma of the prostate. Cryobiology 11: 218–221.
3. Blackwood CE, Cooper IS (1972) Response of experimental tumor systems to cryosurgery. Cryobiology 9: 508–515.
4. Faraci RP, Bagley DM, Marrone JC, Beazley RM (1975) In vitro demonstration of cryosurgical augmentation of tumor immunity. Surgery 77: 433–438.
5. Gursel E, Roberts M, Veenema RJ (1972) Regression of prostatic cancer following sequential cryotherapy to the prostate. J Urol 108: 928–932.
6. Mochizuki T (1981) An experimental study of passive cancer immunotherapy by infusion of the immune lymphocytes. J Jpn Surg Soc 82: 193–202 (in Japanese).
7. Ohkuma T, Ikekawa T, Tanaka S (1980) Cryoimmunointensification therapy with cryosurgery and adjuvant immunopotentiators. In: Proceedings, IV World Congress of Cryosurgery, Sanremo, Italy, pp. 99–112.
8. Ohkuma T, Otagiri K, Ikekawa T, Tanaka S (1982) Augmentation of antitumor activity by combined cryodestruction of sarcoma 180 and protein-bound polysaccharide EA_6, isolated from *Flammulina velutipes* (Curt ex Fr) Sing in mice. J Pharm Dyn 5: 439–444.
9. Shulman S, Brandt EJ, Yantorno C (1968) Studies in cryo-immunology. II. Tissue and species specificity of the autoantibody response and comparison with isoimmunization. Immunology 14: 149–158.
10. Suzuki H, Samura Y, Fujii G (1978) A supermicromethod using whole blood cell culture for evaluating lymphocyte response to phtohemagglutinin. J Cli Exper Med (Tokyo) 105: 882–884 (in Japanese).
11. Tanaka S (1982) Immunological aspects of cryosurgery in general surgery. Cryobiology 19: 247–262.
12. Tanaka S, Ito M, Shinohara, N (1998) Extensive cryosurgery and immunotherapy for advanced bilateral breast cancer. Immunohistochemical assessment and report of a case. Skin Cancer 13: 123–142.
13. Uhlschmid G, Kolb Z, Largiadèr F (1979) Cryosurgery of pulmonary metastases. Cryobiology 16: 171–178.
14. Yantorno C, Soanes WA, Gonder MJ, Shulman S (1967) Studies in cryoimmunology. I. The production of antibodies to urogenital tissue in consequence of freezing treatment. Immunology 12: 395–410.

6. Experimental Cryosurgery of the Adrenal Gland of Animals

Histopathologic Studies and Assay of the Endocrine Function

Shigeo Tanaka with contributions by Tetsuo Ohkuma, and Zenichiro Ishii

6.1 Introduction

Adrenalectomy (2) has been performed as ablative endocrine therapy for advanced breast cancer and prostatic cancer patients (1,4,6). We attempted safe and quick cryosurgical ablation of the adrenal glands in animal experiments. Summarized results on histopathological and functional changes of the adrenal glands after cryosurgery by Tanaka et al. (5,7) are presented in this chapter.

In histopathologic studies of cryodestroyed adrenal glands in dogs and rabbits, light microscopic observation revealed complete necrosis of the zona glomerulosa and zona reticularis of the adrenal cortex 1 week after cryosurgery, and this necrotic state continued throughout the experimental period of 4 months without regeneration of the glands. Adrenal function was followed by radioimmunoassay of the plasma cortical steroid level: cortisol and dehydroepiandrosterone sulfate (DHEA-S), showed a temporarily marked increase in cortisol level immediately after cryosurgery, then decreased and remained at an extremely low level, indicating no compensation, but suggesting cryoimmunological suppression of the function of the contralateral non-treated gland. At the second cryosurgery, that of the contralateral gland, the response was about half, and declined to an undetectable level. However, response to a rapid ACTH test of the bilaterally adrenalectomized dogs showed elevation to the basal plasma cortisol level. These facts indicate that cryodestruction of one side of the adrenal gland substantially lowered the function of the other. But bilaterally adrenalectomized animal still responded to the ACTH test, suggesting a latent, non-detectable level was evoked to a certain level in an emergency, that may be favorable to the adrenalectomized host in man, i.e., at least the ability to respond such stress is reserved.

6.2 Experiment

Animals: Mongrel dogs of both sexes, body weight 7–12 kg, and Japan White rabbits weighing 3 kg were used, and each experimental group consisted of 2 or 3 animals.

Cryosurgery of the Adrenal Gland: Animals fasted for 24 hrs were anesthetized by intravenous injection of 250 mg of amobarbital to the dogs, and 50 mg to the rabbits. Animals were fixed on the operating table in supine position, and the peritoneal cavity was entered through a median incision. A polypropylene conical tube, 50 mm in diameter at the top and 35 mm in diameter at the bottom and 100 mm long, was inserted into the abdominal cavity to retract intestines and to protect adjacent organs, and the left adrenal gland was exposed. The gland was frozen by a liquid nitrogen (LN_2)-driven cryosurgical unit, Linde CE-2B (Frigitronics of Connecticut Inc., USA) with a PR-6 cryoprobe (8 mm outer diameter, with straight freezing tip) equipped with a specially made T-shaped copper probe-tip adaptor (freezing base of 10–20 mm) or a tonsillar adaptor (10 mm in diameter) for the dog, and a copper cylindrical adaptor of 10 mm in diameter for the rabbit. Freezing temperature and time duration for the rabbits and dogs were −60 °C or −160 °C for 2 or 3 cycles, contact method, as described in the legends of the Figures.

Electron Microscopic Changes Immediately after Cryosurgery: The adrenal cortex of a rabbit, immediately after the freezing (−160°C, 2 cycles, 5 + 3 min) was extirpated, fixed in glutaraldehyde, and was divided into 3 sections from the surface to the center of the gland. Figure 6.1 is an electron photomicrograph of a normal adrenal cortex. Numerous strikingly large and sharp ice crystals are recognized in the middle part of the cortex (Fig. 6.2), and drastic mechanical changes in the organelles are seen. At the surface of the gland, cell boundaries are obscure or have disappeared, and rupture of the nuclei is observed. The mitochondria show marked swelling, reduction in matrix density, and disappearance of cristae. Also, the endoplasmic reticulum shows severe destruction of the structure and dissociation of the ribosomes (Fig. 6.3).

Histopathologic Changes after Cryosurgery: 1) Rabbits, 1 week: Figure 4 shows normal adrenal glands. Immediately after 2-cycle freezing, 5 + 5 min, at −60°C, the gland appeared swollen and dark red in color. One week after the freezing, the

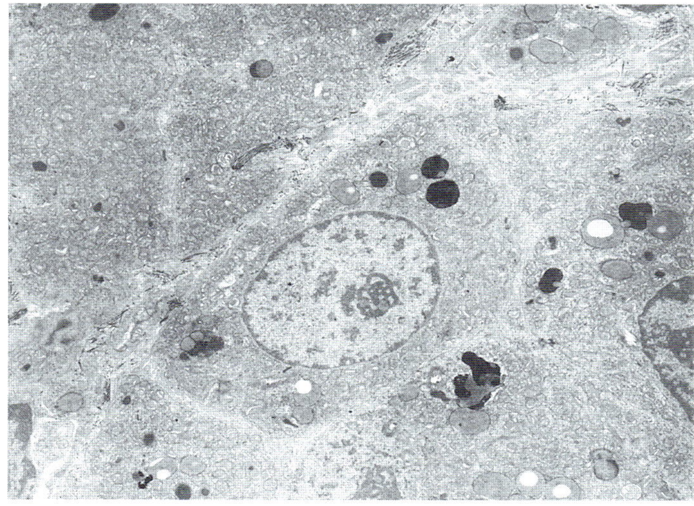

Fig. 6.1. Electron photomicrograph of a normal adrenal cortex of a rabbit

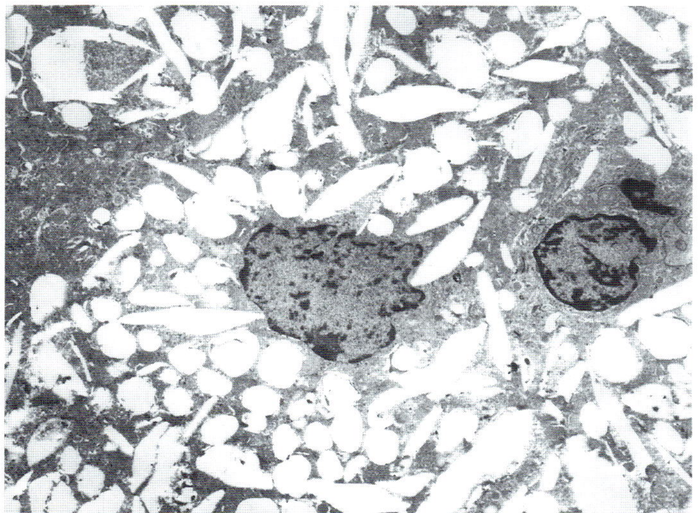

Fig. 6.2. Electron photomicrograph of a middle part of the adrenal cortex of a rabbit, immediately after cryosurgery. −160°C, 2-cycle freezing, 5 + 3 min

zona reticularis was destroyed and stained in deep red with hematoxylin and eosin (H.E.) (Fig. 6.5). Residual cells in the zona glomerulosa were also damaged definitely. The gland was seen almost normal in size, but reddish-brown in color and necrotic. Under the light microscope, the zona glomerulosa showed complete necrosis and the adjacent medulla was almost fading.

2) Rabbits, 3 months: The glands were 3–4 mm in diameter and 2 mm thick and were greyish-yellow in color. Light microscopic examination revealed no regeneration of the glands (Fig. 6.6).

3) Dogs, 2 weeks: Figure 6.7 shows the normal gland, and two-cycle freezing, 5 + 5 min, at −60°C of the glands resulted in a color change from yellow to dark purple immediately after cryosurgery. No bleeding occurred. Laparotomy 2 weeks after cryosurgery demonstrated no intraabdominal adhesion or retroperitoneal hematoma. The treated adrenal glands were hardly distinguishable, but only detected by palpation beneath the lumbo-adrenal vein as an induration. The glands, fibrous and reduced in size, were extirpated and cut into 5 sections for light microscopic studies. Figure 6.8 shows extensive coagulation necrosis from the medulla to the zona fasciculata of the cortex. Though scarce, residual cells are observed in the zona fasciculata and marked vacuolar degenera-

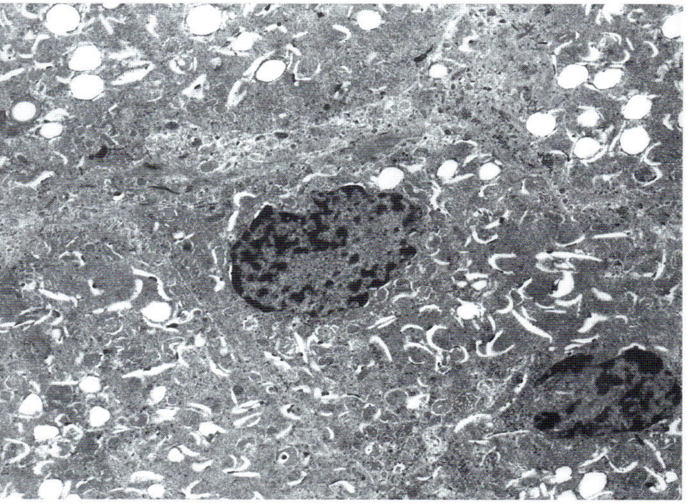

Fig. 6.3. Electron photomicrograph of a surface part of the frozen adrenal cortex of a rabbit, immediately after cryosurgery. −160°C, 2-cycle freezing, 5 + 3 min

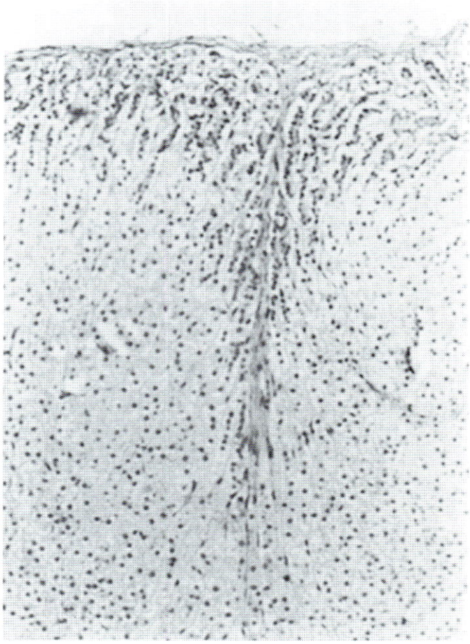

Fig. 6.4. Photomicrograph of a normal adrenal gland of a rabbit (H.E. ×50)

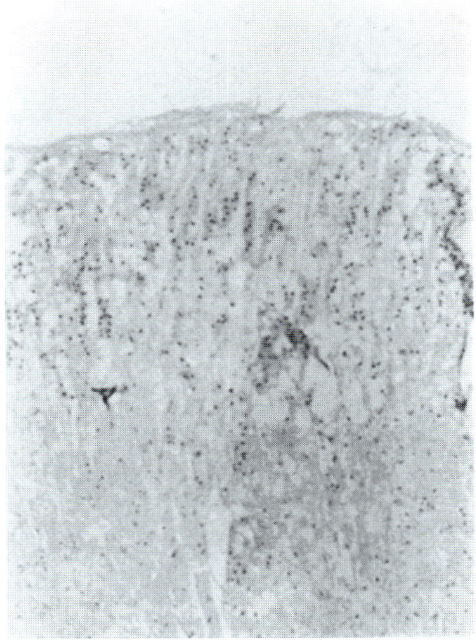

Fig. 6.5. Adrenal gland of a rabbit, 1 week after cryosurgery. −60°C, 2-cycle freezing, 5 + 5 min (H.E., ×50)

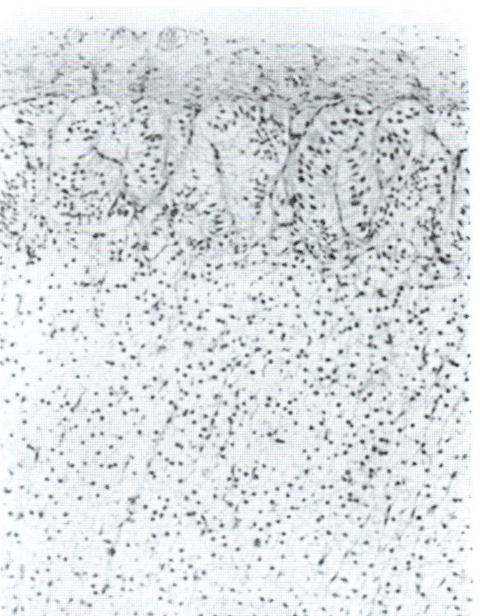

Fig. 6.7. Photomicrograph of a normal canine adrenal gland (H.E. ×50)

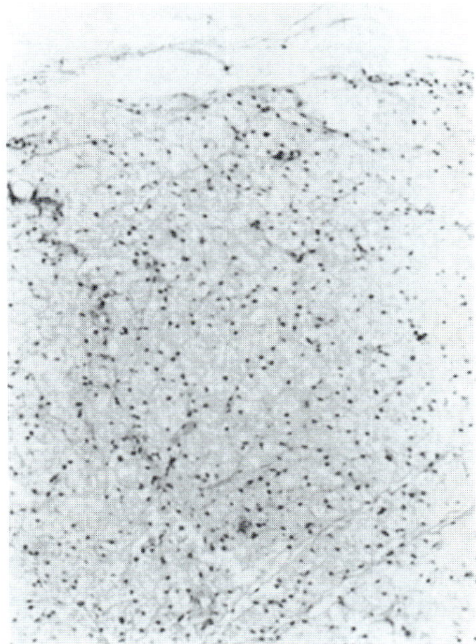

Fig. 6.6. Adrenal gland of a rabbit, 3 months after cryosurgery. −60°C, 2-cycle freezing, 5 + 5 min (H.E., ×50)

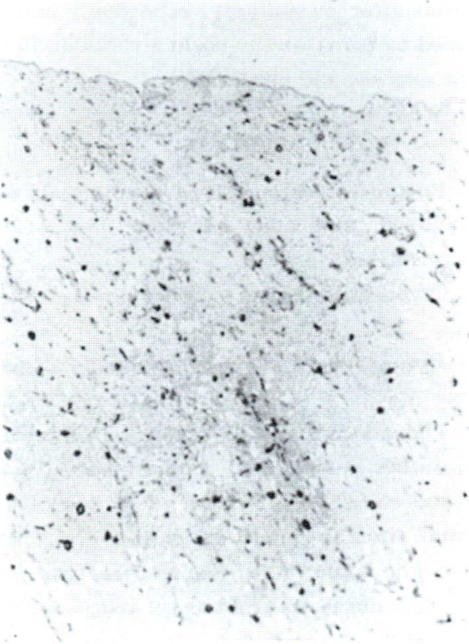

Fig. 6.8. Canine adrenal gland, 2 weeks after cryosurgery. −60°C, 3-cycle freezing, 5 + 5 + 3 min (H.E., ×50)

tion is noticed. The central part of the specimen shows marked degeneration in the zona fasciculata. Coagulation necrosis is seen in all the rest of the specimen.

4) Dogs, 4 weeks: Adrenal glands 10 mm in size prior to cryosurgery, reduced their size markedly to 8 mm 120 days after freezing of the glands, at −60°C for 3 min in each of 2 cycles, with a T-shaped probe-tip adaptor. The glands were hard and fibrous. Figure 6.9 shows a histopathologic view of freeze-treated adrenal glands: Coagulation necrosis, and no normal cells are recognized.

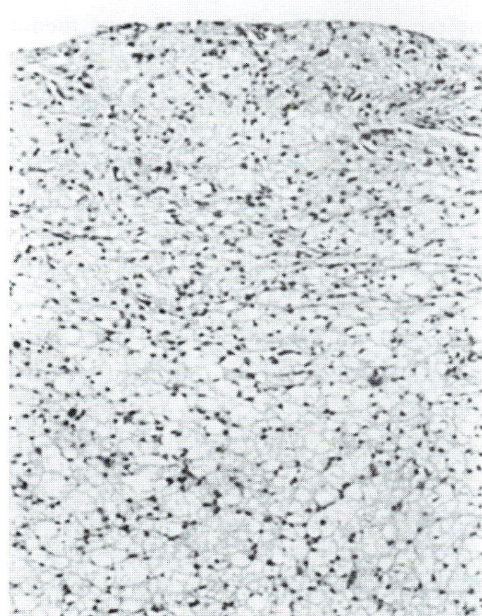

Fig. 6.9. Canine adrenal gland, 4 months after cryosurgery. −60°C, 2-cycle freezing, 3 + 3 min (H.E. ×50)

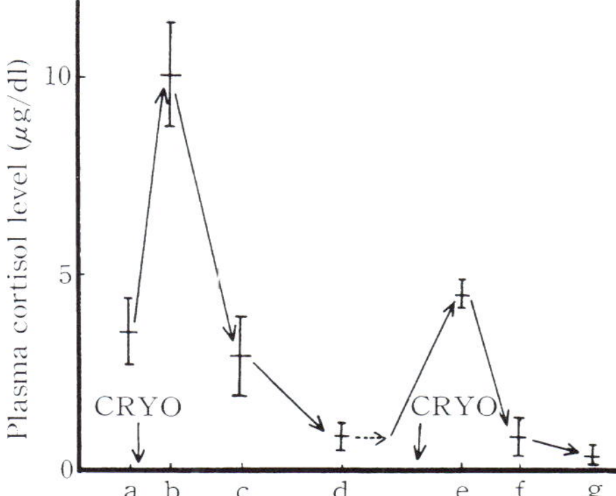

Fig. 6.10. Changes in canine plasma cortisol levels after cryosurgery of the adrenal glands. (a) Normal control. (b) 20–30 min after cryosurgery of the left adrenals ($P < 0.001$, versus (a)). (c) 1–2 days after cryosurgery of the left adrenals ($P < 0.001$, versus (b)). (d) 8–12 days after cryosurgery of the left adrenals ($P < 0.05$, versus (a)). (e) 20–30 min after cryosurgery of the right adrenals ($P < 0.001$, versus (d)). (f) 1–2 days after cryosurgery of the right adrenals ($P < 0.001$, versus (e)). (g) 13–15 days after cryosurgery of the right adrenals ($P < 0.02$, versus (a)). Mean ± SD

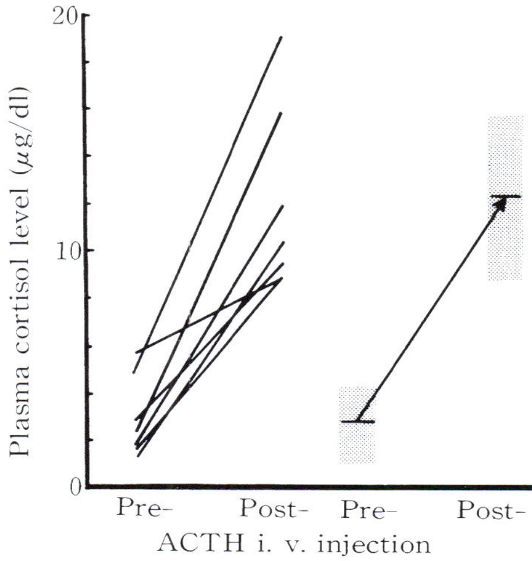

Fig. 6.11. Response of the plasma cortisol level to a rapid ACTH test in the normal dogs. Plasma cortisol level was estimated 45 min after i.v. injection of 0.25 mg of cortrosyn. Mean ± SD

Assay of endocrine function: Thirteen mongrel dogs of both sexes weighing 7 to 12 kg were used. Freezing of the left adrenal gland was performed by the contact method at −60 °C for 1 min in each of 3 cycles. The dogs were given antibiotics (kanamycin sulfate, 250 mg) and 20 mg of bemegride postoperatively. Three weeks later, cryosurgery of the right adrenal gland was performed in the same manner. Average canine body weight prior to cryosurgery, 2 weeks after cryosurgery of the unilateral adrenal gland, and 3 weeks after cryosurgery of bilateral adrenals were 9.2 kg, 8.6 kg, and 10.2 kg, respectively, and the postoperative course was uneventful in all the animals.

Estimation of adrenal function: Radioimmunoassay of plasma cortical steroid level: Cortisol produced by the method of Yoshimi et al. (8) and DHEA-S by Kokubu et al. (3). Rapid ACTH test was done during the time period of 12:30–2:30 p.m. by intravenous injection of 0.25 mg of cortrosyn (a synthetic ACTH, Daiichi Pharmaceutical Co. Ltd., Tokyo) and the plasma was collected 45 min later. In the preliminary experiments, plasma cortisol was estimated on the samples taken 30 min and 60 min after the injection of cortrosyn, and the plasma cortisol level proved to be practically the same in both samples. Statistical analysis was made by the Student's t test.

1) *Basal plasma cortisol level:* Canine basal cortisol levels throughout the experimental period are shown in Fig. 6.10, where the average cortisol level of normal dogs was 3.5 μg/dl. The highest cortisol level of 9.9 μg/dl was noticed after 20 to 30 min of cryosurgery of the left adrenal gland in 11 dogs ($P<0.001$). This elevated cortisol level decreased continuously, to the significantly low value of 0.8 μg/dl 8 to 12 days later ($P<0.05$ versus non-treated control group). After 30 min of cryosurgery of the right adrenal glands in 7 dogs, the plasma cortisol level rose temporarily to 4.5 μg/dl ($P<0.001$), and declined likewise, and 2 weeks later, the lowest level, 0.4 μg/dl, was recorded, and cortisol was not detected in 6 of 7 dogs.

2) *Response of cortisol level to a rapid ACTH test:* Figure 6.11 shows response prior to cryosurgery,

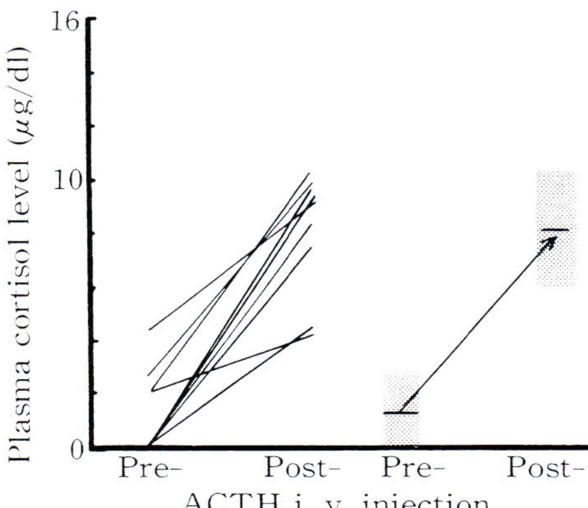

Fig. 6.12. Response of the plasma cortisol level to a rapid ACTH test in the dogs that underwent cryosurgery of the left adrenal gland. Mean ± SD

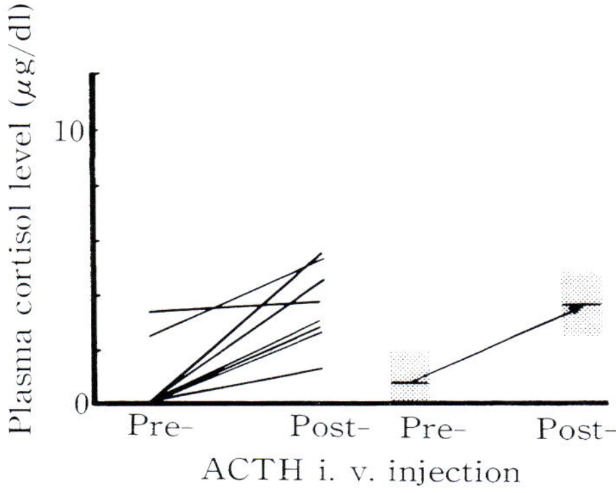

Fig. 6.13. Response of the plasma cortisol level to a rapid ACTH test in the dogs that underwent cryosurgery of the bilateral adrenal glands. Mean ± SD

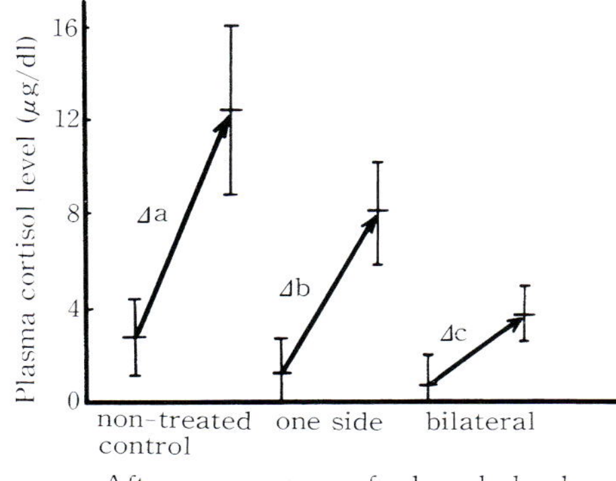

Fig. 6.14. Summary of the rapid ACTH tests, showing depressed adrenal function by cryosurgery. Δ c is significantly different from Δ a and Δ b (P < 0.01)

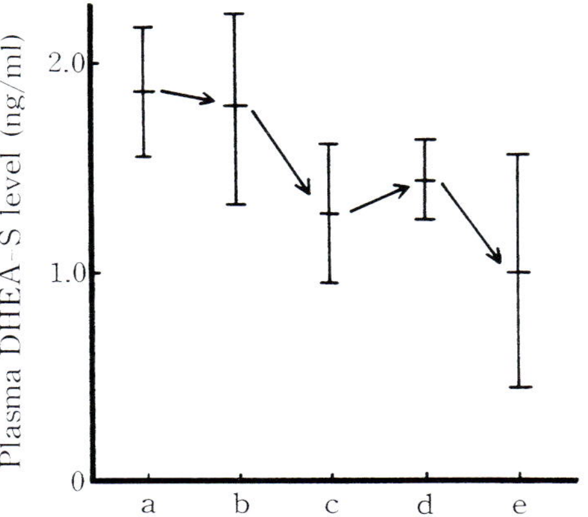

Fig. 6.15. Changes in canine plasma DHEA-S levels after cryosurgery of the adrenal glands. (a) Normal control. (b) 20–30 min after cryosurgery of the left adrenals. (c) 8–12 days after cryosurgery of the left adrenals. (d) 20–30 min after cryosurgery of the right adrenals (e) 13–19 days after cryosurgery of the right adrenals. Mean ± SD (n = 8)

Fig. 6.12 after unilateral cryosurgery, and Fig. 6.13 after bilateral, indicating mean plasma cortisol level elevated to 9.3 μg/dl, 4.9 μg/dl, and 2.9 μg/dl. Figure 6.14 is a summary of the rapid ACTH test. Response to the test was reduced significantly by cryodestruction of the adrenals.

3) *Plasma DHEA-S level:* Changes in the course are depicted in Fig. 6.15. Bilateral cryodestruction reduced the level by 47% versus that of the normal control, 1.87 ng/ml on average. Free DHEA was never detected in the plasma of 8 dogs of a total of 37 in the assays.

4) *Response of DHEA-S level to a rapid ACTH test:* As indicated in Table 6.1, the plasma DHEA-S level increased in 8 of 9 cases by intravenous injection of 0.25 mg of cortrosyn (P < 0.05).

6.3 Comments

In our animal experiments, frozen glands were not absorbed, but remained reduced in size and fibrous throughout the experimental period of 4 months after cryosurgery, and indicated no regeneration of the glands, but leaving only scarce degenerated cells. These degenerated cells, however, left open the question whether they would regenerate. Nevertheless, initial drastic histopatholgic changes are obvious in the electron microscopic studies, in which the mechanical injury by ice crystals is impressive.

Adrenalectomy by cryosurgery (cryoadrenalectomy) is considered to be a safe and quick way to block/ablate the adrenal function. All 13 dogs that had undergone cryoadrenalectomy survived uneventfully throughout the experimental period, although their plasma cortisol levels remained very low, and all 6 dogs with bilateral cryoadrenalectomy survived more than 4 months without administration/compensation of corticoids.

Table 6.1. Canine Plasma DHEA-S Levels

Dog no.			ACTH i.v. injection		Value
			pre-	post-	
Control	7	1.76**	2.58	0.82*	
	11	2.34			
After	5	3.40	2.11	Af1.29	
cryosurgery		6	0.90	1.39	0.49
of the left		7	1.09	2.45	1.36
adrenals	11	0.48	1.95	1.47	
After	5	1.32	2.33	1.01	
cryosurgery		6	2.65	3.87	1.22
of bilateral		12	N.D.***	1.39	1.39
adrenals		13	N.D.	1.14	1.14

*Canine plasma DHEA-S levels were significantly elevated by 0.25 mg ACTH i.v. injection ($P<0.05$, paired comparison).
**ng/ml; ***not detected.

Response to a rapid ACTH test was substantially lowered by cryoadrenalectomy. But even after cryodestruction of both adrenals, the response to a rapid ACTH test was not blocked completely. The response was seen in all of the 6 dogs. The secretion of cortisol following the cortrosyn infection was 31.6% higher than in the non-treated control animals. It is unclear whether the dogs had an accessory adrenal or whether an unfrozen part of the adrenals remained after cryosurgery. However, this response of the cortisol level to a rapid ACTH test might be beneficial in man, because cortisol would be secreted in case of emergency in the patients undergoing cryoadrenalectomy. And, it is possible that the complete ablation of the adrenal function is not clinically necessary, but that cryodestruction of only the adrenal gland on one side may be sufficient.

Technically, cryoadrenalectomy should be performed with extreme caution, not moving the cryoprobe while freezing, to avoid injury of the gland and fragile vessels and postoperative bleeding. It requires only 3 minutes to treat an adrenal gland unilaterally by 2-cycle freezing. Thus it may be applied to patients debilitated by disease, by way, for instance, of the ultrasonically-guided transabdominal approach in the near future.

References

1. Breast Cancer Group in Japan (1973) The effect of endocrine treatment on advanced breast cancer in Japan. Jpn J Cin Oncol 6: 13–18.
2. Huggins C, Bergenstal DM (1951) Surgery of the adrenals. JAMA 147: 101–106.
3. Kokubu T, Hisatomi M, Obuchi R, Mori A, Kamegawa A (1978) The simple methods for radioimmunoassay of unconjugated and sulfate conjugated dehydroepiandrosterone. Folia Endocrinol. Japan 54: 117–130 (in Japanese).
4. McDonald I (1962) Endocrine ablation in disseminated mammary carcinoma. Surg Gynecol Obstet 115: 215–222.
5. Ohkuma T, Tondokoro M, Tanaka S (1982) Experimental cryosurgery of the adrenal gland. (2) Assay of the endocrine function. Low Temp Med 8: 64–69.
6. Osteen RT, Chaffey JT, Moore FD, Wilson RE (1978) An aggressive multimodality approach to locally advanced carcinoma of the breast. Surg Gynecol Obstet 147: 75–79.
7. Tanaka S, Nagata H, Ohkuma T (1982) Experimental cryosurgery of the adrenal gland. (1) Histopathologic studies. Low Temp Med 8: 56–63.
8. Yoshimi T, Tachibana S (1974) Radioimmunoassay for plasma cortisol and aldosterone. Rinshokagaku 3: 53–61 (in Japanese).

Part III

Clinical Cryosurgery

7. The Use of Cryosurgery in Dermatology

Rodney P. R. Dawber

7.1 Skin Cryosurgery

There is more information and experience regarding the effects of cold on the skin than any other organ – both from observation in cold climate and environments and from its many uses, in cryosurgical practice in man and in other animals (1–3). Since the skin has long been known to heal well after cold injury a vast array of conditions have been treated by cryosurgery (Figs. 7.1.1–7.1.11) – often amounting to over-use and mis-use; the comprehensive list (Table 7.1.1) reflects those conditions for which good results have been recorded, though this is not to imply that cryosurgery is the treatment of choice for all these entities (1,4). Cutaneous cryosurgery has come more into the fore during the last 25 years, in part because of improved cryobiological background knowledge, but also because in everyday dermatology, with the ready availability of liquid nitrogen, it has become cheap, quick, easy to perform (5) and can usually be carried out without surgical theatre facilities, and even in the patient's home under certain circumstances.

7.1.1 Mechanism of Damage due to Cold Injury (1,2,3)

Cryosurgery can be loosely defined as the deliberate destruction of diseased tissue by freezing in a controlled manner. Many well recognized events follow the rapid lowering of temperature in biological systems.

7.1.2. Factors Causing Cellular Injury

Extracellular ice: When cutaneous cryosurgery was first introduced, it was thought that the main cause of cell death was the formation of ice in the tissues and the "mechanical disruption" as the ice crystals formed. If cells are frozen *in vitro* extracellular ice forms first; this gradually squeezes the cells together. It has been difficult to demonstrate actual disruption of membranes by this means; however, volume changes in the extra- and intracellular compartments have been measured during freezing and thawing and the conclusion drawn that disruption of cell membranes must occur. It appears that extracellular ice formation alone is not enough to kill cells consistently. The temperature changes during cryosurgery are so rapid that intracellular ice formation is inevitable as well, this being physically extremely destructive.

Hypertonic damage: When extracellular ice is formed in association with cell suspension *in vitro*, the amount of extracellular water decreases, causing an increase in concentration of solutes in the remaining fluid. Changing osmotic gradients between cells and extracellular fluids are therefore produced, which lead to passage of electrolytes out of the cells causing a decrease in cell volume

Table 7.1.1. Some skin conditions treatable by cryosurgery

Acne vulgaris	Leiomyoma
Acrochordon	Leishmaniasis
Adenoma sebaceum	Lentigo maligna
Angiomas	Lentigo maligna melanoma – (Fig. 7a and b)
Angiokeratoma	Lentigo simplex
Angiofibroma	Lichen simplex
Angiolymphoid hyperplasia with eosinophilia – (Fig. 1a and b)	Lupus erythematosus
	Lupus vulgaris
Basal cell carcinoma – (Figs. 2a and b; 3a and b)	Mastocytoma
	Molluscum contagiosum
Bowen's disease – skin and mucosal surfaces – (Fig. 4a and b)	Mucocele
	Neurofibroma
Carbuncle	Nevoid basal cell carcinoma (Gorlin syndrome)
Chloasma (melasma)	
Chondrodermatitis nodularis helicis	Nevus-epidermal -sebaceous
Clear cell acanthoma	
Cryoanesthesia	Palliation
Cutaneous horn	Porokeratosis
Cylindroma	Prurigo nodularis granuloma
Dermatofibroma	Pruritus ani
Digital myxoid cyst	Pseudo-pyogenic granuloma (Syn: Angiolymphoid hyperplasia with eosinophilia)
Eccrine poroma	
Elastosis perforans serpiginosa	Pyogenic granuloma
Eosinophylic granuloma	Rhinophyma
Granuloma annulare	
Granuloma – mycobacterial	Sarcoid
Hidradenoma	Sebaceous hyperplasia
	Squamous cell carcinoma – (Fig. 8a and b; Fig. 9a and b)
Hidradenitis suppurativa	
Histiocytoma	Steatocystoma multiplex
Hyperhidrosis	Syringoma
Ingrowing toenail	Tattoos
	Trichoepithelioma
Keloid	
Kerato-acanthoma	Warts – viral – (Figs. 10a and b; 11a and b)
Keratoses – actinic	
–arsenical	
–seborrhoeic	Xanthelasma

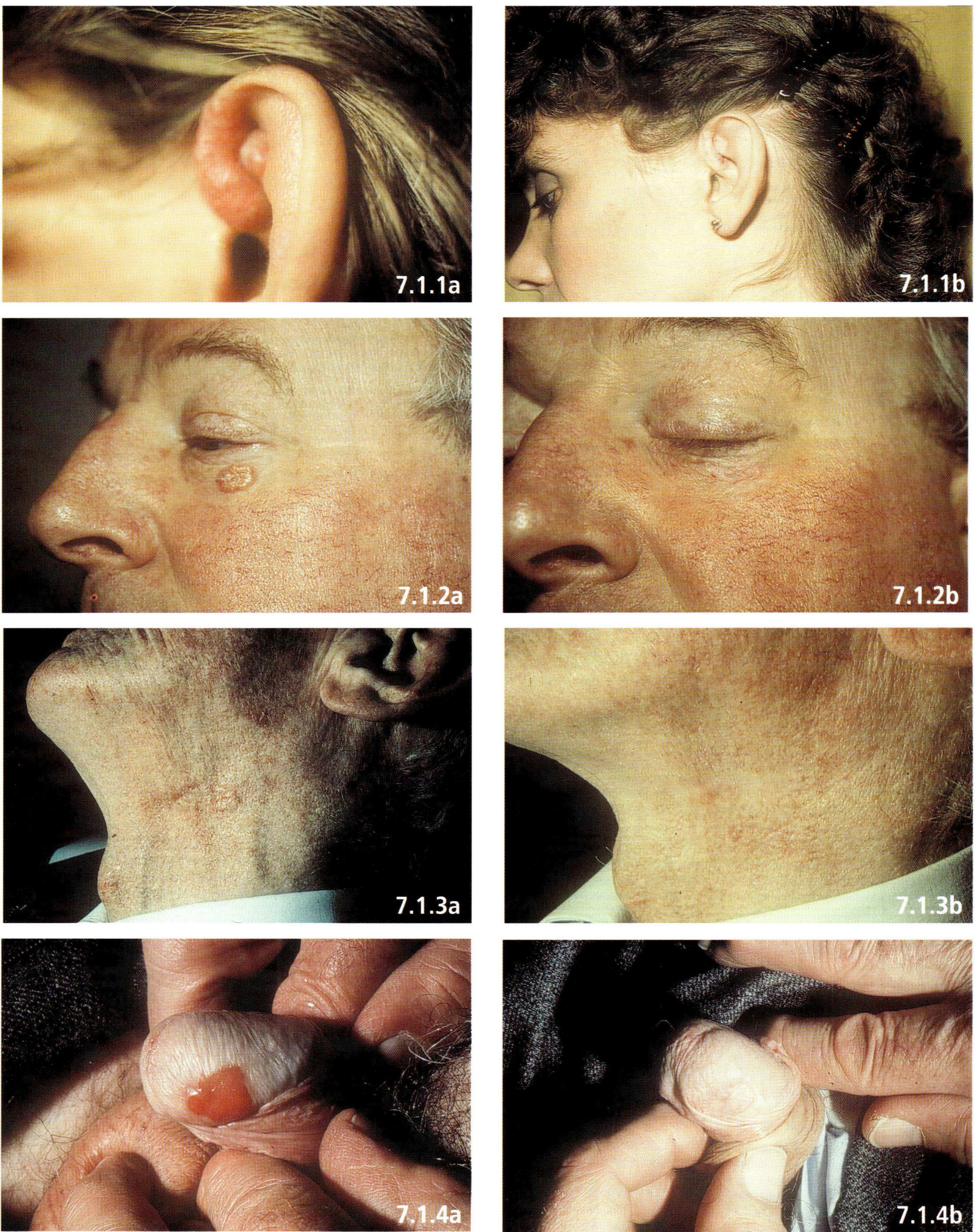

Fig. 7.1.1. Angiolymphoid hyperplasia with eosinophilia (**a**) before and (**b**) after cryosurgery. **Fig. 7.1.2.** Nodular basal cell carcinoma (**a**) before and (**b**) after cryosurgery. **Fig. 7.1.3.** Basal cell carcinoma in X-ray ''damaged'' skin (**a**) before and (**b**) after cryosurgery. **Fig. 7.1.4.** Erythroplasia of Queyrat of glans penis (**a**) before and (**b**) after cryosurgery.

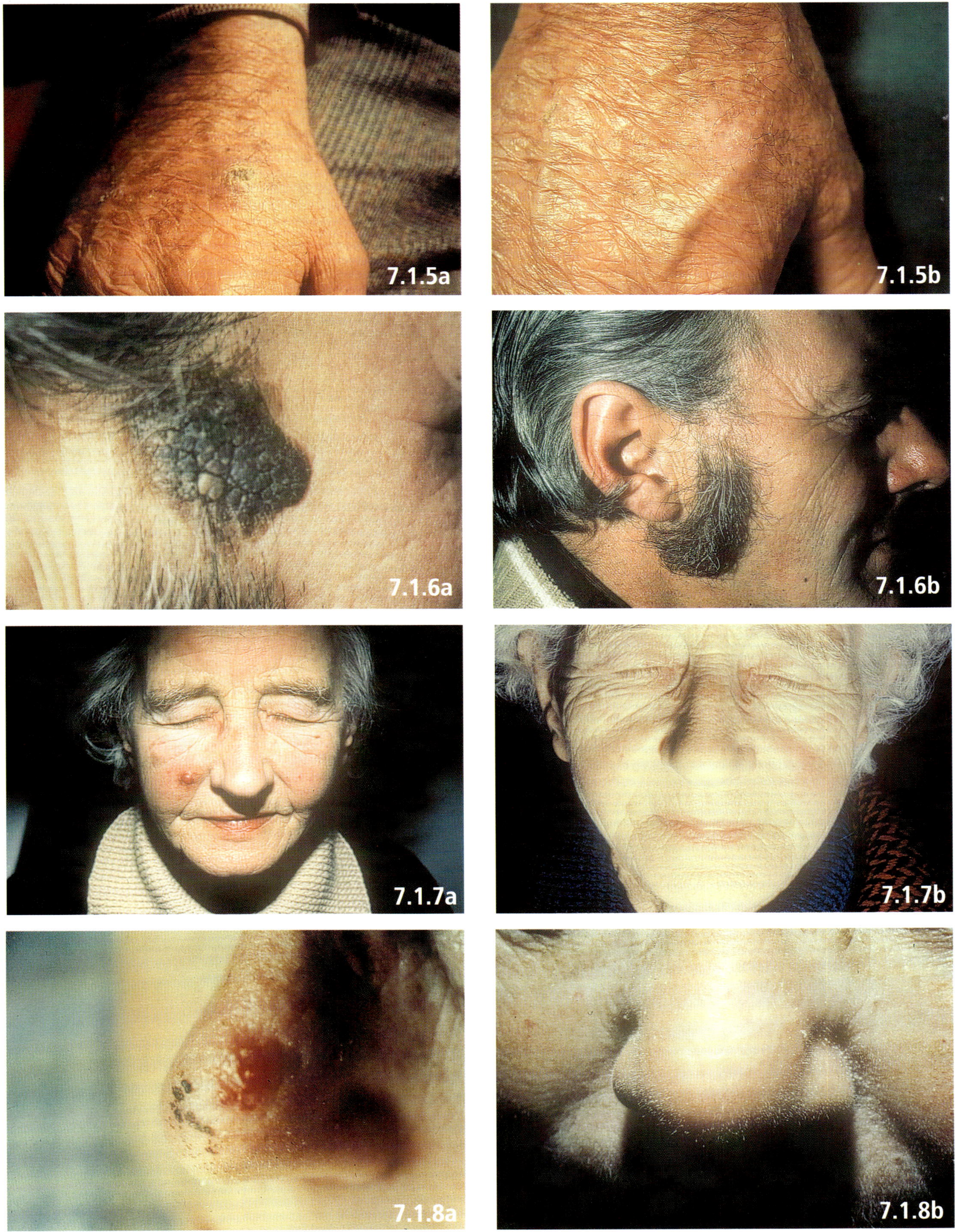

Fig. 7.1.5. a, b Solar keratosis treated by cryosurgery. **Fig. 7.1.6.** Seborrhoelc keratosis **(a)**; after cryosurgery **(b)** there has been some hair loss. **Fig. 7.1.7.** Lentigo maligna melanoma **(a)** – treated cryosurgically **(b)**. **Fig. 7.1.8. a, b.** Nasal squamous carcinoma.

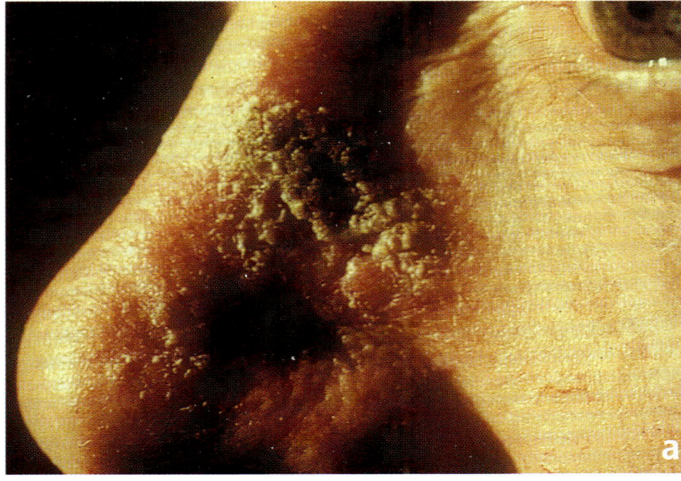
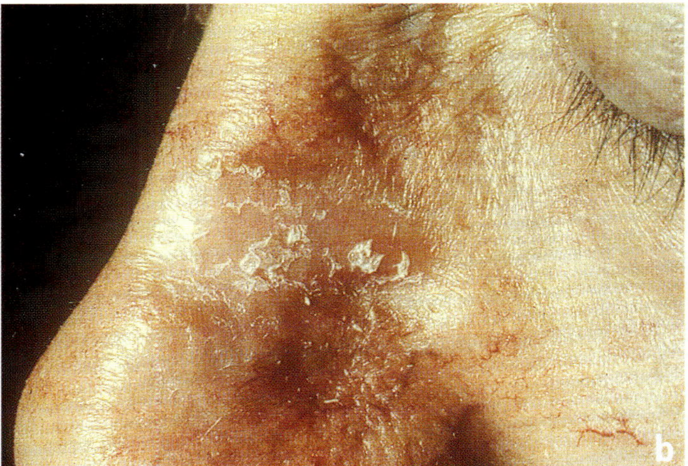

Fig. 7.1.9. Nasal skin squamous carcinoma – extensive superficial type (**a** and **b**)

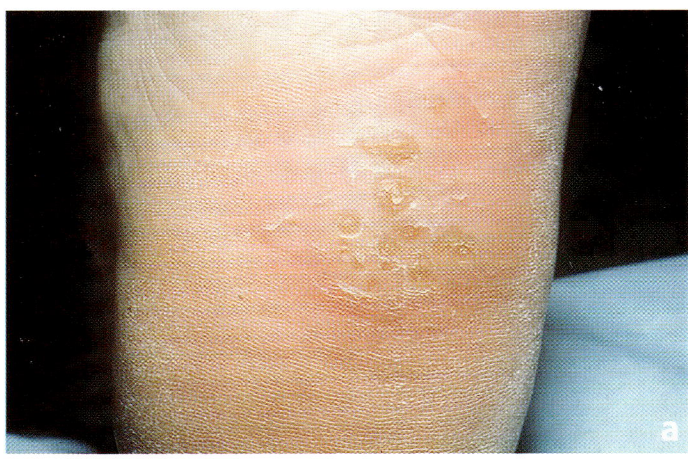
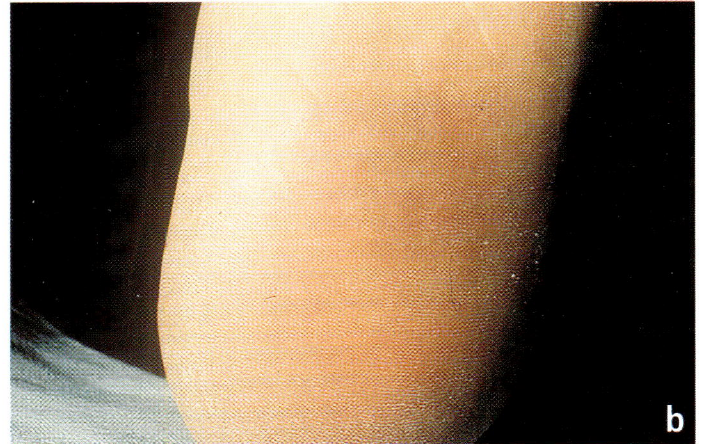

Fig. 7.1.10. Grouped plantar warts (**a** and **b**)

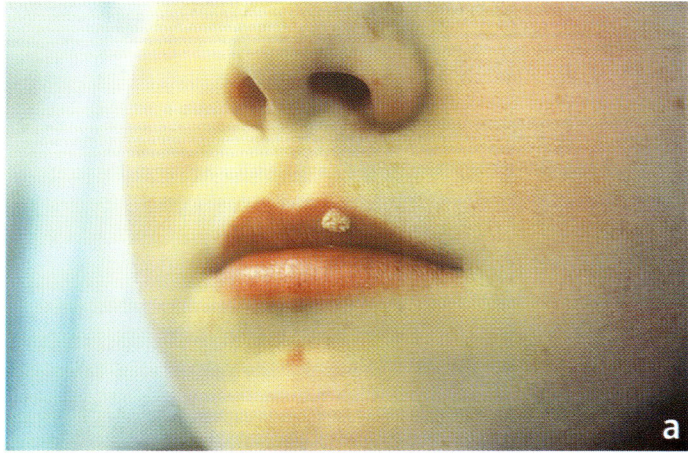
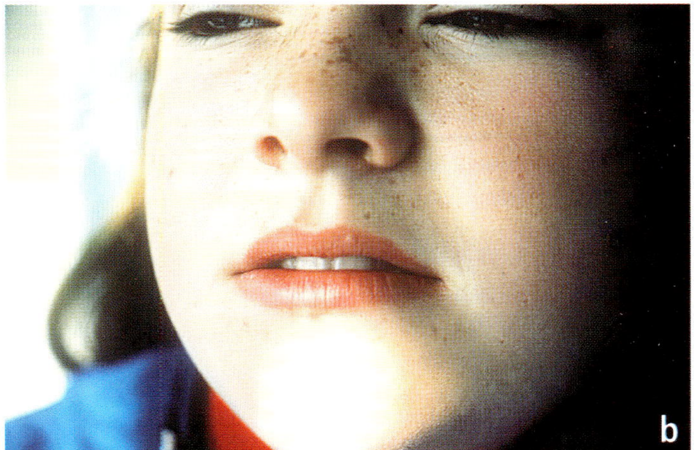

Fig. 7.1.11. Digitate wart of lip (**a** and **b**)

and a disruption of cell membranes. It has been shown that when a certain concentration is reached, normally intracellular components, for example, haemoglobin in red blood cells, pass out of the cell causing irreversible damage. Rapid electrolyte transfer has also been incriminated as the cause of damage to cell proteins and enzyme systems and it is generally accepted that the temperature gradients produced during cryosurgery cause damage by this means, especially during the reverse process of thawing.

Sensitization: In experiments using red blood cells, it has been shown that gross cell damage is produced even if hypertonic conditions necessary for disruption are not achieved. It has therefore been postulated that this sensitisation damage is the result of disruption of phospholipids in cell membranes, but this has not been confirmed by other workers. It may be that events taking place during thawing, for example reversed osmotic gradients, may give rise to this form of damage.

Intracellular ice: Extracellular ice formation and sensitization damage can only occur when freezing is slow, i.e. when differential freezing in different parts of a system is allowed to occur. When very rapid freezing takes place, intracellular ice formation occurs and it is widely believed that this gives rise to cellular death even though cells assume a remarkably normal appearance immediately after thawing. Damage to cell organelles such as mitochondria and endoplasmic reticulum has been postulated to be the cause of intracellular ice injury. The size of the ice crystals is probably important; the larger the crystals, the greater the damage. Most of the evidence supports the general principle that intracellular ice is lethal. It is probably that re-crystallization of ice during the slow thaw time after cryosurgery is responsible for tissue destruction, this process being as important as the initial freeze in causing cell death.

Circulatory changes: Many authorities feel that the following are as important as the initial freeze/thaw events in causing cell and tissue death: a) the circulatory (capillary and lymphatic) malfunction associated with the early endothelial damage and edema and b) the capillary and venous occlusion seen several days after treatment, leading to anoxia, further cell death and tissue necrosis.

Immunological events: Cryosurgery has been shown to enhance immunological reactivity against tumor cells. Lymphocytes and serum from tumor-bearing animals receiving a single cryosurgical dose have demonstrated greater cytotoxicity to an identical tumor in a syngeneic animal than lymphocytes and serum from an untreated animal. This response has been shown to be tissue-specific and stimulated by the release of tumor-specific antigen either during or after freezing. Other workers have observed the effects of an immune reaction after cryosurgery of tissues such as the prostate. Whether such events are important in human cutaneous cryosurgery remains to be proven.

7.1.3 Equipment and Methods (1, 5, 6)

The commonest equipment in use for routine clinical practice is designed to utilize liquid nitrogen as a refrigerant mainly because of its cheapness and universal availability. It is essential for the treatment of pre-malignant and malignant skin lesions because of its ability to give "consistent cell killing". The simplest technique is the dipstick method. This long-used method employs either a cotton-wool swab (Fig. 7.1.12) or copper disc with insulated handles. The swab or disc is dipped into a robust metal Dewar flask containing liquid nitrogen and then applied to the area to be treated. The time of application depends on the size and nature of the lesions to be treated; to maintain relatively long tissue freezing, repeat dipping and reapplication may be necessary. It is very difficult to standardize this technique in view of the many variables: ambient temperature, the pressure applied, distance the dip instrument travels from Dewar flask to the lesion and "dripping" of liquid nitrogen. This technique is considered to be only suitable for small benign superficial conditions, which includes very many conditions listed in Table 7.1.1. "Artistry" and

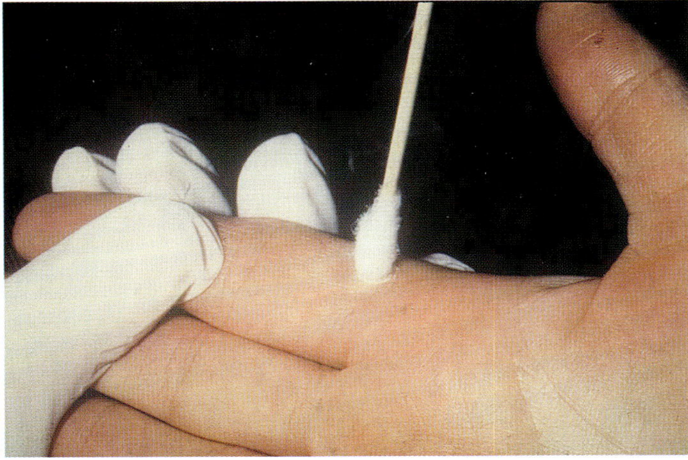

Fig. 7.1.12. Cotton wool bud/stick for cryosurgery

experience are essential if consistently good cure rates are to be achieved with this method; it has been used successfully by dermatologists for many

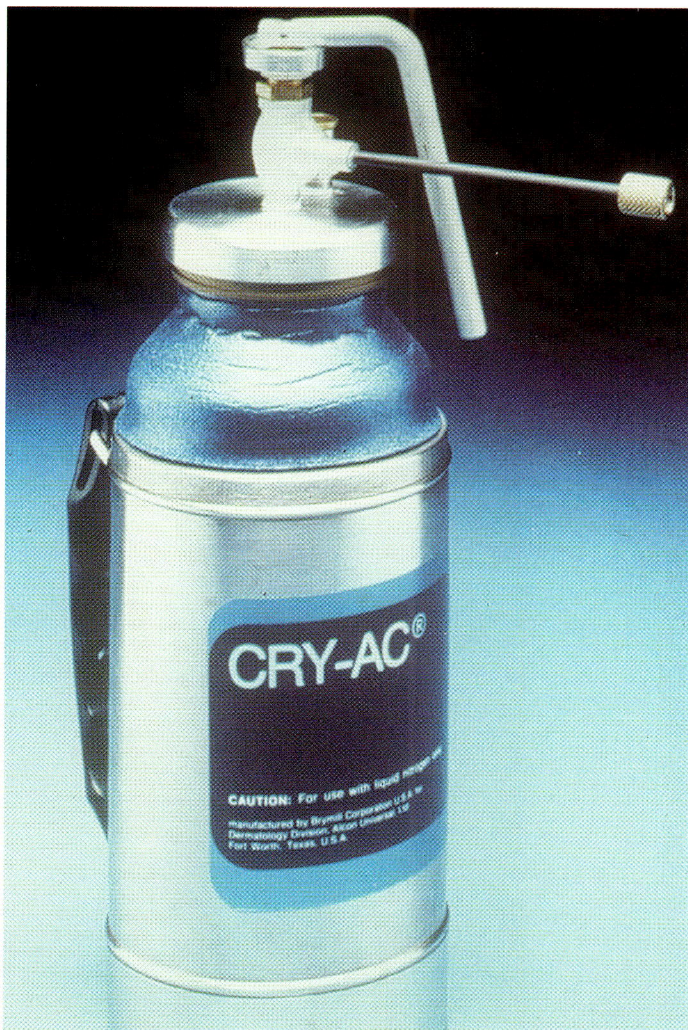

Fig. 7.1.13. Portable liquid nitrogen spray/probe equipment

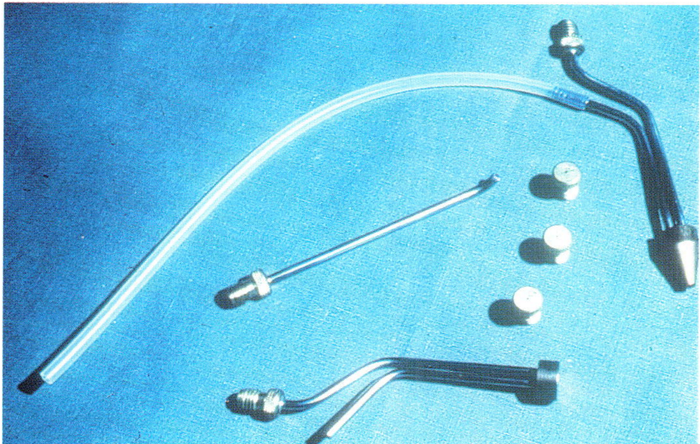

Fig. 7.1.14. Some spray and probes that can be used with the equipment in Fig. 7.1.13

decades. If pre-malignant and malignant integumentary lesions are to be treated, then modern standardized equipment is required (Figs. 7.1.13 and 7.1.14).

For routine outpatient cryosurgery, most dermatologists prefer a small hand-held spray unit or a compact tabletop unit, capable of either spray or cryoprobe application (Figs. 7.1.13 and 7.1.14), the former are by far the commonest used in clinical practice. For details of the various commercially produced units available, the reader is referred to more detailed text (1, 5).

Most units allow for variation in the "width" of the spray and have probe attachments of different sizes to equate with the size of the area to be treated. The probes are generally cylindrical, preferably with flat contact surfaces; they are particularly useful when pressure is needed, for example, with vascular lesions and for areas where "open" spray is a problem around the eye, the mouth and the vagina. Also very small lesions can be treated with pointed probes since spray techniques give too wide an icefield and therefore greater morbidity. Instruments utilizing carbon dioxide snow, or nitrous oxide cooling (Joule-Thomson effect) for dermatological lesions have largely been superseded by liquid nitrogen based methods.

Various items of auxiliary equipment are important if the full range of cryosurgical techniques is to be employed:

Truncated non-conducting cones are frequently employed to limit surface application of the spray. For small lesions, if carefully localized spray is required, auroscope cones can be used. This method gives a very rapid rate of temperature decrease which is *probably* more destructive than the open spray technique. Some recently introduced machines have an attachable "closed cone" that sprays liquid nitrogen into the cone, which is pressed onto the skin.

To protect the orbit of the eye when eyelid tumors are to be treated, a plastic eyelid retractor is essential; if one is not available, a plastic spoon without coarse edges may suffice – this giving adequate "insulation" against chilling effects on the eyes.

7.1.4 Monitoring Devices (5)

If only benign and relatively flat and small premalignant and malignant lesions are to be treated, and liquid nitrogen is the refrigerant, then monitoring equipment is unnecessary – since no physical instrument can measure adequate cell death. The treatment of deep or large tumors requires careful "depth dose" monitoring equipment – these are most commonly a pyrometer – thermocouple combination; some methods employ electrical impedance or tissue resistant-measuring devices which in principle have the advantage of measuring actual freezing; only thin, inexpensive electrodes are needed, and many areas of the tumor can be monitored with a single probe.

In an attempt to standardize the treatment used for different lesions at various sites, and so that we can further our knowledge of the relative sensitivity or resistance of different lesions to cryosurgery, we have adopted a "spot" freeze technique; this enables medical personnel of varying degrees of experience to obtain the same results (1).

The spot freeze technique involves first defining the size of the field to be treated (as with radiotherapy) and then inducing ice formation within that field by liquid nitrogen spray – large lesions are divided into overlapping circles of 2 cm diameter using a skin marker. The liquid nitrogen spray, e.g., C spray of CryAC Units, Brymill Corp, (Figs. 7.1.13 and 7.1.14) is held approximately 1 cm from the skin surface in the center of a 2 cm circle and spraying commences; the white "ice line" is allowed to extend outwards until it fills the circle – this ice field is then "held" for a measured time by continuing the spray with a sufficient jet pressure to maintain the ice line. The measured time will depend entirely on the nature of the lesion; once the time is completed, spraying is stopped and thawing commences. Each 2 cm circle is treated similarly.

A single freeze and thaw is termed a freeze/thaw cycle (FTC); malignant lesions usually receive two, sometimes three, FTCs, the intervening thaw time being at least three times the duration of the initial freeze. Evidently treatment fields of less than 2 cm diameter do not require to be divided up.

The time added after ice field formation must be learned by experience, but will *vary with the size, site and type of pathology*. The record in the hospital notes is usually made, for example, as follows:

LN2 (Liquid Nitrogen)	:	Single ice field : 1	×	15 secs
		Single < 2 cm : 1FTC	×	(Time after ice formed)

This schedule is typical of that used for a small flat plaque of Bowen's disease of the shin. Viral warts may require as little as 4–5 secs, while malignant lesions need up to 30 secs.

Times of less than 30 secs do not usually cause connective tissue distortion and scarring.

We originally tested the adequacy of the spot freeze method in experiments on the flank skin of pigs and shown consistent cell killing and satisfactory temperature levels within the field of treatment. The method is exactly repeatable from patient to patient and site to site; if, following a particular schedule, the treated lesion is not cured, the time of treatment can be lengthened – also whichever doctor sees the case at follow-up, the exact treatment procedure is known and can be specifically modified.

Many other techniques are available involving varying spray methods for treating large lesions and liquid nitrogen probe methods. The important factor is to gain experience with whatever techniques are to be learned by a) experimenting on skin of cheap meats or other animal tissue, e.g., pigs' feet or hock available from most meat retailers; b) working with an animal "model" where possible; c) observing experienced operators in practice. This is particularly important if malignant lesions are to be treated since much of the therapeutic failure with small basal and squamous epitheliomata can be ascribed to poor technique.

As with all surgical treatments, accurate diagnosis is essential before cryosurgery is used: this evidently does not mean biopsy of all lesions prior to freezing, since clinical diagnosis will often be adequate, particularly with benign lesions (Table 7.1.1) and many basal cell carcinomas (Figs. 7.1.2 and 7.1.3). As with radiotherapy, wrong diagnosis may lead to "blurring" of physical signs, for example with melanotic lesions, and may facilitate tumor spread before the diagnosis becomes obvious.

7.1.5 Setting up a Cryosurgery Clinic (1)

When setting up a cryosurgery clinic in hospital or a primary care practice, it is important to take the time to make preliminary arrangements and to check back-up services. Such preparations can help to ensure that delays or even mistakes are avoided. An eight-point plan can be proposed for setting up such a clinic.

- Arrange training for medical and nursing staff.
- Arrange a regular supply of liquid nitrogen.
- Make arrangements for histology reports.
- Organize equipment and facilities for biopsies when appropriate.
- Apportion clinic time for the medical and nursing staff.

- Obtain consent and provide information handouts for patients.
- Keep good records of treatment.
- Decide follow-up policy.

Cryosurgery is a relatively new art or subspecialty in hospital practice. Not all hospital dermatology departments undertake cryosurgery. Some that do, limit themselves to treating benign lesions.

Primary care physicians have used cryogens such as carbon dioxide snow for treating warts for many years. The use of liquid nitrogen is now more widespread. In the UK, this is partly because of reimbursements made for minor surgery procedures listed in the 1990 General Practitioner Contract. It is essential, in these circumstances, that the biological basis for cryosurgery is properly understood.

Simple and benign skin lesions can be treated by a single freeze followed by a natural thaw – a single freeze/thaw cycle.

Malignant skin lesions require a 25–30 second freeze, a minimum 5 minute thaw, followed in most cases by another 25–30 second freeze – a double freeze/thaw cycle (1, 2).

Practitioners in hospital or in primary health care starting out in cryosurgery can first gain valuable experience by attending dermatological surgery workshops. Here aspects of skin surgery and cryosurgery techniques can be learned using pigs' feet as models. Where dermatology departments have cryosurgery clinics, sitting in on such clinics is of great value to practitioners building up their experience in the cryosurgery field. Clearly, such practitioners should gain practical experience in treating benign lesions before progressing to treatment of malignant lesions. In the setting up and running of a cryosurgery clinic, the nurse plays a crucial role. Even when the doctor carrying out the cryosurgery has explained the procedure, its effects and outcome to the patient, the nurse has a role in further communication and reassurance to the patient. The nurse's skills are invaluable during the procedure and vital in the aftercare of the wound, whether in a hospital clinic or in primary health care. It is therefore important to encourage nurses to attend cryosurgery workshops or meetings with their medical colleagues. This ensures that their skills can be used to the full and an efficient cryosurgery service can be offered.

Nurses carrying out nurse-led cryosurgery clinics for the treatment of warts and other benign skin lesions must be adequately trained and fully competent. No treatment should be undertaken if the diagnosis of the lesion is in doubt. Back-up medical care must always be available.

Liquid nitrogen is now readily available. Most hospitals have storage capacity and suitable containers or storage flasks for use in a cryosurgery clinic. Fewer primary health care centres, however, have storage facilities for liquid nitrogen.

It is essential to organize a reliable source of liquid nitrogen if one is to run a regular cryosurgery clinic in primary medicine. This can be done in one of several ways. If a primary care physician can provide a suitable portable storage flask and protective container, the local hospital is usually happy to provide the liquid nitrogen required at a reasonable cost. Companies involved in the supply of cryosurgery equipment offer a built-in supply service at an annual cost for the liquid nitrogen and for the rental of storage equipment. For the practitioner who is very involved in cryosurgery in primary health care, a large 35 liter or 50 liter storage flask is available which can be topped up at appropriate intervals on a cost per liter basis by a local supplier.

The basis of good, safe cryosurgery is pretreatment histopathology where malignancy is suspected or the clinical diagnosis is in doubt. Before one undertakes cryosurgery in primary care medicine, therefore, it is necessary to confirm that good histopathology services are available. Any specimen submitted should be sent in a container of buffered formalin, normally provided by the hospital pathology department. The container must be properly labelled and the pathology request card should include the following information.

- Name, date of birth and address of patient.
- Name and address of doctor.
- Short history of lesion.
- Site and type of biopsy.
- Histology required.

Biopsy packs: The contents of a biopsy pack are often a matter of personal choice. Table 7.1.2 lists the contents of a suitable biopsy pack. In addition the following may be necessary: a No. 15 scalpel blade for full thickness, incisional biopsy, or a 2 or 3 mm biopsy punch if a punch biopsy is considered suitable. Chlorhexidine gluconate 0.05 per cent is a suitable solution (25 ml sachet) for preparation and cleansing of a biopsy site.

Local anesthetic: The "safe dose" of local anesthetic for skin infiltration is 20 ml of lignocaine (1 per cent) or 10 ml of lignocaine (2 per cent). The

Table 7.1.2. Contents of a typical biopsy pack

1 Scalpel handle (Bard-Parker) No 3
1 Spencer Wells forceps
2 Curved mosquito forceps
1 Pair of straight pointed scissors
1 Pair of strabismus scissors
1 Kilner of Mayo needle holder
1 Non-toothed dissecting forceps
1 McIndoe's fine dissecting forceps
1 Gillies skin hook
1 Volkmann's spoon (medium)
5 Cotton-wool balls
10 Gauze swabs (7.5 cm × 7.5 cm)
5 Regal swabs (10 cm × 10 cm)
2 Theater towels
Biopsy punches (2–6 mm diameters)

addition of adrenaline reduces toxicity by half thus doubling the safe dose, i.e. 40 ml of lignocaine (1 per cent with adrenaline 1 in 200,000), 20 ml of lignocaine (2 per cent with adrenaline 1 in 200,000).

Also available is a very useful pre-filled dental cartridge containing 2.2 ml lignocaine 2 per cent with adrenaline 1 in 80,000. A similar cartridge containing 2.2 ml of prilocaine (4 per cent) equivalent to lignocaine (2 per cent without adrenaline) can be used for digital anesthesia. Both local anesthetic cartridges fit into a dental syringe to which can be fitted a fine, flexible dental needle which makes cutaneous anesthesia easier, with fewer puncture sites than with the conventional, rigid needle.

Lignocaine 2.5 per cent, prilocaine 2.5 per cent (EMLA) cream or Ametop may be used for surface anesthesia, particularly when treating warts or molluscum contagiosum in younger children. EMLA should be applied two hours before treatment; Ametop may give adequate anesthesia within 30 mins.

Suture material: Polyglycolate or polygalactin absorbable sutures for subcutaneous use. Ethilon 4/0 (W319), Ethilon 3/0 (W320) or Ethilon 6/0 (W507). Alternatively there is Prolene 4/0 (W539) – these are all non-absorbable sutures for cutaneous use. Other pieces of equipment essential to the cryosurgeon are a magnifying lens to define the full extent of the lesion, a marker pen to outline the field to be treated and a simple ruler to record the size of the lesion.

Set aside clinic time for the doctor and nurse. If an efficient, well-equipped cutaneous surgery/cryosurgery clinic is to be run in the best interest of both doctor and patient, it is essential to set aside specific time which is both adequate and suitable: "suitable" in that it must be a time at which a trained nurse can assist and that all the equipment necessary is available; "adequate" in that it will be sufficient for treating the number of patients intended. As a guide, in a 2–3 hour session 8–10 patients might be treated, depending on their lesion type. The frequency of the clinics will obviously depend on the demand- possibly weekly in hospital and monthly in primary health care.

Consent: However good the doctor's rapport with a patient, consent cannot be implied when undertaking cryosurgery. The consent form need not be elaborate, but for legal purposes must be signed by the patient (or guardian if the patient is a child) and the doctor carrying out the procedures. Before seeking consent, it is very important to explain to the patient the details of cryosurgical treatment in terms of:

Aims of the treatment:

- The possible effects from the treatment in terms of initial swelling and other side-effects.
- The subsequent changes and care of the treated area.
- The probable cosmetic outcome of treatment.
- The follow-up arrangements, especially when dealing with malignant lesions.
- In addition to discussing the procedure with the patient, a simple handout explaining the effects of treatment is very helpful and reassuring to the patient.

Record keeping: For legal, audit and research purposes accurate records should be kept regarding each cryosurgery procedure carried out. Details should include:

- Name, date of birth and address of the patient.
- Date of treatment.
- Type of lesion, size and site.
- Local anesthetic used.
- Any sutures used when carrying out a biopsy.
- Exact procedure carried out (e.g., double 25 second freeze/thaw cycle using liquid nitrogen cryospray), nozzle size and distance from skin.
- Complications, if any.
- Topical application and dressing used.
- Nurse assistant present.
- Doctor carrying out the procedure.
- Space for definitive histopathology should also be available. All these details are best kept in a proper cryosurgery/surgical procedures book.

Separate records of each patient should also be kept for reference and subsequent follow-up.

Follow-up care: All patients undergoing cryosurgery treatment must have follow-up appropriate to the lesion that has been treated. Initial wound care following cryosurgery can well be looked after and supervised by the clinic nurse. However, the doctor embarking on cryosurgery would benefit from being involved at this stage in order to observe the progress of treatment. Any problems or side-effects should be recorded. It is instructive and helpful for both doctor and patient to check the cryosurgery wound at 6–8 weeks. This provides a useful opportunity to assess the clinical and cosmetic outcome of treatment and to discuss any problems with the patient. Until one becomes familiar with the outcome of cryosurgery in the treatment of malignant lesions, in addition to the checks outlined above it is a good policy to review patients at 6, 12, 18 months and 2 years. These reviews are to assess the outcome and to exclude any recurrences. Patients should also be encouraged to report to their primary care physician at any time should they be concerned about changes at the treatment site or any new skin lesions.

Nurse-led cryosurgery service: Several points need to be made before commencing a nurse-led cryosurgery clinic:

Why do you want a nurse to perform cryosurgery?
Who is going to train the nurse?
What time-scale for training is being allowed?
Will the nurse-led clinic receive secretarial support?
Does the nurse have indemnity coverage either from a union or hospital trust?
What nursing roles will the nurse have to give up in order to run a cryosurgery service?
Will it benefit the patients if a nurse runs a cryosurgery clinic?

The profession of nursing is undergoing immense change. The introduction of extended roles and nurse practitioners is coinciding with a reduction in junior doctors' hours and an emphasis on their training. The boundaries between the two disciplines are becoming "blurred" in many areas including dermatology.

Cryosurgery is relatively easy, quick and cheap to perform whether in a primary or secondary health care setting. It is a field in which nurses can become expert practitioners. Already many nurses successfully run cryosurgery clinics, treating patients with a variety of conditions. However if nursing is to remain dynamic, then thought must be given to the training needs of nurses new to the specialty.

Accountability: The Patients Charter (1991) in the UK encourages patients to exercise their rights to high quality care; it is therefore vital to ensure the appropriate training and competence of individuals carrying out dermatological procedures. Nurses are governed by the UKCC (United Kingdom Central Council for Nursing, Midwifery and Health Visiting) and bound by their Code of Professional Conduct. Similar statutes are evolving in other countries. Registered nurses are personally accountable for their practice which must therefore be sensitive, relevant and responsive to the needs of individual patients. The range of responsibilities which fall to individual nurses should relate to their personal experience, education and skill. In 1992 the UKCC published the Scope of Professional Practice document. It states that, in any role the nurse must be satisfied that all aspects of practice are directed to meeting the needs and serving the interests of patients. Also, the registered nurse must:

Endeavour to achieve and develop knowledge, skill and competence to respond to those needs and interests.

Acknowledge any limits of personal knowledge and skill and take steps to remedy any relevant deficits in order to meet the needs of patients.

Make sure that any enlargement or adjustment of the scope of practice must be achieved without compromizing or fragmenting existing aspects of patient care.

Recognize and honor the direct or indirect personal accountability for all aspects of professional practice.

In serving the interests of patients and the wider interests of society, avoid any inappropriate delegation to others which compromises those interests.

This last statement means that managers cannot expect nurses to take on new roles without adequate training and nurses must, in the interest of their patients, say if they are not happy with any area of their workload. In effect, the nurse as an accountable practitioner has the right to agree to do anything and refuse to do everything!

Training: Training for undertaking cryosurgery should be given by an appropriately qualified practitioner. This may be a consultant dermatologist in the case of hospital based nurses or a primary care physician with a specialist interest in dermatology in the case of community based staff. Theoretical knowledge should be consolidated with a period of observation in a cryosurgery clinic. Once the nurse and trainer are confident of the nurse's ability, the nurse should then undertake a period of supervised practice. The length of time of this practice will vary, depending on the confidence and skill of the nurse and the level of competence achieved. Having identified an appropriate mentor/supervisor for the period of supervised practice, an initial assessment, using the clinical assessment criteria (Tables 7.1.3 and 7.1.4) is made. The grades are entered in the grids provided underneath the specific competencies for the given skill and this is then dated and signed. When it is deemed mutually appropriate between mentor and learner, following a period of supervision, a secondary assessment is performed. The new grades are entered into the grid and then an arrow inserted to denote an increase or decrease in grade for the secondary assessment.

Case selection: All patients should see a doctor initially to confirm diagnosis prior to treatment. Legally nurses cannot diagnose a patient's condition. Once the diagnosis has been confirmed either by diagnostic biopsy or on examination by a dermatologist or a primary care physician with experience in dermatology, the patient can be referred on to be treated by the nurse.

Table 7.1.3. Clinical assessment criteria; nurse-led service

	Level of achievement	Grade
Novice	Cannot perform this activity satisfactorily to participate in the clinical environment.	0
	Can perform this activity but not without constant supervision and some assistance.	1
	Can perform this activity satisfactorily but requires some supervision and assistance.	2
Competent Practitioner	Can perform this activity satisfactorily without assistance and/or supervision.	3
	Can perform this activity satisfactorily without supervision or assistance with more than acceptable speed and quality of work.	4
	Can perform this activity satisfactorily with more than acceptable speed and quality and with initiative and adaptability to special problem situations.	5
Clinical Expert	Can perform this activity with more than acceptable speed and quality, with initiative and adaptability and can lead others in performing this task.	6

Table 7.1.4. Nurse competencies for performing cryosurgery

Demonstrates knowledge of the structure and function of the skin	Understands the indications for performing cryosurgery	Selects and prepares appropriate equipment for cryosurgery
Effectively prepares the patient physically and psychologically for the procedure	Can state the possible complications of local anesthetic administration and their significance	Selects a suitable size nozzle for the cryogun and discusses reasons for that choice
Safely and effectively performs the cryosurgery using a Cry-ac flask	Demonstrates knowledge of freeze/thaw cycles and their function	Can state possible complications of cryosurgery
Can select appropriate dressings for the site and conveys any after care required to the patient effectively	Demonstrates knowledge of use of steroids and their side-effects and their use post cryosurgery	Demonstrates accurate recording of events in patient's record and the operation register

Date of initial assessment: ....

Signature of mentor/supervisor: ....

Date of secondary assessment: ....

Signature of mentor/supervisor: ....

Date of tertiary assessment: ....

Signature of mentor/supervisor: ....

Date of subsequent assessment: ....

Signature of mentor/supervisor: ....

Example: Is able to correctly and safely fill and prepare the cryospray equipment for use.
–initial assessment = 1
–secondary assessment= 2
The tertiary assessment is performed as above.

When learners are identified as having reached grade 3 for all the competencies, they are deemed safe to practice without supervision. The number of assessments required to reach grade 3 will be individual. Prior to independent practice the learner must inform the clinical nurse manager of their intent to practice.

The learner must at all times uphold the UKCC Code of Professional Conduct.

Consent: There are several issues surrounding patient consent, not the least of which is whether it is really necessary. The procedure should be fully explained prior to obtaining the patient's written consent. The nurse carrying out the cryosurgery should be the one to obtain the patient's consent.

Patient care: Patient education is an important part of the nurse's role. The nurse will be able to advise the patient on wound care and any further treatment that may be required, ideally giving written guidelines on post cryosurgery care. The patient should know how to contact the department again, if necessary.

Prescribing: Some practitioners use local anesthetic before cryosurgery. In those cases Lignocaine 1% will be administered. Following cryosurgery Dermovate ointment is sometimes used to reduce the post-inflammatory reaction. Nurse prescribing is not yet standard practice in either the hospital or primary care setting: local policies will need to be drawn up. It is advisable to work closely with your local pharmacist. The training program will need to include the use and side-effects of both local anesthesia and topical steroids.

Monitoring and auditing: To ensure that the service is effective in meeting the needs of patients, it will need to be monitored. This can be done in several ways. The number of visits required to treat viral warts effectively can be audited. The recurrence rate for viral warts can be monitored. There must be a commitment on the part of both the nurse and the nurse manager to continuing education, by attendance at relevant study days and courses. The nurse's performance and training needs should be monitored and appraised six-monthly.

Resource implications: To be most effective, the nurse should perform cryosurgery in a designated clinic. There should always be a trained doctor available for advice while the clinic is in progress. The development of nurse-led cryosurgery clinics can help relieve the pressure on waiting lists for outpatient appointments. There is often improved continuity of care for patients especially if they had previously normally attended a large teaching hospital department.

7.1.6 Treatment of Malignant Skin Lesions (7–11)

Theoretically, as with X-irradiation, all skin malignancies could be treatable by appropriate cryosurgical techniques; but like radiotherapy, in clinical practice certain tumor types have been found to be amenable to ''cold killing'' with high cure rates and relatively low morbidity indices (Tables 7.1.5 and 7.1.6). The malignancies which are often treated by cryosurgery are basal cell carcinoma (BCC) (4,12,13,14,15) (Figs. 7.1.2 and 7.1.3), squamous cell carcinoma (SCC) (16) (Figs. 7.1.8 and 7.1.9), carcinoma in situ (Bowen's disease) of skin and adjacent epithelial surfaces (16), lentigo maligna (Hutchinson's freckle) and some cases of lentigo maligna melanoma (1,6,17) (Fig. 7.1.7a and b). In general, malignancy requires two freeze/thaw cycles to ensure consistent cell killing and good success rates. Apart from the examples to be mentioned, it is mandatory to perform a biopsy to obtain tissue diagnosis prior to treatment.

Table 7.1.5. Tumors and patients most suitable for cryosurgery

Types of skin cancer
Superficial basal cell carcinoma
Nodular or ulcerated basal cell carcinoma
Basal cell nevus syndrome
Small, well-differentiated squamous cell carcinoma arising in actinic keratoses
Selection of tumors
Tumors under 2 cm in diameter, with the exception of multicentric superficial basal cell carcinomas which are usually wide-spreading
Tumors with definable margins
Tumors overlying cartilage and bone (avoiding chondronecrosis, lacrimal obstruction and mutilating surgical excision)
Infected tumors
Recurrent tumors from previous radiotherapy
Selection of patients
Patients of all ages, but especially those of poor risk for surgery and for general anesthesia
Patients with a history of infectious jaundice or other serologically transmitted diseases

Table 7.1.6. Tumors less suitable for cryosurgery

Tumors over 2 cm in diameter
Recurrent tumors (with the exception of post radiotherapy)
Tumors with a high recurrence rate, e.g., tumours situated on the nasolabial fold and periauricular areas
Tumors of the feet and lower legs where the time of healing can be protracted
Tumors with the histopathological diagnosis of morphoeic or sclerotic, metatypical or mixed type

Those who are only used to using cryosurgery for benign lesions (4), should start by treating tumors which might otherwise be treated by curettage and cautery or simple excision and primary closure; also until greater skill is acquired, sites which have the highest recurrence rates whatever the method of treatment (bar Mohs' surgery) are best avoided – inner canthus, nasolabial folds and periauricular lesions. In general, one can state that the ear, eyelid and cartilaginous parts of the nose are relatively good sites for cryosurgery because cartilage necrosis is not likely with routine methods; also connective tissue damage and distorting scars are rare (1,18).

Basal cell carcinoma (3,4,7): Superficial spreading BCC or the type often seen on the trunk in the elderly (sun exposure not a factor), lesions of the basal cell nevus (Gorlin's) syndrome and small lesions on X-ray damaged skin (Fig. 7.1.3a and b), are treatable with a single freeze/thaw cycle, i.e. there is less inflammatory morbidity from this than with the two freeze/thaw cycles as used most frequently in the rodent ulcer or cystic types mostly seen on the face (Fig. 7.1.2a and b). With careful case selection, cure rates of greater than 97 per cent can be obtained. Particularly gratifying are the cure rates and excellent cosmetic results obtained for lesions on the nose and the ear. The latter is important because only rarely does BCC invade the underlying cartilage (1). This type of tumor tends to spread horizontally, superficial to the cartilage; squamous carcinoma however, may invade and therefore, if cryosurgery is used after healing and cure, a structural defect may remain forever.

Squamous carcinoma (SCC) (7, 16): It is the author's opinion that correctly used cryosurgery is the treatment of choice for carcinoma-in-situ (Bowen's disease) of the skin, some types of external genital lesions in the female and penis erythroplasia of Queyrat (Fig. 7.1.4a and b); of considerable advantage regarding genital skin Bowen's disease is that the freezing methods used do not cause connective tissue scarring and contracture is a major advantage. Vulval dysplasia (VIN) of Human Papilloma Virus (HPC) type responds poorly.

Well differentiated squamous carcinomas related to sun damage (Figs. 7.1.8 and 7.1.9) require two freeze/thaw cycles to avoid treatment failure, frequent recurrences, or late onset metastases.

Unlike BCC, squamous carcinoma more often invades underlying tissues such as cartilage; lesions on the ear are thus better not treated by freezing. Even though good cure rates can be obtained, loss of ear cartilage and poor cosmetic results are common. The clinical signs of squamous carcinoma in the early stages are less clear cut than BCC.

Therefore prior to treatment of SCC, accurate diagnosis is crucial – evidently this leads to the conclusion that very small lesions are better treated by excision biopsy if primary closure is possible.

Lentigo maligna (LM) and lentigo maligna melanoma (LMM) (Fig. 7.1.7a and b). Dermatologists have in practice been using various freezing techniques for LM and LMM for many decades; anecdotal reports have always appeared good. Dawber & Wilkinson published a series with long follow-up observations confirming the long held view that aggressive cryosurgery gives satisfactory cure rates (7). It is important to note that cryobiological research has confirmed the ease with which normal melanocytes are killed by short freezes as used in clinical practice (19) – fully justifying pilot studies in malignant melanoma or the good prognostic group such as biopsy-proven early MM. Studies are continuing in other types of melanoma (17).

Because of the marked inflammatory reaction that follows cryosurgery for malignant lesions, it is important to give the patient a suitable advice sheet (Table 7.1.7).

Palliation: Over 150 years ago the value of freezing temperatures applied to surface malignant lesions was known – decreasing the size of primary and secondary (often fungating) malignancies in the skin; also pain in such tumors was often decreased and any chronic bacterial infection usually improved or was cured. In parts of the world where surgical facilities and radiotherapy are not available, such palliative methods are still useful, since

Table 7.1.7. Advice sheet following cryosurgery for malignant lesion

• **Patient Information Sheet Cryosurgery**

After cryosurgery the treated area will swell and weep considerably, but this can be reduced by the application of clobetasol propionate 0.5 per cent cream and a gauze dressing which should be held in place by adhesive tape; the cream can be reapplied daily for 4–5 days to minimize the early redness, swelling and soreness.

The wound should form a hard, dry, black adherent crust after 10–14 days. It may be anything from a week to a month or more before it separates to leave a pink scar that ultimately becomes white.

There should be relatively little pain after the procedure, but aspirin 300–600 mg, 4–6-hourly can be taken if required. In the case of aspirin intolerance, paracetamol (acetaminophen) may be used instead. Severe pain or swelling may indicate the presence of secondary infection, when a course of antibiotics may be prescribed by your doctor.

If any problems arise in connection with you cryosurgery, please contact your doctor
(Telephone No: .... Extension: ......).

liquid nitrogen is a better "killing" refrigerant than the 19th century salt/ice mixtures. Kuflik (3,10) has shown that it is still a useful principle to use for many "incurable" malignant skin lesions. Liquid nitrogen is so widely available around the world in hospitals, veterinary and other biological units (mostly for tissue preservation) and other industries that even in less advanced countries, liquid nitrogen can usually be obtained.

7.1.7 Some Advantages, Side-Effects and Disadvantages (18)

The patient usually feels a burning sensation during freezing and thawing. Any pain experienced is usually transient due to the anesthetizing effect of freezing. Local anesthesia is not required for short freeze times but may be indicated when treating malignant lesions or for patients thought to have a low pain threshold. Deep treatments on the forehead may occasionally produce migraine-like headaches, and periungual treatment produces relatively greater discomfort than other digital sites.

Some degree of erythema and edema is to be expected with cryosurgery treatments and in areas where the skin is lax – periorbital skin (Fig. 7.1.15), lips, labia majora and penis – edema may be pronounced. Prolonged freezing schedules may produce blister formation (Fig. 7.1.16); even short freeze times may cause such changes in atrophic skin.

Because this acute inflammation was thought to be unnecessary to obtain good cure rates, for many years the author advocated pre- and post-treatment (3–5 days) anti-inflammatory therapy with soluble Aspirin 300–600 mg up to four times daily or Ibuprofen 800 mg twice daily; and Dermovate (clobetasol propionate) cream daily to the treated area. The value of this has been confirmed by objective assessment. Some authorities recommend systemic corticosteroids to minimize the acute inflammation.

Obviously many of the conditions listed in Table 7.1.1 as being curable by cryosurgery are also amenable to other surgical methods; the modality chosen will often depend on the skills available in the department to which the patient has been referred. Cryosurgery has the advantage over all other modes of being quick, cheap and easy to learn and to carry out; usually sterile surgical facilities are not required and treatment can

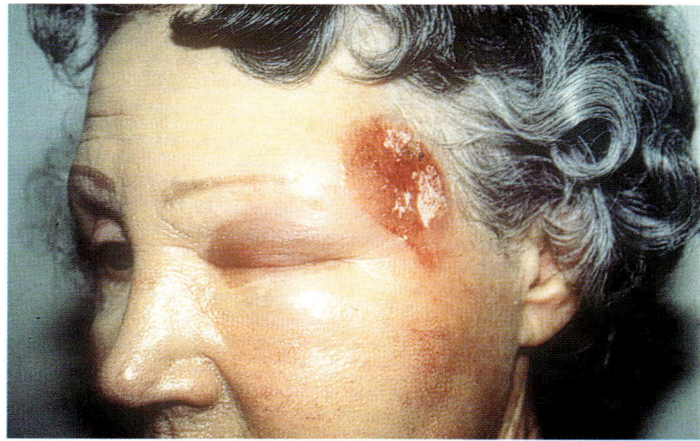

Fig. 7.1.15. Oedema following cryosurgery to a left temple basal cell carcinoma

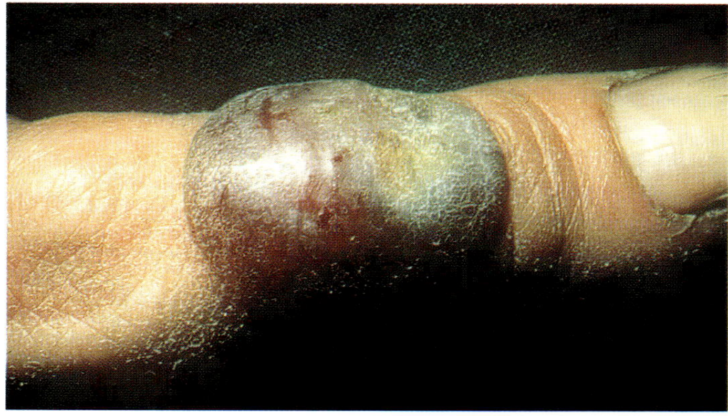

Fig. 7.1.16. Blister formation due to liquid nitrogen spray cryosurgery

be initiated even in the presence of bacterial infection, e.g., ingrowing toenail. The fact that post-treatment connective tissue distortion does not generally occur (1) makes cryosurgery advantageous where scarring would be progressively troublesome, e.g., perianal, penile, vulval and periorbital skin; also over joints where a full range of movement can be expected to be retained even after treatment of malignancy with two or three freeze/thaw cycles.

Cartilage necrosis is extremely rare after freezing; therefore ear, eyelid and many nasal lesions give good cosmetic results after cryosurgery. It should be remembered that the only consistent exception to this dogma is cartilage already invaded by tumor – even if good cure is obtained, a cartilage defect may occur, e.g., squamous carcinoma of the ear.

Anything but the shortest freeze schedules will give pigment changes in the treatment area (19) – hyperpigmentation with very short freezes and at the edge of more aggressively treated areas. Hypopigmentation occurs after prolonged freezing, e.g., approximately 10 secs after ice field formation, and may be permanent; therefore cryosurgery is less valuable in patients with racially dark skin – e.g., Asian or Black African (Fig. 7.1.17) and "exposed part" lesions in Caucasian whites who tan darkly on sun exposure.

In general, cryosurgery is not recommended for the treatment of lesions on sites with coarse terminal hair (20). Hair follicles are easily damaged by cryosurgery and permanent alopecia is not uncommon (Fig. 7.1.6).

Temporary impairment of sensation in the treatment area is common after freezing; only rarely will the patient be aware of this. Such nerve ending damage can be expected to disappear within a few months, apart from after "malignancy regimes" using two or three FTCs. At sites such as the lip margin, permanent sensory loss may give important functional impairment, but in other sites it is generally of no significance. Though nerve trunk damage and "distant" sensory and motor loss have been recorded they are rare and reversible, usually within a few months.

A rare side-effect of cryosurgery is delayed bleeding; this may be due to granulation tissue formation (Fig. 7.1.18) as in pyogenic granuloma, or from erosion of a small artery. The former may require no more than pressure to abort it, or chemical hemostasis or electrocautery; a patent bleeding artery requires tying off with an appropriate suture.

It is now evident that cryosurgical equipment and skill are essential in all dermatology and surgical departments which regularly treat lesions, benign and malignant, of the type noted in Table 7.1.1. (4, 21–23) There are many skin conditions in which excision, radiotherapy and cryosurgery may be alternative modes of treatment under consideration – clearly for many of these lesions, cryosurgery is now the treatment of choice.

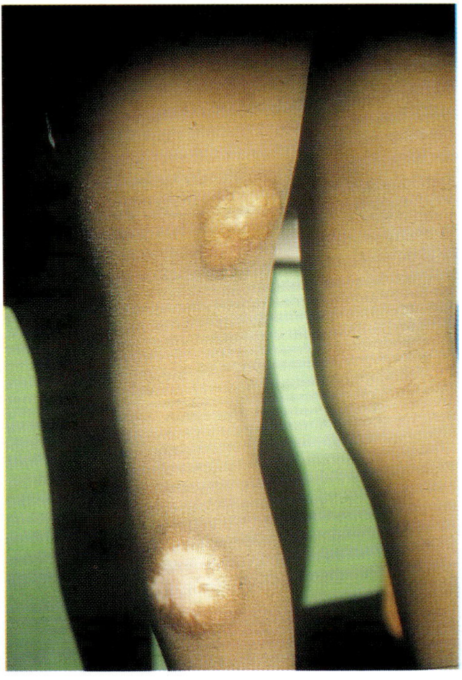

Fig. 7.1.17. Pigment change (permanent) – due to cryosurgery for tropical sore Leishmaniasis

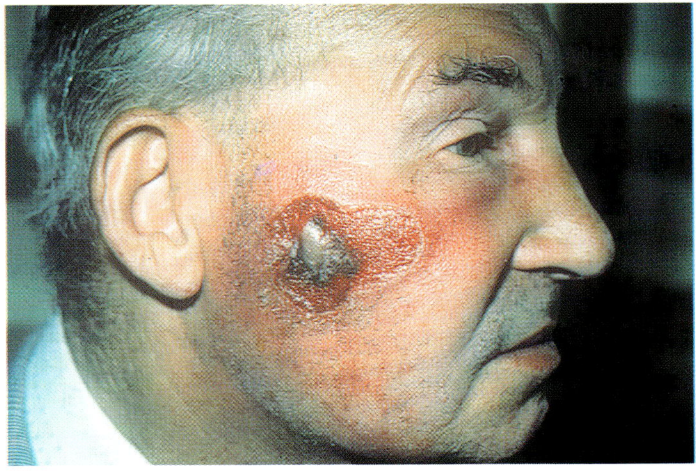

Fig. 7.1.18. Granulating wound with some necrosis following liquid nitrogen spray cryosurgery for a large basal cell carcinoma

References

1. Dawber RPR, Colver G, Jackson A, Pringle F. Cutaneous Cryosurgery. Martin Dunitz, London; 2nd edition, 1997.
2. Torre D, Lubritz RR, Kuflik EG. Practical Cutaneous Cryosurgery. Norwalk, Conn: Appleton and Large, 1988.
3. Kuflik EG. Cryosurgery updated. J. Amer. Acad. Dermatol. 31: 925–44, 1994.
4. Drake LA, Ceilley RI, Cornelison RL et al. Guidelines of care for cryosurgery. J Amer Acad Dermatol 31: 648–653, 1994.
5. Torre D. Cryosurgical Instrumentation and Depth Dose Monitoring. Advances in Cryosurgery. Clinics in Dermatology 8: 48–60, 1990.
6. Sinclair RD, Tzermias C, Dawber RPR. Cosmetic Cryosurgery: In: Cosmetic Dermatology. Eds. Baran R, Maibach HI. Martin Dunitz, London. 12 (10) 541–550, 1998.
7. Sinclair RD, Dawber RPR. Cryosurgery of Malignant and Premalignant Diseases of the Skin. Australasian J Dermatol 36: 133–142, 1995.
8. Gage AA. Cryosurgery of Advanced Tumors: Advances in Cryosurgery. Clin Dermatol 8: 86–95, 1990.
9. Kuflik EG, Gage AA. The five-year cure rate achieved by cryosurgery for skin cancer. J. Amer Acad Dermatol 24: 1002–4, 1991
10. Kuflik EG, Gage AA. Results of Cryosurgical Treatment for Skin Cancer. NY, Igaka-Shoin, 243–54, 1996.
11. Graham GF. Advances in cryosurgery during the past decade. Cutis 52: 365–72, 1993
12. Mallon E, Dawber RPR. Cryosurgery in the treatment of basal cell carcinoma. Dermatologic Surgery. 22: 854–8, 1996.
13. Biro L, Price E. Cryosurgical management of the basal cell carcinoma of the eyelids. J Amer Acad Dermatol 23: 316–7, 1990.
14. Telfer NR, Colver GB, Bowers PW. Guidelines for the management of basal cell carcinoma. Brit J Dermatol 141: 415–423, 1999.
15. Spiller WE, Spiller RF. Treatment of basal cell carcinoma by curettage and cryosurgery. J Dermatol Surg Oncol 3: 443–7, 1997.
16. Holt PJA. Cryosurgery for skin cancer. Brit J Dermatol 119: 231–240, 1988.
17. Brietbart EW. Cryosurgery in the treatment of cutaneous malignant melanoma. Clinics Dermatol 8: 96–100, 1990.
18. Dawber RPR. Cryosurgery: In, Complications in Dermatologic Surgery. Ed: Harahap M. Springer-Verlag, Berlin. Ch. 4: pp 40–50, 1993.
19. Burge SM, Bristol M, Millard PR, Dawber RPR. Pigment change in human skin after cryosurgery. Cryobiology 23: 111–6, 1986.
20. Burge SM, Dawber RPR. Hair follicle destruction and regeneration in guinea pig skin after cutaneous freeze injury. Cryobiology 27: 155–63, 1990.
21. Sheridan AT, Dawber RPR. Laugier-Hunziker Syndrome: Treatment with cryosurgery. J Eur Acad Dermatol Venereol 12 (2), 146–8, 1999.
22. Zouboulis CC, Blume U, Buttner D, Orfanos CE. Outcome of cryosurgical treatment of patients with keloids and hypertrophic scars. Arch Dermatol 129: 1146–51, 1993.
23. Rusciani L, Rossi G, Bono R. Use of cryotherapy in the treatment of keloids. J Dermatol Surg Oncol 19: 529–34, 1993.

7.2 Segmental Cryosurgery of Zacarian and Fractional Cryosurgery for Skin Cancer

Jose C. Almeida Gonçalves with a contribution by J. Abel Amaro

7.2.0 Introduction

Cryosurgery has been demonstrated to be an excellent alternative for the treatment of benign, premalignant and malignant lesions of the skin (1, 2). It is a practical, safe, effective and inexpensive modality. For small tumors, cryosurgery can usually be performed in a single session, in the out-patient clinic, without anesthesia, or, in some instances, under local anesthesia. Larger lesions require two or more sessions. When treating extensive tumors, pain may become intolerable and excessive amounts of local anesthesia may be needed, exceeding the safety limits, particularly in elderly patients. For thick lesions the procedure may be simplified by previous "debulking" (3, 4). For superficial lesions, measuring several centimeters, it is advisable to divide them into several segments and freeze one segment at a time. This technique, known as segmental cryosurgery, was devised by Zacarian (2) and has been used independently – under different names – by several authors in the treatment of benign, pre-malignant and malignant lesions of the skin.

When compared with single-session cryosurgery for extensive tumors, the segmental treatment has the following advantages: 1) it permits the treatment of large lesions, under local anesthesia, with less discomfort to the patient; 2) it allows better monitoring of the freezing field and the freeze/thaw times; 3) it carries a smaller risk of deep necrosis, with involvement of underlying structures; 4) there is less morbidity in the healing process and smaller risk of hypertrophic or retractile scars. The main disadvantage is the need for several visits to the outpatient clinic, which may have a negative impact on the patient's compliance.

Each lesion must be treated according to its histological type and clinical behavior. The different segments of the lesion can be treated consecutively, one by one, in the same session, or just one segment in each visit, at intervals of several days – when the exudative period has subsided – or several weeks after complete healing of the previously treated lesion. Overlapping of the freezing fields is recommended when treating malignant lesions.

7.2.1 Segmental Treatment of Benign Lesions

Large epithelial nevi, with a linear pattern, are a good indication for segmental cryosurgery. Nevertheless, these lesions respond variously to cryosurgery, depending on their water content and, in some cases, their irregular texture and thickness. Lubritz (5) cites Zacarian and Graham who treated several epithelial nevi segmentally, in successive sessions, with significant improvement, but without complete eradication. Lubritz (5) himself reported a large and thick epithelial nevus treated segmentally with remarkable improvement. One of us (JAA) also treated an extensive epithelial nevus, on the back of a 12-year-old girl, with marked improvement. The lesion was divided into several rectangles that were treated one by one, in successive sessions, over about 16 months. Most parts of the lesion were treated by cryosurgery and the remaining peripheral portions of the nevus were vaporized by CO_2 laser.

Castro-Ron (6) reported a large congenital *angiokeratoma*, on the lateral aspect of the left thigh, in a 3-year-old girl, treated segmentally with partial success. He also treated an extensive *capillary lymphangioma*, on the right lower back, in a 16-year-old girl, by segmental freezing, in multiple consecutive sessions with a very satisfactory result.

Keloids can be improved by segmental cryosurgery alone, or in combination with intralesional steroids. Graham (7) reported the case of a 19-year-old man, with extensive keloids on the face, chest and back as sequelae of acne. He had been previously treated by surgery, under general anesthesia, with partial recurrence 4 months later. The lesion was divided into several areas that were frozen repeatedly, in combination with intralesional steroids, with good to excellent results.

Graham also used segmental cryosurgery to treat large areas on the face with multiple *acne scars* (7). She divided the field into several rectangles, of about 4 cm × 2 cm, and froze each one with a fine spray. The freezing times varied from 5 to 15 seconds per section. She warned about the risk of excessive freezing in this benign condition, which could produce atrophy or pigmentary changes.

7.2.2 Segmental Treatment of Pre-Malignant Lesions

The management of large plaques of *leukoplakia* in the mouth can be a difficult problem. Cryosurgery is, probably, the best treatment for these pre-malignant lesions. We treated successfully an extensive leukoplakia of the palate, in a 52-year-old Black woman from Angola, with many years of inverse smoking habit (Figs. 7.2.1 and 7.2.2). The lesion was divided into several sections of about 2 cm × 2 cm that were frozen, one by one, over a period of about nine months. We used a long cryoprobe (Frigitronics) together with a hydrophilic gel (K-Y® lubricating jelly, Johnson & Johnson) for better adhesion. The treatment was painful but the patient was very co-operative, tolerating it quite well. Local anesthesia was used only in the areas close to the teeth. One thicker area in the right side, between two molars, was unusually resistant to cold. A punch biopsy was taken and the histological examination disclosed an invasive squamous-cell carcinoma. The tumor was surgically excised and the patient submitted to adjuvant radiotherapy. She was well after more than 16 years of follow-up.

Large sun damaged areas with *multiple actinic keratoses* are a good example of field carcinogenesis (Figs. 7.2.3–7.2.4). All this skin must be regarded as a pre-malignant condition. The recommended procedure is to freeze the entire field and not just an actinic keratosis each time. Segmental cryosurgery is indicated in such cases. We used this technique to treat multiple actinic keratoses in two

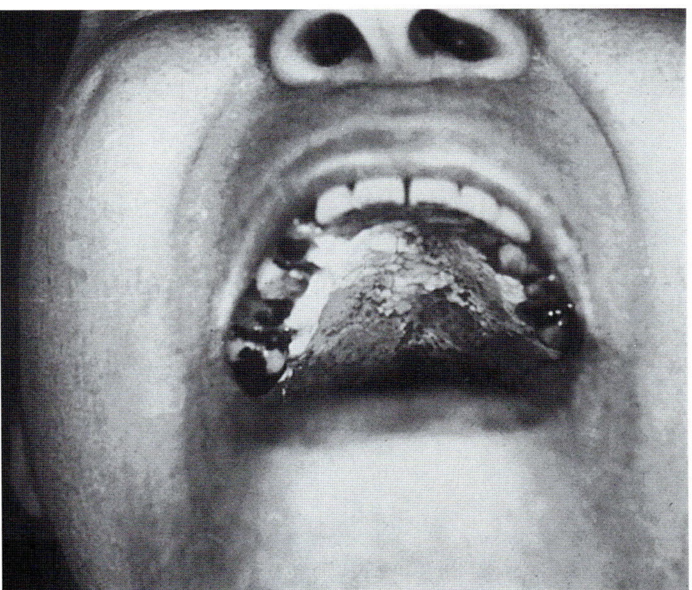

Fig. 7.2.1. Leukoplakia of almost the entire oral mucosa

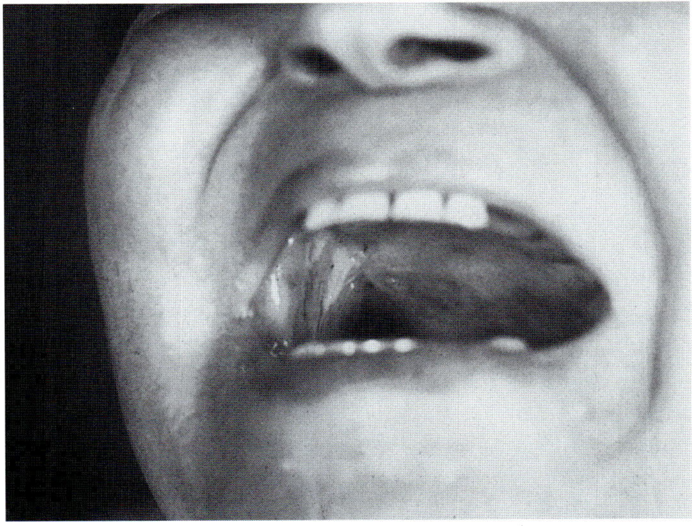

Fig. 7.2.2. After segmental cryosurgery

male patients with extensive baldness and severely damaged scalp due to long lasting sun exposure. After dividing the area in a rectangular web we froze each section with open spray technique, two or three sections each time. The freezing times ranged from 15 to 45 seconds, depending on the thickness of the existing keratosis. Complete clearing of the scalp was achieved in both patients.

7.2.3 Segmental Cryosurgery of Malignant Lesions

Segmental cryosurgery is usually indicated for the treatment of large lesions of *basal cell carcinoma* (BCC) - especially the superficial type – some *squamous cell carcinomas* (SCC), *Bowen's disease* and *lentigo maligna*. Figures 7.2.5–7.2.7 show the method in a BCC of the ala nasi. In the first treatment, one half of the tumor was treated with two freeze/thaw cycles with adequate safety margin. One month later the cancer was considerably reduced and was then definitively treated. Zacarian (2) reported an "extensive rodent type of erosive basal cell carcinoma" invading the nose and cheeks of a 51-year-old male, which was segmentally treated. This patient could not tolerate anesthesia and, therefore, could not be treated by plastic surgery. Then he was sent to a radiotherapist, who declined to treat him because of the extent of the lesion. Finally he was referred for cryosurgery. Segmental treatment was performed, step-by-step, in four separate freezings at the different sites, over a period of four months. The result was excellent, in spite of a recurrence, one year later, which was frozen again, with definitive cure. Zacarian (2) also reported another case of extensive multifocal BCC of the right ear, in a 66-year-old patient, that was successfully treated

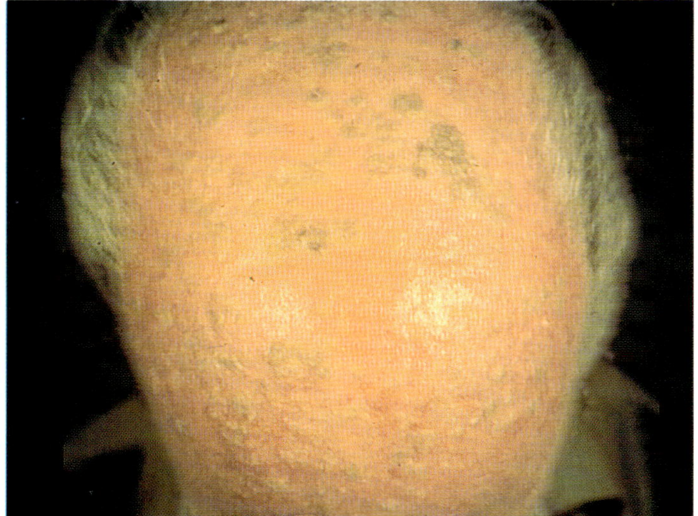

Fig. 7.2.3. Multiple keratoses of the scalp

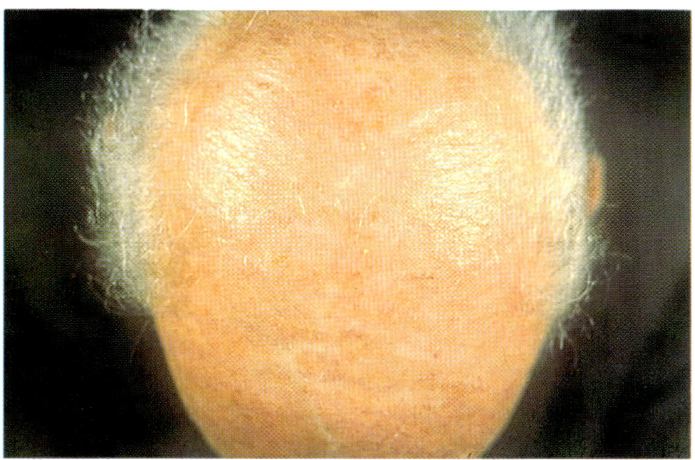

Fig. 7.2.4. After segmental cryosurgery

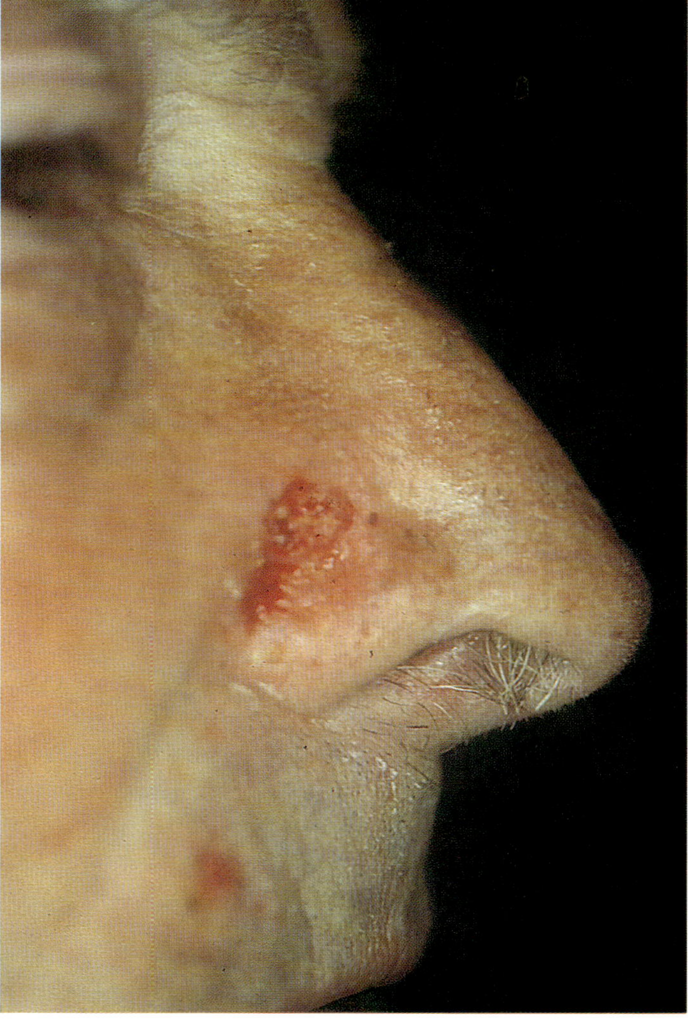

Fig. 7.2.5. BCC, measuring 20 mm × 10 mm, after 4 years' evolution

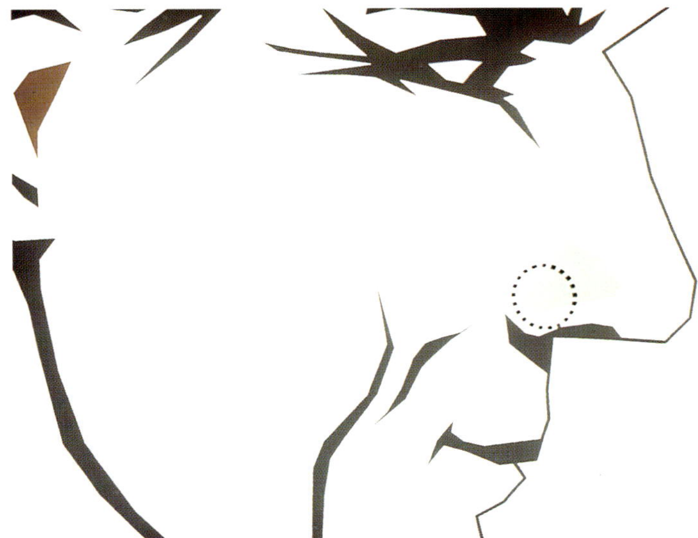

Fig. 7.2.6. Schematic drawing of the first cryosurgical procedure, with 2 freeze-thaw cycles and large safety margin around the tumor

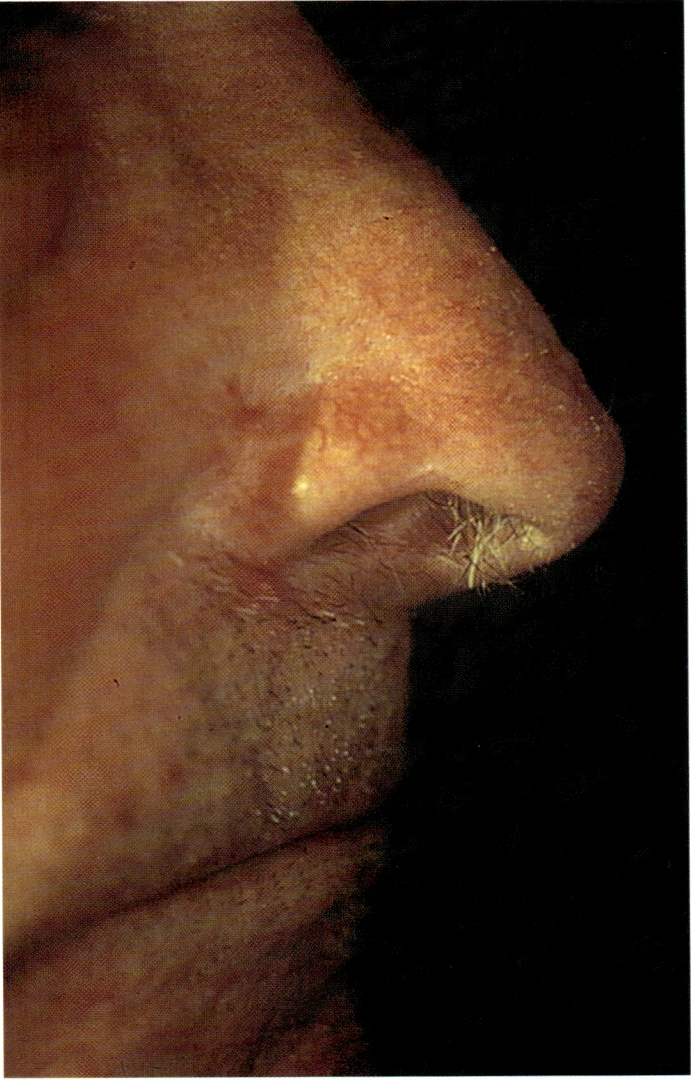

Fig. 7.2.7. One month later, the tumor was reduced to 10 mm × 9 mm. A definitive cryosurgical treatment was performed. No recurrence for 4 years

by segmental cryosurgery. This technique is particularly indicated for the treatment of large superficial tumors of the trunk, where conventional surgery would need extensive grafts or flaps, usually with poor cosmetic results. These lesions are best frozen in quadrants or in halves, as recommended by Zacarian (2), who reported a "6 cm BCC of the back appearing as a large, solid, infiltrated plaque". He divided the tumor into two halves and froze first the upper half during three minutes. The lower half was frozen 6 weeks later. As Zacarian pointed out, "overlapping onto the half of the tumor that was previously frozen is of no concern". Gage (8) reported a technique for the treatment of advanced tumors that can be considered a variety of segmental cryosurgery. He stated that in tumors that are "too large to be frozen in a single application the probe must be used in multiple sites, with careful attention to freezing at the borders of the tumor". Spiller W. and Spiller R. (9) also recommended what they called the "serial treatment" in selected cases of extensive BCC. They reported a large (5 cm × 3 cm) recurrent and invasive basal cell carcinoma of the forehead, treated sequentially by sections, combining curettage, electrodesiccation and cryosurgery. They also emphasised that "the borders between areas frozen at different times should be overlapped to destroy cancer cells that may have grown into the edges of healed scar." These authors (10) also reported a 79-year-old man with a large, 9 cm × 9 cm, recurrent BCC of the scalp, treated segmentally by curettage and electrodesiccation followed by cryosurgery, according to a pre-established diagram. The different sections were treated sequentially at intervals of two to four months. The result was quite impressive since they achieved clinical cure without any bone necrosis. Albright (11) reported an extensive and recurrent basal cell carcinoma of the right side of the head, in a 75-year-old woman, involving about 95 cm^2 of the face, which was successfully treated by aggressive cryosurgery in six "overlapping fields" over a period of one month. The treatment was done under local anesthesia as an office based procedure. Kuflik (12,13) also reported several cases of extensive basal cell carcinoma of the face and trunk treated by segmental cryosurgery, with good to excellent results. Figures 7.2.8 and 7.2.9 show a large BCC of the upper lip, measuring 18 mm × 15 mm, of an elderly patient, aged 92 years. The difficulty in treating tumors at this location without deformity, even by plastic surgery, is well known. She was treated by 3 segmental cryosurgical procedures at monthly intervals. The cosmetic result was remarkable. Figures 7.2.10 and 7.2.11 show a BCC of the border between the orbital and infra-orbital regions, with 3 years' evolution, and 4 years after segmental cryosurgery. Figures 7.2.12–7.2.15 compare the advantage of segmental cryosurgery over the single cryosurgical procedure carried out in two BCCs at the same location.

Large lesions of *lentigo maligna* in critical anatomical areas deserve consideration for segmental cryosurgery, particularly in elderly patients, when general anesthesia involves considerable risk, or when conventional surgery may be too mutilating. Among 30 cases of lentigo maligna, Zacarian (14) reported a large one in an 83-year-old woman that developed over a 13-year period, involving the forehead, bridge of the nose, medial canthus, infraorbital region and cheek. He treated the tumor in two separate stages with a six-week interval. Each session consisted of double freeze-thaw cycles of 3 and 6 minutes, respectively. In spite of the extent of the lesion, he achieved clinical cure without significant sequelae, namely epiphora or ectropion of the lower eyelid. Graham (15) also reported a recurrent lentigo maligna involving the helix of the right ear, in a 61-year-old-man, who refused surgical amputation but consented to be treated by cryosurgery. She froze first the anterior aspect of the tumor, for 90 seconds, by open spray of liquid nitrogen, with a thaw time of about 3 minutes. The posterior part of the lesion was large and was treated two months later. It was divided into four sections. The freezing times were from 60 to 90 seconds, with thaw times varying from 1 min 35 seconds to 3 min 35 seconds.

Over the last 26 years, we have successfully treated 90 patients with extensive lentigo maligna

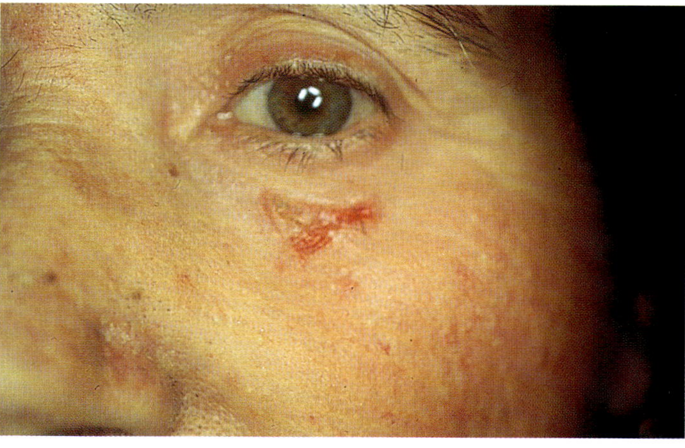

Fig. 7.2.10. A BCC after 3 years' evolution in a 58-year-old woman

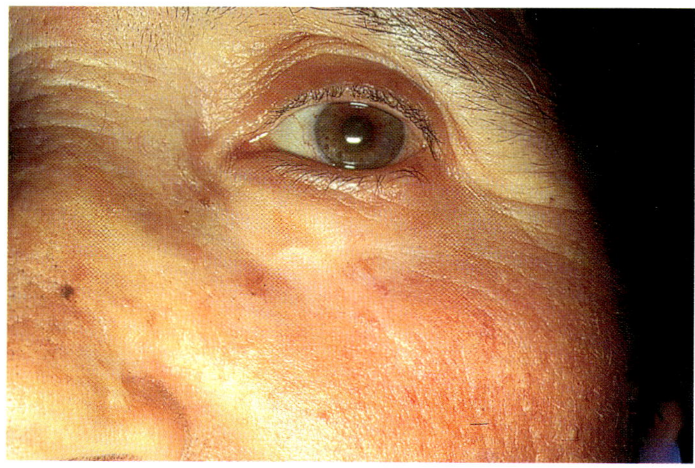

Fig. 7.2.11. Four years after segmental cryosurgery

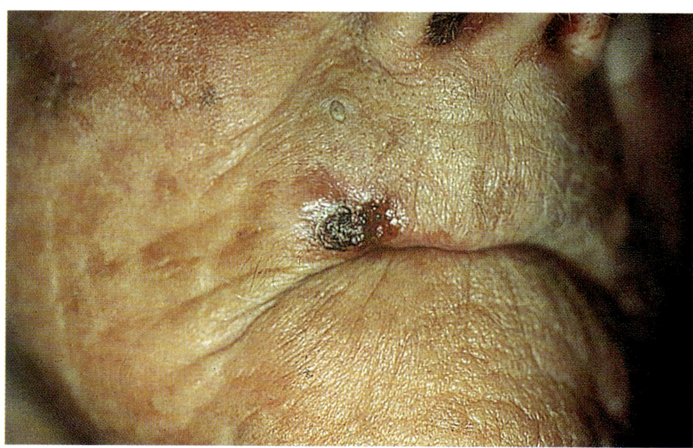

Fig. 7.2.8. An L-shaped BCC on the lip of a 92-year-old patient (18 mm × 15 mm)

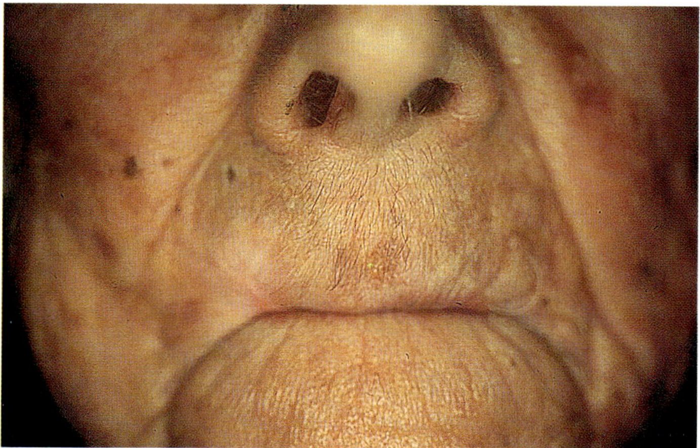

Fig. 7.2.9. After three segmental cryosurgical procedures at monthly intervals, the cosmetic result is remarkable

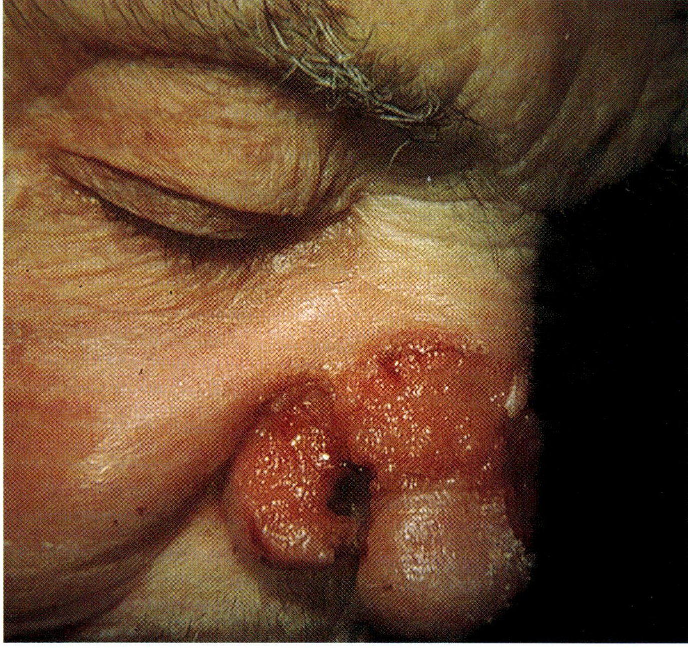

Fig. 7.2.12. A long-standing BCC in a 92-year-old patient. The *ala nasi* had been perforated by the tumor

by cryosurgery, the majority of whom by segmental cryosurgery, and we find that it provides better cosmetic results than the single cryosurgical procedure.

Some authors question the legitimacy of treating lentigo maligna otherwise than with surgery

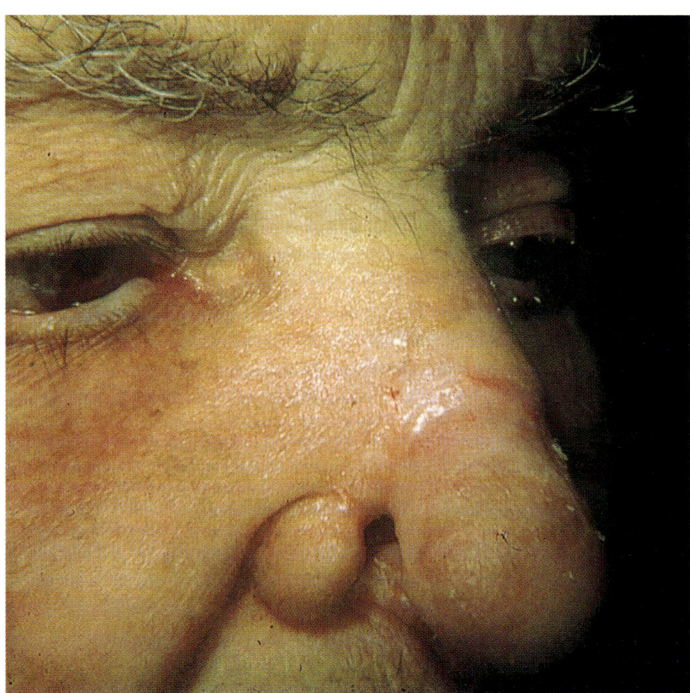

Fig. 7.2.13. Clinical cure after 5 procedures

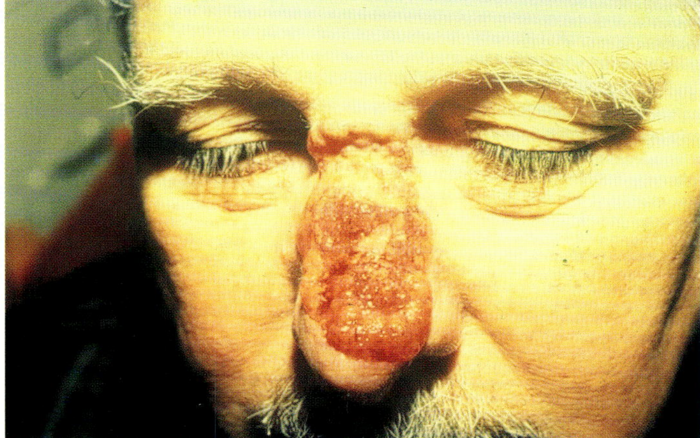

Fig. 7.2.14. A large, neglected BCC

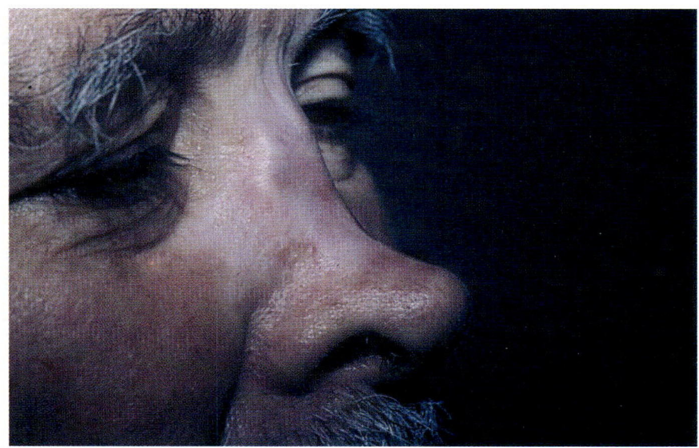

Fig. 7.2.15. After only one cryosurgical procedure, performed on the whole lesion, clinical cure was achieved but with some deformity

(16). In our country, and in our personal experience, there is no therapeutic alternative in almost all cases. These patients are mostly women over 70 years of age –whose lesions are generally extensive but asymptomatic – who peremptorily refuse plastic surgery. Hence, the Portuguese physician must choose between performing cryosurgery and neglecting the lesion, allowing it to evolve.

7.2.4 Fractional Cryosurgery

As we have seen, the segmental cryosurgery of Zacarian represented considerable progress in the treatment of large skin cancers. In 1997, one of us (JCAG) published a paper on a new technique that he called ''fractional cryosurgery'' (17). This was originally devised to deal with BCCs of the eyelids and periorbital areas, which are common lesions on these areas. The value of cryosurgery in treating small periocular malignancies was then well established (18–28). However, for tumors with diameters of 10 mm or more, the usual cryosurgical treatment, with the required safety margin, produces large ulcerations, which may result in variable degrees of retraction of the local structures. In papers published in 1979 and 1982, Biro et al. (19, 20) reported having treated some BCCs of the eyelids larger than 10 mm but in 1990 (21), they stated that they were no longer treating eyelid carcinomas larger than 10 mm. Actually, experienced cryosurgeons have reported some occasional undesirable cosmetic results (19–21, 28). Before devising fractional cryosurgery JCAG treated over 500 carcinomas of the eyelids and periorbital regions, over a period of 30 years, and observed three cases of lagophthalmus (17) in his own experience. The surgeon must be careful when choosing the treatment modality for lesions on the forehead and medial part of the face, where even minor alterations in the features can have considerable physiognomic consequences.

Zacarian's segmental cryosurgery (2) is an excellent method for large, elongated lesions, but it is less adequate for roundish lesions. When treating very advanced cancers, namely of the vulva and breast (see chapter "Cryosurgery of advanced external cancers", in this book) the resulting extensive ulcerations heal by second intention with amazingly good, smooth scars, particularly when those ulcerations are surrounded by mobile skin, as is the case of the breast and vulva of elderly women. During the cicatrization process, the surrounding skin "moves" towards the healing ulceration, as if being pulled by it, and the final scars are not very different from those after conventional surgery. The skin around the eyelids is very mobile, especially in elderly people, which suggested the possibility of developing a technique applicable to periorbital carcinomas larger than 10 mm in diameter. The first 20 cases of periocular BCC treated by this new fractional cryosurgery technique were published in 1997 (17). Subsequently, the technique was applied to carcinomas of the head and neck (including some squamous cell carcinomas), whose size or location could originate local retraction and the resulting modification of physiognomic features, after a single cryosurgical treatment. JCAG's further experience is herein reported.

7.2.5 Surgical Protocol

The lesion is measured and photographed, a biopsy is taken and the apparent contour of the tumor is drawn with ink. Local anesthesia is administered with a 3% mepivacain hydrochloride solution. We prefer a dentist's syringe with a very thin needle, which is less uncomfortable for the patient. A hydrophilic gel is applied over the tumor to ease the taking off of the calories. In accordance with the size of the target area, a cryoprobe is selected and applied, at ambient temperature, to the center of the lesion. The cryoprobe is then chilled internally by the liquid nitrogen and becomes adherent to the skin, thus freezing the tissues.

The first cryosurgical procedure is not intended to freeze the whole neoplasm. The first freezing reaches the apparent limits of the tumor, without safety margin, or, if it is large, the freezing is applied only to its center. The extent of the frozen tissue is clinically assessed. Temperature monitoring is not essential if the surgeon has enough experience, but can be done with advantage.

This first cryosurgical procedure consists of one or two freeze/thaw cycles, according to the following criteria:

a) for tumors on the eyelids, one cycle, always;
b) around the eyelids – one cycle for thin lesions, and two cycles for thick lesions;
c) for tumors at other locations, two cycles.

The resulting ulceration heals slowly, over the following 3–4 weeks. After healing, the lesion is reduced in size or, at least, in thickness, and its measurements are compared with the initial ones and recorded. If the measurements indicate that, clinically, there is no longer danger of retraction, the second procedure is performed in the standard way – two freeze-thaw cycles, with adequate safety margin. If the tumor is still too large, the initial procedure is repeated. The aim of this technique is to obtain successive reductions of the tumor, with as many procedures as necessary, until it achieves a size that permits the complete freezing with safety margin, without risk of retraction.

After the first procedure all tumors generally reduce in size or, at least, in thickness. However, sometimes, no visible tumor remains and, in such cases, the surgeon must not be misled by the clinically apparent cure, and must assume that the carcinoma is not biologically cured – the safety margin had not been frozen – and it is mandatory to carry out two freeze-thaw cycles in the location of the treated tumor, with adequate extent so as to treat the intended safety margin.

7.2.6 Patients

Seventy-eight patients were treated by fractional cryosurgery (34 men and 44 women). Their ages ranged from 30 to 99 years (mean of 71 years). The duration of the disease was: less than five years (30 patients), between five and nine years (15), 10 or more years (7) and undetermined (26). The location of the tumors is indicated in Table 7.2.1.

Sixty-eight patients suffered from primary BCC, one from a recurrent BCC, treated by cryosurgery elsewhere, and nine from SCC. All diagnoses were histologically confirmed. The tumors' major axes measured: between 9 mm and 14 mm (32), between 15 mm and 19 mm (27), between 20 mm and 26 mm (16) and between 32 mm and 45 mm (3). That is, 43 were <16 mm and 35 were >16 mm.

The clinical classification of the BCCs was: nodulo-ulcerative (40), nodular (23), pigmented (3), cicatrizing (1), sclerosing (1) and ulcerated (1). Histologically, all tumors were solid and undifferentiated. The clinical classification of the SCCs was ulcerative (5), nodulo-ulcerative (3) and nodular (1). The histological classification was undifferentiated (3), well differentiated (2), with low grade of differentiation (1), and unclassified (3).

7.2.7 Results

In the first cryosurgical procedure, 41 patients were submitted to a single freeze-thaw cycle, 36 to two cycles and 1 to three. The latter suffered from a thick nodulo-ulcerative SCC, the safety margin having not been frozen in the first procedure. The number of subsequent cryosurgical procedures varied as follows: one in 38 patients, two in 23, and three to six in 17 patients.

In some rare cases a segmental cryosurgery was done in one or two extremities to reduce the size of the cancer before fractional cryosurgery.

Table 7.2.1. Location of the tumors

Periocular regions	No. of patients	Other regions	No. patients
Upper eyelid	6	Nose	4
Lower eyelid	14	Nasal/infra-orbital fold	3
Medial canthus	14	Nasal/oral fold	3
Nasal/orbital fold	1	Infra-orbital	5
Orbital/infra-orbital fold	11	Zygomatic	8
Supra-orbital	1	Forehead	3
Orbital/zygomatic	1	Temporal	1
		Neck	2
		Ear	1
Subtotal	48	Subtotal	30

All patients were clinically cured. All nine patients who suffered from squamous cell carcinoma had no evidence of disease in periods of between one and six years (mean of 3.2 years) of follow-up. Three patients died of unrelated disease after three years of follow-up. Of 69 basal cell carcinomas, eleven cases recurred between six months and three years after the last cryosurgical procedure.

In order to study the cause or causes of this high recurrence rate, the computer database was analyzed for size, location and clinical type of the BCCs. Table 7.2.2 shows the relationship between the major axes of the BCCs and the recurrences. These measurements permit the division of the BCCs into three groups: a) smaller tumors (31), whose diameter was between 9 and 14 mm, with no recurrences; b) medium sized tumors (22), with diameters between 15 mm and 19 mm, with three recurrences; c) large tumors (16), measuring between 20 mm and 35 mm, with eight recurrences. All recurrences were on the border of the scars. The location of the recurrent tumors was: forehead (1), infra-orbital region (2), fold between the orbital and infra-orbital regions (1), neck (1), zygomatic region (2), temporal region (1) and medial canthus (3). The clinical types were nine nodulo-ulcerative, one nodular and one ulcerative. The location and clinical type of the tumors do not seem to have influenced the recurrence, whereas their size does bear a significant relationship to that rate.

Five patients were submitted again to cryosurgery, five to conventional surgery, and one to radiation therapy (17). One patient died of unrelated disease, two years after conventional surgery without evidence of disease. All the others continued without symptoms of disease between one and seven years (mean of 4.2 years) after the respective treatments.

The early sequelae were the usual ones after cryosurgery in these areas: considerable edema of the treated side of the face and sometimes also of the contralateral side, although less intense; serous discharge; moderate conjunctivitis, but never subconjunctival hemorrhage. In some cases, the edema was prevented with a short course of systemic corticosteroids, as was found by Kuflik and Webb (29). Scab formation and sloughing off

Table 7.2.2. Basal-cell carcinomas and recurrences

Major axes (mm)	No. of patients	No. of recurrences
9–14	30	0
15–19	22	3
20–35	16	8

were observed, as usual. The late sequelae were: in some cases, local depigmentation with subsequent slow recovery; in one case, where the BCC was located on the edge of the lower eyelid, there was loss of cilia; in another BCC, measuring 18 mm × 12 mm and located on the medial canthus, strangely enough, a very small retraction of the upper eyelid developed one centimeter outside the external limit of the treated carcinoma; in another BCC of the lower eyelid, a very small retraction disappeared without any treatment, one year after cryosurgery. There was a marked scar in one patient. No lagophthalmos was observed.

The cosmetic results were excellent. In most cases no scar was observed and in the cases in which a small scar was apparent after treatment, it disappeared completely one year later. Figures 7.2.16 and 7.2.17 show a large SCC before and after treatment. The BCC shown in Fig. 7.2.18 would be difficult to treat with any method. An aggressive, deep cryosurgery was quite efficient and produced only a small scar.

7.2.8 Discussion

The use of the cryoprobe is as effective as that of liquid nitrogen spray to treat small cutaneous tumors. Like Biro and Price (quoted (26)) we prefer the cryoprobe to treat small tumors, because it does not require temperature monitoring, it makes it easier to control the limits of the freezing and, on the whole, it is less time consuming. We quite agree with Elton's view that "experienced cryosurgeons, in most cases, are able to assess the depth and adequacy of a tumor freeze by palpation, lateral spread and thaw time" (7). On the other hand, for bulky and advanced cancers (see chapter "Cryosurgery of advanced external cancer" in this book), we always use the thick liquid nitrogen spray with thermocouple monitoring.

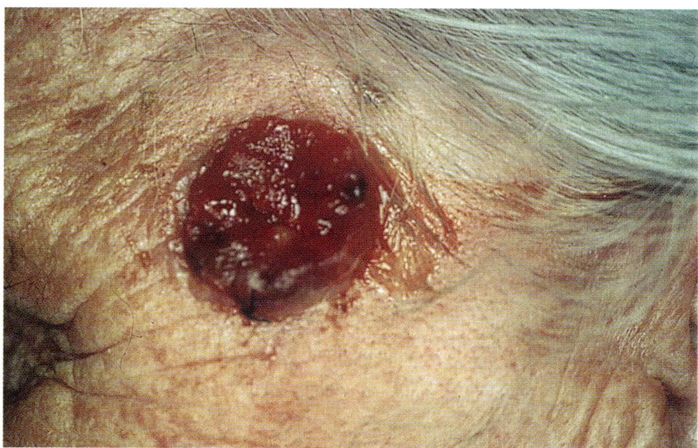

Fig. 7.2.16. A SCC of unknown evolution in a 99-year-old patient, measuring 25 mm × 25 mm

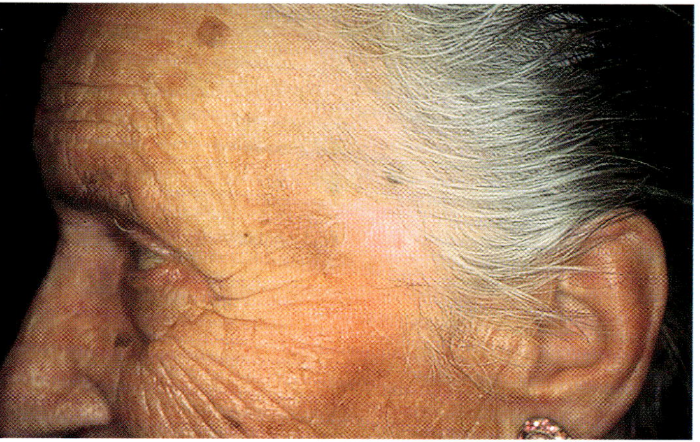

Fig. 7.2.17. After the first fractional cryosurgery, the cancer decreased in thickness and size to 20 mm × 10 mm. The second procedure was the definitive one, with adequate safety margin. She lived three more years without recurrence.

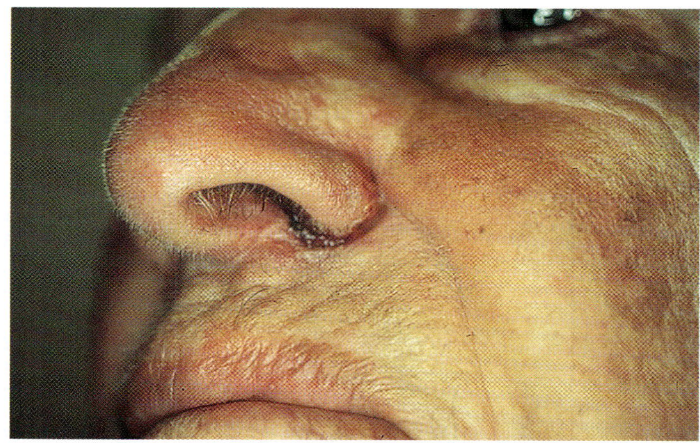

Fig. 7.2.18. A BCC on the fold between the nose and upper lip – a very difficult site for cryosurgical treatment – measuring 18 mm × 13 mm

"Debulking" before freezing is a well-accepted method that significantly improves the cure rate, as was, once more, shown by Gloria Graham (9). It was not applied in the first study (17) because, since it was a therapeutic research technique, the "debulking" would have produced an additional confounding factor when assessing the results of the method. After the first 20 published cases, "debulking" was used when necessary.

When the first results were published, attention was drawn to the following important points: "in the present technique, one must be even more aware of the danger of insufficient freezing of the

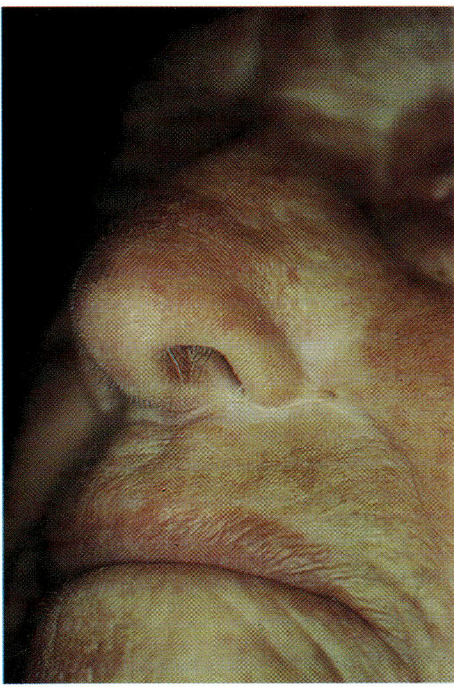

Fig. 7.2.19. One year after two aggressive procedures of fractional cryosurgery

tumors than usually, because the cosmetic results are so outstanding that it is often difficult to be precise as to the site and limits of the treated neoplasm. This is particularly important when, after a cryosurgical procedure carried out only up to the apparent limit and without safety margin, the tumor seems cured, when observed one month later. In such cases, one must not be misled by the apparent cure and must assume that the tumor is not biologically cured and always perform two freeze-thaw cycles with adequate safety margin on the original tumor site. This substantiates the need for thorough recording of the anatomic location and measurements of the tumors, and systematic photographing, under the same lighting and keeping the same distance between subject and camera. Moreover, when in doubt of an apparent cure, biopsies must be performed'' (17).

The recurrence rate of 5.7% in BCCs measuring 9 mm–19 mm is slightly higher than we are used to, but it is still acceptable. Nevertheless, eight recurrences in 16 treated tumors, measuring 20 mm–35 mm is too high. When devising a new technique, it is normal to obtain results that are not completely satisfactory until the protocol has been submitted to long experience and corrected. If eight treated patients suffering from BCC measuring 20 mm–35 mm have no evidence of disease, this proves that it is possible to cure tumors of this size and location; but eight similar patients whose tumors recur, prove that the protocol needs reviewing. There were no recurrences in the treated SCCs measuring 14 mm–45 mm, surely because an adequate safety margin was applied.

The retrospective database analysis showed that the safety margin practiced on large BCCs was insufficient. The causes that can explain the recurrences are: the excellent cosmetic results considerably impaired recognition of where the limits of the treated cancer were. Moreover, the outgrowths of the larger BCCs are longer than those of the smaller ones and were underestimated. Hence, two main modifications to the protocol for large BCCs have been made: 1) Wider safety margins, identical to those used for SCCs; 2) until recently, transparencies were used for the patients' records. In our country, the processing of transparency photographs takes too long a time, those being delivered too late to be useful in assessing the location of the tumors. We are now using digital photographs, because they can be immediately processed on paper and attached to the patient's clinical records, as a reminder of the tumor limits. Thus, we are able to more accurately freeze the safety margin.

Cancers of the medial canthus can become very dangerous if they invade the orbit. All tumors at this location should be carefully examined, and those invading the caruncle must not be accepted for cryosurgery (11). Fourteen BCCs on the medial canthus were treated by fractional cryosurgery. Three, with diameters of 15 mm (2) and 16 mm (1), recurred after six months and one and two years, respectively. The latter, when recurred, showed invasion of the lachrymal caruncle. It was treated and cured by radiotherapy, and followed up for seven years without recurrence. The other two were again treated by cryosurgery and showed no evidence of disease after 5 and 6 years.

In cases where the punctum of the lachrymal drainage system was frozen, occlusion did not occur. Bullock et al. (18) and Liu et al. (32) carried out clinical and experimental work that proved that the lachrymal drainage ducts and canaliculi are not easily occluded by freezing, which, in contrast, happens frequently with conventional surgery. This is a real advantage for cryosurgical treatment of cancers of the inner part of the lower eyelid edge.

The advantages of cryosurgery over conventional surgery in the management of eyelid cancer have long been established (17–28). However, experienced cryosurgeons are well aware of the fact that when treating eyelid tumors greater than 10 mm, less acceptable cosmetic results are to be expected. We consider it highly improbable to treat such lesions, with diameters between 11 mm and 13 mm, by conventional cryosurgical methods, without some degree of retraction, and between 14 mm and 35 mm without lagophthalmos. Fractional cryosurgery prevents these adverse effects.

A point that should be stressed is that, with this fractional technique, the final scar bears no relation to the size of the original tumor, but does, in fact, correspond to the size of the lesion preceding the final procedure. Most scars are imperceptible and the cosmetic results are much superior to those obtained by plastic surgery.

The advantage of both segmental and fractional cryosurgery is that they permit the scope of cryosurgery to be enlarged and provide the possibility of treating larger cancers at the out-patient clinic, with less risk and at lower cost. Another important advantage is the possibility of treating high risk patients for whom there is no other adequate alternative.

References

1. Cahan WG. Cryosurgery of malignant and benign tumors. Fed Proc 1965; 24 (Suppl 15): 241–248.
2. Zacarian SA. Cryosurgery for cancer of the skin. In: Cryosurgery for Skin Cancer and Cutaneous Disorders. Zacarian AS (Ed). St Louis: CV Mosby Co. 1985; 96–162.
3. Kuflik EG. Debulking large tumors. J Dermatol Surg Oncol 1982; 8: 431–433.
4. Kuflik EG. Debulking the lesion before cryosurgery. J Dermatol Surg Oncol 1986; 13: 235–236.
5. Lubritz RR. Cryosurgical approach to benign and precancerous tumors of the skin. In: Cryosurgery for Skin Cancer and Cutaneous Disorders. Zacarian SA (Ed). St Louis: CV Mosby Co. 1985; 41–58.
6. Castro-Ron G. Cryosurgery of angiomas and birth defects. In: Cryosurgery for Skin Cancer and Cutaneous Disorders. Zacarian SA (Ed). St Louis: CV Mosby Co. 1985; 77–90.
7. Graham GF. Cryosurgery for acne. In: Cryosurgery for Skin Cancer and Cutaneous Disorders. Zacarian SA (Ed). St Louis: CV Mosby Co. 1985; 59–76.
8. Gage AA. Cryosurgery for difficult problems in cutaneous cancer. Cutis 1975; 16: 465–470.
9. Spiller WF, Spiller RF. Treatment of basal-cell carcinomas by a combination of curettage and cryosurgery. J Dermatol Surg Oncol 1977; 3: 443–447.
10. Spiller WF, Spiller RF. Cryosurgery and adjuvant surgical techniques for cutaneous carcinomas. In: Cryosurgery for Skin Cancer and Cutaneous Disorders. Zacarian SA (Ed). St Louis: CV Mosby Co. 1985; 187–198.
11. Albright SD III. Case report: Prolonged cure of extensive primary and recurrent cancers of the skin by aggressive cryosurgery. J Dermatol Surg Oncol 1983; 9: 231–234.
12. Kuflik EG. Segmental cryosurgical treatment. J Dermatol Surg Oncol 1987; 13: 235–236.
13. Kuflik EG, Gage AA: Segmental treatment. In: Cryosurgical Treatment for Skin Cancer. Chap 7, Kuflik EG, Gage AA (Eds) New York/Tokyo: Igaku-Shoin, 1990; 107–108.
14. Zacarian SA. Cryosurgery of lentigo maligna. In: Cryosurgery for Skin Cancer and Cutaneous Disorders. Zacarian SA (Ed). St Louis: CV Mosby Co. 1985; 199–214.
15. Graham GF, Stewart R. Cryosurgery for unusual cutaneous neoplasms. J Dermatol Surg Oncol 1977; 3: 437–442.
16. Cohen LM. Lentigo maligna and lentigo maligna melanoma. J Am Acad Dermatol. 1995; 33: 923–933.
17. Gonçalves JCA. Fractional cryosurgery – A new technique for basal cell carcinoma of the eyelids and periorbital area. Dermatol Surg 1997; 23: 475–481.
18. Bullock JD, Beard C, Sullivan JH. Cryotherapy of basal cell carcinoma in oculoplastic surgery. Am J Ophthalmol 1976; 82: 841–847.
19. Biro L, Price E, Brand A. Basal cell carcinomas on eyelids: Experience with cryosurgery. J Dermatol Surg Oncol 1979; 5: 397–401.
20. Biro L, Price E, Brand A. Cryosurgery for basal cell carcinoma of the eyelids and nose: Five-year experience. J Am Acad Dermatol 1982; 6: 1042–1047.
21. Biro, L, Price, E. Cryosurgical management of basal cell carcinoma of the eyelids: A 10-year experience. J Am Acad Dermatol 1990; 23: 316–317.
22. Fraunfelder FT, Zacarian SA, Wingfield DL. Results of cryotherapy for eyelid malignancies. Am J Ophthalmol 1984; 97: 184–188.
23. Fraunfelder FT. Cryosurgery of eyelid: Conjunctival and intraocular tumors. In: Cryosurgery for Skin Cancer and Cutaneous Disorders. Zacarian SA (Ed). St Louis: CV Mosby Co. 1985; 259–273.
24. Kuflik EG. Cryosurgery for basal cell carcinoma on and around the eyelids. J Dermatol Surg Oncol 1978; 9: 911–913.
25. Kuflik EG. Two primary basal cell carcinomas on an eyelid. J Dermatol Surg Oncol 1983; 9: 439–441.
26. Kuflik EG. Cryosurgery for carcinoma of the eyelids: A twelve year expedience. J Dermatol Surg Oncol 1985; 11: 243–246.
27. Kuflik EG, Gage AA. Treatment of eyelid Lesions. In: Cryosurgical Treatment for Skin Cancer, New York/Tokyo: Igaku-Shoin. 1990; 189–200.
28. Caujolle JP, Clevy JP, et al. la cryochirurgie dans le traitement des épithéliomes baso-cellulaires des paupières. J Freeze Ophtalmol, 1989; 9: 231–4.
29. Kuflik EG, Webb W. Effects of systemic corticosteroids on post-cryosurgical edema and other manifestations of the inflammatory response. J Dermatol Surg Oncol 1985; 11: 464–468.
30. Elton RF. Epilogue. In: Cryosurgery for Skin Cancer and Cutaneous Disorders. Zacarian AS (ED). St Louis: CV Mosby Co. 1985; 313–22.
31. Graham GF. Statistical analysis in cryosurgery of skin cancer. Clinics in Dermatology. Advances in Dermatology. Breitbart EW, Elzbièta Dachow-Siwiéc (Eds). New York/Amsterdam/London. Elsevier. 1990; 101–7.
32. Liu D, Natiella J, Schafer A et al. Cryosurgical treatment of the eyelids and lacrimal drainage ducts of the rhesus monkey: course of injury and repair (letter). Arch Ophthalmol 1984; 102: 934–9.

7.3 Cryosurgery for Epithelial Skin Cancers

Peter Nordin

7.3.0 Introduction

Already in the middle of the nineteenth century Arnott (1851) made use of refrigeration in the treatment of malignant tumors. He employed a mixture of ice and saline, which provided temperatures of −24°C. White (1901) was the pioneer in using an extremely cold refrigerant – liquid air. Whitehouse (1907) presented a liquid air spray method, which was, however, difficult to use in practice. At the same time carbon dioxide (carbonic acid) snow (−79°C) was introduced. After 1945 liquid nitrogen (−196°C) became increasingly popular. Only the cotton-wool swab method was used until the 1960's, but it was suitable only for treating superficial benign lesions. In 1963 Cooper described a unit in which liquid nitrogen circulated through a metal probe, which was used mainly for different internal tumors. At the same time pressurized liquid nitrogen spray machines were developed (Zacharian). In the cryosurgical treatment of skin cancer today the most commonly used equipment is a small hand-held liquid nitrogen spray/probe unit. Liquid nitrogen with a boiling point at −196°C is the most reliable refrigerant as it gives consistent cell destruction.

In the choice of treatment for a skin cancer there are different therapeutic possibilities, of which cryosurgery is only one. It is always important to choose the most convenient and safe treatment.

In order to facilitate the choice of therapy of a cutaneous malignancy there are today in many countries *skin tumor clinics* served by a dermatologist and a surgeon or another operating specialist. This collaboration is often very productive, leading to a balanced judgement.

A small tumor can be easily excised but in other malignancies one would consider other treatments, such as curettage-electrodesiccation, radiotherapy, photodynamic therapy, or Mohs' micrographic surgery (MMS). When adequate equipment and proper technique are used, cryosurgery is an efficacious and cost effective therapy of selected skin cancers. However, it has to be emphasised that treatment of malignant lesions with cryosurgery requires an experienced physician.

7.3.1 Cryobiology

The effect of low temperature on living tissue depends on different factors: the rate of temperature fall and rewarming, the solute concentrations, the length of time the cells are exposed to a temperature in the 0°C to −50°C range, and the coldest temperature reached in the target tissue. Rapid cooling, which produces intracellular ice formation, is desired. Slow cooling merely produces extracellular ice formation, which is not sufficiently damaging to the tissue in cancer therapy. Slow thawing with an increased concentration of electrolytes and recrystallization is also damaging to the cells. Vascular stasis and finally failure of the microcirculation contribute to the cell damage.

A double freeze-thaw cycle further increases the tissue destruction. Cellular elements are more sensitive to cold than stromal components, such as connective tissue, cartilage and bone. Melanocytes are more susceptible than keratinocytes and their destruction can lead to depigmentation.

In the cryosurgical treatment of epithelial skin cancers, it has been shown that a temperature of −50°C is required to freeze the skin completely. Earlier, −20°C was often used as a target but this temperature proved to be inadequate.

7.3.2 Equipment

As mentioned before, liquid nitrogen is the only effective cryogen in the cryosurgical treatment of malignant tumors. Moreover it is inexpensive, easily available and versatile, and it is the coldest.

In routine clinical practice liquid nitrogen spray equipment has become the most frequently used device. The most popular units are small hand-held, metal or plastic vacuum flasks with four spray tips, diameters ranging from 0.375–1 mm (labelled A, B, C and D). Spray tips B and C are most commonly used. (The author always uses nozzle B.) Additional equipment used in cryosurgery includes cryoprobes, spray-limiting cones of various size, protective items, temperature monitoring devices, stop-watches, curettes of different size, scissors, punch, scalpel or razor blade, electro-surgical unit, local anesthetic and hemostatic agents (50 percent iron chloride solution). The equipment used by the author is shown in Fig. 7.3.1.

7.3.3 Techniques of Cryosurgery

The aim when treating a malignant skin tumor must be that the first treatment should be the last one, irrespective of therapeutic method used. In order to accomplish this with cryosurgery the tumor has to be frozen sufficiently so that no malignant cells persist.

During the first decades of modern cryosurgery (1960–1970), the goal was a tissue temperature of −20°C to −25°C at the base of the tumor. However, during recent decades there has been a trend towards a more aggressive treatment with lower temperatures in the range from −40°C to −60°C, and a greater use of debulking techniques. To achieve adequate depth of cryonecrosis in malignancies, at least in high risk areas, one should carry out a double, sometimes even triple, freeze-thaw cycle. The freezing time depends on the technique used. With a spray freezing intermittently, about 60 seconds are needed, with the spot freeze method about 30 seconds, and after a careful curettage an even shorter freeze time will be

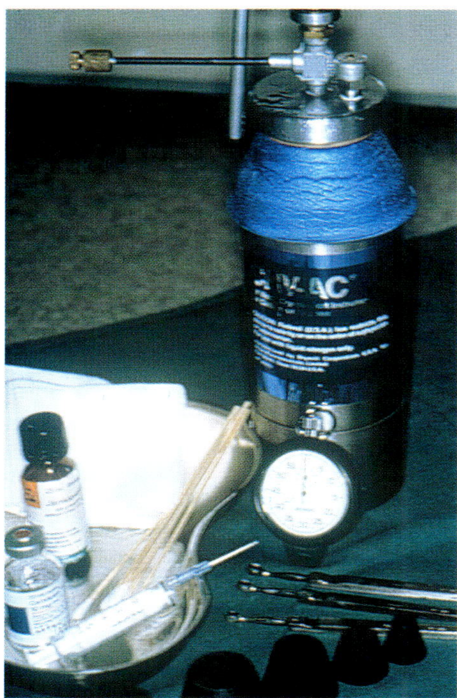

Fig. 7.3.1. The cryosurgical equipment employed by the author

adequate for a 1 cm lesion. The freeze time will increase for a larger tumor. In a malignancy larger than 2 cm the freezing may be divided and applied in sections of the tumor.

Some cryosurgeons employ thermocouples in order to register the exact temperature (−50°C to −60°C) at the base of the tumor. 28- to 30-gauge needles are inserted into the skin so that the tip lies beneath or lateral to the tumor and the temperature can be monitored at this spot. In larger lesions more than one thermocouple is needed. Some minor error is inherent in the temperature recording system, but the equipment is sufficiently accurate for cryosurgical purposes. Temperature measuring is especially useful for deeper tumors and those in critical locations. It is especially valuable for the inexperienced cryosurgeon and when the technique is being taught.

Many cryosurgeons do not measure the temperature because an interrelationship exists between the freeze time, the lateral spread of freeze and tissue temperature, and the adequacy of treatment is based on these. Ideally a special cryosurgery chart could be used (Fig. 7.3.2) with registration of total freeze time, lateral spread of freeze (should be >5 mm), halo thaw time (should be >60 seconds) and total thaw time.

Local anesthesia is rarely used in the cryosurgical treatment of superficial lesions, but in deeper and larger tumors it is often used prior to cryosurgery.

Protection in the freezing of vital organs is often needed. Particularly the eyes have to be protected, and a plastic retractor (Jaeger) or a tongue blade is often sufficient. In the ear canal and in the nostrils soft cotton is appropriate.

When performed properly the different techniques have shown excellent 5-year cure rates of 97–98% (Kuflik, Zacarian, Graham, Holt, Nordin).

Zacarian, Kuflik and Gage advocate the use of a double freeze-thaw cycle that is often preceded by curettage. Torre and Graham have used both single and double freeze-thaw cycles, alone or in combination with shave excision or curettage. Mallon and Dawber have shown that basal cell carcinomas (BCCs) away from the head and neck respond equally well to a single freeze-thaw cycle. Nordin et al. have used a thorough curettage followed by cryosurgery (CC) in a double freeze-thaw cycle in areas at high risk for recurrence, such as the nose and the external ears, with excellent 5-year results.

7.3.4 Patient and Tumor Selection

Before treatment of a malignant tumor a primary decision must be made concerning the aim of the therapy, namely, cure or palliation. The second decision will be which type of treatment will be the most appropriate in this particular patient. The age and state of health of the patient are important. The histopathological type of the tumor, established by one or more punch biopsies, the size of the lesion, and its location are other factors of importance in the choice of therapy. Therefore a correct choice among therapeutic alternatives is essential.

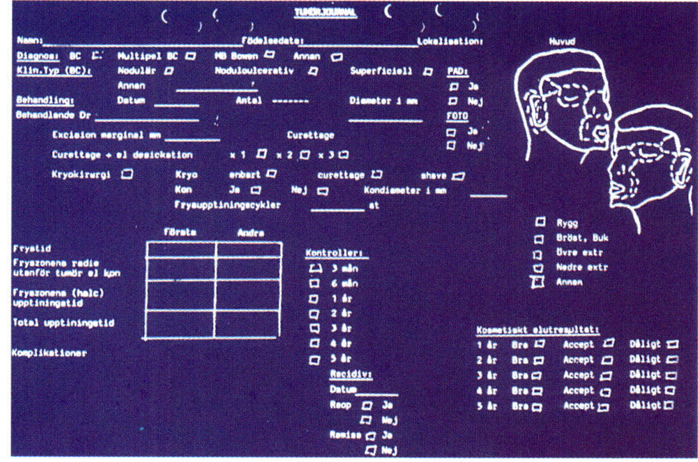

TUMÖRJOURNAL

Namn: Födelsedata: Lokalisation: Huvud

Diagnos: BC Multipel BC MB Bowen Annan

Klin.Typ (BC): Nodulär Noduloulcerativ Superficiell PAD: Ja Nej

Annan

Behandling: Datum Antal Diameter i mm FOTO Ja Nej

Behandlande Dr

Excision marginal mm Curettage

Curettage + el desickation x 1 x 2 x 3

Kryokirurgi Kryo enbart curettage shave

Kon Ja Nej Kondiameter i mm

Frysupptiningscykler st

	Första	Andra
Frystid		
Fryszonens radie utanför tumör el kon		
Fryszonens (halo) upptiningstid		
Total upptiningstid		

Komplikationer

Kontroller: 3 mån, 6 mån, 1 år, 2 år, 3 år, 4 år, 5 år

Recidiv: Datum; Reop Ja Nej; Remiss Ja Nej

Rygg, Bröst, Buk, Övre extr, Nedre extr, Annan

Kosmetiskt slutresultat:

1 år	Bra	Accept	Dåligt
2 år	Bra	Accept	Dåligt
3 år	Bra	Accept	Dåligt
4 år	Bra	Accept	Dåligt
5 år	Bra	Accept	Dåligt

Fig. 7.3.2. A special cryosurgery chart (in Swedish) with registration of total freeze time, lateral spread of freeze, halo thaw time and total thaw time. Type of tumor, and its location and size before and after curettage, is also registered. Dates of treatment, follow-up and recurrence are shown

7.3.5 Indications for Cryosurgery

In general, depending on the cryosurgical technique used, most BCCs – except the morphoeiform types and the recurrent BCCs with secondary sclerosis – are effectively treated with cryosurgery. Many squamous cell carcinomas (SCCs)– especially well-differentiated SCCs arising in actinic keratoses and SCC *in situ* – are also well suited for cryosurgical treatment. Because of high cure rates, very acceptable cosmetic results, and cost effectiveness with this procedure, cryosurgery is the treatment of choice for a wide range of skin cancers. Those tumors overlying cartilage on the nose and ears are often most suitable for cryosurgery, even if they are located in high risk areas. Cartilage is resistant to freezing injury and the architecture of the organ is preserved.

Superficial BCCs, which are often multiple, are ideally treated with an open spray technique in a single freeze-thaw cycle (Fig. 7.3.3) and many tumors can be treated at a single out-patient visit.

In the treatment of a skin cancer on the face, it is important to be aware of two facts: First, and most important, the risk for recurrence in the so called H-zone is about twice that in other locations (Fig. 7.3.4). In this area the tumor may grow with "silent" outgrowths in different tissue planes. Second, the cosmetic result after healing by second intention will be best on concave surfaces (Fig. 7.3.5).

Tumors with a high risk for recurrence are often less suitable for cryosurgery alone. Suggested therapy for these malignancies is set forth in Table 7.3.1. However, for an experienced cryosurgeon even tumors at difficult sites, such as the ear, eyelids and nose, are relatively well suited for cryosurgery.

In many epithelial tumors, recurrent as well as primary, the borders are not seldom clinically ill-definable. This is especially true when a malignancy is located over cartilage or bone, where it may grow radially along the perichondrium or the periostium. In such a case excisional surgery – relying on the visual delineation of the extent of involvement of the tumor – must include a sufficient amount of normal-appearing tissue to ensure tumor-free borders. When available, MMS is the preferred treatment for these tumors.

However, in the primary non-morphoeiform BCCs with ill-definable borders a combination of a careful curettage followed by cryosurgery in a double freeze-thaw cycle could be an alternative. The curettage may reveal lateral and deep extensions of the tumor that were not obvious clinically. The curettage will differentiate "soft" tumors from normal tissue and leave normal dermis, cartilage or bone. The curetted material is preferably sent for histopathological examination. When the tumor area is frozen with a perilesional halo of at least 5 mm, the ice front will extend through most of the

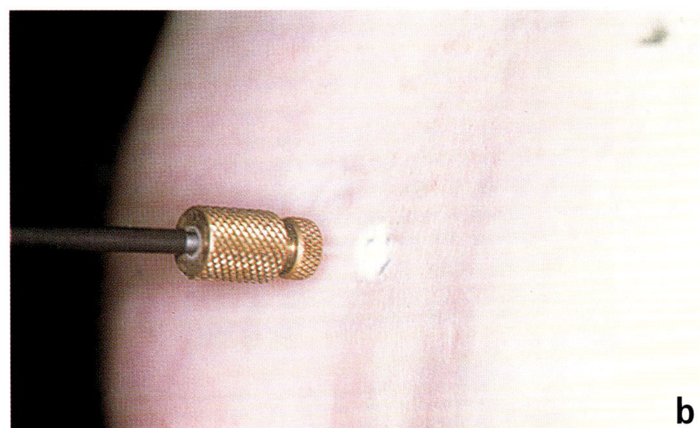

Fig. 7.3.3. An example of a small superficial BCC treated with liquid nitrogen - open spray technique in one freeze-thaw cycle. **a** Before treatment the margins have been marked with ink. **b** Freezing. **c** The result obtained after freezing for 7 seconds with a lateral spread of freeze of about 5 mm

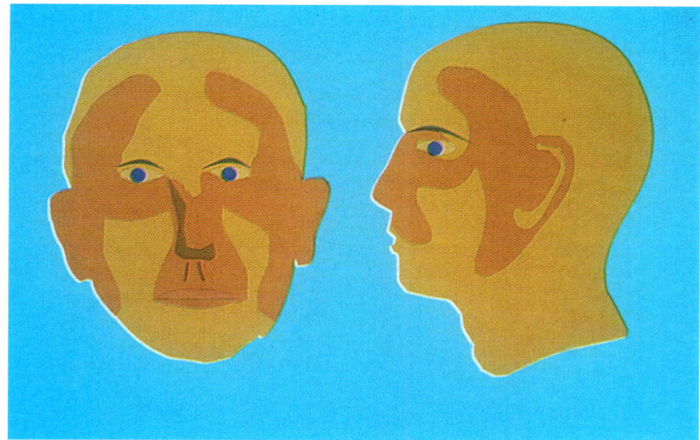

Fig. 7.3.4. The so called H-zone of the face is a high-risk area for recurrence, where the tumor can grow with "silent" outgrowths in different tissue planes

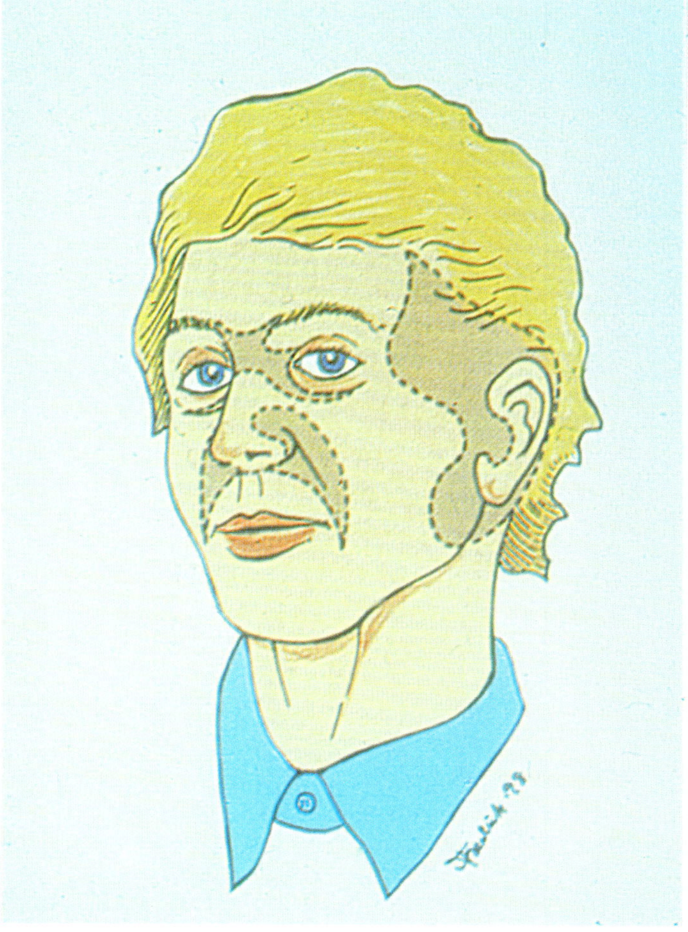

Fig. 7.3.5. The cosmetic result will be better on concave than convex surfaces of the face

tissues, including cartilage and bone. Very rarely a BCC, but sometimes a SCC, invades cartilage or bone. Any remaining tumor outgrowths after the curettage will be erased by the liquid nitrogen without destroying the stromal tissue, such as connective tissue, cartilage or bone (Fig. 7.3.6). This is especially true when the freeze time does not exceed 30 seconds. This makes CC a suitable treatment even for infiltrative and micronodular BCCs. Furthermore, preservation of these tissues is of great importance in the healing process for a good cosmetic result. About a year after CC the scars are hypopigmented but so soft that any recurrence is easily noted. This is in contrast to defects reconstructed by flaps, where recurrences are hard to observe. Some examples of patients with different epithelial skin tumors treated with CC are seen in Figs. 7.3.7–7.3.11.

Cryosurgery for tumors on the lower leg and scalp is followed by a prolonged healing time. It is important to take this fact into account in the choice of therapy. However, cryosurgery is not contraindicated in these locations.

Recurrent (previously treated) tumors have a lower cure rate than primary tumors, irrespective of treatment modality; cryosurgery is no excep-

Table 7.3.1. Suggested treatment of facial epithelial skin cancers with a high risk of recurrence

Tumor type or site	Excisional surgery	Mohs micrographic surgery	Cryosurgery	Curettage-cryosurgery
Morphoeiform BCC	+	++	–	–
Recurrent non-sclerotic BCC	+	++	(+)	+
Recurrent sclerotic BCC	+	++	–	–
Basosquamous cancer	+	++	–	+
BCC with ill-definable borders	(+)	++	–	+
BCC > 2 cm	+	++	–	+
Tumors on nasolabial fold, inner canthus, periauricular area	+	++	–	(+)
Tumors on lips close to lip red	++	++	–	–
Tumors on eye lid	(+)	+	+	+
SCC, moderately or poorly differentiated	+	++	–	–
SCC, well differentiated	++	++	(+)	++

BCC Basal Cell Carcinoma, *SCC* Squamous Cell Carcinoma

tion. However, Kuflik and Gage (1997) have reported excellent results in 54 selected patients with recurrent BCCs. They recommend the use of thermocouples in these tumors.

In the case of palliative therapy of inoperable malignancies, cryosurgery has its place in the therapeutic armamentorium, even if complete destruction is not achieved. Kuflik (1985) has shown that cryosurgery is a useful therapy for "incurable" skin cancers.

Cryosurgery is particularly useful in patients receiving anticoagulants, those allergic to anesthetics, and those with pacemakers.

7.3.6 Contraindications

There are no absolute contraindications for cryosurgery except known cold intolerance. However, many aggressive skin tumors (e.g., morphoeiform and recurrent BCCs) as well as tumors at certain sites are preferably treated with other methods for higher cure rates and better cosmetic results (Table 7.3.1).

7.3.7 Tissue Response and Postoperative Care

After freezing, the tissue responds in a predictable way with erythema, vesiculation, edema, exudation and sloughing, and the wound will heal by second intention. During the exudative stage the wound requires frequent washing with soap and water, and dry gauze dressings are changed 3–5 times daily. The wound will begin to dry up after 5–14 days – depending on tumor size – and an eschar develops. It is allowed to dry and fall off spontaneously, but sometimes its edges have to be lifted with a pair of scissors. Lesions after cancer treatment on the head and neck generally heal after 4 to 6 weeks. Large malignancies and those on the trunk and extremities may require longer healing times, sometimes up to 3 months.

Edema, particularly periorbital, can be ameliorated with wet compresses, a superpotent corticosteroid cream, or a few days' course of systemic corticosteroids.

Systemic antibiotics are rarely needed but may be used prophylactically in patients with certain other diseases.

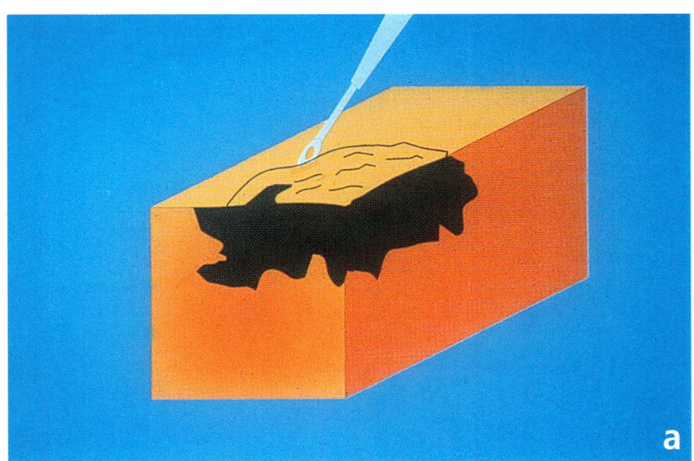

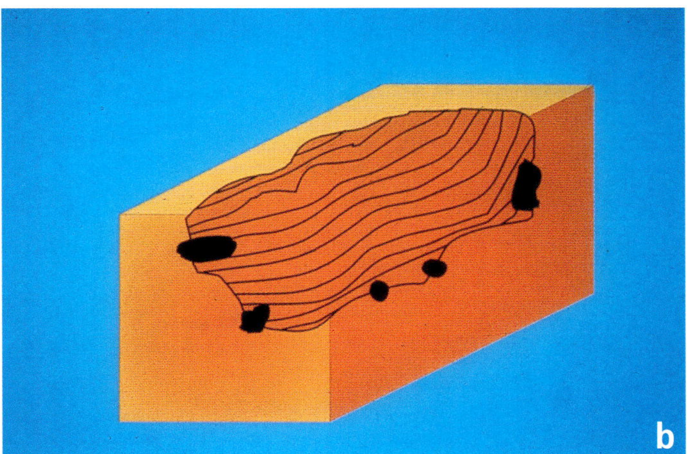

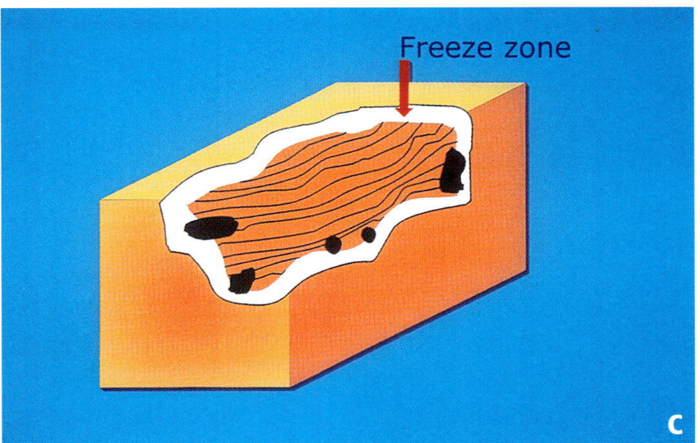

Fig. 7.3.6. A general outline of curettage followed by cryosurgery of a BCC. **a** Curettage. **b** After a careful curettage there are still tumor extensions left behind not reached by the curettes. **c** Freezing with liquid nitrogen with a lateral spread of freeze of about 5 mm in two freeze-thaw cycles provides lethal tissue temperature to eliminate tumor offshoots

7.3.8 Complications

It is important to be aware of and inform the patients about the usual and expected postoperative tissue response. The incidence of complications after cryosurgery is low. They may be classified as temporary and permanent. Pain during and

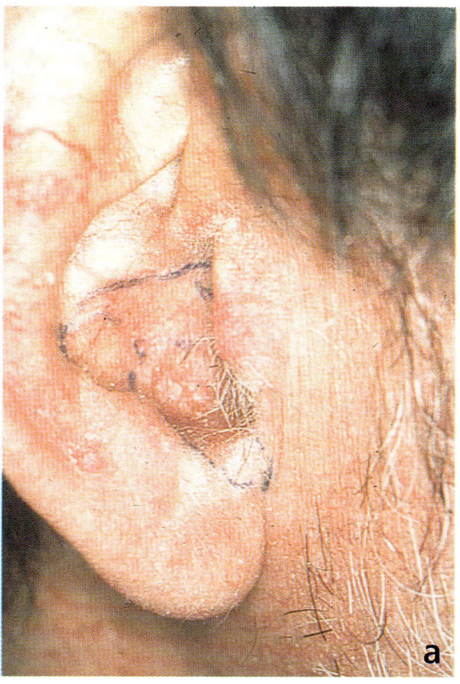

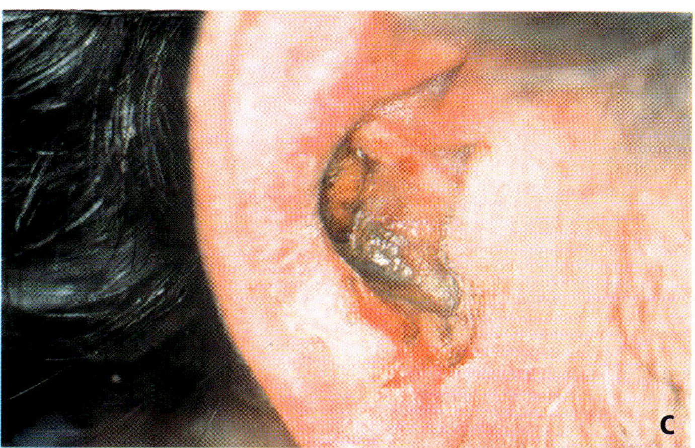

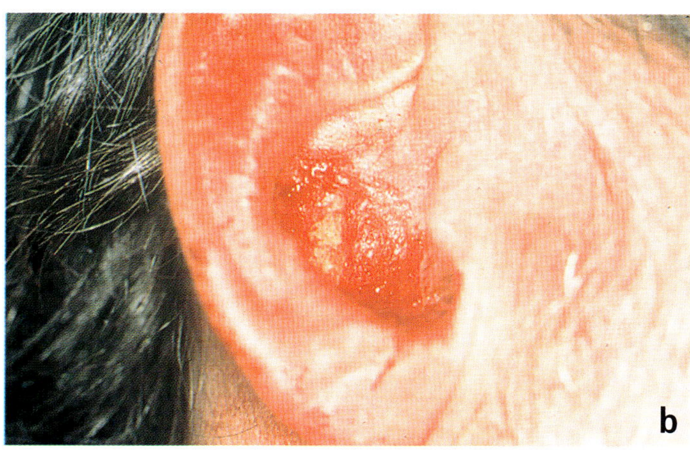

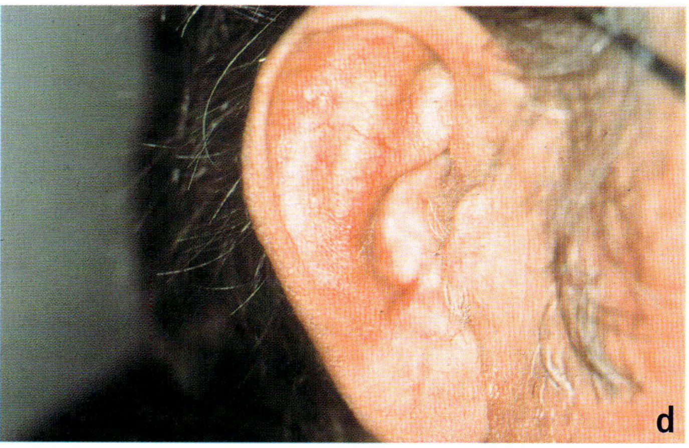

Fig. 7.3.7. Treatment with curettage-cryosurgery of a recurrent - after two incomplete surgical excisions - basal cell carcinoma of the concha of the right ear. **a** Before treatment the estimated diameter was about 10 mm. **b** After a thorough curettage the maximal diameter was 30 mm and in places the tumor grew down to the cartilage, which, however, was not affected. **c** After 2 weeks an oozing wound but no pain. **d** The result obtained after 5 years

immediately after cryosurgery is common. It may be quite intense but it is usually transient. Certain anatomical sites are more likely to produce pain – particularly the distal part of fingers, parts of the ears, lips, temples and the scalp. Edema, especially periorbital, is also very common. The more infrequent temporary complications are seen in Table 7.3.2, and the permanent complications are seen in Table 7.3.3.

7.3.9 Recurrence and Follow-up

The reason for failure to cure a malignancy with cryosurgery may be attributed to poor technique with insufficient treatment. It may also be due to an imperfect assessment of the tumor type and its extension. As mentioned earlier (Table 7.3.1), certain types of skin cancers are unsuitable for treatment by cryosurgery. Recurrences are also more common following treatment of malignancies in certain areas of the face, such as the inner canthus, the nasolabial fold and the periauricular area.

Most recurrences following cryosurgery develop during the first 2 years, but they may appear many years later. Torre has reported a recurrence after 12 years. In the follow-up it is often convenient to examine the patient 1–2 weeks after cryosurgery, then after 3, 6 and 12 months and, when possible, yearly for 5 years or more. At these visits it is also important to look for new skin tumors as about 40 percent of patients treated for a BCC after 5 years have got a new BCC, as shown by Robinson (1987) and others.

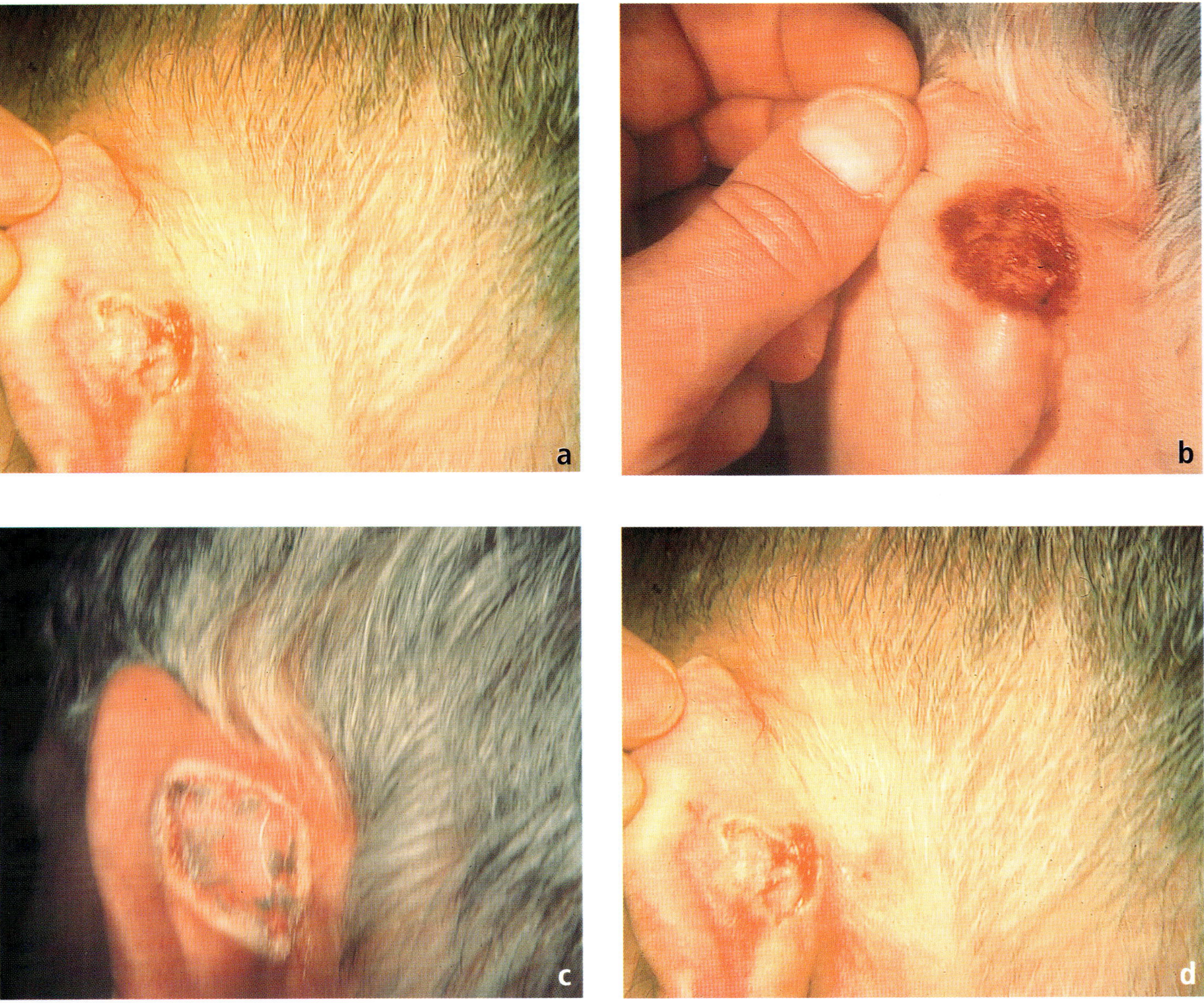

Fig. 7.3.8. Curettage-cryosurgery for an ill-defined ulcerated BCC on the dorsal aspect of the left ear. **a** Before treatment. **b** After a careful curettage with different-sized curettes the extension of the tumor is larger than expected, and also has four deeper cavities reaching the cartilage. **c** The tumor area frozen with liquid nitrogen. **d** The result obtained after 6 years

7.3.10 Results

As briefly mentioned above, cryosurgical treatment – with different techniques – of epithelial skin cancers, mainly BCCs, has given excellent 5-year cure rates of 97–98 percent.

Zacarian (1983) reported a cure rate of 97.3 percent after treatment of 4,228 malignancies, and in 1991 he presented similar results in 5,400 tumors. Kuflik and Gage (1991) presented a series of 3,540 new epithelial skin cancers with a 5-year cure rate of 98.4 percent. Graham (1990) has reported similar excellent results with a cure rate of 98.2 percent after treatment of 3,593 skin tumors. Holt (1988) presented a 5-year cure rate of 97 percent in 279 malignancies. Most of these tumors in the different series were treated with open-spray technique, sometimes preceded by debulking of the cancer. Nordin et al. (1997) used a combination of a careful curettage followed by cryosurgery in the treatment of 61 primary BCCs on the nose and found only one recurrence after 5 years of follow-up. In 1999 Nordin reported similar 5-year results, having used the same technique on epithelial skin cancers of the external ear.

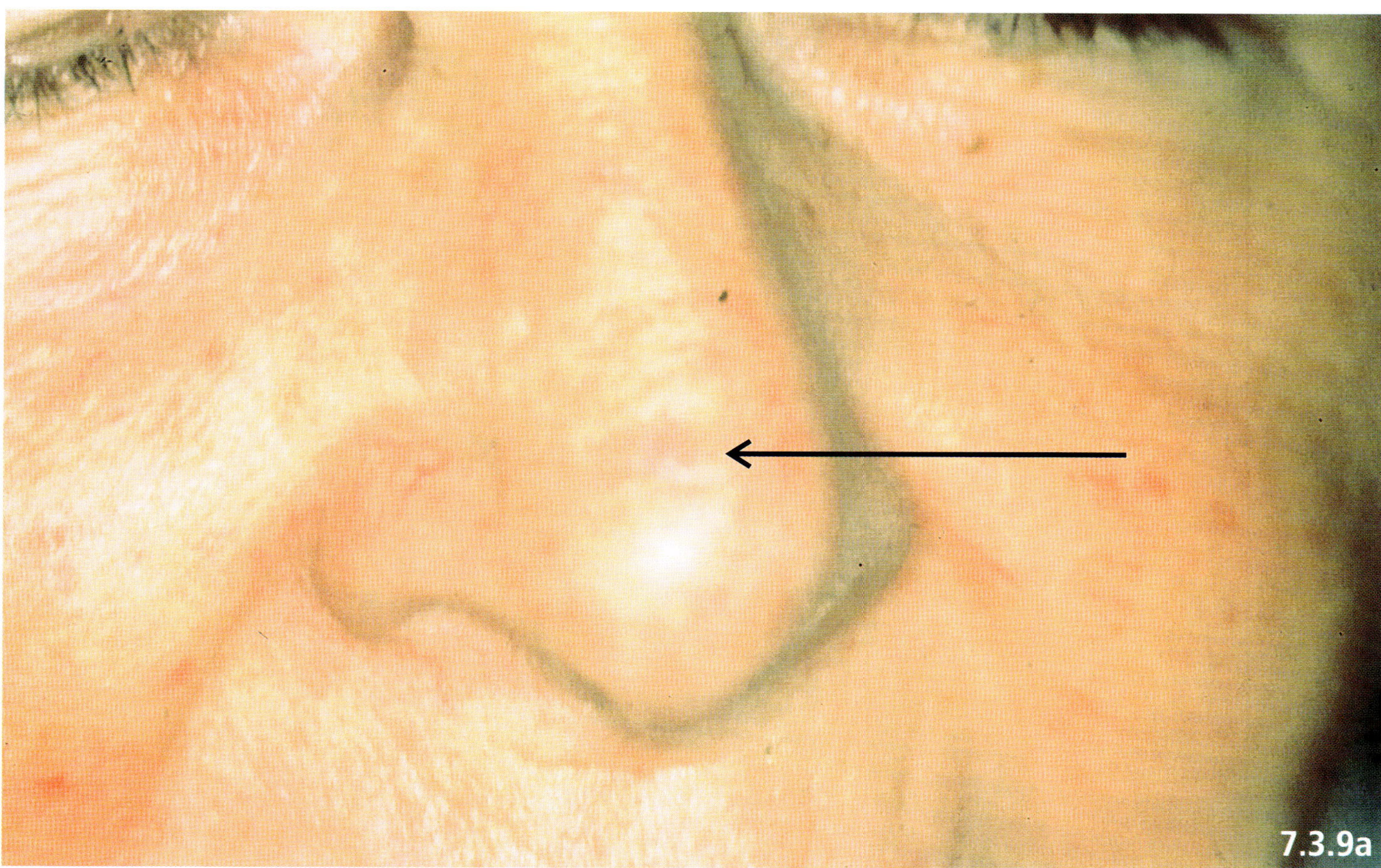

Fig. 7.3.9. Treatment with curettage-cryosurgery of an ill-defined discrete BCC with a diameter of about 10 mm on the bridge of the nose. **a** Before treatment. **b** A meticulous curettage is performed, and the lateral extension of the tumor is found to be much wider than expected. **c** The tumor area frozen with liquid nitrogen with a lateral spread of freeze of about 5 mm. **d** After 1 month there is still a slightly oozing wound but no pain. **e** The result obtained after 5 years

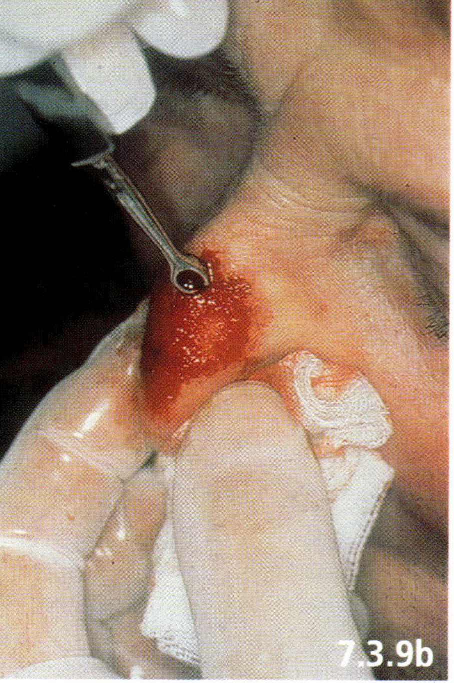

Table 7.3.2. Temporary complications of cryosurgery

Frequent complications
Pain
Edema
Infrequent or rare complications
Headache affecting forehead, temples and scalp
Delayed bleeding
Nitrogen gas insufflation
Infection
Syncope
Febrile reaction
Blister formation
Pyogenic granuloma
Pseudoepitheliomatous hyperplasia
Hyperplastic scarring
Hyperpigmentation
Neuropathy or paresthesia
Cold urticaria
Milia
Bone necrosis and arthralgia – mainly terminal phalanx of interphalangeal joints
Nail dystrophy

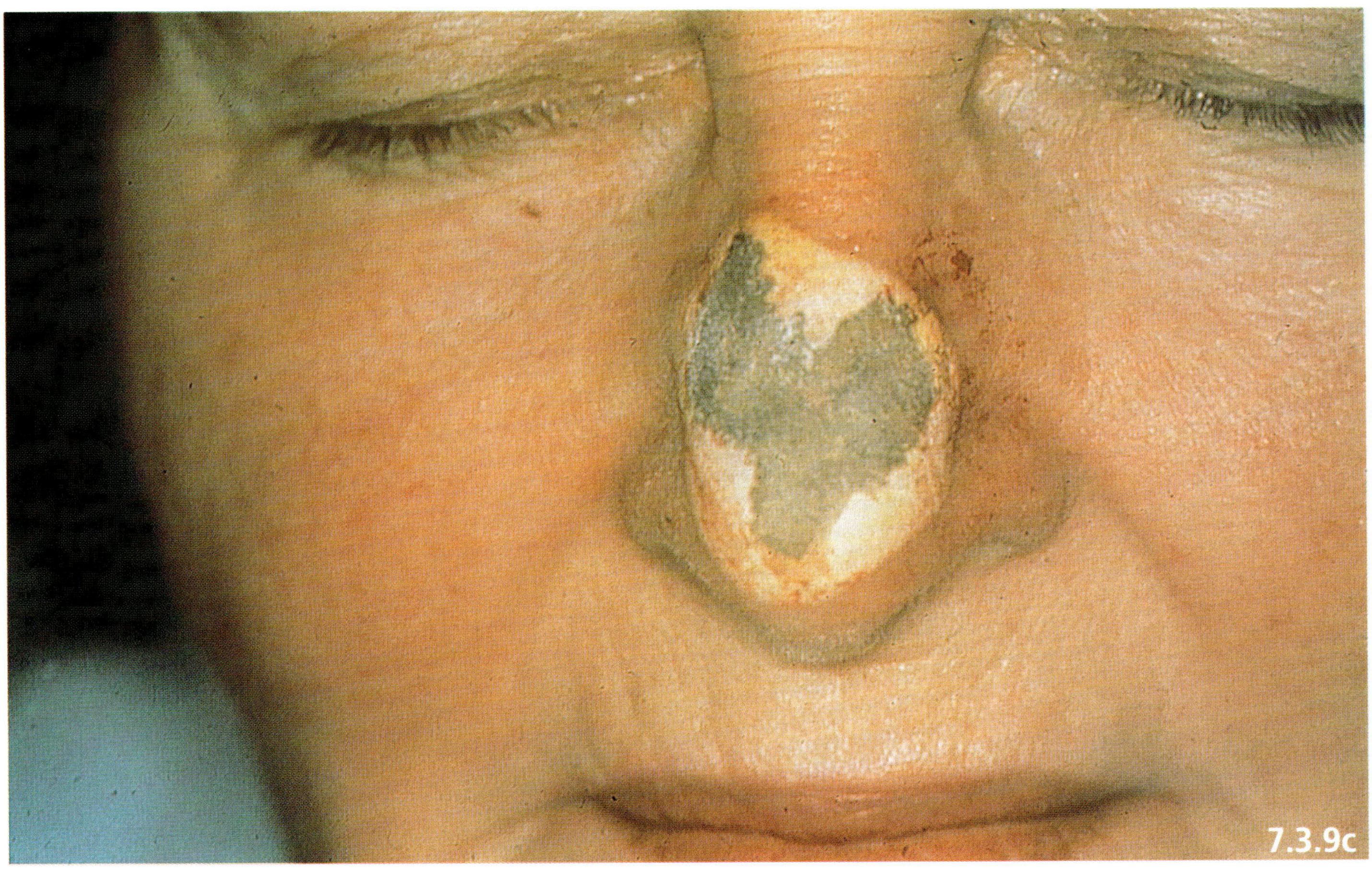

7.3.9c

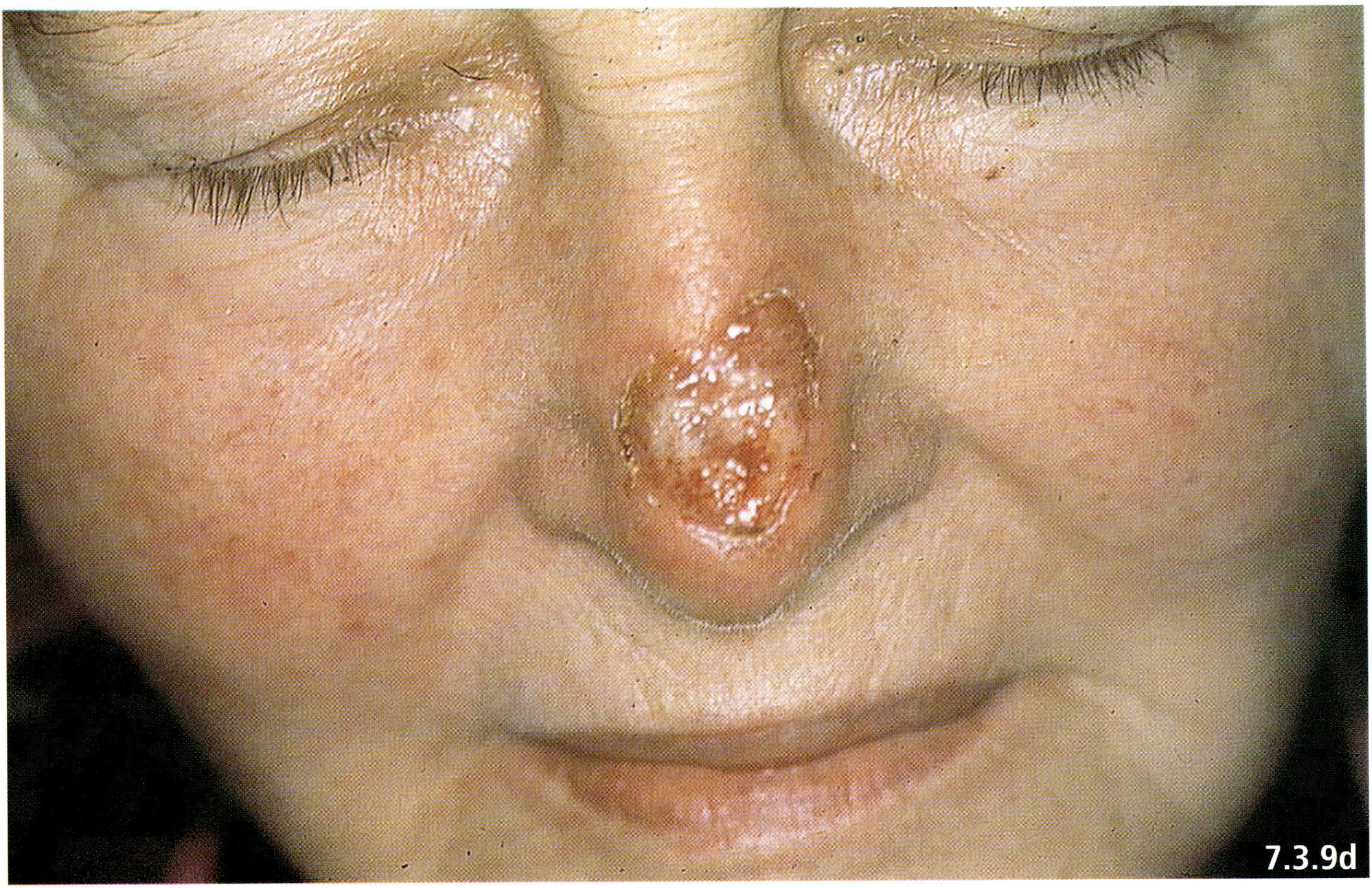

7.3.9d

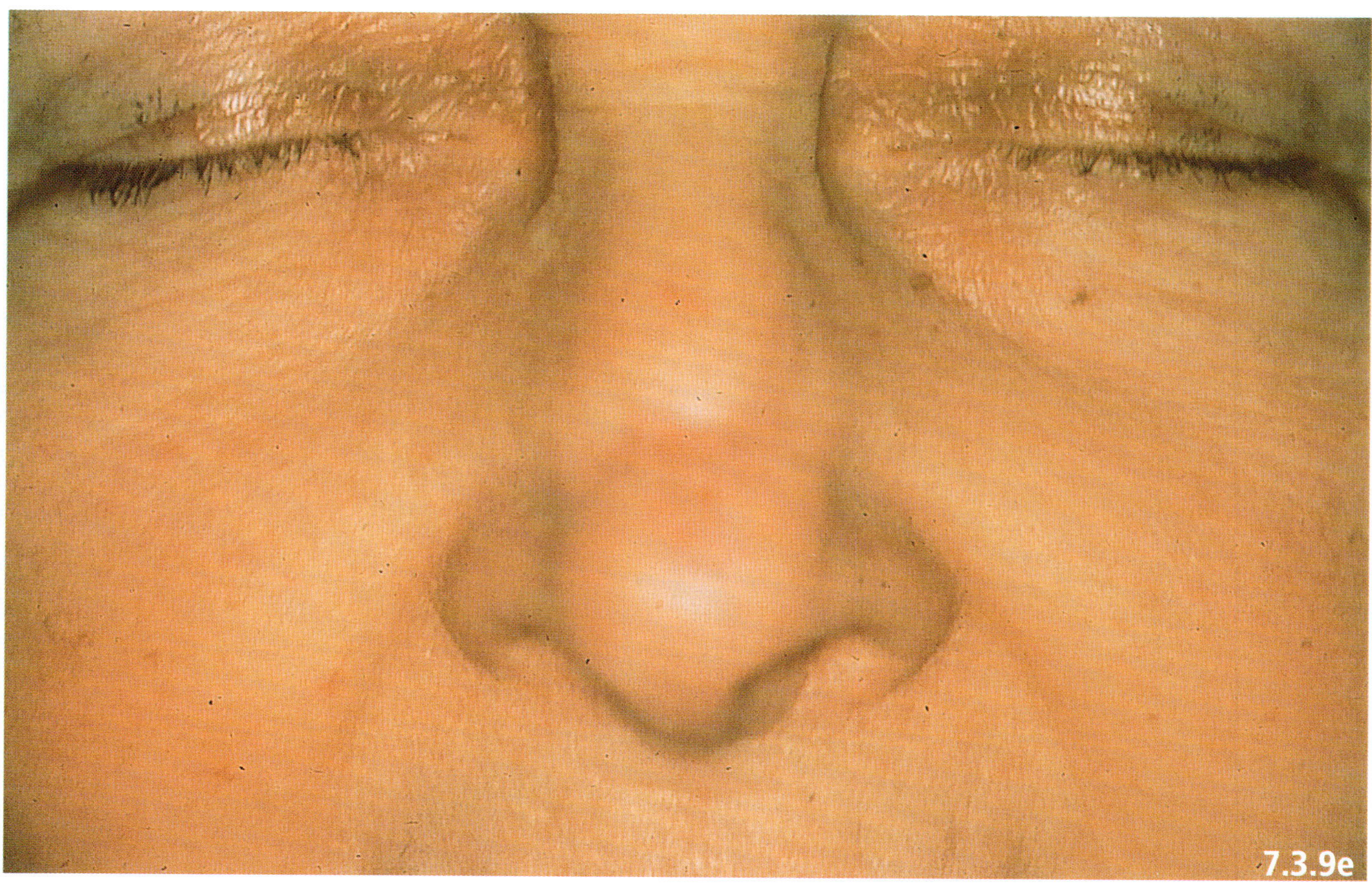

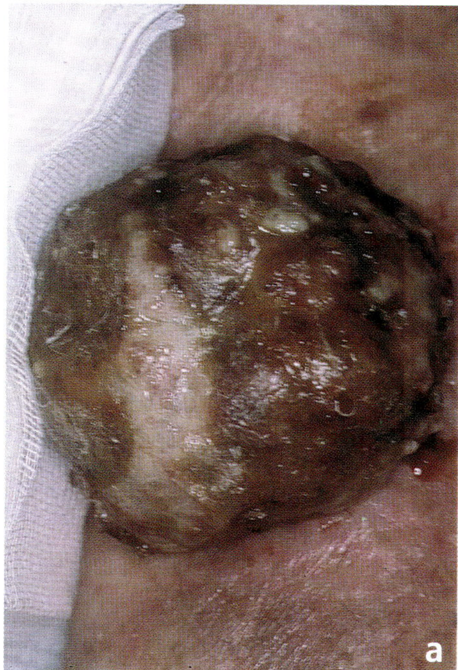

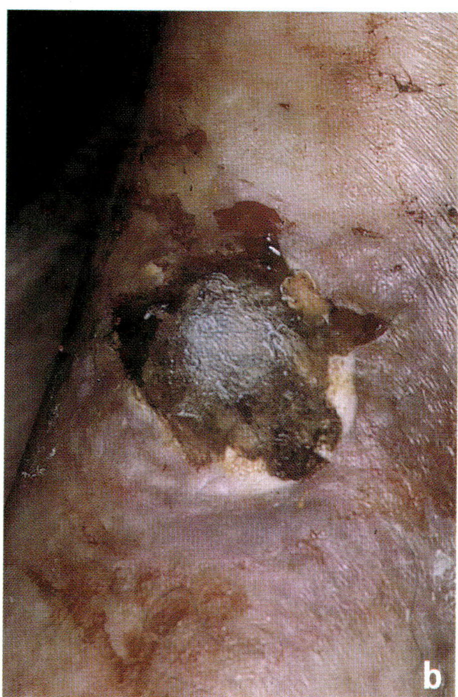

Fig. 7.3.10. Treatment with curettage-cryosurgery of an about 5 cm SCC on the right lower leg of a 90-year old woman, who refused surgery. **a** Before therapy. **b** After a careful curettage and freezing with liquid nitrogen. **c** After 3 weeks a slightly oozing wound. **d** The result obtained after 1 year

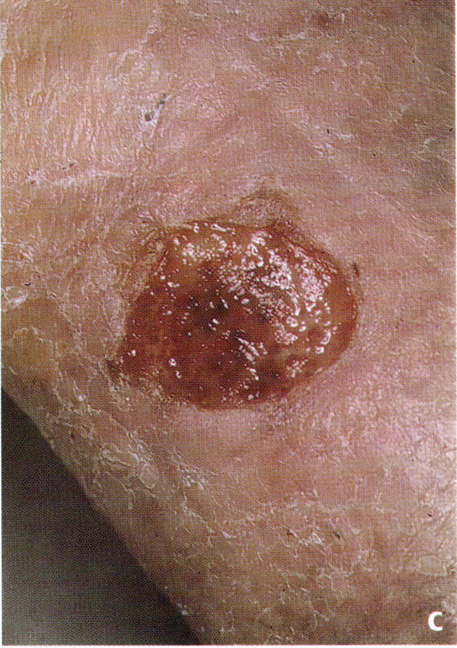

Fig. 7.3.10c

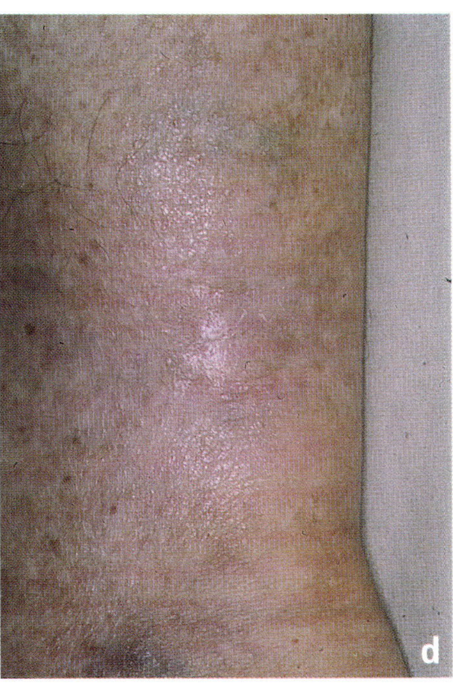

Fig. 7.3.10d

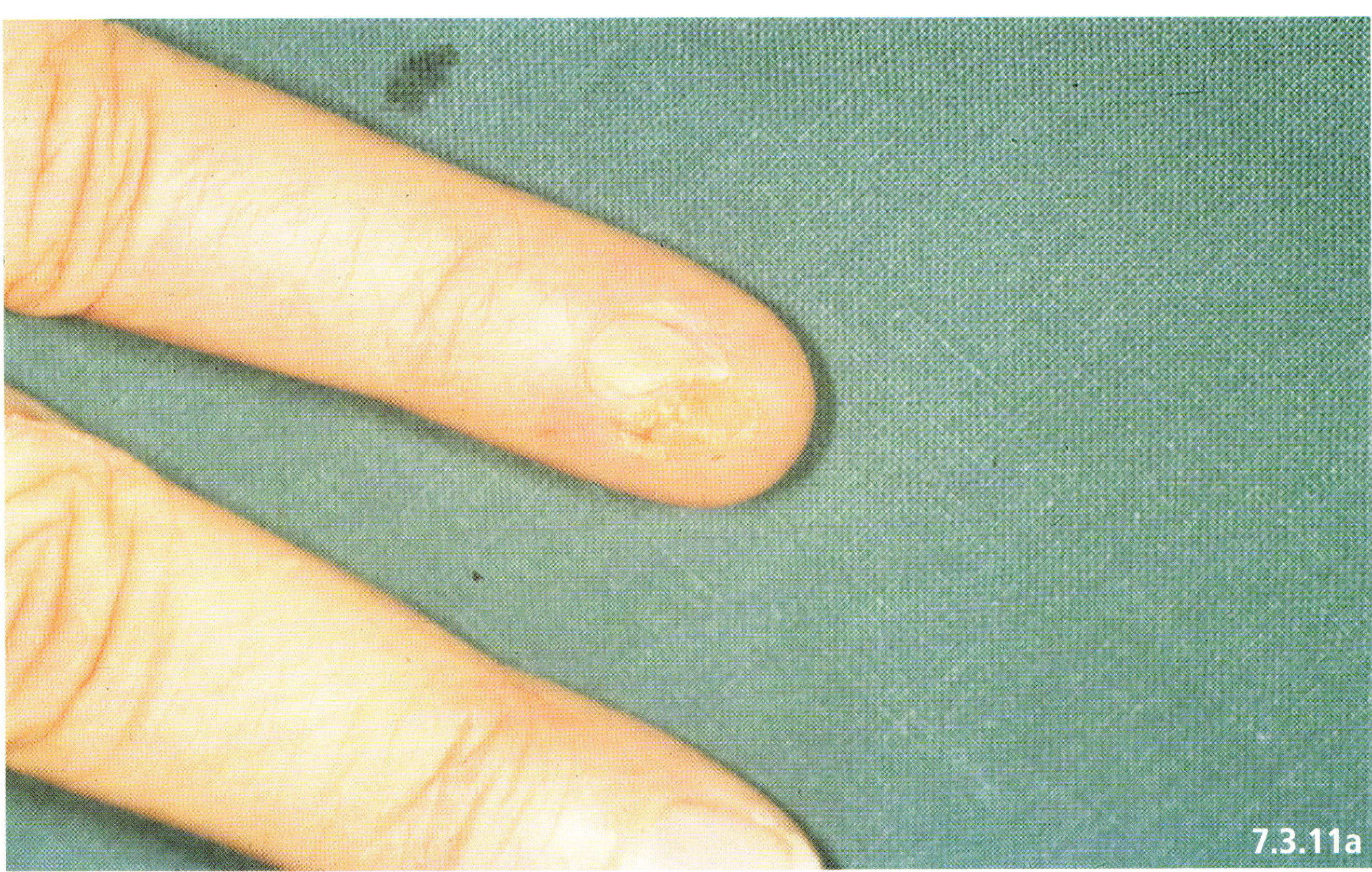

Fig. 7.3.11. Curettage-cryosurgery of a recurrent (incompletely excised) SCC *in situ* (Bowen's disease) on the subungual area of the left ring finger of a female pianist. **a** Before treatment. **b** After a meticulous curettage the tumor was found to occupy all the subungual area. **c** After freezing with liquid nitrogen - open spray method in a double freeze-thaw cycle. **d** The finger after 2 weeks. **e** The result obtained after 6 months, dorsal aspect. **f** Volar aspect

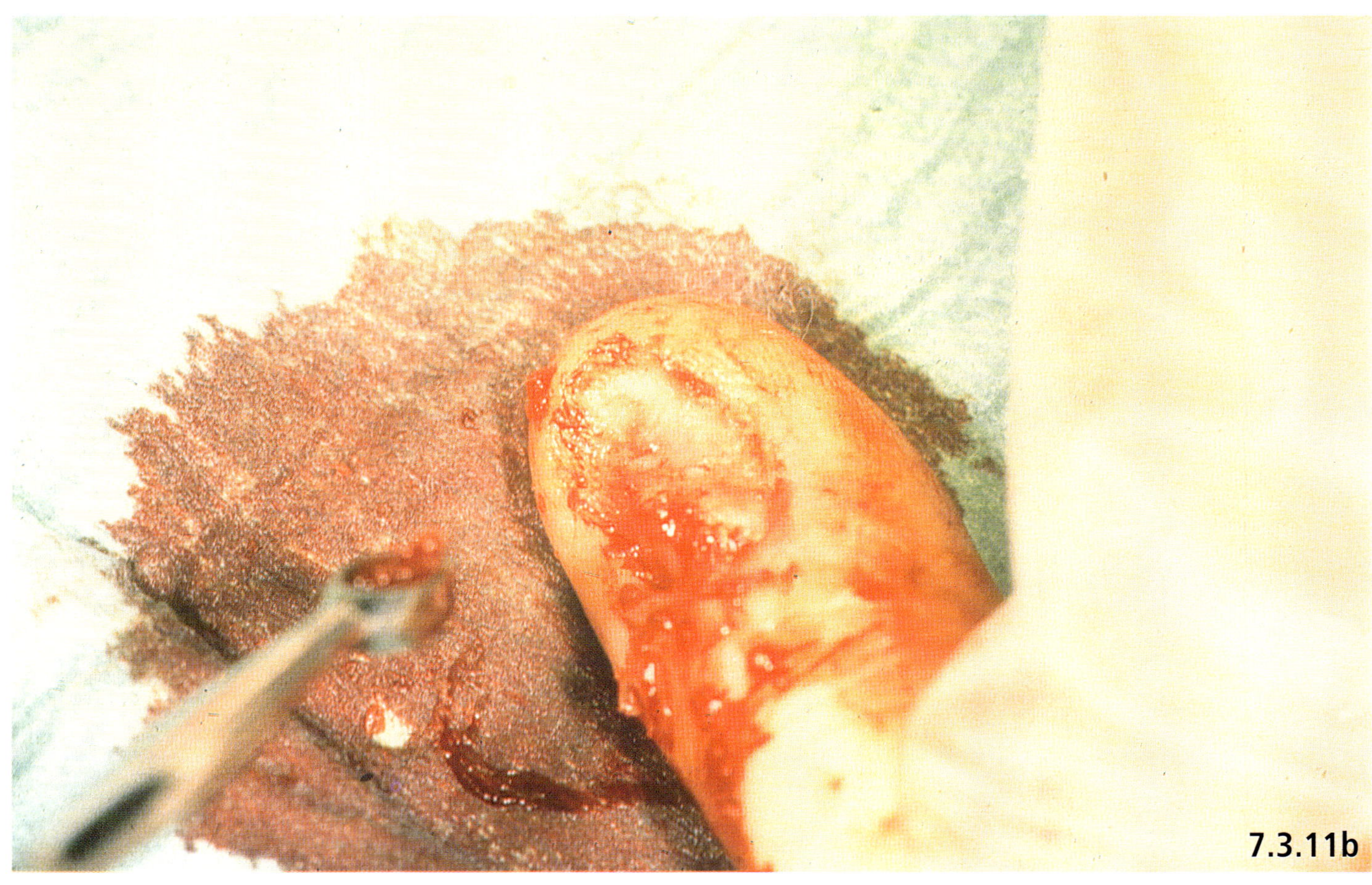
7.3.11b

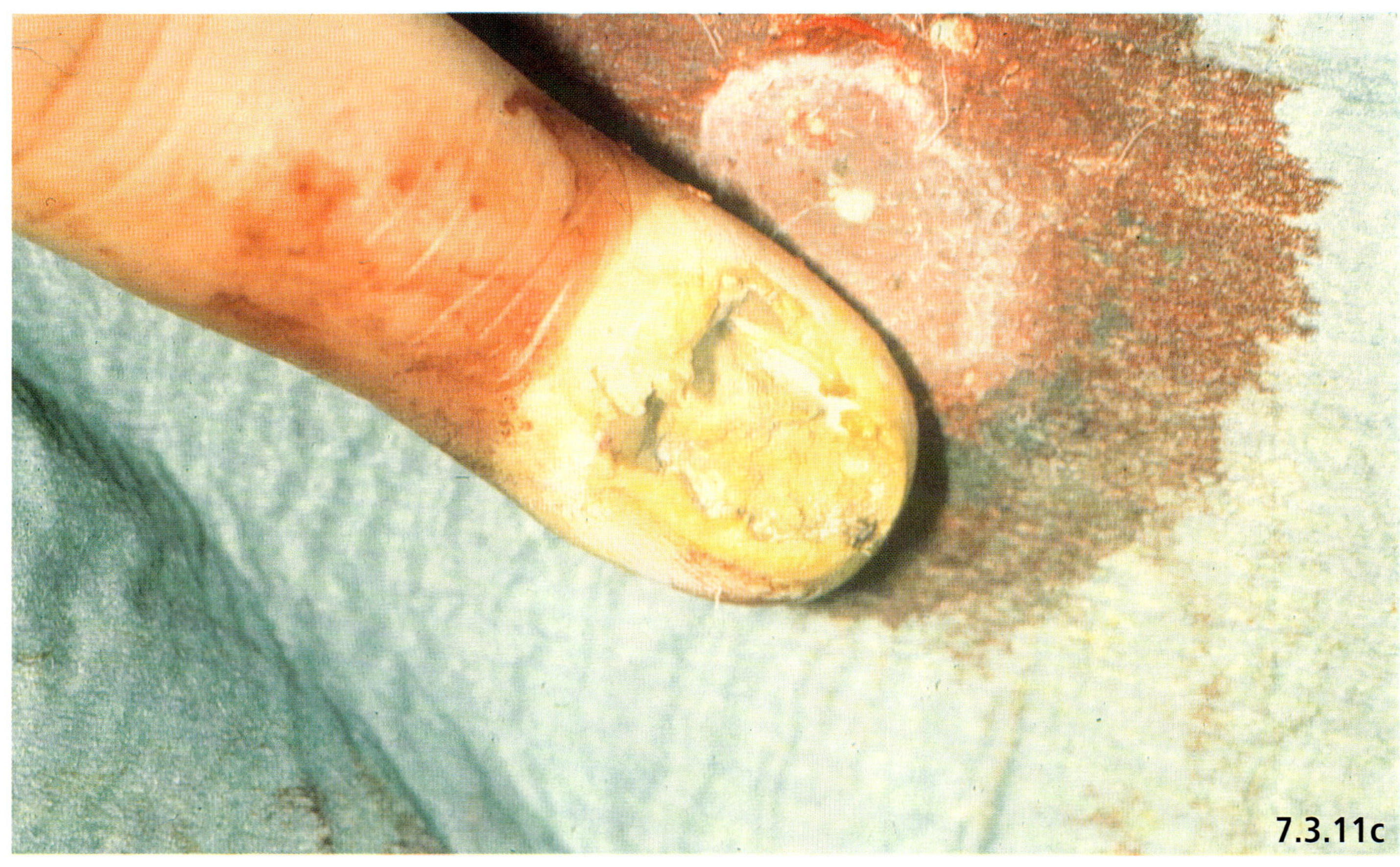
7.3.11c

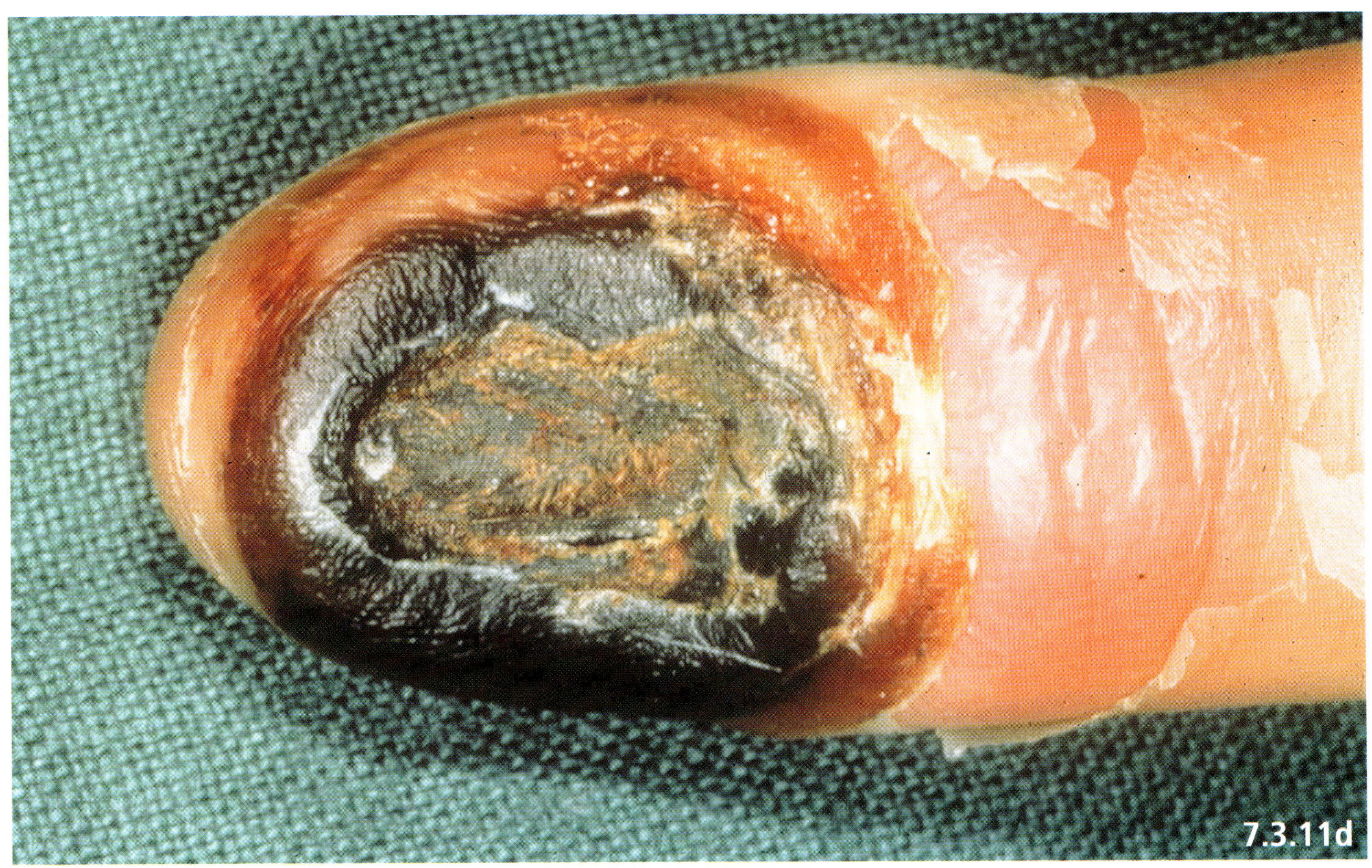
7.3.11d

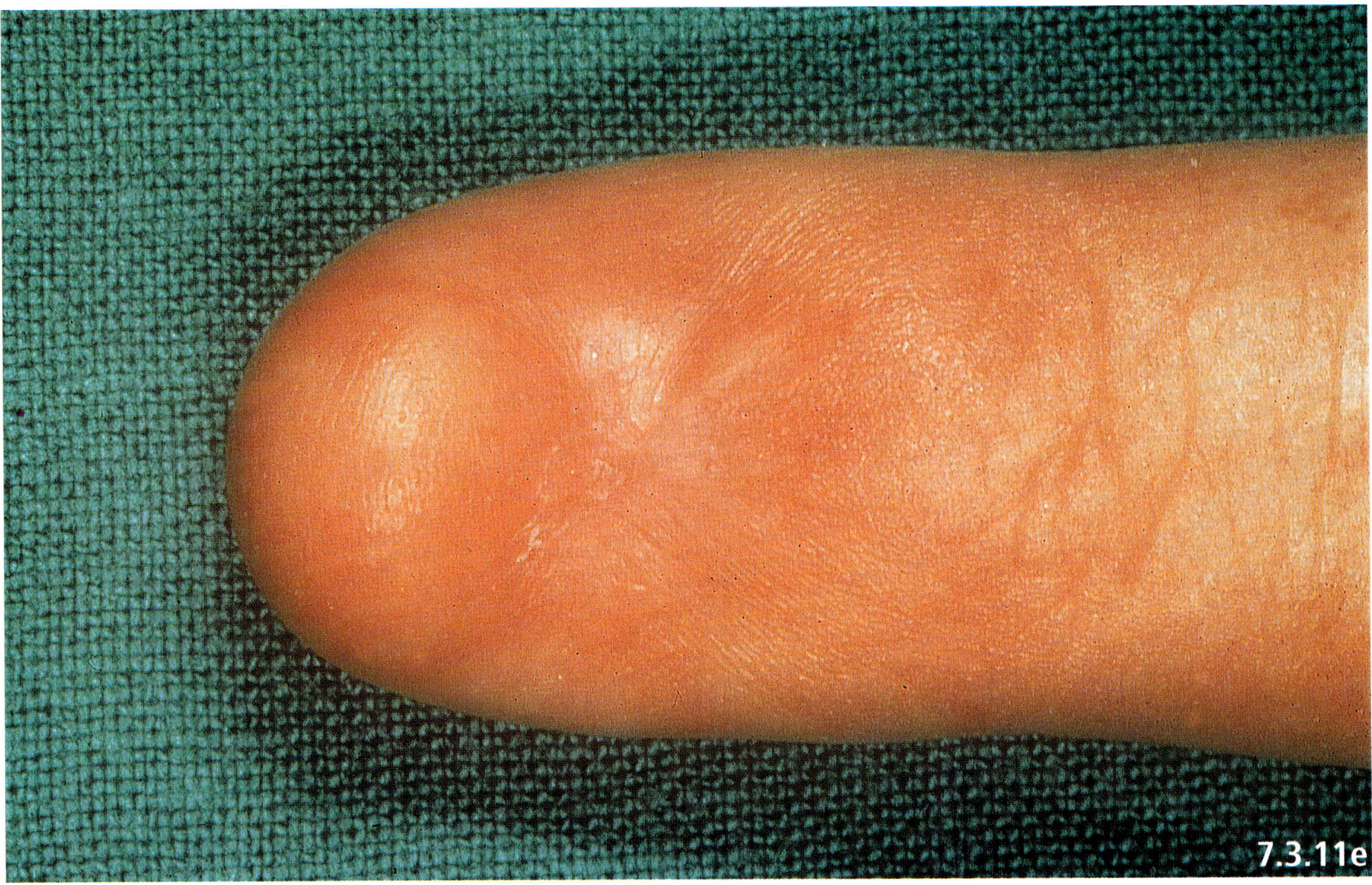
7.3.11e

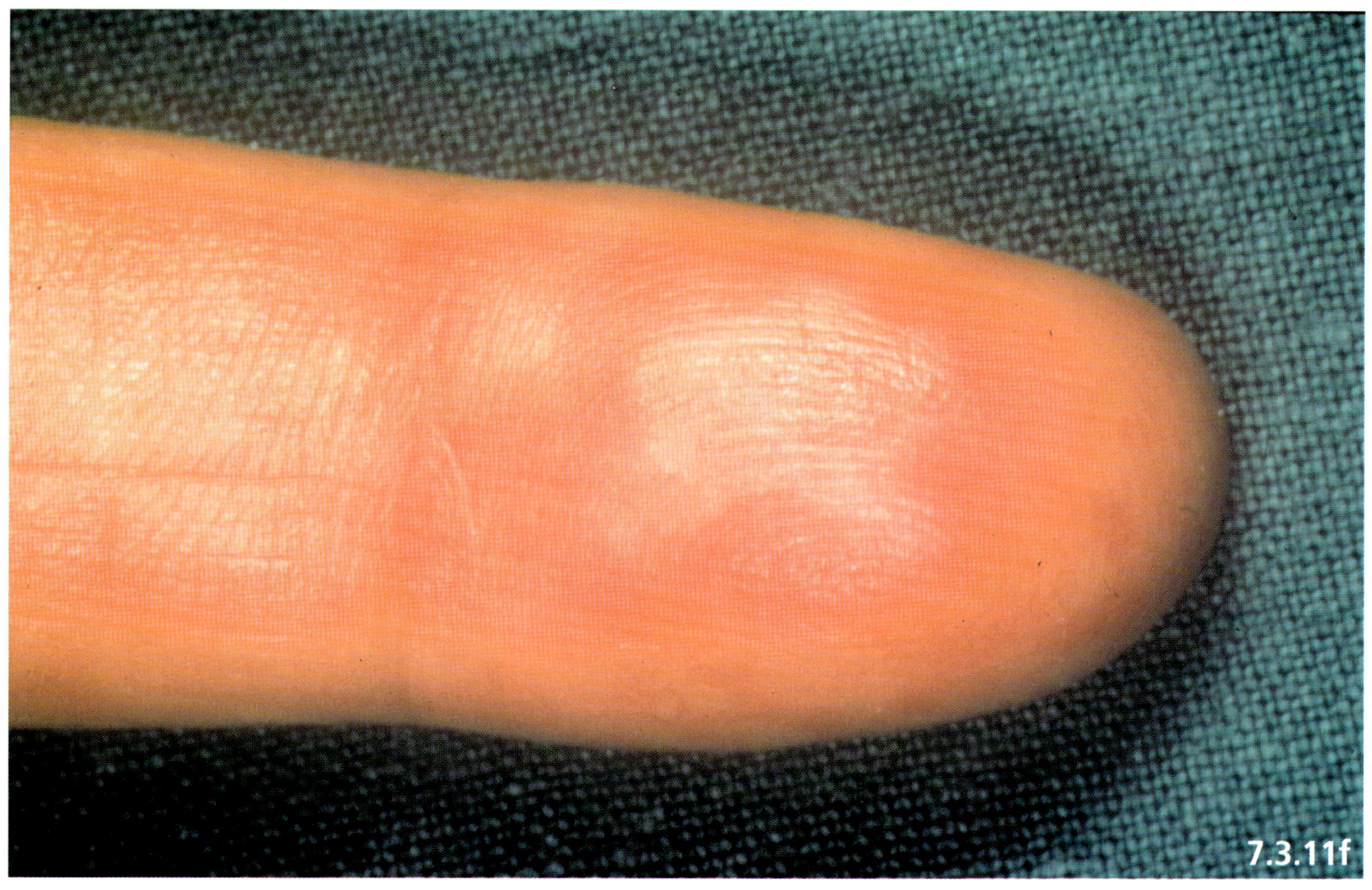

Table 7.3.3. Permanent complications of cryosurgery

Retraction of tissue (lips, eyebrows, ala nasi)
Tissue defects (notching of the ear and ala nasi)
Ulceration
Tendon rupture
Alopecia
Ectropion and notching of eyelids
Hypopigmentation
Scarring

Table 7.3.4. Advantages and disadvantages of cryosurgery, especially in combination with curettage

Disadvantages	Advantages
Lack of histopathological tumor margins	Tissue sparing
Healing by second intention	Not very resource demanding
Weeping wound 1–2 weeks	Cheap
	Quick
	Safe

Cure rates for recurrent tumors are lower. However, Kuflik and Gage (1997) have reported results that compare favorably with other methods in the treatment of selected recurrent BCCs.

7.3.11 Cosmetic results

The scars after cryosurgery are often hyperplastic during the first year but thereafter they are flat but hypopigmented with good or acceptable cosmesis. A recurrence is easily seen in such a scar. In general, the cosmetic result is better on concave than on convex surfaces (Zitelli 1983).

Advantages and *disadvantages* of cryosurgery are seen in Table 7.3.4.

7.3.12 Final comment

In summary, it could be said that cryosurgery, alone or preceded by a careful curettage, is an excellent alternative treatment modality for different epithelial skin tumors. Therefore, cryosurgical equipment should be available in all dermatology departments where there is outpatient treatment of skin cancers. However, it has to be emphasized that tumor selection is important and the treatments must be performed in a thorough and adequate way in order to obtain good results.

Acknowledgements

I am grateful to Mr. Bo Stenquist, Mohs' Surgeon, and Dr. Kjell Hersle, Consultant Dermatologist, for their valuable comments.

References

1. Abide JM. The meaning of surgical margins. Plast Reconstr Surg 1984; 73: 492–496.
2. Albom MJ. Surgical gems, the management of recurrent basal cell carcinoma. Please no graft or flaps at once. J Dermatol Surg Oncol 1977; 3: 382–384.
3. Albright SD. Treatment of skin cancer using multiple modalities. J Am Acad Dermatol 1982; 7: 143–171.
4. Colver GB, Dawber RPR. Cryosurgery – the principles and simple practice. Clin Exp Dermatol 1989; 14: 1–6.
5. Dawber RPR. Cold kills! Clin Exp Dermatol 1988; 13: 137–150.
6. Dawber RPR. Cryosurgery: complications and contraindications. Clin Dermatol 1990; 8: 108–114.
7. Elton RF. Complications of cutaneous cryosurgery. J Am Acad Dermatol 1983; 8: 513–519.
8. Gage AA. What temperature is lethal for cells? J. Dermatol Surg Oncol 1979; 5: 459–464.
9. Graham GF, Clark LC. Statistical analysis in cryosurgery of skin cancer. Clin Dermatol 1990; 8: 101–107.
10. Graham GF. Cryosurgery. Clin Plast Surg 1993; 20: 131–147.
11. Hendrix Jr, JD, Parlette HL. Micronodular basal cell carcinoma. A deceptive subtype with frequent clinically undetected tumor extension. Arch Dermatol 1996; 132: 295–298.
12. Holt PJA. Cryotherapy for skin cancer: results over a 5 year period using liquid nitrogen spray cryosurgery. Br J Dermatol 1988; 119: 231–240.
13. Jacobs GH, Rippey JJ, Altini M. Prediction of aggressive behaviour in basal cell carcinoma. Cancer 1982; 49: 533–537.
14. Kuflik EG. Cryosurgery updated. J Am Acad Dermatol 1994; 31: 925–940.
15. Kuflik EG. Cryosurgery for palliation. J Dermatol Surg Oncol 1985; 11: 867.
16. Kuflik EG, Gage AA. The five-year cure rate achieved by cryosurgery for skin cancer. J Am Acad Dermatol 1991; 24: 1002–1004.
17. Kuflik EG, Gage AA. Recurrent basal cell carcinoma treated with cryosurgery. J Am Acad Dermatol 1997; 37: 82–84.
18. Kuflik EG. Segmental cryosurgical treatment. J Dermatol Surg Oncol 1987; 13: 235–236.
19. Kuflik EG. Cryosurgery for tumors of the ear. J Dermatol Surg Oncol 1985; 11: 1165–1168.
20. Levine HL, Bailin PL. Basal cell carcinoma of the head and neck: identification of the high risk patient. Laryngoscope 1980; 90: 955–961.
21. Lindgren G, Larkö O. Long-term follow-up of cryosurgery of basal cell carcinoma of the eyelid. J Am Acad Dermatol 1997; 36: 742–746.
22. McIntosch GS, Osborne DR, Li AK, Hobbs KE. Basal cell carcinoma: a review of treatment results with special reference to cryotherapy. Postgrad Med J 1983; 59: 698–701.
23. Mallon E, Dawber RPR. Cryosurgery in the treatment of basal cell carcinomas: assessment of one and two freeze-thaw cycle schedules. Dermatol Surg 1996; 22: 854–862.
24. Nordin P, Larkö O, Stenquist B. Five-year results of curettage-cryosurgery of selected large primary basal cell carcinomas on the nose: an alternative treatment in a geographical area underserved by Mohs' surgery. Br J Dermatol 1997; 136: 180–183.
25. Nordin P. Curettage-cryosurgery for non-melanoma skin cancer of the external ear: excellent 5-year results. Br J Dermatol 1999; 140: 291–293.
26. Robins P. Chemosurgery: My 15 years of experience. J Dermatol Surg Oncol 1981; 9: 779–789.
27. Robinson JK. Risk of developing another basal cell carcinoma. Cancer 1987; 60: 118–120.
28. Robinson JK, Pollack SV, Robins P. Invasion of cartilage by basal cell carcinoma. J Am Acad Dermatol 1980; 2: 499–505.
29. Rowe DE, Carroll RJ, Day Jr, CL. Mohs' surgery is the treatment of choice for recurrent (previously treated) basal cell carcinoma. J Dermatol Surg Oncol 1989; 15: 424–431.
30. Rowe DE, Carroll RJ, Day Jr, CL. Long-term recurrence rates in previously untreated (primary) basal cell carcinoma: implications for patient follow-up. J Dermatol Surg Oncol 1989; 15: 315–328.
31. Roenigk R, Roenigk H. Current surgical management of skin cancer in dermatology. J Dermatol Surg Oncol 1990; 16: 136–151.
32. Shepherd JP. The effect of low temperature on dermal connective tissue components. Oxford, University of Oxford, 1979; Thesis.
33. Shriner DL, McCoy DK, Goldberg DJ, Wagner Jr, RF. Mohs micrographic surgery. J Am Acad Dermatol 1998; 39: 79–97.
34. Spiller WF, Spiller RF. Treatment of basal-cell carcinomas by a combination of curettage and cryosurgery. J Dermatol Surg Oncol 1977; 3: 443–447.
35. Strum HM, Leider M. An editorial on curettage. J Dermatol Surg Oncol 1979; 5; 532–533.
36. Torre D. Cryosurgery of basal cell carcinoma. J Am Acad Dermatol 1986; 15: 917–929.
37. Torre D. Cryosurgical instrumentation and depth dose monitoring. Clin Dermatol 1990; 8: 48–60.
38. Zacarian SA. Cryosurgery of cutaneous carcinomas: an 18-year study of 3022 patients with 4228 carcinomas. J Am Acad Dermatol 1983; 9: 947–956.
39. Zacarian SA. Cryosurgery in the treatment of skin cancer. In: Friedman RJ, Rigel DS, Kopf AW, eds. Cancer in the skin. Philadelphia: WB Saunders. 1991; 451–465.
40. Zitelli JA. Wound healing by secondary intention. A cosmetic appraisal. J Am Acad Dermatol 1983; 9: 407–415.

8. Cryosurgery of Advanced External Cancer

J. C. Almeida Gonçalves with contributions by J. Abel Amaro, and Cecília Moura

8.0 Introduction

Our criterion to consider a cancer as advanced is not primarily related to its size, but to the degree of difficulty or impossibility of eradicating it. In fact, location, histological type and degree of local or metastatic spread to other anatomical structures are more important than the actual dimension.

Shigeo Tanaka stated in 1992 that "the most important problem in cryosurgery is standardization of the technique" (61). This short sentence touches the core of the difficulties with the new cryosurgical techniques. Protocols are always exhaustively described in books and papers on conventional surgery. Unfortunately, this is not so frequent in papers on the advances in cryosurgery. The inevitable consequence of an abridged description of a protocol is that it is not reproducible by readers. Thus, results are too dependent on the individual experience of the particular physician and of his own approach to cryosurgery. An exhaustive, careful and didactic description of all cryosurgical protocols, in papers and textbooks, is essential when a new technique is reported. This is why we have tried to describe cryosurgical protocols in great detail, both those of other authors or our own.

In spite of the vast possibilities of cryosurgery, it is not frequently used to treat large cancers because, until recently, it was generally believed that massive tumors could not be frozen to actual cancericidal temperatures. Old textbooks stated that freezing a neoplasm larger than 3 centimeters was not possible. Indeed, this is not so, and it is possible to efficiently freeze bulky and advanced cancers with lethal temperatures, if one has the adequate technique. Those opinions are surprising, when one considers that, more than 30 years ago, William G. Cahan did remarkable pioneering work on cryosurgical treatment of massive recurrent cancer (5–8). When examining the record of his experience collected over 5 years of cryosurgery practice (6), one marvels at the mass of knowledge he obtained in such a short period, his grasp of what was then a new technique and a new science, how he thoroughly understood the possibilities of cryosurgery and, last but not least, his inventiveness, creating techniques that were the basis for future developments (6). When, 6 years later, he published a chapter in the book of which he was one of the editors (7), he had treated 400 cancers, eighteen of which were massive and/or recurrent. He described one of his techniques: A "way of dealing with the problem of extensive local cancer is to excise a large portion of the bulk of the tumor and freeze near its base". This was the principle of "debulking" that later became so important (see chapter "Segmental cryosurgery of Zacarian and fractional cryosurgery" in this book). We now believe that the "debulking" was simultaneously devised and practiced by other authors independently.

Cahan noted, surprised, "how infrequently the necrotic areas become secondarily infected" (6) and that "the slough was discarded, leaving a clean granulation base which healed by re-epithelialization or a thin pliable scar" (6). To ease the freezing he advised that, "in some sites, tributary vessels may be temporarily compressed or even permanently ligated so that the vascularity of the tissues is reduced" (6). When he began to treat advanced cancer, he confessed, in his very humane way, that "the clinical trials were not selected at first but were efforts born of therapeutic desperation. Many of the patients in this category were hopelessly sick with their cancer, which had proved resistant to surgery, irradiation, chemotherapy, cautery, or combination of these. The patients and their physicians sought any reasonable method for help and, as a consequence, the patients were in debilitating states with far-advanced tumors" (5). He drew attention to the need for careful placing of thermocouples to permit accurate control of the progress of the freezing. He carried out experiments with spontaneous carcinomas in mice and dogs, including breast cancer (5–8). His techniques and writings constituted the basis for those who devoted themselves to treating advanced cancers.

In his protocols Cahan used probes with two cryosurgical techniques: *contact freezing* and *penetrating freezing*. In the latter, he introduced the probe directly inside the massive tumor to obtain a deeper and more efficient freezing. In some cases, he used two probes simultaneously, deriving the liquid nitrogen from two separate cryogenic systems (8). To control the hemorrhage that can result from the penetration of the probe in the *penetrating freezing technique*, he used gelfoam, rolled into a small tight cylinder that was inserted as a tampon into the ice-lined hole after the probe was withdrawn. The tampon was allowed to remain in place (7). To estimate the effective extent of the freezing, he used many thermocouple needles inserted at intervals, radially, around the probe, but he honestly recognized, in 1966, that "in spite of the available monitors, most freezing has been checked by sight and palpation, and a fair amount of it in bulky tumors is by 'blind flying' " (6). Later on, he improved his monitoring technique by the application of more thermocouples, some at the clinical limit of the tumor, some deeply located in the vicinity of organs and tissues adjoining the cancer, so that if any dangerous fall in temperature occurred, as freezing progressed, the process could be discontinued before damage was done. He stressed the importance of "thinking in three dimensions" and of anticipating inadvertent damage to vital neighboring organs (7). He also discovered that one could cryosurgically treat part of a bulky tumor and repeat successively the cryosurgical procedures on the same lesion, after the sloughing off of the necrotic tissue resulting from the previous procedure, until complete eradication was achieved or, at least, an acceptable palliative result was obtained (8). This finding was of the utmost importance and opened the way to cryosurgically treat very massive neoplasms that could not be frozen in one procedure. From the oncological point of view, this is not inconvenient because cryosurgery does not promote metastasizing. He wrote that he employed three techniques to treat massive cancers:

a) the use of probes, either single or in combination, applied on the surface or inside the tumors;
b) the spraying of the refrigerant on the tumor;
c) surgical excision of the bulk of the tumor, followed by a combination of a) and b).

The first author of this chapter – JCAG, who initiated the treatment of advanced external cancers in Portugal – would like to affirm his deep admiration for the wonderful, pioneering and creative work of William G. Cahan.

To our knowledge, the British K. Lloyd-Williams was the first European surgeon to perform cryosurgery on advanced cancer. He was a brilliant and inventive physician who had a very open and fascinating personality. He devised several cryosurgical techniques, among which was the *cryobiopsy* – biopsy after local freezing (46,47), and treatments for cancer and hemorrhoids. For the larger tumors, he preferred multiple-pointed probes that were introduced inside the lesions, which was further progress in relation to Cahan's penetrating technique with one or two probes. Unfortunately Lloyd-Williams did not publish very much and we do not know the details of most of his surgical protocols and results.

South American dermatologists and surgeons obtain excellent results with reduced technical resources. Stolar and Turjansky developed a technique that performs prior "debulking" by conventional surgery or radiofrequency (59,71–74), either by removing the cancer without safety margin or, if this is not possible, reducing it to a thin, non-bleeding layer that is subsequently frozen, using a hand held device (CRY-AC, Brymill Corporation). With this apparently simple technique, but with great surgical competence, they also succeed in eradicating large cancers that would be inoperable by conventional surgery. Many of their good results have been repeatedly presented at congresses of cryosurgery but have not been published in detail. Their skill and good results are remarkable, even with large cancers. Their techniques are largely followed by many physicians in Argentina and other South American countries. This demonstrates a phrase that we heard during the discussion at a recent congress: "More important than the apparatus are the people who are behind it" (Figs. 8.1–8.5).

In the 1988 meeting of the American College of Cryosurgery, in Orlando, Castro-Ron presented the solution he had found to treat some very large scalp cancers, for which he did not have adequate equipment. He used an empty beer tin can, removed its top, put a piece of rubber around the opening, to protect his fingers, filled it with liquid nitrogen and applied its base on the surface of the

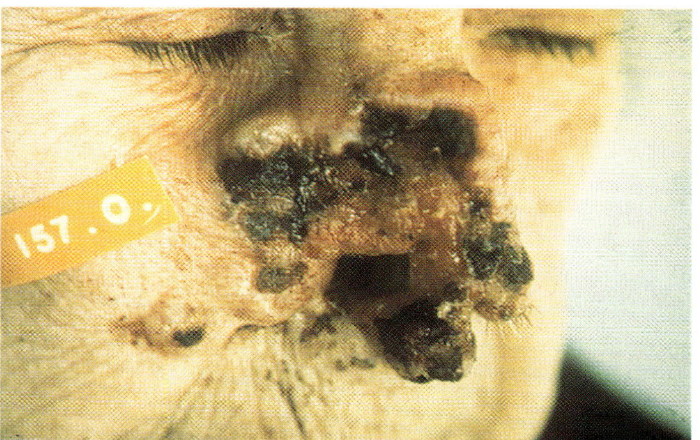

Fig. 8.1. Long-standing, terebrating, recurrent BCC post surgery and post radiotherapy, in an 80-year-old woman. (Courtesy of Turjansky and Stolar)

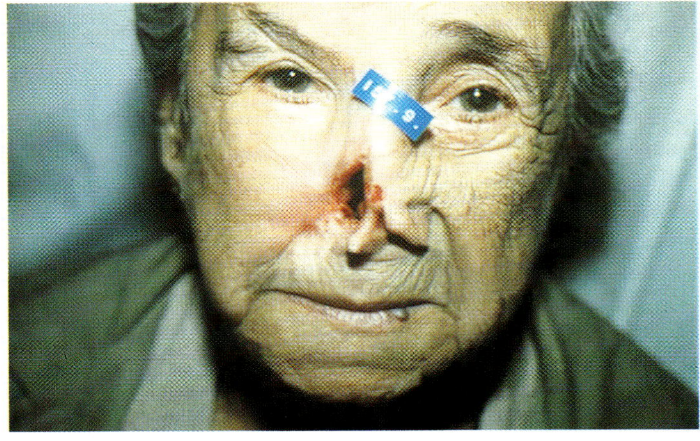

Fig. 8.2. Same patient: after three freeze/thaw cycles with liquid nitrogen spray

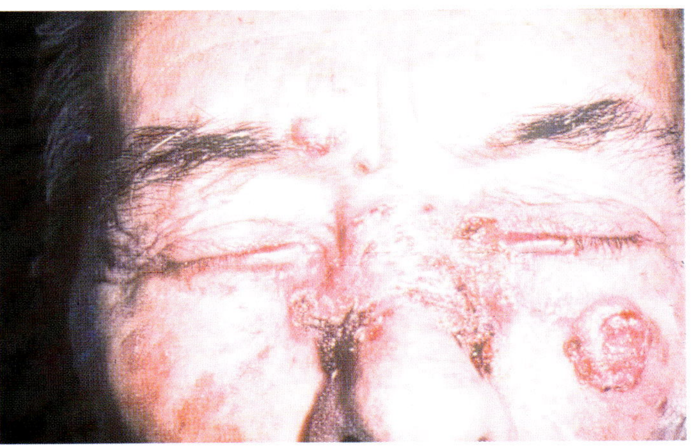

Fig. 8.3. BCC and SCC on the face of a 78-year-old woman who also suffered from cardiac disease. (Courtesy of Stolar and Turjansky)

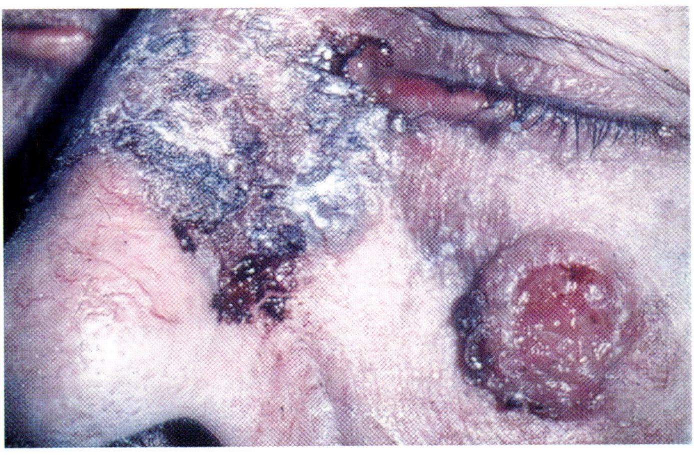

Fig. 8.4. Close-up of Fig. 8.3

cancers. He obtained their apparent cure, with one or more of such original and imaginative cryosurgical procedures.

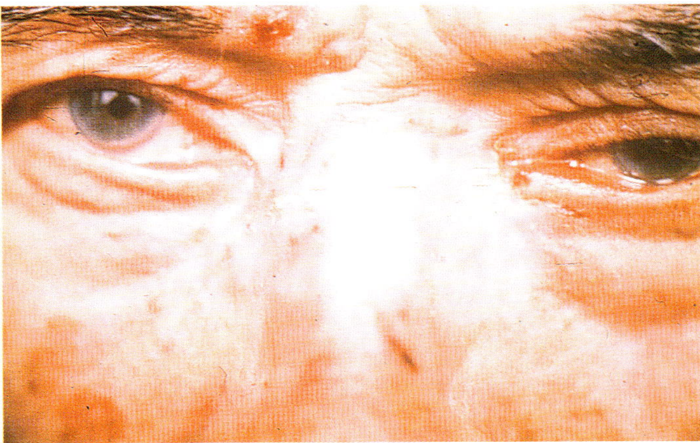

Fig. 8.5. Same patient, two years after cryosurgery

Kuflik explored the possibilities provided by segmental cryosurgery (41–44) and treated large skin cancers (see chapter on segmental cryosurgery).

Through 1995, Tanaka treated by cryosurgery 424 malignancies, 43 of which were skin cancers (60–69), some of them advanced, achieving a high cure rate. The protocol used was similar to that he used to treat breast cancer (see ''Cryosurgery of breast cancer'').

Andrew A. Gage has been doing noteworthy work on the cryosurgical treatment of advanced cancers of the skin and mouth (12–14). He always uses liquid nitrogen and prefers the probe contact to the spray, considering the cryoprobe techniques to provide a predictable and more controllable area of necrosis, even in the treatment of large cancers. He reserves the spray technique for extensive superficial skin cancers and considers the running off of liquid nitrogen drops from the frozen surface of the lesion and the risk of insufflation with gas, or even fatal embolism, when it is applied on ulcerated and undermined neoplasms, as a considerable disadvantage. Sometimes he employs both techniques simultaneously for selected large and bulky cancers, but rarely uses the penetrating freezing technique, due to the risk of uncontrollable hemorrhage. Nevertheless, he recognized the difficulty in freezing large tumors with a single application, recommending immediate and successive applications of the probe, until complete freezing of the lesion, plus an adequate safety margin of apparently normal tissue, is achieved. He stressed that the firm pressure of the probe against the tissue is essential for reducing the heat supply to the tumor provided by the circulation. He used the penetration freezing only in selected cases of bulky tumors, aiming to obtain closer contact with the tissue and to produce more extensive and deep-freezing. The risks of the penetrating technique can be minimized by the use of cryosurgical equipment provided with a heating system at the head of the probes, which has the advantage of combining rapid and deep freezing with the hemostatic effect of heating. However, he generally carries out previous debulking of large tumors by partial surgical or electrocutting excision in order to obtain effective freezing at the base of the tumor. He reserved the open spray technique for the treatment of multiple, small skin carcinomas and for extensive superficial skin cancers.

Sometimes he employed both techniques – spraying and contact probe – simultaneously for the treatment of selected advanced cancers of the skin and oral cavity. Between 1964 and 1975 he treated 84 selected cases of oral cancer, preventing bone-sacrificing operations. Morbidity was minimal. In stage I disease, the 5-year-survival rate was 83%; in stage II, it was 50%. The results in more advanced stages were inferior in terms of survival, but the distressing symptoms ceased and good palliation was obtained (14). In special problematic cases he combined cryosurgery with other therapeutic modalities, such as classic surgery, radiotherapy and chemotherapy.

In the chapter "Segmental cryosurgery of Zacarian and fractional cryosurgery for skin cancer" of this book, cryosurgery of lentigo maligna is referred to. There are not many references to cryosurgical treatment of other stages of malignant melanoma. The sensibility of its cells to cold and the probability of immunological effect of cryosurgery would suggest a larger use of the technique. It is foreseeable that the results could be better than those of conventional surgery. E. W. Breitbart has done persistent research in this field (3, 4). He mentions that the destruction of melanoma cells induced by cold occurs between −5°C and −7°C; conversely, the destruction of connective tissues requires temperatures under −20°C. Breitbart always studies the tumor by ultrasonography and follows the progress of the freezing by the same method. After the first freezing, he performs the cryobiopsy and the fragment is placed in formalin while it is frozen. The cryobiopsy traverses the entire tumor and is taken at its deepest point, as indicated by ultrasonography. The advantages are: there is no crushing or tissue laceration during extraction and the microscopic measurements of the melanoma are equivalent to its actual size. The introduction of the fresh biopsy tissue into formalin causes some shrinkage and the resulting measurements of the Breslow level are not equivalent to those in live tissue. He treated 43 primary malignant melanomas with very good results (3). In 1989, he compared immunologically eight patients with melanomas in stage II (TNM classification, UICC 1987) who were treated by cryosurgery with eight patients also suffering from melanoma in the same stage and with similar characteristics, treated by conventional surgery (4). Lymphocyte populations in the peripheral blood, namely, T-cells, T-helper cells, HLA-DR-positive cells and the ratio helper/suppressor T-cells were studied in both groups, before treatment and on the second, sixth and twentieth day after treatment. The difference was striking. Those values increased in all patients treated by cryosurgery, between 24.1% and 54.9% in relation to mean values, while they were lower than mean values in all patients treated by conventional surgery, about 25% less than the values of these measures before treatment. The ratio T-Helper/suppressor cells was 23% higher than mean values in the first group and 25.5% lower in the second (76).

Multiple previously documented examples showed that melanoma patients treated by cryosurgery had longer disease-free periods between treatment and recurrence. It was also demonstrated that in some patients with a good immunological state, after freezing one or more metastases there was regression of other non-treated metastases.

To our knowledge, this was the first study that presented immunologically measured data that confirmed clinical studies on the booster immunological effect of cryosurgery on melanoma patients (76). The probable explanations are: cryosurgery modifies the cellular membrane and the surface antigens due to protein denaturation; and the intracellular antigens that were not in contact with the immunological system are freed and can work as autoantigens. From this process can also result the liberation of associated intracellular tumoral antigens that originate a specific immunological reaction, contributing to the destruction of the primary tumor and its metastases. The real advantage of cryosurgery is that the necrosed tumor remains in place, originating antibodies, in contrast to conventional surgery (76).

Itoh and Tanaka treated 10 patients suffering from malignant melanoma, staged between I and IV (UICC 1990). In all cases a cryobiopsy was performed. Three tumors were surgically removed after cryosolidification and seven melanomas were submitted to cryosurgery. Four patients were alive at the time of publication with follow-up between 5 and 16 years. Itoh and Tanaka concluded: 1)

"Cryosurgery should be the first choice therapy for stages I and II. Cryosurgery is particularly indicated for head and neck, and mucosal lesions in anatomically critical sites. 2) Cryosolidification of the suspicious tumor is mandatory, not only when performing biopsies, but also when doing conventional wide excision as the first treatment. 3) For stages III and IV, cryosurgery may be a choice for palliation. A beneficial effect owing to cryoimmunology reaction may be expected" (40,76).

Turjansky and Stolar prefer conventional surgery to treat malignant melanoma but, in case of poor health conditions or patient refusal, they do not hesitate to treat these cancers by cryosurgery (71). Neither do we. Until 1995, they had treated 74 cases of lentigo maligna and malignant melanoma (73). Regrettably, we have not had access to a detailed description of their experience.

8.1 Perilesional Protection Prior to Cryosurgery of Advanced Cancer

When treating advanced external cancers or bulky neoplastic masses, we follow three rules: efficient protection around the lesions; the use of a thick spray of liquid nitrogen, supplied by an apparatus with high pressure through a nozzle, measuring 1 mm in diameter; and accurate control of the advance of the ice front on the surface and in the interior of the mass. Alternatively to the thick spray of liquid nitrogen some authors use multiple penetrating probes with an apparatus that has a high capability to quickly remove heat from the neoplastic tissues (56,77). The difficulty in freezing large and bulky cancers is to obtain cancericidal temperatures in the entire tumoral mass. If a single non-penetrating cryoprobe is used, the progress of the freezing decelerates; a few minutes later, the freezing stops, having attained about 2 cm in depth; only rarely is it useful to freeze for more than 10 minutes (12). If spray is used, the conversion of liquid nitrogen into gas becomes incomplete as the surface of the lesion becomes frozen, and droplets of liquid nitrogen run off, freezing surrounding structures (12). For small tumors, intermittent spraying, or reducing the pressure inside the cryogenic apparatus, lessens that inconvenience, but it also shortens the freezing time and diminishes the capacity to achieve deep freezing. To cope with this problem, one of us (JCAG) developed – with the collaboration of Biodermis Corporation – an adherent reinforced silicone sheet (Cryosil®) with a hole equivalent to the size of the tumor plus the safety margin, permitting the use of continuous spray that assures a quick freezing (26).[1]

When feasible, prior reduction of the tumoral mass – so-called "debulking"– is a good technique that considerably improves the cure rate (29,35–37,41–44). With really large and advanced cancers that are very irrigated, particularly if they are friable, non-solid and fungating, debulking by conventional surgery can be difficult or even impossible, due to the difficulty in controlling hemorrhage. In these cases, debulking must be done by cryosurgery.

JCAG devised some protocols to deal with these situations, as will be detailed below. In order to achieve cancericidal temperatures inside bulky tumors a thick spray must be applied for long periods. To prevent dripping of liquid nitrogen and freezing of skin around the target – the tumor plus the safety margin – the drops must be stopped with efficient perilesional protection. Some surgeons protect the skin around the tumor with a Vaseline embankment (67,68). We also do this for medium sized tumors but, for advanced ones, we prefer to limit the target with one of the following three methods: a) for cancers located on the head and extremities, we use many layers of common bandages (Figs. 8.6, 8.22); b) for neoplasms on the trunk, a paraffinated gauze bandage that must be folded some fifteen times, creating a smooth and flexible "plaque" that is stitched onto the edge of the target (Fig. 8.26, 8.27, 8.29, 8.47); c) for any location, the placement of a large reinforced, adherent silicone sheet (commercially available for small cancers) with a central hole cut into it, in accordance with the size of the target (Fig. 8.8).

Our procedure for any advanced external cancer is based on the above general principles, but specific adaptations are required for each neoplasm, according to its individual characteristics and location. The important consequence of the careful physical limitation is that the limits of the cryonecrosis are accurate and predictable (Figs. 8.9, 8.32, 8.48). The cryosurgeon can use liquid nitrogen spray continuously, and for as long as necessary, between 15 and 60 minutes and can thus concentrate on monitoring the progress of the ice front. Ultrasonography is important to a previous definition of the real size of the tumor and to control the advance of the freezing, in real time. Regrettably we never had access to this equipment in the institutions where we worked.

[1] Cryosil ®, distributed by Biodermis Corporation, 3078E Sunset Road, Suite #1, Las Vegas, NV 89120, USA.

8.2 Cryosurgery of Advanced Cancer of the Extremities

Squamous cell carcinomas (SCC) of the extremities occur mostly on the dorsa of the hands of outdoor workers. When these tumors are left to their natural evolution they become adherent to important underlying structures, and amputation is the usual treatment. Reference to cryosurgery of such cancers in the literature is scarce. In 1980, O. Martins et al.

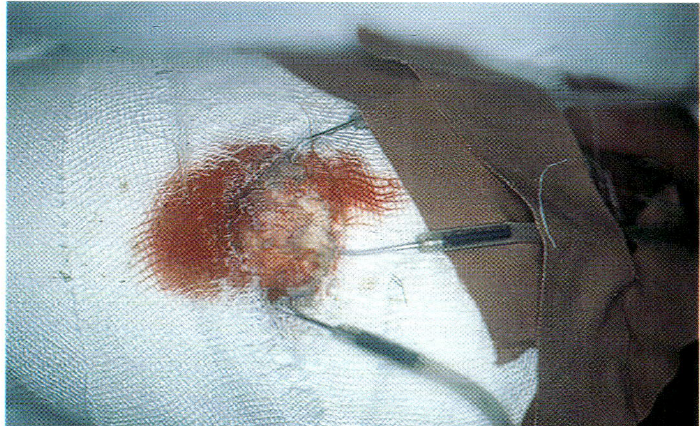

Fig. 8.6. Perilesional protection for tumours of the hand

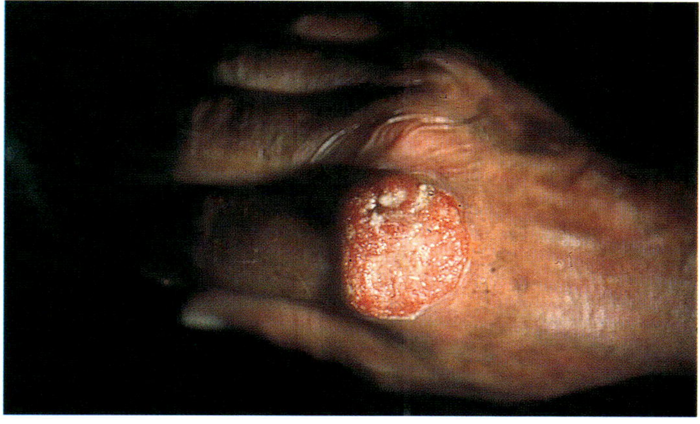

Fig. 8.7. Adherent SCC over the second metacarpophalangeal joint

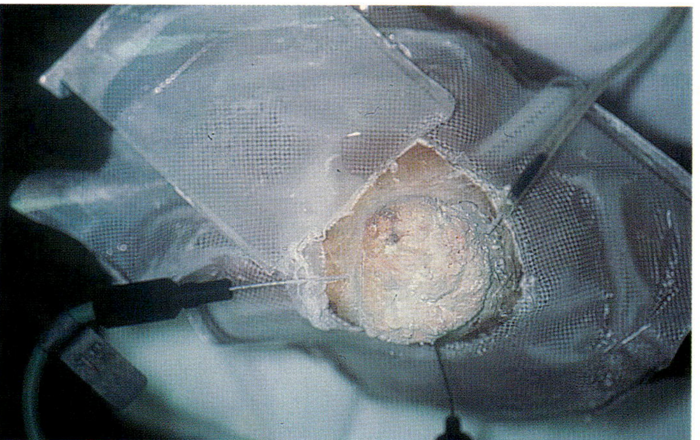

Fig. 8.8. In this case the perilesional protection was done with adherent silicone sheets (Cryosil®).

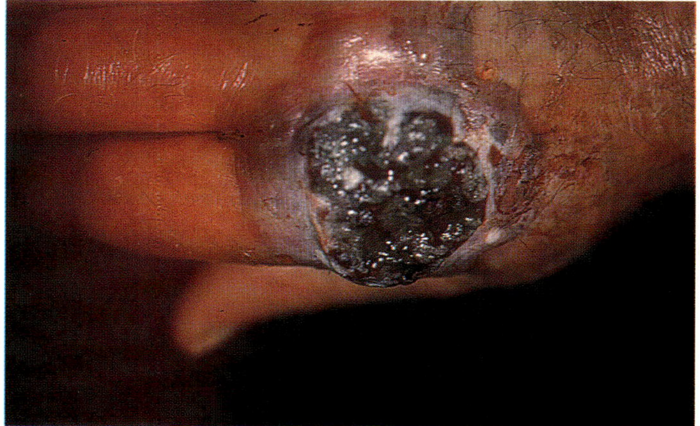

Fig. 8.9. Same patient as in Figs. 8.7 and 8.8, 24 hours after cryosurgery

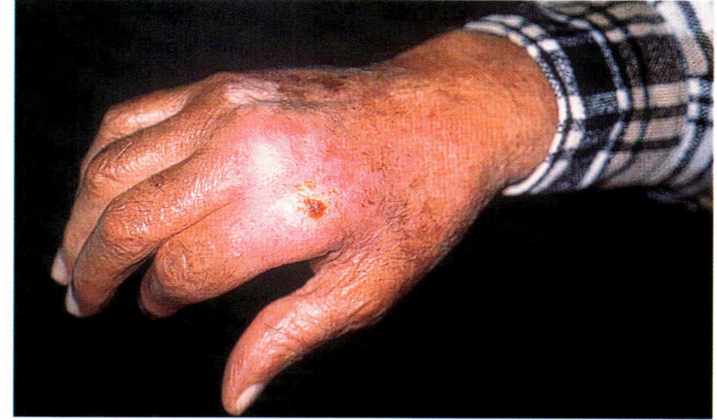

Fig. 8.10. Same patient, five months later

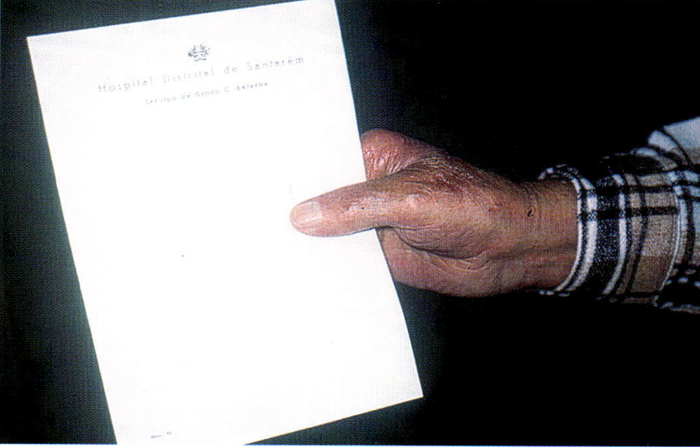

Fig. 8.11. Same patient: the functions of the hand were maintained

published the cryosurgical treatment of an SCC of the dorsum of a hand, measuring three centimeters. It was successfully treated after debulking (53). Through 1995, Turjansky and Stolar treated 2480 malignant lesions of the extremities (72), which is 20% of the location of all malignancies they have treated. Twelve of these cancers were proposed for amputation that could be prevented. They always use debulking by radio frequency and cryosurgery with liquid nitrogen spray from hand-held devices.

In 1986, one of us (JCAG) published his cryosurgical technique to deal with these dangerous cancers (17), treatments having started in 1978. The method has since been used by him and by his collaborators. The *surgical protocol* (Figs. 8.6–8.11) is as follows: Anesthesia can be general, nerve block or caudal, depending on the tumor location and the patient's general condition. Adherent silicone sheets (Cryosil®) (Fig. 8.8) or bandages are firmly applied around the tumor and safety margin (Fig. 8.6). The number of layers depends on the physical type of the bandage and must be sufficient to prevent the freezing of normal skin and stop the running droplets. Usually, we do not use debulking for cancers of the extremities. Thermocouples are introduced inside the cancer, under its apparent inner limit and under its borders (Fig. 8.8). An open, thick spray, obtained from an apparatus with high pressure, is used (Frigitronics CE-4). Inside the tumor the temperature attained is low, around −50°C, but at the edge of the tumor and at the underlying structures it is important to have temperatures higher than −20°C in order to spare those structures. Lymphadenectomy is carried out when adenopathies are seen. Necrosis is completed in about 6 days and the necrotic tissue is easily removed with scissors. Any suspect site is biopsied and, if necessary, cryosurgery is repeated. The resulting ulceration is permitted to heal by second intention, which occurs within four to eight weeks. As a rule, no grafting is performed because healing by second intention facilitates the detection of possible persistence or recurrence. Moreover, the cosmetic results are very good and grafting or other plastic correction is not necessary (Figs. 8.12–8.13).

We treated 30 SCCs of the extremities of 23 patients (23). All cancers were so advanced that amputation had been proposed. Nine patients were male and 14 were female, and almost all were rural workers. Their ages were between 55 and 93 years (mean 76.5). Only five were under 70 years of age. Eighteen patients had a single cancer and five had multiple lesions. Twenty-five patients had lesions on the upper limbs and five on the lower limbs. Nineteen carcinomas were on the dorsa of the hands. One was at the root of the fourth and fifth fingers and the proposed surgery had been amputation of both fingers. Three were on the leg and two on the foot. The time of evolution was between 1 and 6 years, but, in many patients, it could not be determined due to the poor memory common in elderly people. The tumors were primary in 21 patients, and recurrent after conventional surgery in two. Their major axes were between 25 mm and 130 mm in length. The smaller one was over the articulation of the second metacarpophalangeal joint. In all patients with a single tumor, it was invasive and adherent to the underlying planes; in the patients with multiple lesions, at least one was invasive. A skin graft was carried out only in one patient who had a cancer on the heel. Debulking was performed in one of our first patients who had a large cancer on the tenar region, by cryosurgery. One week later, another cryosurgical procedure was performed with definitive eradication of the cancer.

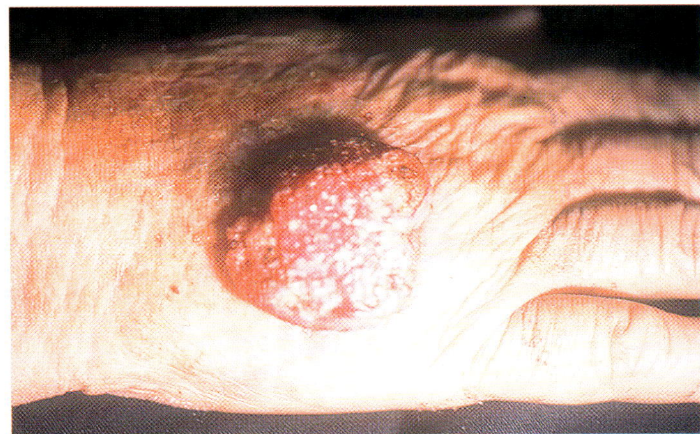

Fig. 8.12. Large SCC before treatment

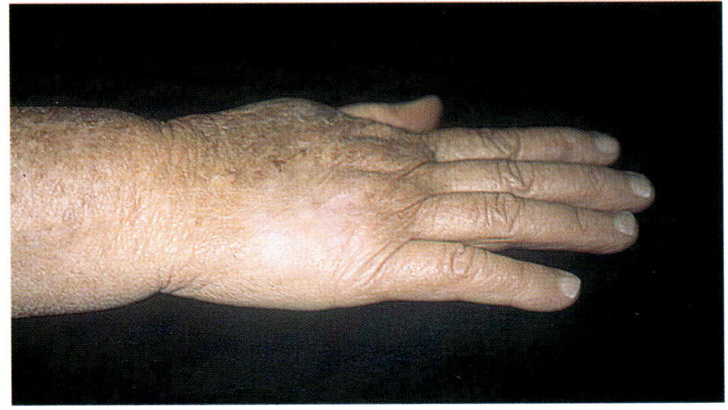

Fig. 8.13. Same patient, three years after cryosurgery

Eighteen patients had their malignancies cured and physical function was maintained, in follow-ups between 1 and 8 years. In a few cases the extensor tendons of the dorsum of the hand were exposed after removal of the cryonecrosed tumor. We expected that these exposed tendons would be destroyed or, at least, hindered in their function. In fact, this did not happen. They were slowly covered by granulation tissue and, after healing, their function was maintained without any impairment. Our first patient was treated with an inadequate cryosurgical technique, due to lack of experience, and the extremity had to be amputated. Two carcinomas persisted after cryosurgery and produced metastases, and the patients eventually died. In two others, cryosurgery was unable to cure the cancers and the patients were treated by another technique devised by one of us (JCAG) – chemosurgery with zinc chloride paste (20). These patients suffered amputation of two fingers by this method, but the remaining fingers permitted a functional hand.

Besides the advanced cancers that had been proposed for amputation, we also treated 21 SCCs of the extremities, measuring between 20 mm and 50 mm that could also have been treated by conventional surgery. Eighteen patients were without evidence of disease – between six months and nine years after cryosurgery – and three had recurrences soon after.

The advantages of cryosurgical treatment in these cases are: smaller tumors can be treated in the outpatient clinic, which takes one fifth of the time necessary to carry out conventional excision and grafting and, last but not least, we consider that, very probably, the cure rate of the cryosurgically treated patients is higher than that achieved by conventional surgery.

The value of debulking is well established (35–37,41–43,29) and we usually do it in other malignancies, but not in advanced cancers of the extremities. As we use a high-pressure source of liquid nitrogen with a nozzle 1 mm in diameter, a previous complete debulking would expose healthy structures to a strong spray, resulting in too quick a freezing that would risk damage to them. With our technique of perilesional protection and thick spray, it is possible and easy to freeze a whole tumor of approximately 100 cm^3. The cancer mass is quickly frozen to cancericidal temperatures, but controlled and slower freezing of the interface between the tumor and the underlying structures must be obtained. Furthermore, when frozen, the tumoral mass becomes a cooling source capable of freezing the slender peripheral extensions of neoplastic tissue. Kuflik wrote "good results from cryosurgery occur because cellular components are more susceptible to cold injury than are stromal components" (44). This explains why it is possible to destroy the cancer and to spare the fibrotic underlying structures.

It is extremely important to carefully control the advance of freezing when it approaches the edge of the tumor, in order to prevent irreparable damage to the underlying structures. Less attentive practice may result in amputation, the prevention of which is the very aim of this method.

The overall results and prevention of amputation in 18/23 patients supports the position that cryosurgery is the best treatment for advanced cancer of the extremities.

8.3 Cryosurgery of Advanced Carcinoma Arising in Pilonidal Sinus

Among the complications of a long-standing sinus pilonidalis, malignant degeneration of the cyst wall or of the sinus tract is rare around 0.1% (1). The resulting cancer is usually a squamous cell carcinoma (SCC). Generally, the patient seeks medical advice at a late stage, because he is used to the discomfort of the chronic oozing produced by the cyst, and he can present with an advanced malignancy (we have never observed pilonidal sinus untreated for decades in women).

We treated by cryosurgery five men aged between 50 and 75 years (mean 59.6 years). All patients had suffered from a long-standing sinus pilonidalis with multiple episodes of infection and suppuration. The precise length of time during which their cysts were present before malignant transformation could not be ascertained in three patients, but was in all cases longer than 25 years. In two, it was 33 and 53 years, respectively. The time of evolution was known in only one patient – around 2 years. The histological diagnosis was SCC in all patients, two being classified as well differentiated. One carcinoma was primary; all the others had recurred after conventional surgery and radiotherapy (21, 25, 32).

Surgical protocol: (Figs. 8.14–8.17) Anesthesia was general in four patients and epidural in one. When four of these patients were treated – between 1980 and 1991– the target was limited with surgical cloths tightly applied with adhesive tape (see Atlas of Cryosurgery). In the last patient, treated in 1996, this was done with folded paraffinated gauze bandages. Thermocouples were applied inside the tumors, under the probable interface between the

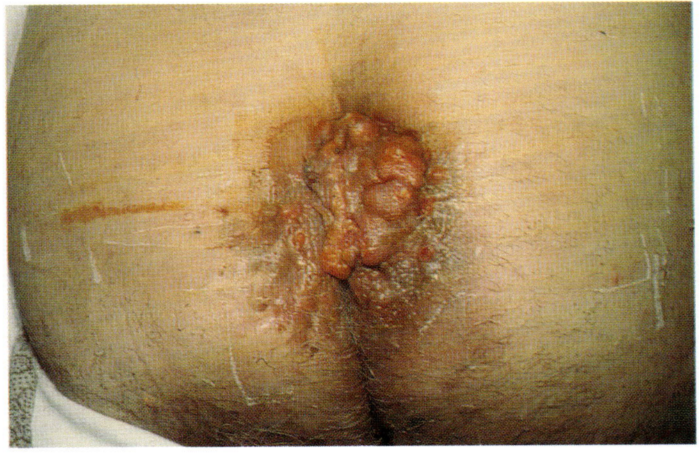

Fig. 8.14. Primary, invasive, inoperable SCC, adherent to the sacrum

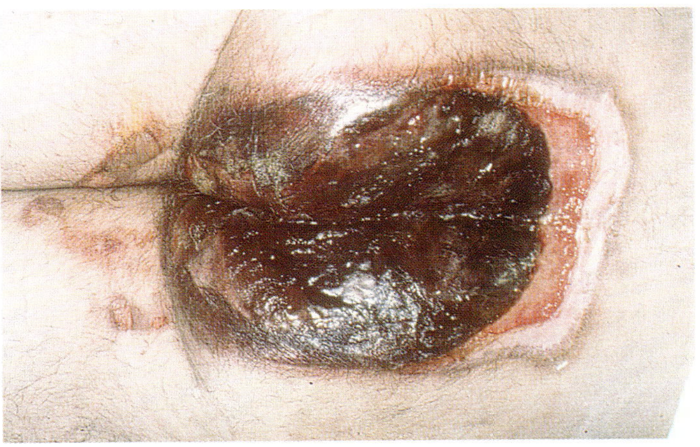

Fig. 8.15. Same patient: large necrosis after the first cryosurgery, which was intended as debulking

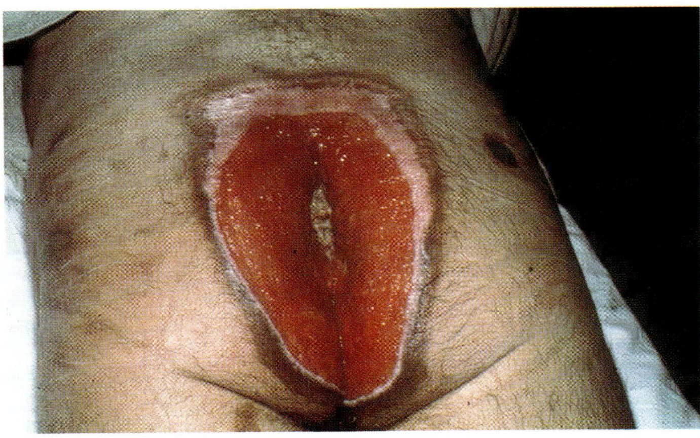

Fig. 8.16. Same patient, after debulking; the remaining cancer was adherent to the sacrum

malignancy and the underlying structures, and under their apparent clinical limits. All cancers were submitted to two freeze/thaw cycles with thick spray from a high-pressure apparatus (Frigitronics CE-4) down to –70°C. In one patient a single cryosurgical procedure (with two freeze/thaw cycles) was performed. In the others, the tumors were too bulky and the first cryosurgical procedure was intended as massive debulking. The necrotic tissue was removed over the two or three weeks following cryosurgery. Approximately one month later, another cryosurgical procedure was performed to eradicate the remaining cancer. The results were: three patients had no more evidence of disease for between seven and fourteen years; one had a recurrence 8 years later and was again submitted to an aggressive cryosurgery and subsequent plastic surgery and is well at the time of writing, four years after the last intervention; the fifth patient, who had an enormous tumor, measuring 150 mm × 60 mm, had no local recurrence but died of metastasic disease 10 months after the cryosurgical treatment.

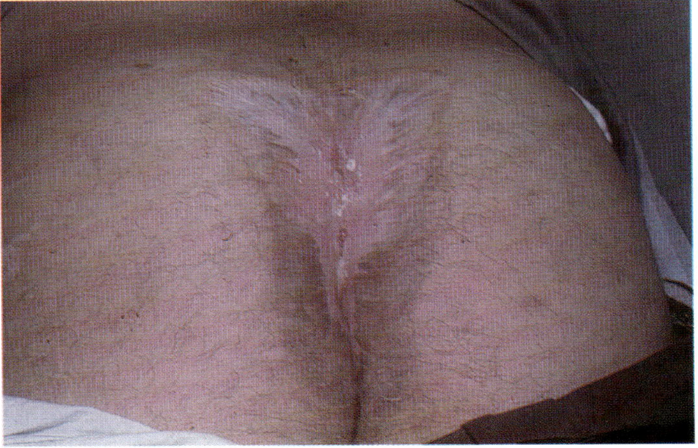

Fig. 8.17. Same patient: a second cryosurgical treatment eradicated the tumor. After healing

These cancers develop in people who have a tendency to neglect their illnesses and who seek medical advice too late. Complete removal by conventional surgery is difficult, because the tumor soon becomes adherent to the sacrum and coccyx, originating arduous or impossible eradication. Cryosurgery offers the possibility of carrying out real tissue sterilization, without destroying bone. The local eradication achieved in all patients demonstrates the value of cryosurgery in such advanced cancers.

8.4 Cryosurgery of Advanced Basal Cell Carcinoma Invading Orbital Structures

When a basal cell carcinoma (BCC) originating in the eyelids or the canthi invades the orbit, it becomes a serious situation with high mortality.

In such cases, the usual surgical treatment is exenteration of the orbit. The only reference we found in the literature was that of Cahan who successfully treated by cryosurgery a huge SCC that deeply invaded the orbit. Plastic reconstruction was performed one year later (7). Stolar and Turjansky also successfully treated one BCC invading the orbital structures (Figs. 8.18–8.20).

One of us (JCAG) treated six patients with long-standing, terebrant basal cell carcinomas, deeply invading the orbital structures, with loss of sight of the invaded eye. One was a primary cancer (see *Atlas of Cryosurgery*, 2001) and five were recurrences after multiple surgical and radiation procedures. All the recurrent tumors were referred to him by the departments of head and neck surgery or radiation therapy and were considered unsuitable for further conventional treatments. These cases were presented in congresses of cryosurgery (31), but this is the first time that they are published. Three men and three women were

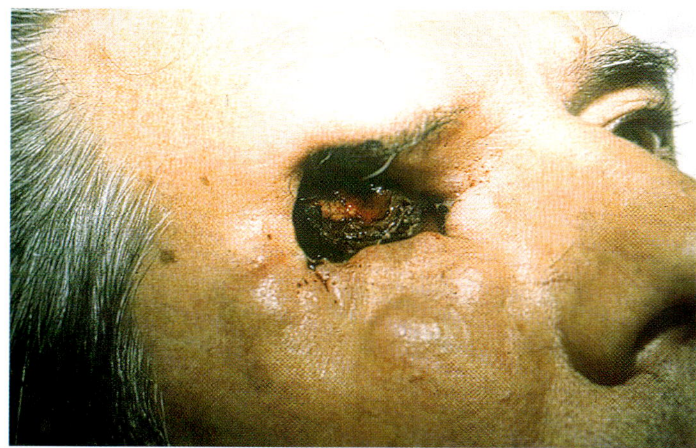

Fig. 8.18. Long-standing, invasive, inoperable BCC of the orbit that recurred after exenteration. (Courtesy of Stolar and Turjansky)

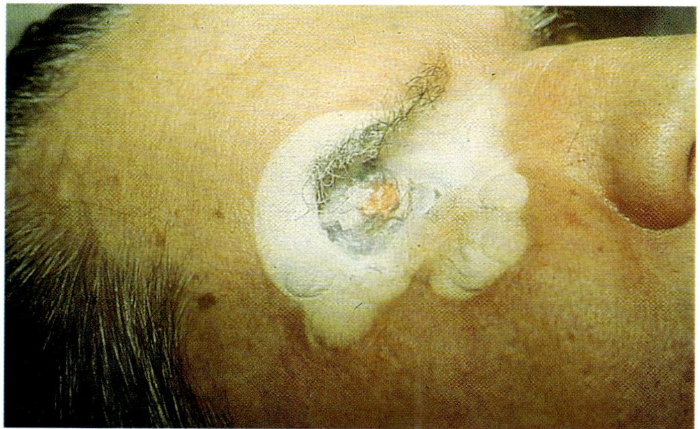

Fig. 8.19. Same patient, immediately after cryosurgery by spraying

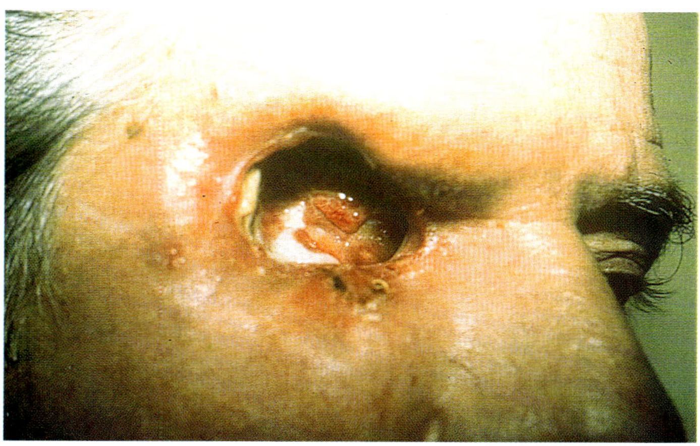

Fig. 8.20. Same patient, after healing

treated. Their ages varied between 60 and 89 years (mean 69.1 years). The time of evolution varied from 6 to 30 years (mean 20 years). At the time of treatment of these patients, we had no access to CAT scanning or magnetic resonance imaging. At present exhaustive CAT or MRI studies should be done.

The *cryosurgical protocol* (Figs. 8.21–8.23) was:

All patients received general anesthesia. In the first five patients neither debulking nor enucleation were performed. In the sixth, only the exophytic part of the tumor was removed by electrocutting. After the anesthesia was induced, the whole head was firmly bandaged with many layers, except for the orbital region and an adequate safety margin (Fig. 8.22). The purpose of the bandages was to efficiently stop the drops of liquid nitrogen that run off during freezing. Several thermocouples were inserted into the tumor (Fig. 8.22). The extremities of two other thermo-

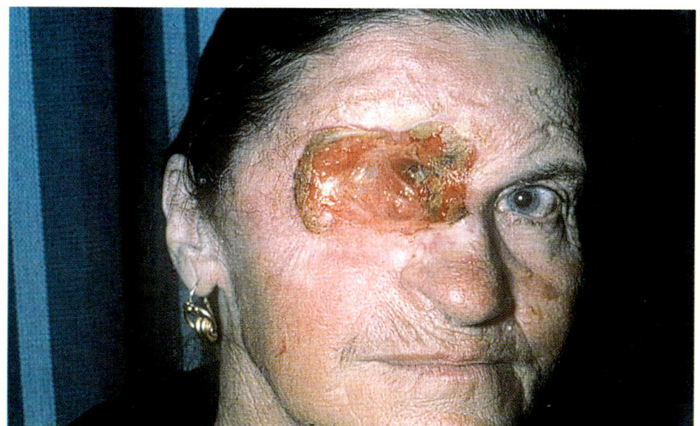

Fig. 8.21. Invasive and recurrent BCC after several radiation sessions

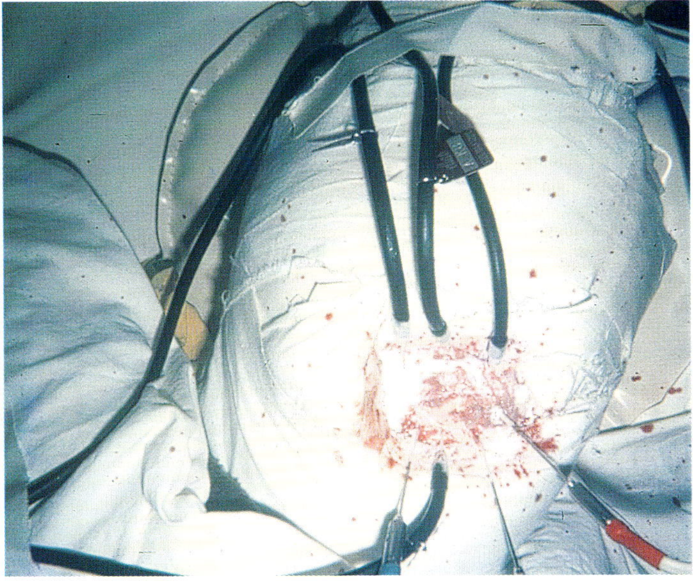

Fig. 8.22. Same patient: the whole head was protected with bandages, leaving only the orbital region exposed

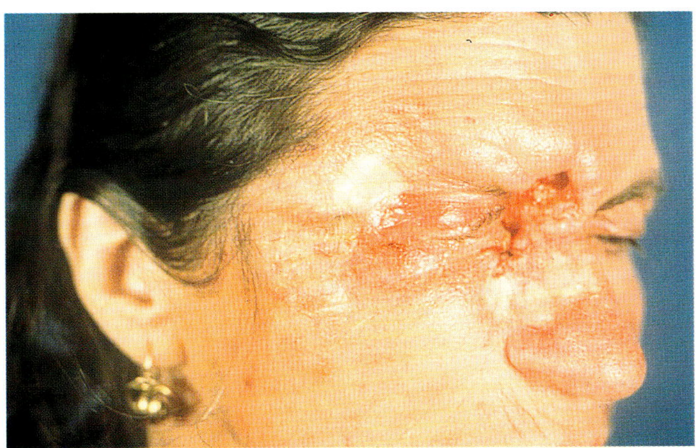

Fig. 8.23. Same patient, one year after clinical cure. She was well 13 years after cryosurgery

couples were placed against the orbital plate. The freezing was carried out with a continuous spray of liquid nitrogen from an apparatus with high pressure (Frigitronics CE-4). Freezing of the external neoplastic tissue was done as quickly as possible, but the advance of the ice front inside the orbit was carried out more slowly while always monitoring the temperatures, particularly those of the two thermocouples applied against the orbital plate. These should not be excessively cooled in order to prevent possible damage to the brain. Two freeze-thaw cycles were carried out. The temperatures achieved in the neoplastic tissues were between −50 and −60°C (Figs. 8.21–8.25).

In the days thereafter, the edema was considerable (see *Atlas of Cryosurgery*, 2001). The necrotic

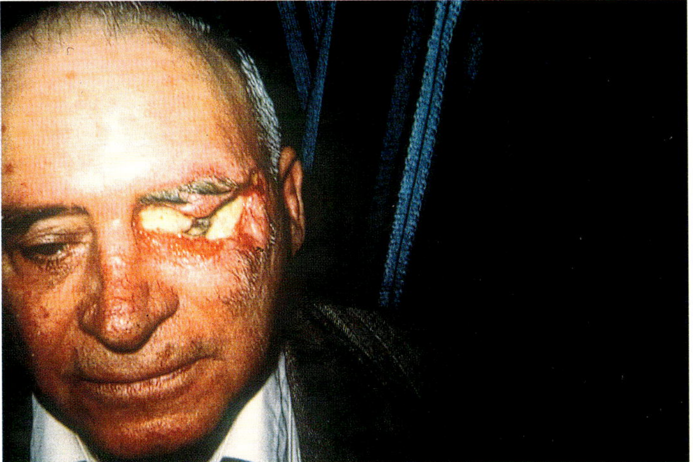

Fig. 8.24. Invasive BCC of the orbit, recurrent post surgery and post irradiation

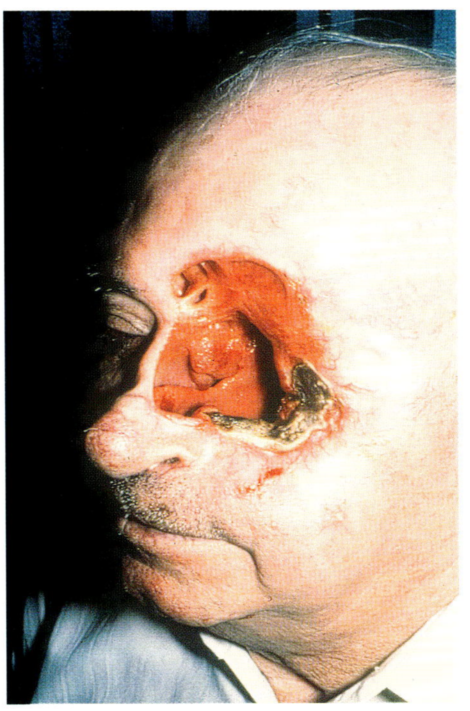

Fig. 8.25. Same patient: the tumor was controlled but not cured. Small recurrences inside the orbit were successively treated with cryoprobe contact. The patient died, three years later, of unrelated disease

tissue was slowly removed over about six weeks. The healing was by second intention. No plastic reconstruction was done in any patient.

The *results* of cryosurgery were:

a) in all patients, the pain ceased with the operation; b) two patients were cured and followed up for 13 years, without recurrence; c) in two patients, the cancer persisted but with acceptable palliative result, with survival of 2 and 3 years, respectively: d) two patients died shortly after cryosurgery. One was an 89-year-old woman, who soon died from heart disease, the other was a 65-year-old man who became mentally confused immediately after cryosurgery and died of bronchopneumonia one month later. Necropsy was not done, but it is probable that there was brain damage through the orbital plate.

Figures in the *Atlas of Cryosurgery* (2001) show a 60-year-old patient who suffered from a terebrant BCC of the orbit. She had a tumor of the nose that recurred three times, the last time six months before our examination, when it invaded the orbit. The temperatures during freezing were −30°C in the first cycle and −50°C in the second. The time of freezing in the first cycle was 22 minutes and the thaw time was 30 minutes. She had no recurrence for 13 years.

Fortunately, dreadful cases of invasive BCCs of the orbit are becoming more and more rare with the progress of medical care in our country, and so JCAG has not treated any new cases in the last 16 years. The reason he did not publish these cases is that he wanted to proceed to a modified protocol, that is herein suggested for those who may come across a similar case: First, carry out enucleation, but leaving tissues about one centimeter thick on the orbital walls. Perform cryosurgery separately, because when done immediately after conventional surgery it can provoke uncontrollable hemorrhage. Protect the head with bandages, as indicated. Apply thermocouples on the orbital walls, and two more against the orbital plate on the roof. Shield the orbital roof with some tightly applied pieces of paraffinated gauze some 5 cm × 5 cm. Solidly freeze the other three aspects of the orbital cavity, with two or three freeze/thaw cycles to −50°C. Remove the gauze that protected the upper wall of the orbit and slowly freeze-thaw twice the tissues on the roof of the orbit, carefully following the progress of the temperature of the two thermocouples applied against the orbital plate, and do not permit it to go under −12°C/−15°C. Over the following year no plastic surgery should be performed, because it would hinder detection of eventual recurrences. It can be performed after one or two years, if there has been no recurrence.

8.5 Cryovulvectomy for Advanced Cancer

Neglected cancer of the vulva causes great discomfort and, as it progresses, considerable suffering. It is surprising that so many patients seek medical advice so late. As time passes, treatment becomes more and more difficult. In the past, some authors tried palliative cryosurgical treatment of advanced vulvar cancer, using cryoprobes, with reduced benefit (9,45,70). Indeed, the cryoprobe cannot freeze the tumors deeply enough (12,13). In 1970, H. Günther presented a communication on "Cryosurgery of vulvar carcinoma" at a congress of gynecology in East Germany (38). The abstract does not give very much information. It seems that he used a technique not very different from ours. We did not find any other publication of his and tried to contact him through the German Embassy in Lisbon, without success. In 1976, Wallach treated a vulvar carcinoma with four segmental cryosurgical procedures, and with final conventional surgery (75), with success. J. Sommer et al. treated 146 cases of advanced vulvar cancer by cryosurgery, between 1971 and 1986 (57). The carcinomas were defined as inoperable by conventional surgery, but neither staging of the tumors nor clear and objective description of the protocol was given. It was said only that the exophytic part of the cancer was removed by electrocutting and that each tumor was treated over 10 minutes. From the text and from the accompanying photos it becomes evident that no vulvectomy was ever attempted and that only tumorectomy was carried out. There were five pulmonary embolisms, one of them lethal. The cure rate was 38.4%. The lack of staging and of a good description of the surgical protocol makes the comparison with other series difficult. In 1982, A. Favard et al. treated four advanced vulvar cancers by cryosurgery, with different individual protocols, succeeding in clinically curing two patients and obtaining a good palliative result in the other two (11). Stolar and collaborators treated seven cases of vulvar carcinoma in situ with three freeze/thaw cycles with liquid nitrogen spray obtained from a hand-held device (CRY-AC, Brymill Corporation) without recurrence. Three ulcerated SCC of the vulva were removed by conventional surgery. After adequate hemostasis three freeze/thaw cycles using Torre's cone-spray technique were administered to the ulcerated surface. There was no evidence of disease in the next four to six years. Three cases of recurrent Paget's disease after conventional surgery were treated with three freeze/thaw cycles also using the cone-spray technique. The patients were well after 10 years of follow-up. Six cases of adenocarcinomas of the endometrium metastasized to the lower third of the vagina were treated with acceptable palliative results (10, 59, 71–74). In these cases the combination of radiofrequency and cryosurgery was used.

In 1974, one of us (JCAG) began the treatment of advanced vulvar cancers with cryosurgery and, step by step, developed a controlled and predictable cryovulvectomy (19,22,24,30). In a book such as this one, we consider important a detailed description of surgical protocols to facilitate the work of those who want to perform the described techniques, without the benefit of personal instruction.

Cryovulvectomy is indicated for advanced cancer. A vulvar cancer is considered advanced if it is not possible to excise it by conventional surgery with adequate safety margin and/or if the metastases cannot be removed. Staging is basic to planning the treatment and to subsequently evaluating the results.

Surgical protocol (Figs. 8.26, 8.28–8.34): General or epidural anesthesia is optional. At present, protection of the tissues surrounding the cancer and its safety margin is done with a paraffinated gauze bandage, folded fifteen times, which yields a smooth and flexible "plaque" (Fig. 8.26). Three such plaques measuring about 17 cm and one measuring 10–12 cm are prepared (Fig. 8.27). The plaques are applied against the skin, on the contour of the area to be frozen and their inner limit is stitched to the skin (Fig. 8.29). The larger plaques are applied as follows: one across the middle of the pubis; two generally in the genitocrural folds, but, when needed, they are moved inward or outward, according to the size and limits of the cancer; the smaller plaque is applied transversely near the posterior vulvar commissure. The inner edges of the plaques are stitched to the skin, leaving

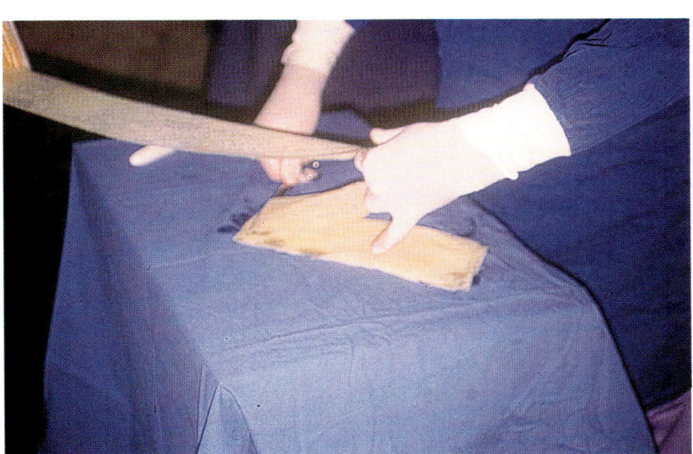

Fig. 8.26. A paraffinated bandage is folded to create a flexible "plaque"

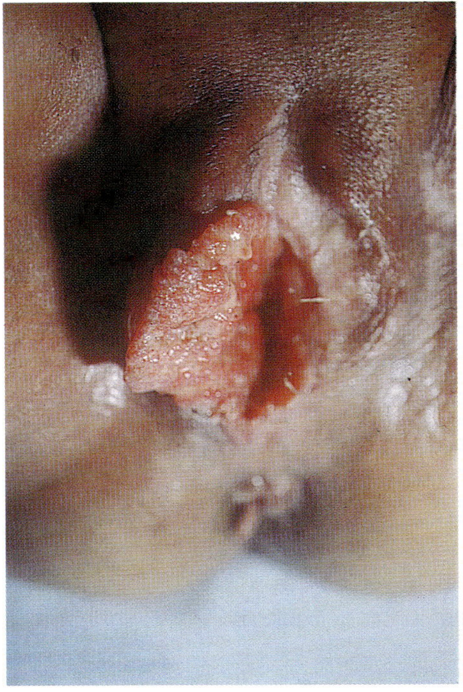

Fig. 8.28. Inoperable SCC of the vulva (illustration of protocol – Figs. 8.28–8.34)

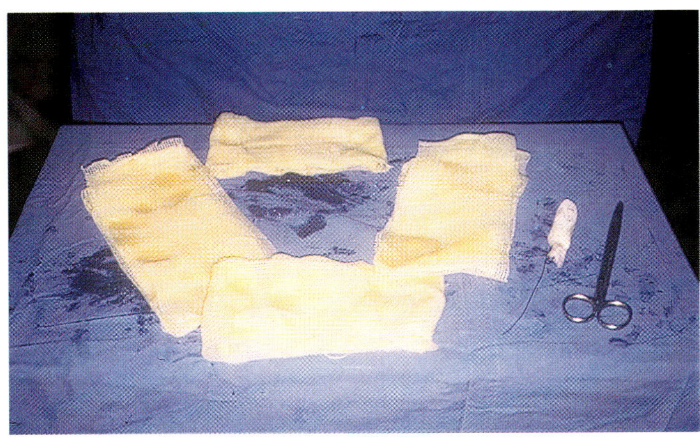

Fig. 8.27. Four such "plaques", three measuring about 17 cm and one between 10 and 12 cm are prepared for the treatment of vulvar cancer

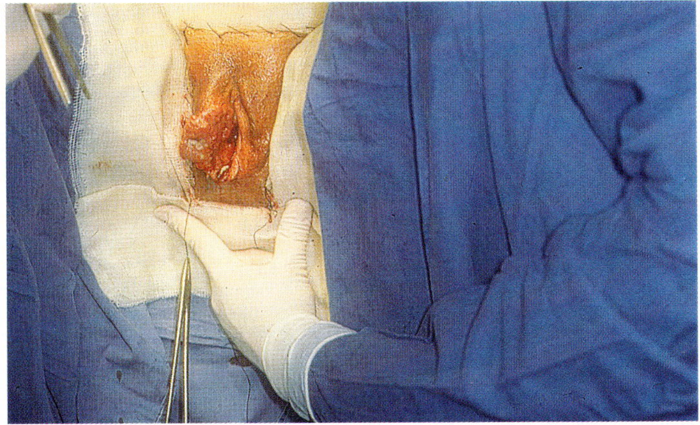

Fig. 8.29. The paraffinated folded bandages are stitched around the cancer and safety margin

exposed the target – the cancer and its safety margin. This provides a predictable and accurate limit of the freezing. Tissue temperature is monitored by 8–12 thermocouples, whose location is important (Fig. 8.30). They must be strategically placed, one against the pubic symphysis to prevent excessive local destruction. The others are placed inside the tumor. The extremities of the thermocouples must be inserted between 3 cm and 4 cm below the surface of the tumor. Their placement must be carefully chosen, so as to permit mental estimation of the shape and size of the ice ball at any moment of the procedure. Their actual placement will differ in each individual case, according to the shape, dimension and architecture of the tumor. Cahan stressed the importance of "thinking in three dimensions" and of anticipating inadvertent damage to vital neighboring organs (7). The aim is to create conditions to check the freezing progress, control the low temperatures inside the cancer and prevent excessive destruction. Freezing is achieved with a continuous open thick spray of liquid nitrogen from a high-pressure apparatus (Frigitronics CE-4). When beginning the freezing, one point of the neoplasm is selected and the spray is persistently applied thereon, until an ice ball forms and its inner temperature falls to −60°C to −80°C. The contour of the ice ball is then slowly and progressively widened to encompass the entire vulvar region and the lower half of the pubis. These details are essential to obtain fast and efficient freezing. It would be an error to direct the spray over the entire exposed area, because this would result only in superficial cooling, which is completely ineffective. The tumoral mass must attain temperatures between −50°C and −80°C, but the temperature of the thermocouple adjoining the pubic bone must not go below −15°C to prevent its exposure after removal of the necrotic tissue. To complete the freezing, 30 to 45 minutes are necessary. The region is permitted slow natural thawing, after which a second freeze-thaw cycle is carried out. To begin the second freezing, another point is chosen to prevent the repetition of any strategic mistake that may have been made in the course of the first freezing. After the second thawing, lymphadenectomy is performed, during the same surgical procedure, if feasible. On the following day, the whole area is dark violet and on the contour there are second-degree burn blisters, which should be punctured. In a few more days the region will turn black. About three weeks later, the skin is mummified and there will be a sulcus in the contour, demarcating the necrotic tissues from the normal looking ones. The necrotic tissues are removed around three weeks later and the wound is allowed to heal by second intention. Complete local healing occurs between 9 and 12 weeks. The resulting scar is smooth, painless and without hypertrophy (Figs. 8.26–8.34).

JCAG treated 115 such patients whose ages varied between 37 and 96 years, but who were

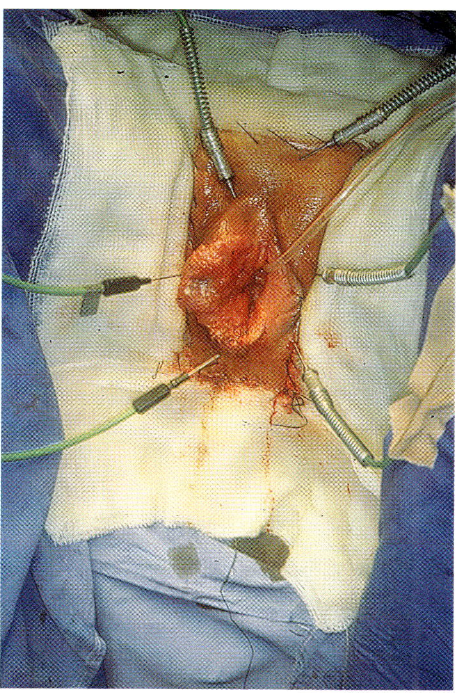

Fig. 8.30. The inserted thermocouples

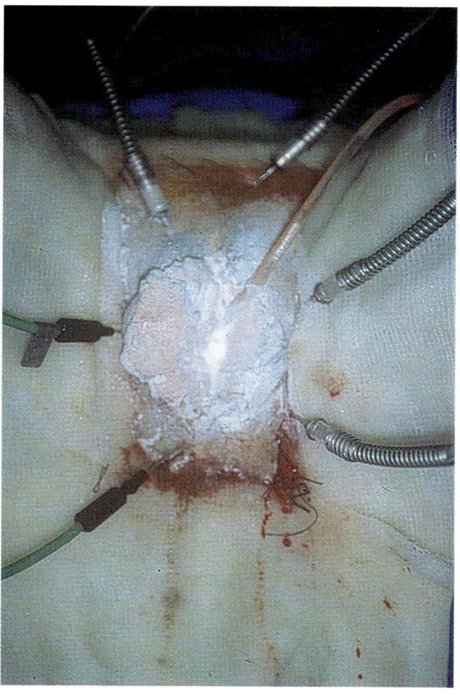

Fig. 8.31. Immediately after freezing

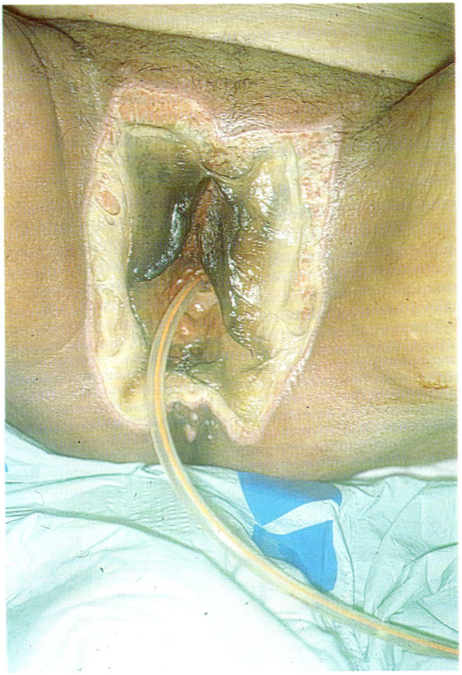

Fig. 8.32. Three weeks later, there was a sulcus around the necrotic tissue

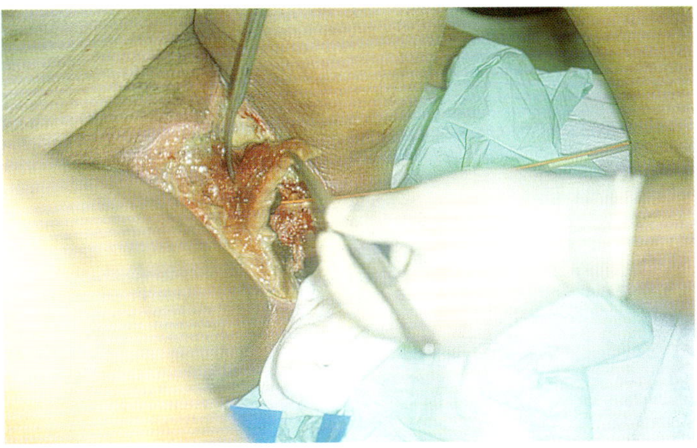

Fig. 8.33. The necrotic tissue was easily and painlessly removed

mostly in their sixties and seventies. The criterion to accept them for cryovulvectomy was the difficulty or impossibility of operating with conventional surgery. The time of evolution of the tumors was between some months and more than six years. Eighty cancers were primary and 35 were recurrent. All the cancers were classified according to the FIGO classification. However, since this is applicable only to primary cases, a difficulty arose. In order to assess the results it was necessary to have homogeneous groups. Thus, he decided to classify the 35 recurrent cases in equivalent "phases", using criteria similar to those established by the FIGO classification for primary cancers. The FIGO classification does not apply to melanoma. The sole case of melanoma was advanced and invasive. For the purpose of staging it was considered equivalent to stage IV of the vulvar carcinoma.

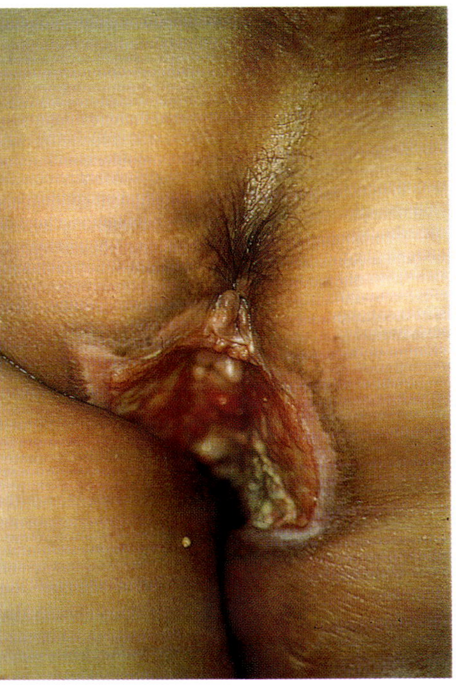

Fig. 8.34. Nine months after cryosurgery. It would have been impossible to surgically remove this primary vulvar SCC without resection of the anus

Histological examination showed 111 squamous cell carcinomas, two adenocarcinomas, one Paget's disease and one nodular and invasive melanoma. Thirty-seven patients (32.2%) presented in stage IV and for these only palliative treatment was performed, which was successful as such. Only 9 patients (7.8%) were in Stage II, and were admitted to cryosurgery, because the tumors were near either the urethral meatus or the anus and it was not possible to surgically remove them with an adequate safety margin. The majority of patients – 69 (60%) – had stage III disease or were in an equivalent "phase" if recurrent.

When devising the cryovulvectomy technique, successive modifications had to be made, in order to prevent complications as they arose. Over time, performance improved considerably and better results were obtained. In the first years of these treatments, 24% of the patients had two, rarely more, cryosurgical procedures. This was reduced when more experience was acquired. There were complications in 22 patients, some of which were due to early lack of experience but contributed to the construction of an improved surgical protocol: exposure of the pubic bone in two cases with necrosis in one, when the thermocouple was not applied against the pubic symphysis; destruction of the perianal region with definitive incontinence; deep burning of the skin of the buttocks due to inadequate perilesional protection; urethral stenosis due to early removal of the catheter; and one case of lethal embolism.

This last-mentioned case is here described in detail to alert fellow cryosurgeons to such accidents. A palliative cryovulvectomy was carried out in a patient with a $T_3N_3M_{1a}$, stage IV, but in good general health. After removal of the necrotic tissue a persistent tumor 3 cm in diameter was observed in the middle of the cryosurgical ulceration. In a Stage III case, a second thorough cryosurgery would have been done, but, in this hopeless case, it was decided to carry out only a tumorectomy to limit surgical aggression. The technique chosen was freezing of the persistent tumor, using the close spray, inside a Torre cone. The first freezing seemed uneventful but, at the beginning of the second procedure, the patient suddenly died. Necropsy showed that death was due to embolism. The conclusion we drew is that Torre cones are good for short freezing of skin tumors with integral skin, but should not be used in long cryosurgical procedures on ulcerated and undermined tumors. It is also preferable not to use them with high-pressure apparatuses. In two cases, the necrotic tissues were removed by electrocutting, intending to hasten their elimination. This proved to have serious consequences. Instead of the usual thin, pliable and painless skin, a hard, irregular and painful scar resulted.

Other complications were unavoidable and can occur again: profuse hemorrhage in 2 cases; rectovaginal fistula in two patients where the cancer invaded the posterior aspect of the vagina; fecal incontinence in two cases where there was deep invasion of the anus; urinary incontinence in 2 cases where there was extensive invasion of the urethra; transient urinary incontinence in 3 cases; abscess in one case; prolapse of the bladder in one; and one case of lethal sepsis. Besides the mentioned deaths, there were two more intra-operative deaths due to cardiac failure in elderly patients. Cryovulvectomy was well tolerated in the remaining patients. A common consequence of cryovulvectomy was cicatricial stenosis of the introitus. Only two patients accepted the suggested plastic correction, which was successful. The advanced age of the patients accounts for the easy acceptance of this occurrence.

None of the patients complained of pain after the operation, but most referred to a tolerable burning sensation during the three postoperative hours, which was easily controlled with mild analgesics. The preoperative pain and discomfort completely ceased after cryovulvectomy, even in patients that were treated palliatively. The complete removal of the necrotic tissues – between 3 and 4 weeks later – depended on their individualization and demarcation. This also applied to the time required for healing – between 9 and 12 weeks. Patients with good hygienic conditions at home can leave the hospital during the fourth or fifth week postoperatively. During the first few weeks after the operation the exudate is enormous. We tried many types of dressing. Experience showed that the best one was a diaper indicated for incontinent people.

Clinical cure was obtained in 47.4% of cancers in stages II and III but in 66% in combination with local irradiation. The difference in percentage was due to metastases. The mortality rate was 1.66%, while with radiotherapy, chemotherapy and surgery it is 7% (30), and many patients suffer continuous pain due to radiodermatitis after radiation. Patients in stage IV received palliative treatment. All pain and discomfort disappeared but, obviously, survival was short (mean of 4 months; range 1–15 months) (Figs. 8.35–8.40).

JCAG's formal training is not that of a general surgeon and, during the first years of the deve-

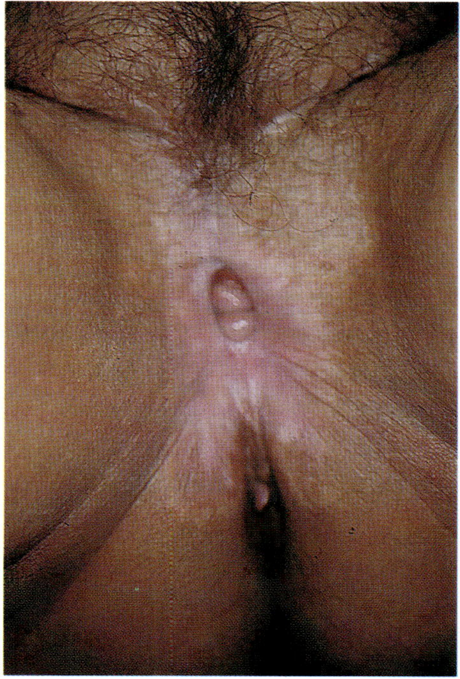

Fig. 8.35. Same patient, four months later. Treatment eradicated the cancer and did not cause incontinence. She was well five years after treatment

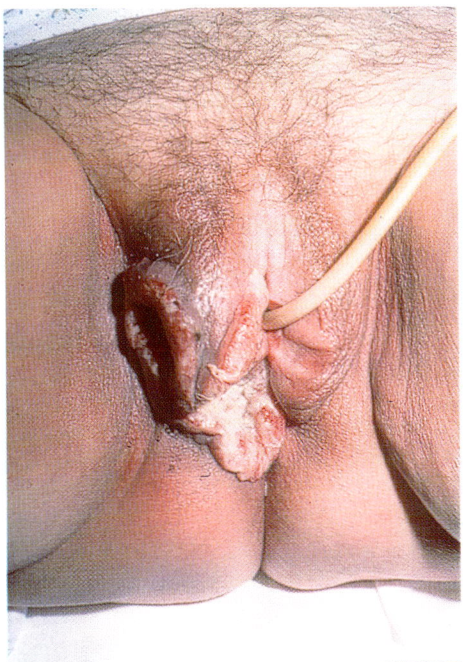

Fig. 8.36. This inoperable SCC had a very unusual architecture

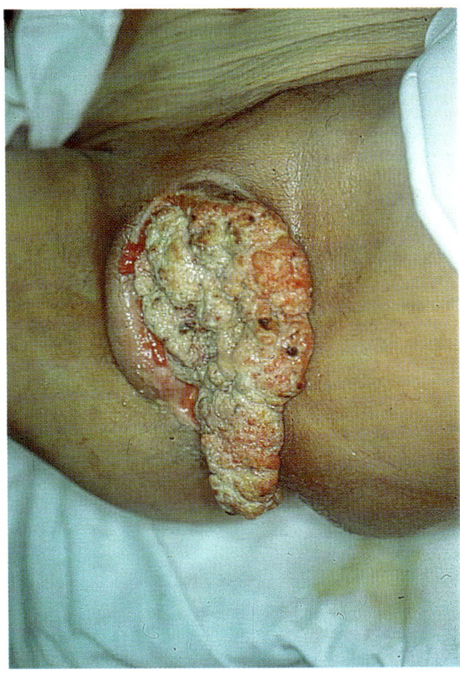

Fig. 8.38. This stage IV SCC invaded the pelvis and was adherent to regional ganglia

lopment of his cryovulvectomy technique, most lymphadenectomies of his patients were performed by one of the two departments of surgery of the Portuguese Institute of Oncology. It is not unusual for therapeutic teams involving different specialities to have some difficulties in their personal and work relationships. In those first years, he had considerable difficulty in obtaining early lymphadenectomies from one of the departments. In 44/69 of those early patients, lymphadenectomy was performed between 2 and 4 months after cryovulvectomy, and in 6 cases the interval was even between 5 and 14 months. Only in 25 cases was it carried out within one month. With a better collaboration from one of the surgical departments the results would have been much better. Only in the last 17 years has he succeeded in obtaining prompt collaboration from the surgeons, and

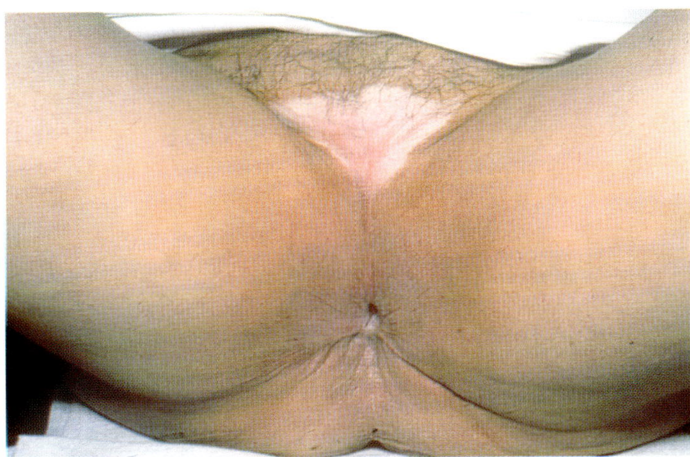

Fig. 8.37. Same patient, three years post cryosurgery

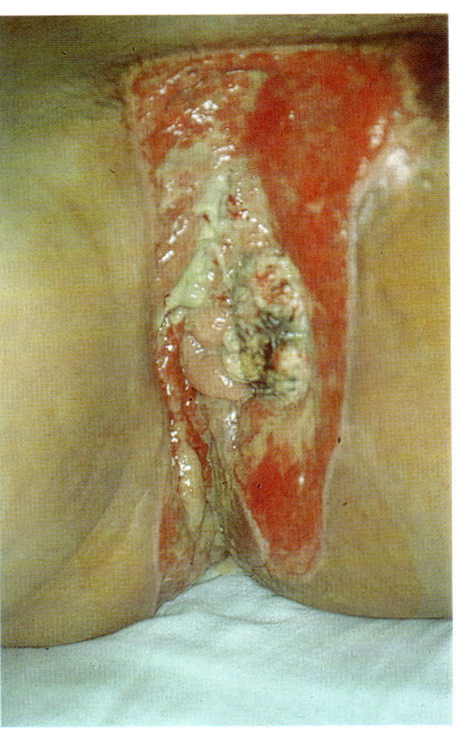

Fig. 8.39. Same patient: palliation was achieved as intended

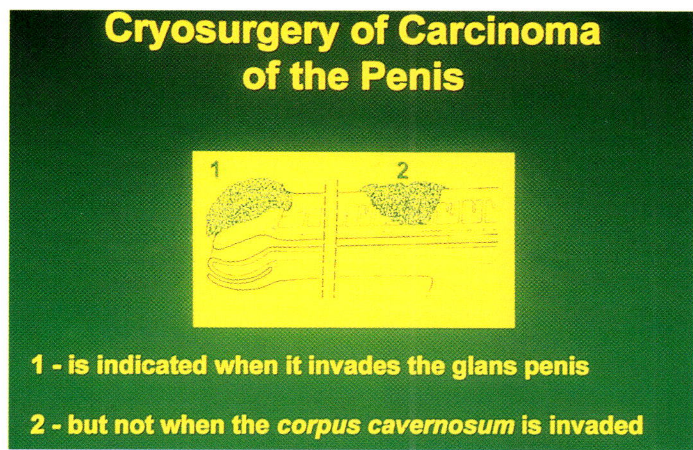

Fig. 8.40. Schematic drawing of the T_2 penile SCC (TNM, UICC, 1999)

cryovulvectomy and lymphadenectomy – when feasible – have been carried out at the same time, with obvious therapeutic advantage. In 19 patients with stages II and III disease, where lymphadenectomy was delayed, 11 were clinically cured (57.9%), in eight patients who had simultaneous lymphadenectomy five had no evidence of disease (62.5%). The difference is not statistically significant, but we consider that timely lymphadenectomy is fundamental in the treatment of vulvar cancer. Many patients have lost their lives due to delayed lymphadenectomy or, in a few cases, to their own refusal to submit to the procedure (22, 30). It is interesting to note that, in the last few years, the number of cryovulvectomies has diminished considerably, because patients present in earlier stages of the disease.

One frequent error in conventional surgery is removing advanced cancers with insufficient safety margins, which should be at least 2 cm outside the apparent limit. In cases where this safety margin cannot be implemented, cryovulvectomy gives better results.

8.6 Cryosurgery of Invasive Penile Cancer

The most frequent treatment for invasive carcinoma involving the glans penis – generally a squamous cell carcinoma – is radical or partial amputation (2,55). Among the therapeutic modalities of conservative treatment for this cancer is cryosurgery. To our knowledge, the first such treatment was performed by P.S.H. Hughes who in 1979 treated two cases of verrucous carcinoma of the penis, with debulking by electrocutting followed by cryosurgery with liquid nitrogen spray and thermocouple monitoring. Both patients were well one year after cryosurgery. One of them was young and the sexual function was preserved (39). In 1982, G. Madej and J. Meyza treated 15 patients with either superficial invasion of the subcutaneous tissues or invasion of the glans penis-corpus spongiosum, measuring between 2 cm and 5 cm. They used contact with a cryoprobe covering the whole surface of the lesion and froze twice for three minutes. All patients were cured, with urinary and sexual functions maintained (52). In the two following years, B. P. Matveev and collaborators published papers in Russian, to which we have no access. They sometimes combined cryosurgery and chemotherapy (54). G. Castro-Ron in 1989 presented in a cryosurgical workshop at Durham five cases successfully treated with the cryoprobe technique. Three tumors were small, one was medium-sized and one was large. Considerable edema developed, but no catheterization was needed. Turjansky and Stolar used a quite different protocol. They excised the cancer with radiofrequency and carried out three freeze/thaw cycles with close spray of liquid nitrogen inside Torre's cones, between 120 and 180 seconds. They treated 12 patients with four recurrences (72).

One of us (JCAG) treated 13 cases of invasive squamous cell carcinoma of the penis, between 1993 and 2000, but at the time of writing only 10 have acceptably long follow-up. Cryosurgery with curative purpose is indicated when the cancer invades the glans penis but not the corpus cavernosum (Fig. 8.40). Therefore, accurate staging of the primary tumor is important and the clinical examination must now be supported by ultrasonography and magnetic resonance imaging.

The *surgical protocol* (Figs. 8.41–8.44) is as follows: Anesthesia is general or regional. The former is used when lymphadenectomy is carried out at the same time. The shape and size of the prepuce is clinically assessed. If the risk of phimosis is foreseeable, due to the edema after cryosurgery, prior circumcision is performed. Catheterization is usually done, which is indispensable when the meatus is to be frozen. When the tumor is too thick debulking can be done. The cryoprobe technique is used. One probe of adequate size is chosen and a hydrophilic gel (K-Y Jelly®, Johnson and Johnson) is applied between the tumor and the probe. If possible, the progression of freezing should be controlled by ultrasound. A safety margin of at least one centimeter is advisable. The criterion for lymphadenectomy is that accepted in urologic oncology (2,55). On the following day, considerable edema develops (Figs. 8.43 and see *Atlas of Cryosurgery*, 2001).

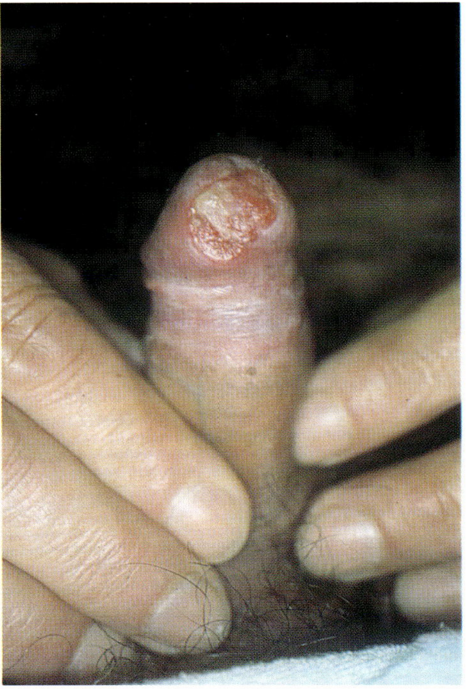

Fig. 8.41. SCC of the glans penis

Ten uncircumcised patients with penile cancer treated cryosurgically are analyzed herein. Nine cancers were primary and one was recurrent. The age of the patients ranged between 44 and 83 years (mean 64.7 years). The time of evolution of the disease was between five months and six years

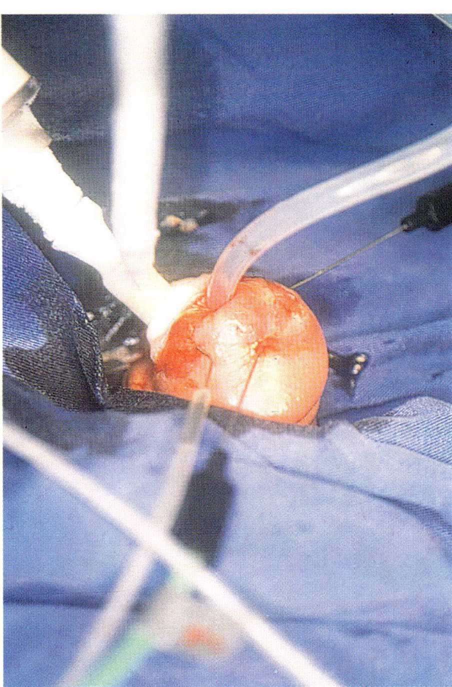

Fig. 8.42. Same patient, during cryosurgery, under thermocouple monitoring

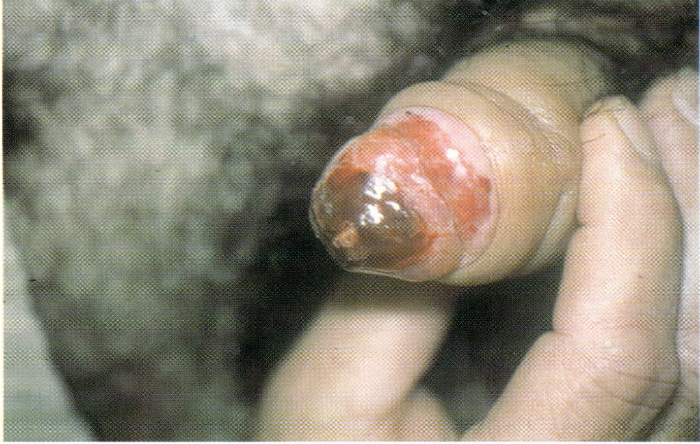

Fig. 8.43. Same patient, three days after cryosurgery

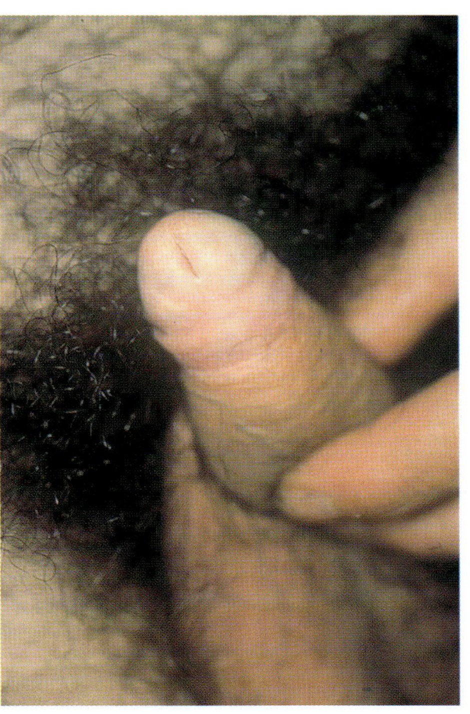

Fig. 8.44. Same patient, after healing

(mean 19 months). Major axes varied between 10 mm and 41 mm (mean 26.4 mm). The histological diagnosis was: nine SCCs – five of which accompanied by lichen sclerosus – and one verrucous carcinoma (tumor of Buschke-Löwenstein). Eight patients were submitted to a single cryosurgical procedure, one patient underwent two and the remaining patient underwent three. Only one cancer was debulked. In five patients, lymphadenectomy was carried out at the same time. Five patients were cured and had no evidence of disease for between two and five years. One had three small local recurrences, always treated by

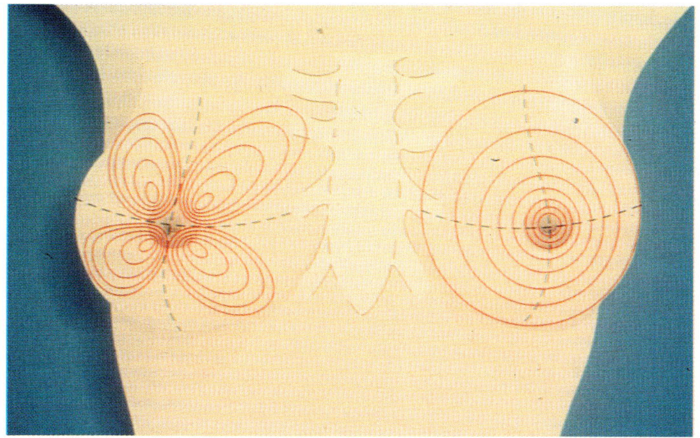

Fig. 8.45. Schematic drawing of "four eggs" freezing technique, of the right breast. On the left is shown what must not be done. Application of the spray over the mammary areola would create a central and superficial snow ball that would make it impossible to freeze the whole breast. (Illustration of protocol – Figs. 8.46–8.49)

cryosurgery. At the time of writing, he is well, two years after the last cryosurgical procedure. One patient who suffered from an SCC, measuring 30 mm × 20 mm, after cicatrization had a small persistence of the tumor at the posterior limit of the glans penis. It was removed by conventional surgery and there is no evidence of disease after three years. One patient who also suffered from lichen sclerosus had either a new local cancer or a recurrent one after five years of apparent cure. In fact, we could not decide between the two, because after this period it could be a new cancer originating from the persistent lichen sclerosus. He underwent another cryosurgical procedure and there is no evidence of disease at the time of writing, after three years of follow-up. One patient abandoned the outpatient clinic and only returned two years later, with a large local recurrence that required amputation. One patient abandoned our department, had successive recurrences and was treated elsewhere, and eventually died nine years post cryosurgery.

In summary: eight patients apparently cured with maintained physiological function, one underwent amputation and one died.

The treatment of superficial penile neoplasms is analogous to similar skin situations and is not referred to in this chapter (2, 55, 58, 71).

The usual treatment of invading SCC of the penis – total or partial amputation – causes considerable psychological suffering and despair. Amputation can be prevented by cryosurgery in many cases, with maintained functional performance. Nevertheless, this is an aggressive and dangerous cancer with a high mortality rate. Staging is essential and the established criteria for cryosurgery must be strictly observed.

8.7 Cryosurgery of Advanced Breast Cancer

Advanced breast cancer causes enormous suffering, tremendous physical discomfort and unbearable anxiety, particularly when the tumor becomes ulcerated and fungating. As a rule, it is very vascular, hence causing abundant capillary exudation, or severe hemorrhage, often difficult to control. Even the ordinary procedure of changing the dressing is a common cause for hemorrhaging. The repeated chronic or acute blood loss often results in moderate to severe anemia. Some cancers attain very large volume. Due to fast growth and to poor local vascularization, necrosis occurs which, combined with bacterial invasion, causes repellent odor that can be so intensely offensive as to become intolerable to relatives and friends. Pain is not a frequent symptom and appears only when deep invasion occurs. As the patient's general condition deteriorates – anorexia and malnutrition having added to the morbid process – she feels increasingly miserable. In many cases, this situation can go on for months.

Conventional surgery and/or radiotherapy are of limited value in advanced local disease and result in high recurrence rates. Chemotherapy is used to complement the local treatment but its value is reduced in advanced breast cancers and has considerable morbidity. When the tumor develops resistance to them, these treatments are no longer useful, frequently contributing to an increase in the patient's suffering.

Among many advanced external cancers cryosurgically treated by Cahan, four were massive recurrent breast cancers (6,7), three of which with good palliative results: the patients' quality of life was improved, due to reduction of the tumoral mass and pain, the disappearance of the fetid odor and of the anemia, although their lives were not prolonged (6); a fourth patient with inoperable breast cancer was treated according to a different protocol. A simple mastectomy by conventional surgery was carried out; the resulting ulceration was treated by cryosurgery with contact probes during the same operation. Some ribs were exposed but clean granulation tissue developed which subsequently accepted a skin graft. The patient died eight months later. The text does not indicate whether there was local recurrence or whether she died from metastatic disease.

Lloyd-Williams also treated advanced breast cancers with good palliative results but unfortunately there are no detailed reports of his cases and of his protocol.

The best known contribution of Patrick Le Pivert to cryosurgery was the invention of bioelectrical low frequency impedance to control the freezing and destruction of cancerous tissues (47–49). But he also created many important techniques for various morbid conditions and treated seven inoperable breast cancers, five in stage III and two in stage IV, with good palliative results (46). His protocol was as follows: After measuring the tumor and delimiting its contour, he divided the tumoral mass into various zones. He introduced one or more electrodes into each zone, some superficially and some deeply. Each zone was successively frozen until an impedance value between 1 and 2 Mega Ohms was obtained, which he had already proved to correspond to cryodestruction. In some cases, the impedance monitoring was supplemented by thermocouple control. The frozen areas were overlapped. After freezing, all the neoplastic tissue was permitted to thaw. Le Pivert carried out two variants of this cryosurgical protocol: one was scalpel surgery immediately followed by cryosurgery (similarly to what Cahan did in the treatment of one case); the other consisted of two cryosurgical procedures, at 3-week intervals. Taking into account the advanced oncological stages, the results were very good: one patient was clinically cured 13 months post treatment and five were alive and well 6 months after the operation.

Shigeo Tanaka did remarkable research on the applications of cryosurgery, in general, in dermatological surgery, on cryoimmunology and on the treatment of advanced cancers by cryosurgery (60–69). The majority of the 424 cancers he treated, until 1995, were advanced. Among them, there were 49 breast cancers – 9 primary and 40 recurrent (68). His surgical protocol was carefully described (68). He generally uses either thermocouples or impedance – in some cases both – achieving tissue temperatures down to at least −50°C to 60°C, or tissue impedance of 500 kΩ (68), and carries out three or more freeze-thaw cycles. He frequently combines liquid nitrogen spray and contact with large probes (60, 62, 63, 68). The surgical protocol varies according to the volume and shape of the cancer. In bulky tumors he uses penetrating probes. He controls the bleeding with oxycellulose cotton and/or coagulant agents. The skin around the tumor is protected with a Vaseline embankment and the frozen areas are overlapping. Necrotomy is carried out 3 weeks later with minimal bleeding and without any pain. His results are satisfactory, taking into account the advanced stage of the disease and the debilitated condition of the patients: the volume of the cancer was always reduced, the foul smell disappeared and the quality of life was considerably improved. Some cures were achieved. Six months after cryosurgery of one advanced, unresectable primary breast cancer, the patient died of pneumonia-like symptoms. The autopsy revealed no remnants either of the tumor or of metastases (66). A very important case of carcinoma erysipelatodes of the breast was described. There were inflammatory skin metastases, widely and rapidly spreading, treated by liquid nitrogen spray. The patient was saved. For this latter case, there was very probably no other feasible treatment (66). The complications mentioned were pleural effusion in some cases and one case of transient renal failure (66). The survival in nine primary cancers was 61.0% and the recurrence cases were 44.4% over three and five years. Lately he has developed a new modality of anticancer treatment: *cryochemotherapy*. Before cryosurgery he introduces an anti-neoplastic agent, such as Mitomycin-C, which is administered inside the breast cancer, in adjacent areas or intravenously, either during the operation or shortly after (67). Results of this new method are still unknown to us.

Gage treated one large, recurrent, fungating and ulcerated breast cancer in successive sessions with cryoprobe contact until control of the tumor bulk was achieved (13).

J. Zaloudík and collaborators treated 23 advanced breast cancers with a cryosurgical apparatus that permits the simultaneous introduction of many cryoprobes and that has a very high capability to remove heat (KCH 5000, Special Medical Technology Co. Ltd.). They freeze 2–3 cm of neoplastic tissue in depth, with necrotomy a few days later. With such repeated debulkings they succeed in destroying even bulky and exophytic cancers. They have obtained survivals of more than three years (77).

In 1987, one of us (JCAG) published his personal technique of carrying out an actual mastectomy by cryosurgery and called it *cryomastectomy* (16, 18, 27). The present *surgical protocol* (Figs. 8.46–8.55) is herein described in detail: The patient is given general anesthesia. The homolateral arm must not be placed along the body, in order to prevent accidental freezing of its skin. Currently, the protection of the tissues surrounding the breast cancer and its safety margin is accomplished with paraffinated gauze bandages folded fifteen times, which creates a smooth and flexible "plaque"

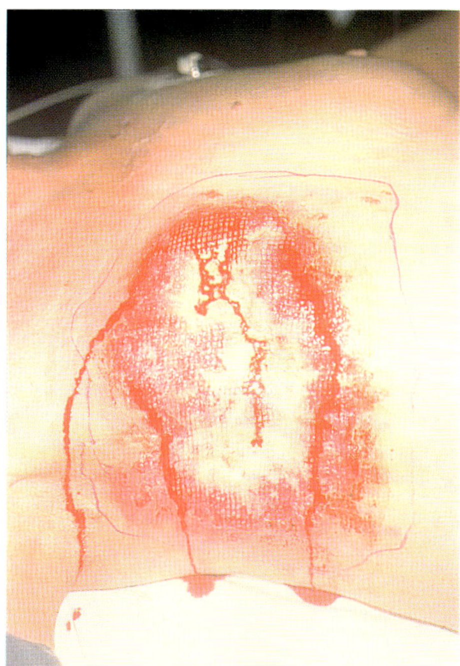

Fig. 8.46. Prior to the operation, the contour of the target – cancer plus safety margin – is marked with ink

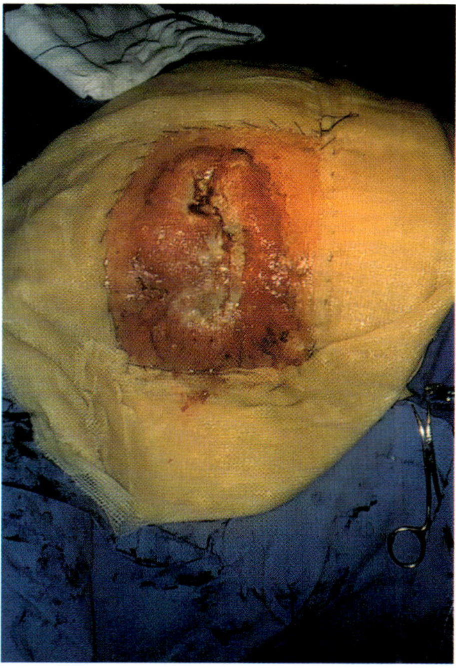

Fig. 8.47. The "plaques" made with folded paraffinated bandages were stitched onto the edges of the target

(Figs. 8.26, 8.47). Depending on the size and shape of the cancer two or more such "plaques", long enough to surround the extent of the area to be frozen, are prepared and applied against the skin. Their inner edges are stitched to the skin (Fig. 8.47). Most advanced breast cancers are bulky and at first evaluation it does not seem easy, or even

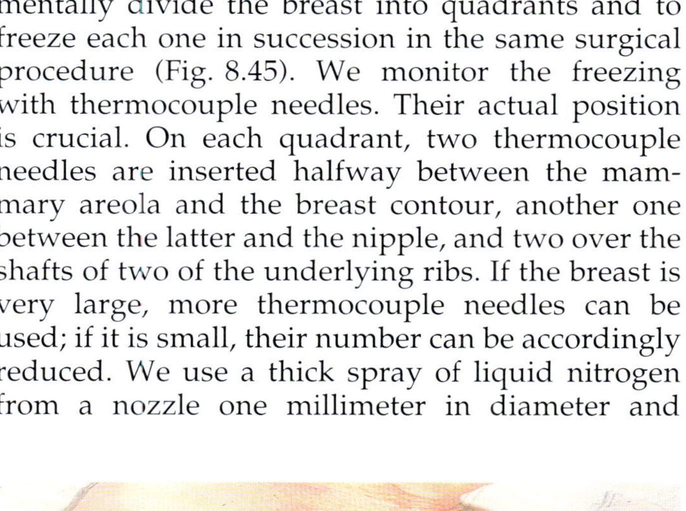

possible, to thoroughly freeze the entire mass. The strategy devised to deal with this difficulty is to mentally divide the breast into quadrants and to freeze each one in succession in the same surgical procedure (Fig. 8.45). We monitor the freezing with thermocouple needles. Their actual position is crucial. On each quadrant, two thermocouple needles are inserted halfway between the mammary areola and the breast contour, another one between the latter and the nipple, and two over the shafts of two of the underlying ribs. If the breast is very large, more thermocouple needles can be used; if it is small, their number can be accordingly reduced. We use a thick spray of liquid nitrogen from a nozzle one millimeter in diameter and

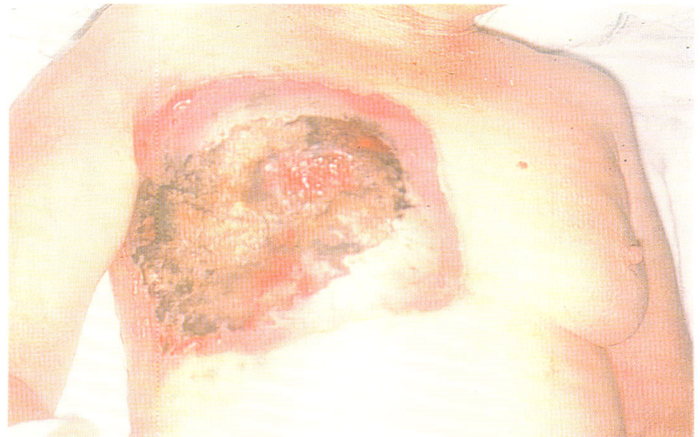

Fig. 8.48. The limitation of the freezing was accurate

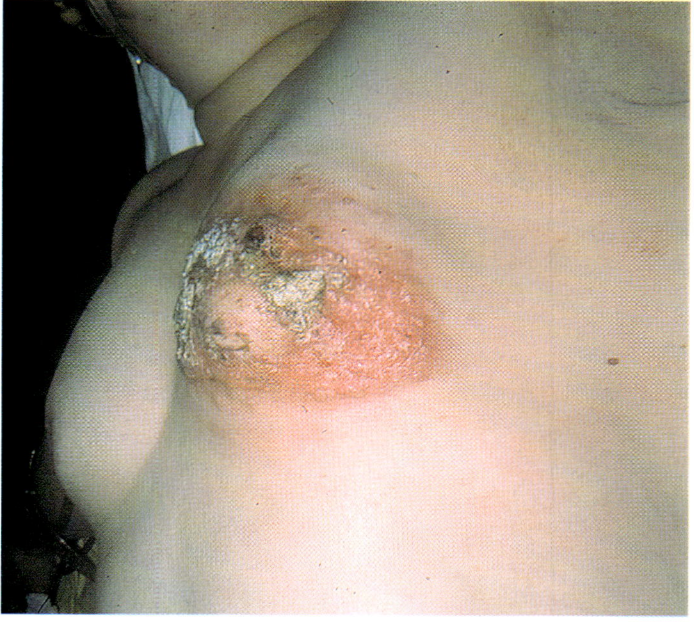

Fig. 8.49. Persistent irradiated breast cancer

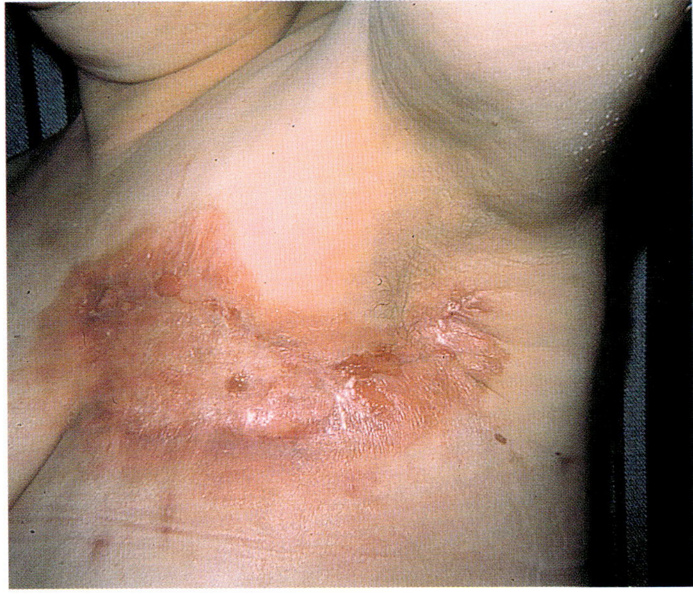

Fig. 8.50. Same patient: clean ulceration after removal of the necrotic tissue

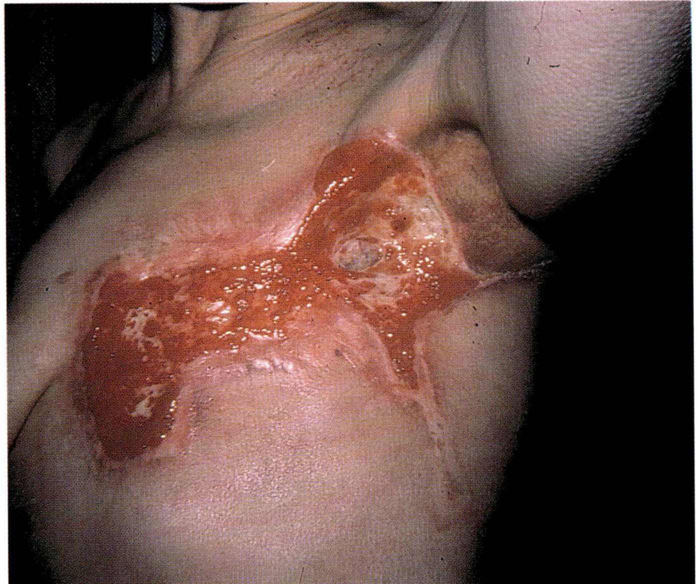

Fig. 8.52. Same patient: after removal of the necrotic tissue resulting from cryosurgery

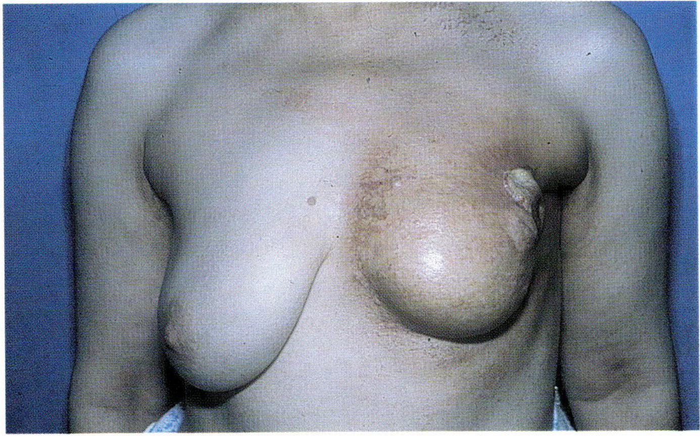

Fig. 8.51. Ulcerated breast cancer, post irradiation and chemotherapy

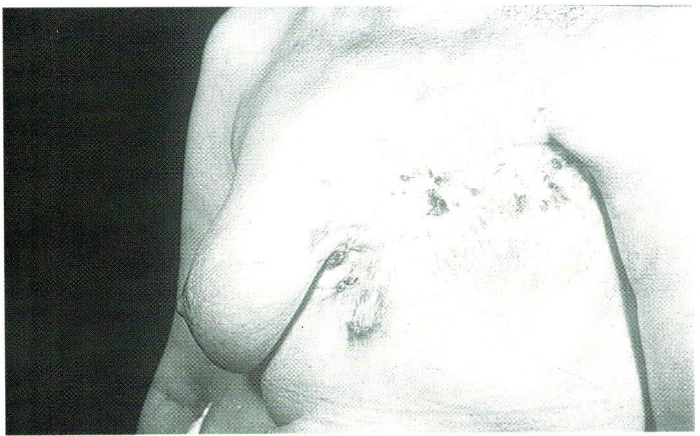

Fig. 8.53. Same patient: after healing, small neoplastic nodules kept appearing around the scar, which were treated with probe contact cryosurgery. The patient survived 6 years

high-pressure equipment (Frigitronics CE-4). Each quadrant is frozen in its turn. The aim of the freezing is to produce, inside each quadrant, an egg-shaped frozen mass with cancericidal temperature within. One point is selected – radially, in the middle of the quadrant and, longitudinally, at the boundary of the inner and the middle thirds of the breast – on which the spray is persistently applied until an ice ball has formed and the temperature has dropped below −50°C, if possible to −70°C. The ice ball is then enlarged, in width and in depth, taking on the intended ovoid shape, always within the same quadrant. This cooling technique is essential and it would be an error to scatter the spray over the whole breast, or even the quadrant, for that would result in slow and superficial cooling which is completely ineffective. During the entire procedure, the cryosurgeon must continuously estimate the three-dimensional shape of the changing mass of the frozen tissues, which must not include the ribs. Thermocouple temperatures must be closely monitored at all times and the temperature over the rib's shaft must not be permitted to go below −12°C. The shaft is very sensitive to freezing and would shatter if frozen, in contrast with compact bones that are very resistant to freezing. When the freezing of the fourth "egg" is concluded, the temperature of the remaining quadrants has meanwhile risen, and the cryosurgery continues until the desired temperature is again obtained. The four frozen volumes of tissue

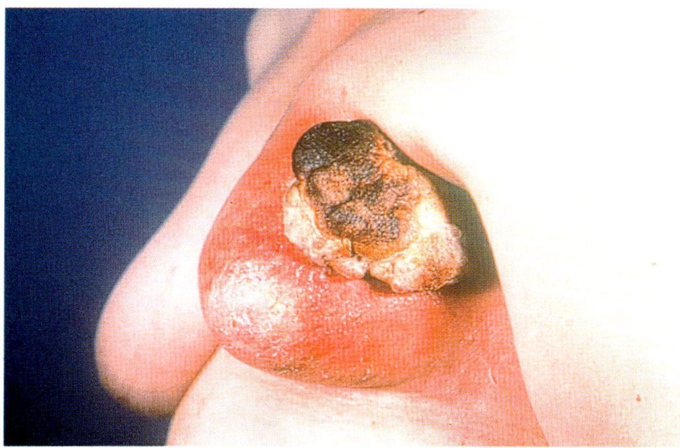

Fig. 8.54. Persistent cancer post chemotherapy and post irradiation

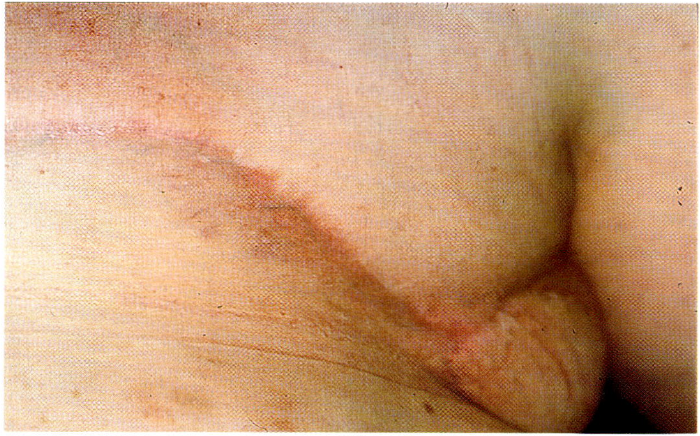

Fig. 8.55. Same patient: the scar after cryosurgery was remarkably similar to one resulting from conventional surgery

have contact with one another, and themselves act as sources of cold, lowering the temperature of the tissues under and among them, so that when spraying is discontinued, the frozen mass goes on modifying its shape until temperature equilibrium is attained. After some time, the entire tumoral mass tends to achieve the same temperature. A real danger with these heat exchanges among tissues with different temperatures is the spreading of the frozen tissue to the base of the breast, so as to include the thoracic wall. It is necessary to dynamically understand this process and to anticipate the dropping of the temperatures on the ribs' surface, before they reach the limit of −12°C. This can be prevented by slowing the freezing when the thermocouples over the ribs register around 0°C, and by discontinuing the freezing before it reaches that limit. Freezing among the bases of the four "eggs" creates a concave frozen surface, in conformity with the shape of the thoracic wall.

The cryosurgical procedure for the first freezing of the whole breast is time-consuming and depends on its size and histological structure – fibrotic areas freeze more slowly. The average freezing time is 45 minutes. In our experience the minimum time was 35 minutes and the maximum 60 minutes. When freezing of the entire breast has been achieved, slow thawing can begin. Generally, complete thawing requires 60–75 minutes. Beginners can be impatient and initiate the second freeze-thaw cycle before thawing is completed. This must not be done. The cancericidal effect of complete thawing is important and the second freezing enhances cellular death if it begins after complete thawing of the previous cycle. A second freezing is carried out, in the same manner, but starting in a different quadrant and following the opposite direction, in order to avoid any strategic error that may have been made in the course of the first freezing. This freezing, generally, takes half the time that was necessary for the first one, due to the vascular damage that resulted from the initial freeze-thaw cycle. The thermocouple needles can only be removed after the second thawing is completed. The total time for the whole surgical procedure, with the 2 freeze-thaw cycles, is between 3 and 4 hours. The same technique applies to recurrent cancers in patients who previously underwent mastectomy by conventional surgery, but the protocol must be individually adapted to the architecture and location of the recurrence.

Absorbent dressing is required and, since there will be abundant exudation in the days following cryosurgery, it must be changed as often as necessary, at least every 12 hours, but sometimes every six hours. Necrotic tissues are removed one week post treatment, with scissors, without any pain or need for analgesia. When the cancer has a fungating part, this can be removed 4–5 days later, thus considerably diminishing the fetid smell; however, the remaining tissue is excised only at the end of one week, when all arteries are thrombosed. Once all the necrotic mass is removed, and if there are no specific contraindications, the patient may be discharged and have the dressings changed in the outpatient clinic. The resulting ulceration heals by second intention, in 8 to 12 weeks, leaving an acceptable scar.

Thirty patients were treated (13 by JCAG, 16 by JAA, and a patient with bilateral breast cancer had one tumor treated by each one of us). Their mean age was 57.2 years (range 23–83 years). The duration of disease was between 1 and 34 years. Three tumors were primary and 27 were recurrent or persistent after other therapeutic modalities before referral. Histologically, the tumors were ductal infiltrating carcinoma (24), lobular carcinoma (3), mucous carcinoma (1), squamous cell carcinoma (1) and one unclassified. Two cancers were primary, four were recurrences after conventional surgery and the remaining recurred after radiotherapy and/or chemotherapy. In one patient, the tumor was bilateral. The tumors were all locally advanced and unsuitable for any other therapeutic approach. Four patients had confirmed ganglionic metastases and one patient had distant metastases. The younger patient was a Black African woman who suffered from a primary inoperable cancer. Prevailing symptoms were large ulcerative tumors with offensive smell and frequent hemorrhage (Figs. 8.50–8.56).

In 15/30 patients, local eradication was achieved. Five patients (16.6%) have no evidence of disease at the time of writing, after three to six years of follow-up. One of these had bilateral breast cancer. Interestingly, one breast was operated by JCAG and the other by JAA – no difference was discernible between the two operated sides. Subsequently, plastic surgery was done. She is without evidence of disease 4 years postoperatively. In 9 other patients a good palliative effect was obtained. One patient is alive at the time of writing but with active disease, and has been followed up for 36 months. In 15 patients the cancer either persisted or recurred. Eight died between 2 and 7 years (mean of 4 years and 9 months) later. The tumors that persisted or recurred were again treated by cryosurgery or local chemosurgery using zinc chloride paste (34), without regaining the previous volume. In the cases where recurrent nodules developed around the scar, they were successfully treated by probe contact cryosurgery, similarly to what was performed by Gill et al. who treated twenty metastatic breast cancer nodules with good results (15). The six patients who died due to metastases had a survival time of between 2 and 24 months (mean of 14.2 months).

One of our earlier patients had a very large breast, and partial debulking was made by electrocutting. Immediately after what seemed an efficient electro-coagulation, the usual cryosurgical procedure was carried out. Profuse hemorrhage occurred after thawing, requiring blood transfusions. Obviously this technique was not repeated. Very probably, if the cryosurgical procedure had been performed in another operation, the accident would not have occurred. After the cryosurgical protocol was established and experience was acquired, the difficulty of freezing a whole breast no longer arose.

The complications were: three patients who bled profusely, requiring blood transfusions; both cryosurgeons (JCAG and JAA) had one case each of exposed and broken ribs at the beginning of their respective activities; one case of pleural effusion; and one case of moderate post-operative pain. The two patients with exposed and broken ribs healed easily with fibrosis and without local recurrence. Both died of metastatic disease 15 months and 7 years later, respectively. Exposure of the thoracic wall and the breaking of ribs can be a serious complication.

In order to carry out an effective cryomastectomy, a good cryosurgical technique and skill in the treatment of massive cancers is required, similar to that of a general surgeon when performing major conventional surgery. Cryomastectomy is not for beginners and is much more difficult to perform than cryovulvectomy. When performing the latter, one has a strong "temperature resistance", due to the fact that the vulva is highly irrigated. The danger of freezing adjoining structures is reduced, if one proceeds cautiously and accurately. Conversely, the breast is less irrigated and colder, thus the limit of freezing is more difficult to control. Moreover, the breast's anatomical site, over the convex surface of the thorax, adds to the difficulty. If an adequate cryosurgical protocol (this or any other) is not carefully followed, the thorax wall may inadvertently be included in the frozen tissues, which in some cases can cause pneumothorax. Another risk is anaplastic conversion after cryosurgery, noted by some authors, which is rare and usually caused by insufficient freezing. This did not happen in any of our 30 patients.

When successful, cryomastectomy achieves complete removal of a cancerous breast and is particularly indicated when surgical excision is no longer feasible. The procedure is well tolerated, even by elderly and sick patients; it always alleviates suffering and provides longer global survival with better quality of life. High cure rates cannot be expected when dealing with such advanced cases. We had 5/30 (16.6%) of patients with no evidence of disease between 2 and 6 years later, which is rewarding. Cryomastectomy can also be combined with other non-surgical oncological treatments.

The actual novelty in this method for advanced breast cancer started with the conception of a simple but very effective method for protecting the skin surrounding the lesion, and continued with the mentioned strategy of dividing the breast into quadrants when freezing. The combination of these two techniques allows the liberal and continuous application of the spray for the needed length of time, thus permitting the accurate prediction of the extent of the frozen surface and of the mass of necrosed tissues. In this manner, lethal temperatures are achieved in large tumoral masses, due to the much higher capability of the spray to remove heat as compared to the cryoprobe.

When performing any physical oncological treatment, be it surgery, cryosurgery, chemosurgery or radiotherapy, the safety margin is the same but the resulting degree of inflammation differs. Scalpel surgery causes moderate inflammation, whereas that resulting from cryosurgery, particularly in the case of advanced cancers, is intense and, probably has a positive influence on the eradication of the peripheral neoplastic extensions. Quite possibly, the exposure of antigens from the cryonecrosed tissues left in situ to the patient's immune system accounts for some of the good results of cryosurgery (4, 76).

There is a tendency to underrate cryosurgery of advanced cancer and to consider it as *merely palliative*. This attitude is ethically incorrect, because even if cryosurgery of such tumors would be *merely* palliative, a palliative tool to deal with such desperate cases would be of the utmost importance. It should, in fact, be stressed that besides its unique advantages as palliation, cryosurgery also cures a significant number of serious and advanced malignancies for which there are no other therapeutic modalities available.

References

1. Abboud B, Ingea H. Recurrent squamous cell carcinoma arising in sacrococcygeal pilonidal sinus tract; report of a case and review of the literature. Dis Colon Rectum, 1999; 42: 525–528.
2. Baez AP and Herrera JR. Invasive Carcinoma of the Penis. Management and Prognosis. Urologic Oncology. Oesterling JE, Richie JP, (Eds). Philadelphia: WB Saunders Co, 1997; 595–617.
3. Breitbart EW. Cryosurgical consideration for melanoma. Cryosurgery for Skin Cancer and Cutaneous Disorders. Zacarian SA (Ed). CV Mosby Co., St. Louis, 1975; 215–236.
4. Breitbart EW. Cryosurgery in the treatment of cutaneous malignant melanoma. Clinics in Dermatology. Advances in Cryosurgery. Breitbart EW, Dachów-Siviéc E (Eds). Elsevier. New York, Amsterdam, London, 1990; 96–100.
5. Cahan WG. Cryosurgery of malignant and benign tumors. Federation Procs. 1965; 24: 241–248.
6. Cahan WG. Five years of cryosurgical experience: Benign and malignant tumors with hemorrhagic conditions. Cryosurgery. Rand RW, Rinfret AP, Leden H von (Eds). Illinois: Springfeld, Thomas, 1966; 388–409.
7. Cahan WG. Cryosurgery: The Management of Massive Recurrent Cancer. Cryogenics in Surgery. Leden H von, Cahan WG (Eds). New York: Medical Examination Publishing Company, Inc., 1971; 182–233.
8. Cahan WG. Cryosurgery of massive recurrent cancer. Panminerva Medica, 1975; 17: 359–361.
9. Chamberlain GVP. Gynecology. Practical Cryosurgery. HB Holdein (Ed). Pitman Medical. London, 1975.
10. Elida MJ, Stolar E, Seone A. Carcinoma epidermoide de vulva estadio II (FIGO). Tratamiento con radiocirugia, cirugía y criocirugía. Rev Soc Arg Patol Tracto Gen Infer Colposco. In press.
11. Favard A, Dauplat J et Giraud B. Cryochirurgie et cancers vulvaires. J Gyn Obst Biol Repr. 1982; 11: 745–9.
12. Gage AA. Cryosurgery of advanced tumors of the head and neck. Cryosurgery for Skin Cancer and Cutaneous Disorders. Zacarian SA (ed). CV Mosby Co., St. Louis, 1975.
13. Gage AA. Cryosurgery of Advanced Tumors. Clinics in Dermatology – Advances in Cryosurgery. Breitbart. EW. Dachów-Siviec. E. (Eds). New York, Amsterdam, London: 1990; 86–95.
14. Gage AA. Cryosurgery for oral cancer. Abstracts ot the 9th World Congress of Cryosurgery, Paris. 1995; 54.
15. Gill W, Long W, Fraser J and Lee P. Cryosurgery for neoplasia. Brit J Surg. 1970; 57: 494–502.
16. Gonçalves JCA. Treatment of Advanced Cancer of the Breast. IV International Congress of Dermatologic Surgery. Granada. 1983.
17. Gonçalves JCA. Cryosurgery of advanced cancer of the extremities. Skin Cancer, 1986; 3: 211–21.
18. Gonçalves JCA. Cryomastectomy for advanced cancer. Skin Cancer, 1986; 4: 283–296.
19. Gonçalves JCA. Cryovulvectomy – A New Surgical Technique for Advanced Cancer. Skin Cancer, 1986; 1: 17–32.
20. Gonçalves JCA. Chemosurgery without systematised microscopic control of advanced cutaneous cancers: II report of two cases of invasive squamous cell carcinoma of the hand. Skin Cancer, 1986; 4: 297–303.
21. Gonçalves JCA. Cryosurgery of advanced carcinomas arising in pilonidal sinus. Skin Cancer, 1987; 2: 183–195.
22. Gonçalves JCA. Criovulvectomia para o cancro avançado. Gin Med Repr, 1989; 2: 61–81.
23. Gonçalves JCA. Cryosurgery of advanced squamous-cell carcinomas of the extremitis. Cryomedicine. Stolar E, Turjansky E (Eds). Buenos Aires. Montserrat. 1992; 73–75.
24. Gonçalves JCA. Cryovulvectomy for advanced cancer. Cryomedicine. Stolar E, Turjansky E (Eds). Buenos Aires. Montserrat. 1992; 265–266.
25. Gonçalves JCA. Cryosurgery of advanced carcinomas arising in the pilonidal sinuses. Cryomedicine. Stolar E, Turjansky E (Eds). Buenos Aires. Montserrat. 1992; 333–334.
26. Gonçalves JCA and Dores. Protection of the skin around small tumors with a silicone sheet (Cryosil,). Abstracts of the 9th World Congress of Cryosurgery Paris. 1995.
27. Gonçalves JCA. Cryosurgery of breast cancer. Cryosurgery. Mechanism and applications. International Institute of Refrigeration. Paris. 1995; 121–6.
28. Gonçalves JCA. The importance of effective protection of perilesional tissues in cryosurgery of advanced cancer. Abstracts of the 9th World Congress of Cryosurgery. Paris. 1995; 56.
29. Gonçalves JCA, Martins C. Debulking of skin cancers with radio frequency before cryosurgery. Dermatol Surg, 1997; 23: 253–257.
30. Gonçalves JCA, Amaro JA and Moura C. Treatment of advanced cancer of the vulva – A comparison of the results by radiotherapy plus chemotherapy versus cryovulvectomy''. First European Congress of Cryosurgery. 2000. San Sebastian. Spain.
31. Gonçalves JCA. Cryosurgery of advanced basal-cell carcinomas invading the orbital structures. Abstracts of the 9th World Congress of Cryosurgery. Paris. 1995; 35.
32. Gonçalves JCA. Cryosurgery of advanced squamous cell carcinoma carcinoma on sinus pilonidalis. Abstracts of the 9th World Congress of Cryosurgery. Paris. 1995; 58.
33. Gonçalves, JCA. Cryosurgery of squamous cell carcinoma of penis, First European Congress of Cryosurgery. San Sebastian, 2000.
34. Gonçalves. JCA. Chemomastectomy for advanced cancer. Skin Cancer, 1987; 2: 49–68.
35. Graham GF, Clark LC. Statistical update in cryosurgery for cancers of the skin. Cryosurgery for Skin Cancer and Cutaneous Disorders. Zacarian SA (ed). CV Mosby Co., St. Louis, 1975; 298–305.

36. Graham GF, Clark LC. Statistical analysis in cryosurgery of skin cancer. In Clinics in Dermatolology. Breitbart E, Dachów-Siwiéc (Ed) Elsevier. New York, Amsterdam, London, 1990; 101–7.
37. Graham GF. Cryosurgery for benign, premalignant, and malignant lesions. Cutaneous Surgery. Wheeland RG (ed). Philadelphia: WB Saunders Co., 1994; 866–7.
38. Günther H. Kryochirurgie des Vulvarkarzinon. Abstracts of the ''Gynekologenkongress der D.D.R'', 1970; 27: 908–9.
39. Hughes PSH. Cryosurgery of verrucous carcinoma of the penis. Cutis, 1979; 24: 43–45.
40. Itoh M, Tanaka S. Cryosurgery for the treatment of malignant melanoma. Skin Cancer, 1995; 10: 43–52.
41. Kuflik EG. Debulking large tumors. J Dermatol Surg Oncol, 1982; 8: 431–433.
42. Kuflik EG. Debulking the lesion before cryosurgery. J Dermatol Surg Oncol, 1986; 13: 235–236.
43. Kuflik EG. Debulking the lesion before cryosurgery. J Dermatol Surg Oncol, 1986; 12: 321–322.
44. Kuflik EG. Cryosurgery updated. J Am Acad Dermatol, 1994; 31: 925–943.
45. Lash AF Gynecologic Malignant Tumors. Handbook of Cryosurgery. (Ed). RJ Ablin. Marcel Dekker Inc New York, Basilea, 1980.
46. Le Pivert P, Le Petit JC, Fraisse J, Cuilleret J, Brizard CP. Cryotumorectomie reglée dans les cancers du sein. Aspect technique et théorique: Éssai d'interprétation. Les Colloques de l'Institut National de la Santé et de la Recherche, 1976; 62: 267–278.
47. Le Pivert P, Binder P, Ougier T. Measurement of intratissue bioelectrical low frequency impedance. A new method to predict pre-operatively the destructive effect of cryosurgery. Cryobiology, 1977; 14: 245–250.
48. Le Pivert P. Cryosurgery: Current issues and future trends. Proceedings of the Tenth International Cryogenic Engineering Conference. Finland, 1984; 551–557.
49. Le Pivert P. The development of cryosurgical instruments for internal medicine. Cryogenic Enginering Conference MIT. Cambridge, Massachussets, 1985.
50. Lloyd-Williams K. General Surgery. Practical Cryosurgery. Holden HB (Ed). London: H.B. Pitman Medical, 1975; 150–163.
51. Lloyd-Williams K. Cryosurgery and its Applications. Current Surgical Practice. Hadfield J, Hobsley M (Eds). London, Edward Arnold, 1978; 2: 243–267.
52. Madej G, Meyza J. Cryosurgery of penile carcinoma. Short report on preliminary results. Oncology, 1982; 39: 350–2.
53. Martins O, Oliveira AS, Picoto AS, Verde F (Extr.5). Cryosurgery of large tumors on the dorsa of hands. J Dermatol Surg Oncol, 1980; 6: 568.
54. Matveev BP, Mikhailovsky AV, Gotsadze DT [Treatment of penile cancer] [Article in Russian]. Vopr Onkol, 1984; 30: 71–6.
55. Rubio-Briones J, Villavicencio H, Regalado R et al. Carcinoma escamoso de pene: protocolo de tratamiento según nuestra experiencia en 14 años. Arch Esp Urol, 1997; 50: 473–480.
56. Schmidt D. Real contribution of cryosurgery in the treatment of advanced breast carcinoma. Abstracts of the First Central European Congress of Cryosurgery. Plzen. Czech Republic. 1996; 13.
57. Sommer J, Renziehausen K, Neuhaser H et al. (Crvv.6) Möglichkeiten und Grenzen der Kryochirurgie des Vulvarkarzinom –12 jährige Therpiegebnisse. Zentbl Gynäkol. 1986; 11: 745–749.
58. Sonnex TS, Ralfs IG, plaza de Lanza M, et al. Treatment of erythroplaisa of Queyrat with liquid nitrogen cryosurgery. Brit J Dermatol, 1982; 16: 581–4.
59. Stolar E, Turjansky E. Tecnicas combinadas (criocirugia y radiofrecuencia) para el tratamiento de las lesiones premalignas y malignas del tracto genital inferior. Cryomedicine 1996. Stolar y Turjannsky (Eds) Buenos Aires, 1996; 259.
60. Tanaka S. Twelve years of cryosurgical experience in general surgery. Proceedings of the IV world Congress of Cryosurgery. Sanremo. 1980; 605–614.
61. Tanaka S. Immunological aspects of cryosurgery in general surgery. In: Biomedical Thermology. New York: Alan R Liss Inc, 1982; 799–814.
62. Tanaka S. General cryosurgery: state of the arts, tends, and prospects. In: 5th World Congress of Cryosurgery, Padilla-Cruz A, Sumida S (Eds). The University Press. University of Philippines System. Quezon City. Diliman, 1983; 45–51.
63. Tanaka S. Development of cryosurgery in Japan: an overview: (II) Basic studies on cryosurgery and instrumentation. Low Temp Med, 1993; 19: 18–23.
64. Tanaka S. General cryosurgery: state of the arts, trends and prospects''. Low Temp Med, 1992; 18: 49–60.
65. Tanaka S. Development of cryosurgery in Japan: an overview: (I) historical review of cryosurgery in Japan. Low Temp Med, 1992; 18: 100–104.
66. Tanaka S. Development of cryosurgery in Japan: an overview: (III) Cryosurgery in general surgery and boundary fields. Low Temp Med, 1993; 19: 42–55.
67. Tanaka S. Development of cryosurgery in Japan: an overview: (IV) Cryoimmunology, problems and future prospects of cryosurgery. Low Temp Med, 1993; 19: 119–128.
68. Tanaka S. Cryosurgical treatment of advanced breast cancer. Skin Cancer. 1995; 10: 9–18.
69. Tanaka S. Cryosurgery of skin cancer and malignancies of the oral cavity. Skin Cancer.1995; 10: 27–35.
70. Townsend DE. Cryosurgery of Advanced Vulvar Carcinoma. Surg Cl N Am. 1978; 58: 97–107.
71. Turjansky E, Stolar E. Lesiones de Piel y Mucosas. Técnicas terpeúticas. Turjansky E, Stolar E Eds) Edama. Buenos Aires, 1995.
72. Turjansky E, Stolar E. CD Rom – Criocirugía y Radiofrequencia en piel y mucosas. Data vision – McGraw-Hill. Argentina, 1998.
73. Turjansky E. Stolar E Criocirugia en cáncer cutáneo. Casuistica. Lesiones de Piel y Mucosas. Técnicas terapeúticas. Turjansky E. Stolar E (eds). Edama. Buenos Aires, 1995; 189–170, 185.
74. Turjansky E, Stolar E. Lesiones malignas en el aparato genital femenino. DC Rom Criocirugía y Radiofrecuencia en piel y mucosas. Multimedia. BDM Criocirugia. Data Vision –mc Graw Argentina, 1998.
75. Wallach RC. Cryosurgery of advanced vulvar cancer. Obstet Gynecol, 1946; 47: 454–458.
76. Weyer U, Peterson I, Ehrke A, Breitbart EW. Immunmodulation durch Kryochirurgie beim malignen Melanom. Onkologie, 1989; 12: 291–296.
77. Zaloudík J, Fait V, Janáková L et al. Palliative cryosurgery of inoperable exophytic tumors with long time survival. Abstracts of the First Central European Congress of Cryosurgery. Plzen. Czech Republic, 1996; 15.

9. Abdominal Cryosurgery

9.1 Liver Cryosurgery for Primary and Secondary Liver Tumors

Nikolai N. Korpan with contributions by Jaroslav V. Zharkov, Iwan S. Tchekman, Franz Beer, and Gerhard Hochwarter

9.1.0 Introduction

Foremost among the most important areas in which cryosurgery is used are primary and secondary curative and inoperable liver tumors. Liver cryosurgery is a new method of treatment, in which the tumorous lesion is ablated in situ by means of a cryosurgical instrument. In recent years a new path has opened up for patients with liver tumors thanks to cryosurgery. No more than 25% of patients with an isolated liver tumor have conventional surgery. Of these, 20–35% achieve 5-year survival.

The different forms of liver cryosurgery are:

- *Liver cryoresection* – the operative excision of pathological organ structures by means of a cold-producing clamp or scalpel
- *Liver cryoextirpation* (*liver cryoablation*) – complete cryosurgical removal of a well demarcated focus or tumor in healthy tissue by way of a trocar or disc shaped cryoprobe (cryoapplicator)
- *Liver cryodestruction* – a surgical intervention with the use of cold to partially remove a tumor in order to reduce the tumor mass
- *Laparoscopic liver cryosurgery* (*minimally invasive liver cryosurgery*) – a cryosurgical procedure for removal of the liver tumor or tumor reduction using laparoscopy and other minimally invasive techniques.

9.1.1 Cryotechnical Operating Methods

Long-term worldwide experience with the use of cryosurgery in advanced stages of liver cancer demonstrates the possibilities and limits of the method.

Open Liver Cryosurgery (Figs. 9.1.1–9.1.5)

Method of Application (Placement)

In the open procedure, cryoextirpation is carried out on the operable liver tumor (liver metastasis)

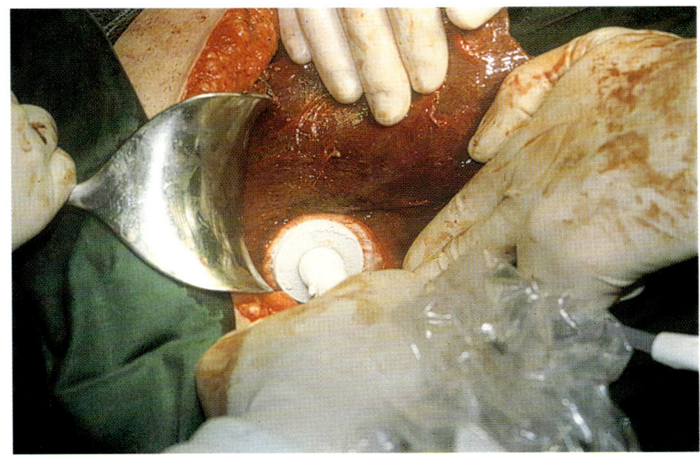

Fig. 9.1.1. Open Liver Cryosurgery: Method of Application (Placement). Female, 47 years old. Multiple large liver metastases from primary breast cancer. The cryoprobe, 30 mm in diameter, is directed into the center of the lesion (liver segment VII) under direct vision

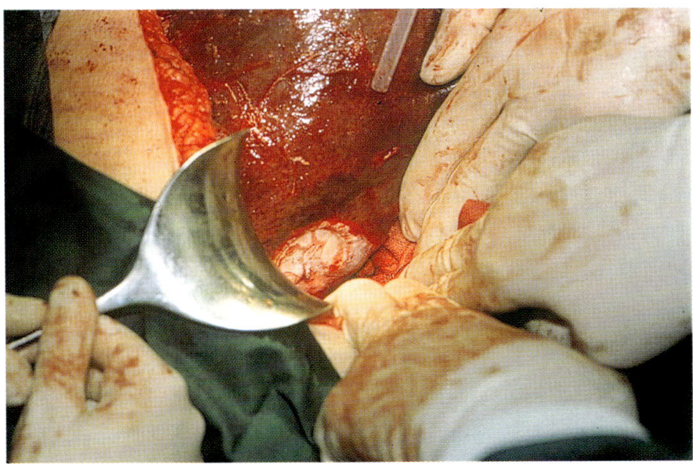

Fig. 9.1.2. Same patient. View of the post-cryosurgical zone, which measures 52 mm in diameter

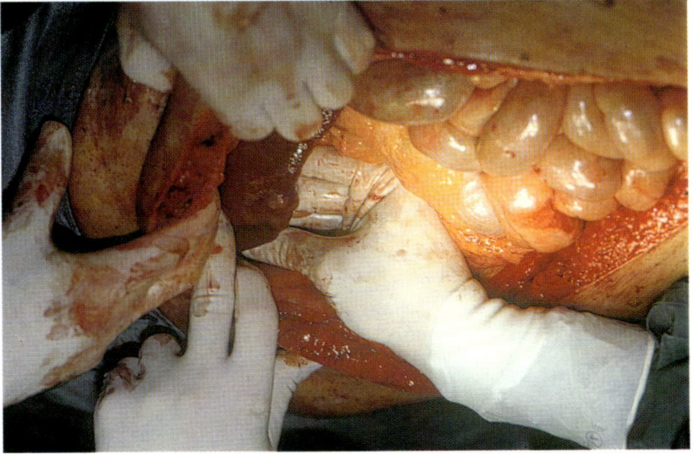

Fig. 9.1.3. Open Liver Cryosurgery: Method of Application (Placement). Male, 69 years old. Multiple large colorectal liver metastases in segment V/VI

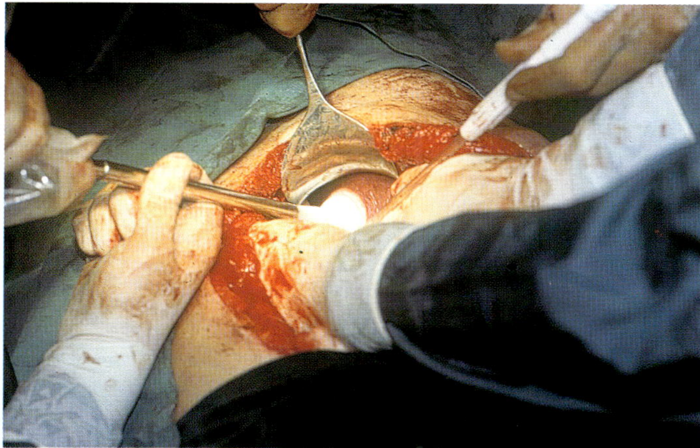

Fig. 9.1.4. The tip of a disc-shaped cryoprobe 50 mm in diameter is applied to the center of the liver metastasis

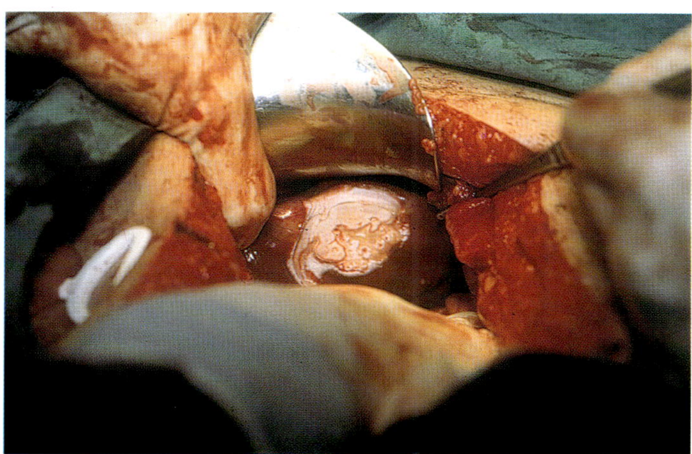

Fig. 9.1.5. Same patient. Typical view of the post-cryosurgical zone, which is 68 mm in diameter. A single freeze-thaw cycle was used at a temperature of −180°C for 7 min

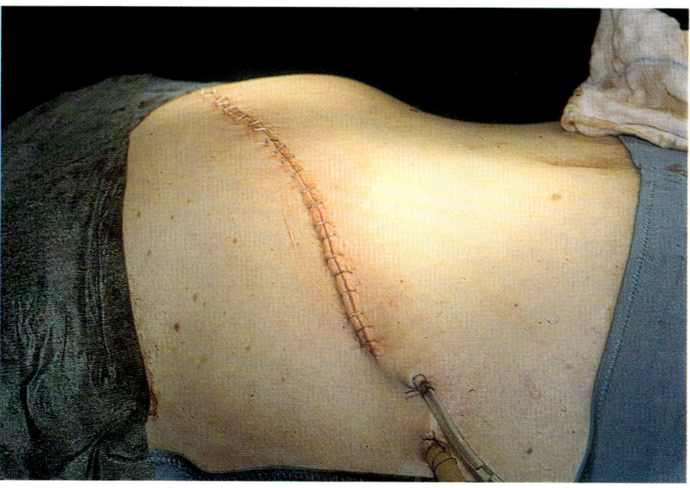

Fig. 9.1.6. Same patient. The abdominal cavity is closed with subhepatic and subcutaneous drainage

or cryodestruction on the inoperable liver carcinoma (liver metastasis) by application of the rounded tip to the tumorous infiltrative liver parenchyma.

In this method different cryoapplicators with diameters between 2 and 20 mm are used. As a rule the cryosurgical procedure is set for 1 to 3 sessions with a duration of 10 sec–3 min. The freeze-thaw cycle is carried out automatically and, in turn, has a duration of 1.1–2.7 min, during which the cryozone reaches a volume of 40–180 cm^3, and has a visually clear demarcation from neighboring structures. The duration of the procedure and the number of treatment sessions must be individually set, depending on the individual clinical picture. The cold shock at a temperature of −170°C to −190°C destroys the cancerous tissue, while healthy tissue is spared because the extent and depth of the cold application can be exactly regulated. The abdominal cavity can be closed with drainage for early postoperative controlled bleeding and bile leakage (Fig. 9.1.6).

Based on experimental studies using different low temperatures in vitro with gelatine solutions as well as in vivo in the animal model with dog livers, the following optimal parameters were determined for cryosurgery of parenchymal organs, including liver surgery:

- Freeze temperature at −180°C to −190°C, with rapid freezing of the tumor required
- Duration of a treatment session: 5–7 min
- 2–3 freeze-thaw cycles
- Spontaneous thawing, which must be carried out very slowly

For advanced liver cancer or for liver metastases, several cryosessions are required in order to carry out overlapping treatments of the entire tumorous infiltrate and to cryodestroy either the entire or a part of the tumor mass.

At the end of the operation, the abdominal wall is closed in layers and a drain placed either subhepatically or subdiaphragmatically. Occasionally it will be necessary because of the interaoperative situation to place a rubber or a Robinson drain.

Needle (Probe) Method: In this method cryoneedles (cryoprobes) of the smallest possible caliber are required in order to spare the parenchyma to the extent possible. The cryoneedle is implanted in the tumor mass, single needles with a diameter of at least 2 mm and maximally 2.2 cm being used. For cryosurgery for larger liver tumors with a diameter of maximally 2–3 cm a synergistic cooling effect can be achieved by the use of several cryoneedles (cryoprobes). When 2 or more cryoprobes are used for liver cryosurgery, the distance between the cryoinstruments is important.

The liver tumor (liver metastasis) is carefully punctured with a thin cryoneedle and immediately next to it a cryoprobe is placed according to the Seldinger technique. Thereafter, depending on the situation, 1–3 freeze cycles are carried out on a small metastasis. Where there is a larger liver metastasis, several thin needles are implanted in the tumor mass under ultrasound monitoring at a distance of 2–3 cm from one another in the form of an equilateral triangle; parallel to this, cryoprobes are placed in the liver parenchyma. After thawing, the cryoprobes are removed and the abdominal wall closed layer by layer.

Since the open cryosurgical operation is less invasive than the procedure for liver resection, the complication rates and postoperative mortality are low in theory, and in practice are very seldom seen. The postoperative course after cryosurgery is mostly problem-free and no complications arise, in contrast with conventional liver resection, where they are common. After the cryosurgical procedure the in-hospital stay of the patient is 5–7 days instead of the 2–4 weeks following conventional surgery. Similarly, the cost factor is much lower than in traditional operations.

There are no known contraindications for patients with liver tumors who are considering cryosurgical procedures.

Laparoscopic Liver Surgery (Fig. 9.1.7 A–C)

With the patient under general anesthesia, a Veress needle is placed in the pneumoperitoneum and the optic endoscope is introduced into the abdominal cavity. After inspection of the abdomen, an incision is made in the right upper abdomen and a 12-mm working trocar introduced under endoscopic vision. Immediately thereafter a laparoscopic cryoapplicator (cryoprobe) is applied to the liver parenchyma in the area of the tumor or is implanted deeply into the tumor mass.

Thereafter the liver tumor (liver metastasis) is cryoextirpated in the usual fashion at a temperature of −180°C to −190°C with spontaneous thawing and freezing. Different special cryoneedles and cryoapplicators are used in this connection.

Percutaneous Liver Cryosurgery

A minimal subcostal incision is made in the right upper abdomen. The cryoinstrument is applied to the liver tumor or a cryoprobe implanted in the tumor mass. At present this procedure is in the experimental stage and is being used only on one patient.

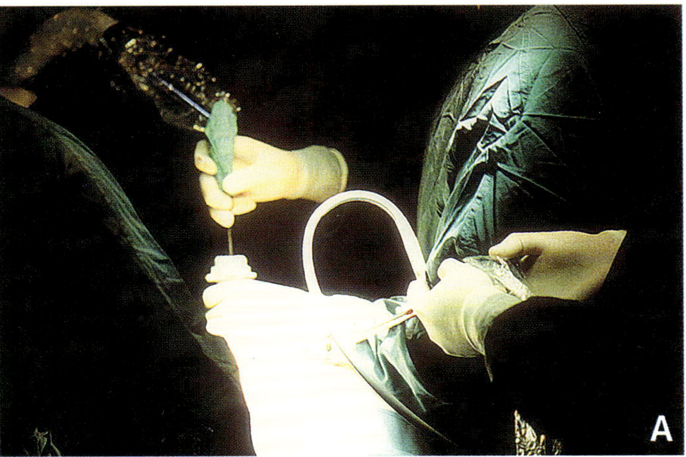

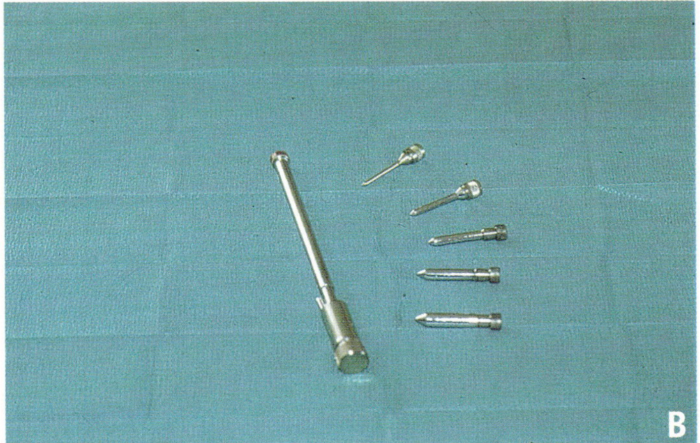

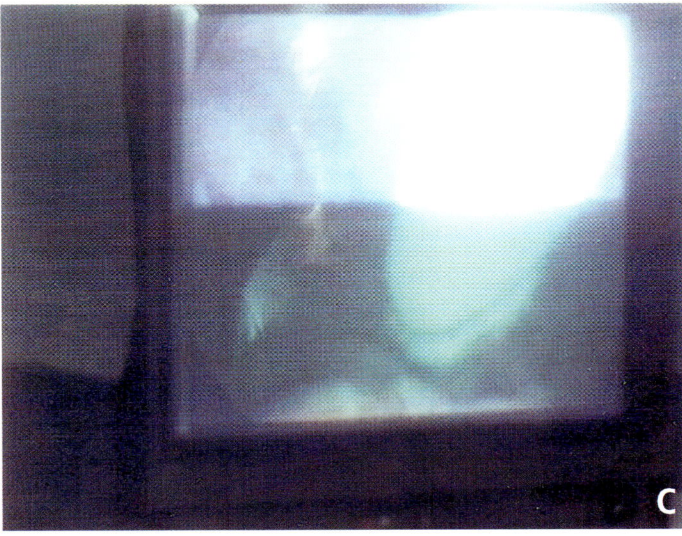

Fig. 9.1.7. A photograph taken during laparoscopic hepatic cryosurgery (**A**). The standard cryosurgical probes that we developed to perform adequate abdominal laparoscopic cryosurgery, including hepatic cryosurgery (**B**). A photograph of laparoscopic cryosurgery performed on superficial liver metastasis (segment IV/V) with one laparoscopic cryoprobe (**C**)

9.1.2 The Present State of Liver Cryosurgery

Sparing open and minimally invasive (laparoscopic) cryosurgical procedures with modern high-performance cryodevices should be used for operable as well as for inoperable malignant tumors with curative intent. The advantages already mentioned elsewhere include the high performance level, the complication-free results of surgery, the high curative results of treatment, the short stays in hospital, the reduced hospital costs, as well as the patient's enhanced quality of life.

9.1.3 Perspectives in the Treatment of Operable and Inoperable Primary and Secondary Liver Tumors

New perspectives are opening for the minimally invasive treatment of malignant tumors. Cryosurgery is of enormous importance for the enhancement of the quality of life and the improvement in survival rate of patients with liver cancer. The destruction of large areas of tissue in the human organism by extreme hypothermia was, after all, the technical demand made on modern cryosurgical devices. At first, however, it was difficult to maintain a constant, programmed temperature of −170°C to −190°C at the tip of the probe without thereby also damaging healthy tissue. These problems have been dealt with in the latest generation of devices, whereby the unimpeded use of cryosurgery in different areas of medicine is guaranteed.

Cryosurgical treatment is successfully used alone with curative intent, as sole or supplementary palliation, or in combination with other systemic or local/regional treatments. Observations at present show that cryosurgical intervention on the liver has been well tolerated by the patients involved.

There is hardly any doubt that both open (conventional) and laparoscopic cryosurgery will be one of the standard methods in the treatment of liver tumors.

References

1. Korpan NN, Zharkov JV, Sacher R. A morphological study of cooling rate response in normal animal liver tissue: Cryosurgical Implications. Europ J Clin Invest 1999; 29 (Suppl 1): 22.
2. Adam R, Akpinar E, Johann M, Kunstlinger F, Majno P, Bismuth H. Place of Cryosurgery in the Treatment of Malignant Liver Tumors. Ann Surg 1997; 225 (1): 39–50.
3. Korpan NN. Hepatic Cryosurgery for Liver Metastases. Long-Term Follow-Up. Ann Surg 1997; 225 (2): 193–201.
4. Gage AA, Baust J. Mechanisms of tissue injury in cryosurgery. Cryobiology 1998; 37 (3): 171–186.
5. McKinnon G, Temple WJ, Wiseman DA, Saliken JC. Cryosurgery for malignant tumors of the liver. Can J Surg 1996; 39 (5): 401–406.
6. Korpan NN, Hochwarter G. Pancreatic cryosurgery - a new surgical procedure for pancreatic cancer. Eur J Clin Invest 1997; 27 (Suppl 1): A33.
7. Korpan NN. The use of low temperatures in oncology. In: The low temperatures in medicine (Ed. Ternovoi KS, Gassanov LG) 145–162 (Naukova Dumka, Kyiv, 1988).
8. Korpan NN. Möglichkeiten und Grenzen der modernen Kryochirurgie. In: Was gibt es Neues in der Medizin. Medizinisches Jahrbuch (Ed. Neugebauer H.), 207–213 (Dr. Peter Müller Verlag-Wien, 1996).

9.2 Cryosurgery for Hepatic Tumors

Calvin H.L. Law with a contribution by Ved R. Tandan

9.2.0 Introduction

Tumors of the liver, either primary or secondary, can represent a major challenge to oncologists. The most effective treatment for these tumors remains surgical resection when feasible, but in a majority of situations, tumors of the liver are not amenable to resection. Many patients with primary hepatocellular carcinomas also have an underlying liver dysfunction, thereby precluding the ability to remove much liver parenchyma without significant risk of liver failure in the post-operative setting. Secondary metastases can also present the surgeon with a significant predicament by having multiple metastases that, for anatomic reasons, are not completely resectable. The addition of a local, destructive therapy that would allow maximal destruction of malignant cells while minimizing the destruction of the surrounding normal parenchyma broadens the therapeutic options available for patients with malignancies of their liver.

The introduction of hepatic cryosurgery in 1963 opened up this option of "local ablation" for many patients around the world with hepatic tumors. There is now worldwide experience in using cryosurgery in the settings of hepatocellular carcinoma, colorectal metastases, and neuroendocrine metastases. Additional more limited experience is also available for other hepatic tumors as well.

9.2.1 Experimental Basis for Cryosurgery of Liver Tumors

Several important animal experiments laid the foundation for the use of cryosurgery for liver tumors. This foundation is based on (1) the feasibility and (2) the ablative ability of hepatic cryosurgery. A variety of animal models were used by different authors to demonstrate these two criteria.

Healey et al. (1), then later Dutta et al. (2,3) demonstrated in a series of dog models that cryosurgical destruction of liver tissue could be achieved without adverse effect on long term liver function. However, there were significant problems in both series. In Healey's series, there was a significant death rate (11/34 of the animals) from major hepatic vein injury. In Dutta's series, the major problem was with the development of fatal intraparenchymal cracks in the liver during the thawing phase of the cryosurgery. These problems would later be addressed by improvements in the instrumentation (vacuum insulated cryoprobes) and in instrument placement (intraoperative ultrasound). However, the experimental feasibility of hepatic cryosurgery was established.

Ravikumar et al. published a series of experiments that served as a model demonstrating the efficacy of cryosurgery in ablation of metastatic colorectal cancer (4). There were four series of experiments based on a rat model. The first series of experiments involved the implantation of colon cancer isografts in bilateral rat thighs. One thigh was subjected to cryosurgery while the other thigh acted as a control. Cryosurgery resulted in complete tumor destruction while the control side continued to have viable cells. In the second series of experiments, the colon cancer isografts were randomized to undergo single, double or triple freeze/thaw cycles. Recurrences occurred in the single cycle group only. In the third series of experiments, the colon cancer isografts were pretreated with cryosurgery then implanted. Eight of nine isografts failed to show growth. Fourth, the rat model was changed to implanted colorectal liver metastases and then they were randomized to cryosurgery (two cycle), resection or sham laparotomy. In this last series, the overall results for both cryosurgery and resection were similar. These sets of experiments helped to establish that (1) cryosurgery was ablative to colorectal cancer cells with a two cycle freeze/thaw sequence, (2) cryosurgery left almost all cells unviable, and (3) there was potential for the cryosurgical ablation to be as effective as surgical resection.

9.2.2 Clinical and Technical Aspects of Cryosurgery for Liver Tumors

Patient Selection: In general, patients who are excluded from hepatic resection by a few criteria should be considered for hepatic cryosurgery. Table 9.2.1 outlines the general selection criteria used for hepatic cryosurgery. Cryosurgery should be offered only where resection cannot be attained for a specific lesion or in combination with resection to achieve complete ablation. Definite candidates are those patients with anatomically unfavorable disease and those with multiple lesions, which may be bilateral or may involve resection of too much functional hepatic parenchyma. However, it is important to remember that open cryosurgery involves much the same stresses as other operations requiring a major laparotomy and thus the patient must be a candidate for this as well.

Table 9.2.1. General selection criteria for cryosurgery of liver tumors

1. No evidence of extra-hepatic disease.
2. Patients not suitable for resection alone.
3. Tumors whose size is amenable to cryosurgery ($\leq$6 cm).
4. No comorbidities preclude the required procedure.

The patient should have a good respiratory reserve since the most widely used technique is to perform hepatic cryosurgery via a right subcostal incision. This incision may lead to post-operative mechanical respiratory limitations. In addition, it is common to develop a sympathetic pleural effusion after hepatic cryosurgery (5) although the overall respiratory complications are less severe than with liver resection (5). Another limitation is the presence of ascites or advanced liver disease that would preclude the patient's ability to tolerate a laparotomy. This limitation is partially addressed by a laparoscopic approach.

Although the cryosurgery offers an ablative alternative in situations where resection is precluded by number of lesions or by anatomic location of lesions, the principle of both procedures is still to offer the patient a complete "ablation" of all known lesions. Thus the patient should have an extensive work-up to rule out extra-hepatic disease. Detailed imaging should be organized for every patient considered for hepatic cryosurgery. For metastatic colorectal cancer, any evidence of unresectable extrahepatic metastases would be considered an absolute contraindication to cryosurgery and thus detailed examinations of the chest, abdomen, and pelvis with helical CT scan-

Table 9.2.2. Contraindications to hepatic cryosurgery

- Gross ascites
- Active Coagulopathy
- >50% hepatic replacement with tumour
- Extra-hepatic disease (relative contraindication in neuroendocrine tumours)
- Invasion of major vessel (portal vein or IVC)
- Unresectable lesion >6 cm diameter

ning are preferred. A recent colonoscopy to rule out recurrent or metachronous disease would also be required. The same principle would also apply to hepatocellular carcinoma. In this case, detailed helical CT scan imaging of the chest and abdomen and a bone scan would be preferred. An exception to this principle is in the setting of metastatic neuroendocrine tumor. A labeled octreotide scan is a very helpful addition to standard cross-sectional imaging, and evidence of unresectable extrahepatic disease would be a relative contraindication to hepatic cryosurgery for neuroendocrine metastases. However, symptomatic patients may benefit from tumor burden reduction or "debulking" surgery (6).

Several limitations still remain mainly due to the technique of cryosurgery at its present development. Current technology still limits the size of lesion that can be completely destroyed by cryosurgery, although careful planning of multiple probe insertion points and the use of overlapping "ice balls" can achieve ablation diameters of 10 cm. However, the target lesion should be encompassable with 1 cm margins. Cryoablation of greater than 30–40% of hepatic parenchyma is associated with increasing risk of complications, so that cryosurgery is limited to lesions involving less than 50% of the hepatic parenchyma. Another limitation is the proximity of major bile ducts. Though the major vessels are "protected" by blood flow that prevents freezing of the vessel wall, no such protective mechanism exists in the bile ducts. Therefore, lesions near the confluence of the bile duct would not be amenable to cryoablation if they were to be encompassed within the proposed area of cryoablation.

Pre-Operative Work-Up: Cryosurgery involves a significant physiological impact to the patient. Even with the introduction of laparoscopic techniques, most patients undergo a significant laparotomy similar to that required for a hepatic resection. Thus, pre-operative work-up must be as rigorous as that typically used for a patient undergoing a major operation. In addition, many patients will be brought to the operating room for both a hepatic resection and cryosurgery.

Rigorous investigations to determine the patient's candidacy for cryosurgery should be accomplished as described above. The patient should also have a biochemical work-up that includes evaluation of the complete blood count, coagulation parameters, liver function and renal function. In addition, preoperative measurement of tumor markers such as CEA (colorectal metastases) and alpha-feto protein (hepatocellular carcinoma) can be useful in prognosis (7) as well as to follow the response to therapy.

9.2.3 Details of Cryosurgery of the Liver

Pre-incision Preparations: The patient is brought to the operating room and positioned supine. General anesthesia is induced and endotracheal intubation established. This is followed by the establishment of arterial pressure catheters, central venous pressure monitoring (especially if considering a combined resection and cryosurgery) and core temperature probe (esophageal temperature probe). An upper (with or without a lower) body warmer device is secured to the patient. Onik et al. had compared patients undergoing hepatic cryosurgery with or without a body warmer device and found that patients with the body warmer device were warmer (35.3 versus 34.2°C, $p < 0.0001$) and had a lower temperature drop (0.73 versus 1.81°C, $p < 0.0001$).(8). A Foley catheter is placed to monitor urine output. A temporary nasogastric tube is placed to decompress the stomach. The abdomen is then prepped with surgical prep from nipple line down to hypogastrium and draped widely.

Exposure and Preparations for Cryosurgery: Access is established initially with a right subcostal incision positioned two finger breadths below the costal margin (the laparoscopic approach will be explained in the subsequent chapter). Once the presence of extrahepatic disease or untreatable hepatic disease is ruled out by a careful laparotomy and intraoperative ultrasound, the incision is extended as needed for exposure. Typically, we use a bilateral subcostal incision, or in some cases a "hockey stick" incision is used to spare the patient bilateral rectus muscle disruption. The "hockey stick" incision is a right subcostal incision with a midline extension up to the xiphoid without injury to the left rectus muscle. We have found that this latter incision can provide adequate exposure to an average sized left lobe with the assistance of a fixed table retractor such as the Thompson® or the Omni® retractor. The liver is initially mobilized by dividing the falciform ligament back to the inferior vena cava, which allows the placement of fixed table retractors that can allow for "lifting" of the costal margins and allow maximum exposure of the liver. This maneuver can be critical to exposing the posterior segments of the right lobe. The rest of the liver mobilization is achieved by taking down the right and left triangular and coronary ligaments. On the right side, the inferior vena cava can also be adequately exposed up to the entrance of the right hepatic vein to allow for vascular control later in the case. The porta hepatis should be exposed to allow for careful inspection for portal nodes and to allow for a subsequent Pringle maneuver as needed. Care should be taken not to injure an aberrant left hepatic artery as one exposes the medial border of the porta hepatis along the lesser curve of the stomach. An intra-operative ultrasound probe is now used to visualize the tumor(s) to be treated and visualize its relationship to the major vessels and bile ducts (if visible). Planning of the route with which to approach the tumor is done carefully with the priority maneuver being to avoid spearing the major vessels. The proposed surface entry point of the cryoprobe is then scored with electrocautery. If histological confirmation had not yet been achieved, tissue is now taken with a core needle biopsy under ultrasound guidance.

Application of the Cryoprobes: Under ultrasound guidance, the cryoprobe is directed in the direction of the chosen route into the lesion. Once the tip of the probe is confirmed to be in the middle of the lesion, the freezing process is initiated. Ultrasound imaging is used intermittently during the freezing process to monitor progress as well as to ensure that a 1 cm margin is ensured around the lesion. The 1 cm margin is based on the same reasoning that is used in resection, namely that less than 1 cm margins are associated with a higher local recurrence rate (9). The ultrasound image of the advancing edge of the ice ball is striking and appears as a hyperechoic shadow with posterior acoustic shadowing (see Fig. 9.2.1). Once the hyperechoic shadow reaches the 1 cm margin point, the circulation of liquid nitrogen is interrupted to allow for the thawing cycle. The receding of the ice ball can be seen on intraoperative ultrasound and when this line recedes back 1 cm (i.e. the margin), the next freeze cycle is initiated. The reason for the incomplete thawing is to reduce the complication rate (further detailed below). The probe is left in place during the second thawing cycle until the temperature at the probe has risen to −20 degrees Celsius. The track left by the probe is then packed with a hemostatic agent such as Surgicel®. Each cycle should take approximately 8–15 minutes depending on the size of the ice ball being created.

Three other situations deserve special mention. Deep-seated lesions, such as those in the posterior right lobe, may be better approached with com-

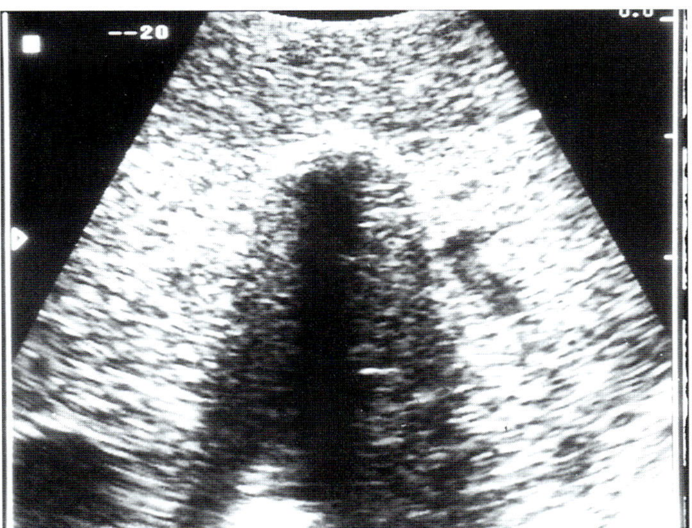

Fig. 9.2.1. Ultrasound image of ice ball

mercially available guidewire-dilator kits. Using ultrasound guidance the wire is introduced to the middle lesion followed by a sheath and dilator. The stiffer dilator is removed and the cryoprobe is placed within the sheath. The sheath is removed and the procedure is completed as detailed above. Deep lesions seated closer to larger vessels may require the addition of a Pringle maneuver which involves a non-crushing occlusion of the porta hepatis. A second situation occurs when a lesion(s) cannot be completely encompassed by one probe alone. In this case, the aim is to place these probes eccentrically and position the probes so that the outer extent of the expected cumulative ice ball is out to the requisite 1 cm margin. The probes will have overlapping areas of freezing, with the priority being the establishment of an adequate margin around the tumor. The freezing process can then be carried out simultaneously via the probes as detailed above. The final situation involves taking greater care when the lesion is in proximity to other organs especially the gallbladder, colon, duodenum, stomach and diaphragm. Adequate mobilization (or cholecystectomy if needed) of the adjacent organ must be initiated prior to the freezing process to avoid unnecessary risk of injury.

At the conclusion of the cryosurgery and removal of the probes, hemostasis must be ensured and then closed suction drains are placed in the areas of dependent drainage (subphrenic and subhepatic). The incision is closed with continuous, two layer heavy gauge absorbable suture (in patients with underlying chronic liver disease, we tend to use non-absorbable sutures).

9.2.4 Intra-operative Pitfalls

Injury to Major Vessel: There are two mechanisms by which a major vessel can be injured by cryosurgery. The first is the potential for thrombosis if the major vessel is within the zone of freezing and the second is a direct injury during the placement of the probe. As mentioned, intraoperative ultrasound should be carefully used to map out a probe route that avoids the major vessels, which may lie in close proximity to the lesion. As for the former mechanism, thrombosis of a major vessel is unusual since blood flow through it gives the vessel a protective "cold sink". However, injury to a vessel may occur despite this, especially in instances where the use of a Pringle maneuver is employed and reduces the "heat sink" protection of blood flow. If there is not adequate mobilization prior to this, vascular control may be difficult to achieve. Therefore, the porta hepatis, the inferior vena cava and the hepatic veins where they join the inferior vena cava should be identified prior to cryosurgery in cases where the lesion is close to a major vascular structure. Attempting to explore the hepatic parenchyma while there is still active and rapid bleeding will result in grave consequences.

Inadequate Cryoablation: Intraoperative ultrasound must also be used to measure the size of the lesion at its greatest diameter. The size of the ice ball must be 1 cm beyond the tumor translating to a diameter at least 2 cm greater than the greatest dimension of the tumor. Therefore, both initial measurement and accurate placement of the probe is essential to avoid inadequate cryoablation.

Post-probe Removal Bleeding: After freezing there can be a significant blood loss from either the probe tract or from cracks in the parenchyma of the liver. In most cases, bleeding will occur during the thaw cycle of the procedure. Bleeding (unless it is massive) can be controlled with a combination of compressive maneuvers. Hemostatic material can be used to pack the tract tightly but care must be taken not to induce parenchymal fracture during packing. Manual compression of the probe tract can also be successful in arresting the hemorrhage but persistence of upto 20 minutes of compression may be needed to achieve control.

Parenchymal Fracture: Surface cracks can also occur secondary to the freezing process especially in situations where a large area is being frozen using multiple probes. It can also occur during probe removal especially if one torques on the probe while trying to remove it. Preventative measures include waiting for the probe to reach at least −20°C and a soft rotational action on probe removal may help decrease the chance of parenchymal fracture. If subsequent bleeding occurs, it can be controlled with sutures, packing or hemostatic agents.

9.2.5 Post-operative Care and Complications

Routine precautions and post-operative care for the patient with a laparotomy are employed. This would include chest physiotherapy, adequate pain control using epidural analgesia or patient controlled analgesia devices (PCA), and monitoring of urine output. Standard bloodwork would include a postoperative complete blood count, electrolytes, renal function (creatinine and blood urea nitrogen), coagulation factors (INR, PTT), and liver enzymes (AST, ALT, ALP, GGT, BILI).

Cryosurgery can induce certain significant complications. Complications can be classified into intraoperative, immediate and delayed. Understanding and recognizing these complications will allow one to initiate treatments that can help ameliorate the consequences of the complications.

Intraoperative complications were partially discussed above and are mainly related to hemorrhage. These include probe placement-related major vascular injury, probe removal bleeding and parenchymal fracture. A further intraoperative complication that can occur with cryosurgery is hypothermia. As previously mentioned, this complication can be ameliorated with the use of body warmer devices. If a significant cryosurgery is being offered (for example, multiple lesions or one large lesion), the use of two body warmers for the upper and lower torso is advisable. Myoglobinuria can also manifest intraoperatively at the time of the thaw cycle. It is discussed below.

Immediate complications include those that can occur during the early post-operative period after the cryosurgery. These can include acute renal failure, biliary fistula, hepatic abscess, coagulopathy, transient biochemical derangements, pleural effusion, acute respiratory distress syndrome and the most serious, the "cryoshock" phenomenon (10).

Pleural effusion is a common complication and is thought to be a sympathetic process reacting to the inflammation caused by the cryoablation of the liver tumor. Some authors have elected to treat this with tube thoracostomy (11) while others have found that most are asymptomatic and spontaneously resolve (5). Treatment will be based on the amount of respiratory compromise caused by the effusion. For example, those patients with preoperative chronic obstructive pulmonary disease will have a greater degree of respiratory compromise from the effusion.

Biliary fistula results from damage to the endothelial lining of a bile duct adjacent to the area of hepatic cryosurgery. We consider lesions close to the bifurcation to be a contraindication to hepatic cryosurgery because of this risk. The risk of this has been reported from 0.5% (10) to 10% (5). Controlling the biliary drainage and eliminating any distal biliary obstruction are the mainstays of treatment. These strategies established 100% healing of biliary injuries in the series from Weaver et al. (12,13). Prophylactic measures proposed include the use of metallic stents (to allow for contiguous re-epithelialization after injury) (5) as well as intra-biliary circulation of warmed saline (14). The potential biological "protective" effect on an adjacent tumor warmed by this saline irrigation technique has not been explored. A potentially life threatening biliary complication is arteriobilious fistula formation leading to hemobilia (15).

Hepatic abscess can occur early or late and occurs in the area of necrosis caused by hepatic cryosurgery. The incidence in the series from Siefert et al. is low (0.6%) (10). Interestingly, Sarantou et al. (5) reported one abscess occurring 3 months post-cryosurgery following a dental procedure. Treatment involves antibiotics to the appropriate organism and to drain the abscess cavity percutaneously. Hepatic abscess drainage can occasionally complicate a pleural effusion and cause an empyema as well.

Transient biochemical derangements are the most benign of the complications, involving subclinical rise in liver enzymes, leukocytosis, thrombocytopenia and myoglobinuria. These changes usually resolve over a period of days without clinical consequences. However, these changes can also progress to more severe complications if they do not resolve. Thrombocytopenia may be part of the cryoshock phenomenon (DIC) and myoglobinuria may result in acute renal failure. To monitor these changes, serial bloodwork should be ordered. Myoglobinuria is very common and 94% of 136 patients in the study from Weaver et al. developed this.

The etiology of coagulopathy is multifactorial following hepatic cryosurgery and involves hypothermia, thrombocytopenia or worse as part of the cryoshock phenomenon. Treatment is addressed to each of the factors. Hypothermia is treated with warmers as described above. Thrombocytopenia associated with coagulopathy can be treated with a platelet transfusion or the addition of 1-desamino-8-D-arginine vasopressin (DDAVP). The true etiology of this thrombocytopenia is not determined but there seems to be correlation with the number of freeze-thaw cycles and number of lesions cryoablated (16,17). This must be balanced with the data showing the efficacy of at least a double thaw cycle (4) and thus has led to suggestions to perform a partial double freeze (10) which we have advocated above.

Acute renal failure can be a major problem post hepatic cryosurgery. In the world review by Seifert et al., renal failure accounted for 12% of the mortality in the group of patients who died following hepatic cryosurgery. The etiology is thought to be from the myoglobinuria (which can occur during the thawing cycle) that is complicated by acute tubular necrosis. Similar to thrombocytopenia, observations have been made relating the incidence of acute renal failure to the volume of frozen liver and the number of complete thaw cycles. Prophylaxis is important and adequate diuresis with a judicious combination of fluid infusion and mannitol initiated at the start of the thaw cycle is critical. Weaver et al. (13) also suggested the use of furosemide and urinary alkalinization.

Acute respiratory distress syndrome (ARDS) can also occur following hepatic cryosurgery, and recent work from Blackwell et al. (18) has shown a significant difference in the incidence of lung injury following 35% cryoablation versus 35% hepatic resection in a rat model. Cryoablation resulted in the release of pro-inflammatory factors (NF-kappa-B dependent cytokines) that was detected in both liver and lung tissues, but in the hepatic resection group there was no increase in these pro-inflammatory factors. The authors concluded that the production of specific pro-inflammatory cytokines was a unique feature of cryoablation and not resection.

The cryoshock phenomenon is characterized by multi-organ failure (ARDS, liver failure, renal failure, shock), severe coagulopathy, and disseminated intravascular coagulation (DIC). This is basically a coalescence of the aforementioned complications following hepatic cryosurgery, and in fact many refer to the manifestation of an individual characteristic (e.g., acute renal failure) as an "incomplete cryoshock phenomenon". The etiology of cryoshock phenomenon may be related to tumor lysis. Firstly, many of the characteristics of cryoshock occur proportionally to the amount of tissue destruction. Secondly, lower volume cryosurgery, such as that administered to the prostate, has a much lower incidence of cryoshock phenomenon. The overall prevalence of cryoshock phenomenon was studied by Seifert et al. (10) in a survey of surgeons performing hepatic cryosurgery. In this report, the complication was not common (1%) but the consequences were severe causing death in 29% of patients who manifested the cryoshock phenomenon. It also accounted for 18.2% of the total mortality rate. Treatment is supportive, using the same strategies as described above for the individual components of cryoshock phenomenon (renal failure, coagulopathy, etc.).

Delayed complications occur at a much more distant time after hepatic cryosurgery, usually occurring well after the patient has returned home. More common problems include ventral hernia (common to all laparotomies). Tumor recurrence at a cryosurgical site can also be considered a complication of incomplete ablation. Delayed hepatic abscess can also occur, as mentioned above.

9.2.6 Specific Results of Cryosurgery for Liver Tumors

The use of cryosurgery is now worldwide with the survey (1998) by Siefert et al. reporting 72 centres performing cryosurgery with a total of 2173 patients (19). However, data on the results of hepatic cryosurgery, though promising, are still not sufficient to consider it an alternative to hepatic resection in patients who have resectable disease (20).

9.2.7 Cryosurgery for Primary Liver Tumors: Hepatocellular Carcinoma

Hepatocellular carcinoma is the fifth most common cancer worldwide (accounting for 5.4% of cancers) (21) and is more common in areas of endemic hepatitis such as East Asia. Implicated etiologies are based on a chronic irritation to the liver and include hepatitis B and C, ethanol-induced cirrhosis and exposure to other hepatotoxic chemicals which can be from exogenous exposure or endogenous genetic defects. It is a lethal disease in part because of the combination of neoplastic virulence and the background of hepatic dysfunction, which limits almost every aspect of treatment from resection to chemotherapy. Thus treatments which can ablate a lesion and yet preserve liver function offer an attractive solution to this difficult problem. The ultimate example of this would be transplantation but the availability of organs is the bottleneck in offering this treatment. Cryosurgery offers a solution that preserves hepatic parenchyma while offering tumor ablation.

The data concerning the use of cryosurgery specifically in the setting of hepatocellular carcinoma is unfortunately very heterogeneous. Cryosurgery for hepatocellular carcinoma has been studied (1) in a limited number of patients in most series, (2) for different indications and the outcome analyses combined, and (3) in combination with a variety of other therapies. Table 9.2.3 provides a summary of recent studies looking at the efficacy of hepatic cryosurgery for hepatocellular carcinoma.

The largest experience is provided in Zhou et al.'s report (22). In fact, it has been estimated that China accounts for up to 53.9% of new cases of hepatocellular carcinoma worldwide annually

Table 9.2.3. Cryosurgery for hepatocellular carcinoma – recent studies

Reference	No. of patients	Recurrence rate	Survival/months	5 year survival	Other treatment
Adam R(38) Published 1997	9	NA	63%/24 months	N/A	Resection chemotherapy
Wong WS(24) Published 1998	12	NA	50%/12 months 30%/24 months	NA	Ethanol injection
Crews, KA(39) Published 1997	8	NA	60%/18 months	NA	
Wren SM(40) Published 1997	12	7/12	Mean survival = 19 months	NA	Chemo-embolization
Zhou XD(22) Published 1998	235	NA	78.4%/12 months 54.1%/36 months 39.8%/60 months	39.8%	Resection, hepatic artery ligation, hepatic artery infusion
Bilchik AJ (41) Published 1997	5	NA	NA	NA	
Lam CM (42) Published 1998	4	3/4	NA	NA	

Table 9.2.4. Stratified results of cryosurgery for hepatocellular carcinoma based on Zhou XD et al. (22)

Group	Number	1 year survival	3 year survival	5 year survival
Total patients	235	78.4%	54.1%	39.8%
Small HCC	80	97.2%	77.1%	55.4%
Large HCC (>5 cm)	155	68.7%	42.1%	32.4%
Cryotherapy alone	78	63.9%	40.3%	26.9%
Cryotherapy plus hepatic artery ligation and/or perfusion	58	79.8%	51.7%	39.6%
Cryotherapy of residual tumor plus resection of main tumor	27	73.6%	52.6%	46.0%
Cryotherapy plus resection of frozen tumor	72	98.2%	86.2%	60.4%

(21). With the larger number of patients in that study, the authors were able to analyze their outcomes in a more stratified manner (see Table 9.2.4). They were able to demonstrate that cryosurgery can offer long term control of hepatocellular carcinoma. The overall 5 year survival of 39.8% compares favorably with resection data that shows 41.3% 5 year survival (23). There are no available randomized controlled data comparing resection, transplant and cryosurgery. The majority of the experience with cryosurgery for hepatocellular cancer is also single centre based up to this point.

Caveats of this technique are related to the background of chronic liver disease. A cirrhotic and nodular liver can be exceptionally difficult to ultrasound (even intraoperative ultrasound). Thus, the critical step of watching the ice ball completely form to the correct dimension can be exceedingly difficult and may be a reason that Wong et al. (24) required a further ablative therapy (ethanol injection) after the cryoablation of the tumor. Secondly, one must be sure that the volume of cryoablation performed is within the tolerance of the patient's liver function.

In summary, cryosurgery has a definite role in hepatocellular carcinoma offering an effective ablation with longer term survivals that are comparable to resection in the larger series. However, the data are mostly single institutional and there are certain caveats associated with the effective use of cryosurgery for hepatocellular carcinoma that preclude us from recommending cryosurgery as first line treatment.

9.2.8 Cryosurgery for Metastases: Colorectal Adenocarcinoma

Colorectal adenocarcinoma is a major problem worldwide, being the second most common tumor in developed nations (21). In patients who have had colorectal cancer, approximately one quarter of the patients will develop isolated metastases to the liver but of these patients, only 10–20% will qualify for a resection. However, in the group that undergoes resection, there can be extended survival of up to 50%. Unfortunately, there are still many patients with metastases isolated to the liver who by virtue of anatomy or number of tumors will not be a resection candidate. Cryosurgery offers an alternative treatment for these patients. The questions remaining include the efficacy of and survival after cryosurgery for colorectal metastases to the liver.

A review of the literature in 1997 by Tandan et al. (20) demonstrated the limitations of the data on cryosurgery for hepatic metastases. Limitations of the data that they reported included: (1) only one study assembled a true inception cohort with histologically proven metastases to the liver; (2) outcome assessment was not blinded in any of the studies; (3) no clear indication how many patients were followed up and for how long, making interpretation of the survival rates impossible. This made it impossible to clearly determine the efficacy of cryosurgery compared to resection. However, it was noted that some patients were surviving long term after cryosurgery with approximate 2 year survivals ranging from 30 to 64%. It was clear though that further study would be needed to better define the actual benefit of cryosurgery and also to better define the prognostic factors for hepatic cryosurgery. Since then further data has arrived from Korpan et al. (25), Weaver et al. (13) and Siefert et al. (7).

Korpan's study (25) examined, prospectively over a period of ten years, patients with liver metastases. The patients were randomized into one of two groups. The first group received cryosurgery in some form either alone or in combination with surgical resection. The second group underwent conventional surgery alone (no additional cryosurgery). Both groups then had adjuvant 5-FU/Leucovorin chemotherapy after surgery for the colorectal liver metastases. The total number of patients was 123. Table 9.2.5 summarizes their results. Several important observations were made in their study. Firstly, the five year survival rate in the group who had surgery alone (36%) was consistent with the results of trials using surgery alone for colorectal liver metastases (20–49% (20). Cryosurgery resulted in a significantly higher survival of 44% compared to the group who had surgery alone. From this, the authors concluded that cryosurgery may play a role as an adjunct to resection in the setting of resectable colorectal liver metastases. Secondly, in the cryosurgical group, 14 patients (22%) were discovered to have unresectable disease and subsequently underwent a cryoablative procedure (only) for these lesions. In the non-cryosurgical group, 12 patients were discovered at laparotomy to have unresectable disease and were explored only. The patients who underwent cryosurgery did not have a complete tumor ablation (between 90–97% tumor destruction) but did achieve a higher mean overall survival than those who underwent exploratory laparotomy only (actual survival numbers were not specified in the article).

Weaver et al. (13) further studied the usefulness of cryosurgery in the setting of the unresectable liver metastases. They chose patients who were deemed unresectable due to location and/or number of lesions and excluded patients with >50% liver involvement, cirrhosis, lesions >6 cm and total number of lesions >10. A total of 136 patients underwent 158 cryosurgical procedures. The overall group had a median survival of 30 months. Twenty patients in the series required multiple cryosurgery for recurrent hepatic disease. These results compare favorably to older studies looking at the natural history of unresectable liver metastases (mean survival between 4 to 13 months) and at newer studies looking at survival after aggressive chemoradiation (mean survival 20 months) (26) and hepatic artery infusion (mean survival 13–19 months) (27–29).

Weaver et al. also showed that in patients with pre-cryosurgery CEA levels of >100 ng/dL had a poorer survival (14 months) than the overall group. Seifert et al. (7) explored this issue further by performing a multivariate analysis on their series of 116 patients who had colorectal liver metastases treated with cryosurgery. Their overall median survival was 26 months, comparable to the previously mentioned study. Their analysis of prognostic factors (see Table 9.2.6) may help us further define those who will benefit from cryosurgery.

Currently, resection remains the therapy of choice in patients with colorectal metastases to the liver. However, despite a significant number of patients developing isolated liver metastases, very few in that group are actually eligible for resection. Cryosurgery helps to expand the indications for treatment. Although it is clear that inadequate evidence exists (20) regarding the efficacy of cryosurgery compared to resection, it appears to be an effective adjunct to surgery. Cryosurgery in the setting of unresectable liver metastases expands the indications for surgical intervention and, in those patients with better prognostic indicators, may offer an improved survival in an otherwise incurable situation.

9.2.9 Cryosurgery for Metastases: Neuroendocrine Tumors

Neuroendocrine tumors make up a much smaller proportion of patients presenting with liver metastases. In this group of patients, the natural history is somewhat less virulent but they can often be very symptomatic because of the hormonal production of the neuroendocrine malignancy. Previous studies of aggressive surgical resection for metastatic neuroendocrine tumors of the liver suggest that cure is rare but not impossible and cytoreduction effects a measurable improvement in symptoms and delays need for medical therapy (30–34). Some patients however, do not meet the criteria for resection and in several reports, cryosurgery has been attempted. Table 9.2.7 summarizes the results of larger series of hepatic

Table 9.2.5. Hepatic cryosurgery +/− conventional surgery versus conventional surgery alone data from Korpan (25)

Group	3 year survival	5 year survival	10 year survival
Cryosurgery +/– resection (n = 63)	60%	44%	19%
Conventional surgery alone (n = 60)	51%	36%	8%

Table 9.2.6. Prognostic factors for cryosurgery in colorectal liver metastases (data from Seifert et al. (7))

Favourable Prognostic Factors on Multivariate Analysis (Cox Regression)
Low presurgical serum CEA
Small diameter of cryoablated metastases (<=3 cm)
Absence of untreated extrahepatic disease at laparotomy
Absence of nodal involvement at primary resection
Complete cryotreatment
Good to moderate differentiation of the primary resection

cryosurgery in which metastatic neuroendocrine tumors were also treated.

It is clear that, in most series, very few neuroendocrine metastases were treated with cryosurgery and their major outcomes were not specifically studied. Instead their outcomes were combined with the outcomes for other indications. Two studies (6,35) looked specifically at hepatic cryosurgery for neuroendocrine metastases. These results confirm the efficacy of cryosurgery for non-resectable hepatic neuroendocrine metastases. Though the natural history of neuroendocrine tumors even with metastases confers a much better prognosis overall than hepatoma or colorectal metastases, symptomatology is a known predictor of poor prognosis. In both series, cryosurgery was effective in generating at least a partial decrease in the symptomatology of these patients. These previously symptomatic patients then went on to have long term survival (see Table 9.2.7) which was more consistent with the natural history of asymptomatic patients.

9.2.10 Cryosurgery for Metastases: Other Primaries

There are other neoplasms that metastasize to the liver but their biology is somewhat different than in the cases of colorectal metastasis and neuroendocrine metastases. Often, there is extra-hepatic disease (for example, bone metastases in breast cancer) but liver metastases occur very rarely. Non-colorectal and non-neuroendocrine metastases treated by hepatic cryosurgery have included breast, gastric, melanoma, ovarian, renal, small bowel, and pancreatic. There are too few numbers in any series to allow for any useful analysis.

Even recent data from studies looking at liver resection for breast metastases have been controversial regarding prognostic factors. Maksan et al. (36) found that initial lymph node status was critical but Selzner et al. (37) did not. A review of several studies looking at liver resection for non-colorectal liver metastases also found little agreement on prognostic factors (12).

A patient with a predicted good natural history would benefit the most from any additional and localized therapy to the liver such as cryosurgery. These patients include those with a longer disease free interval, absence of extra-hepatic disease, single metastasis, and long-time stable disease (on or off other therapy such as chemotherapy). In a review by Berney et al. (12) the unanimously agreed upon factor in all studies was the "curative nature of the resection".

Further study will be needed before guidelines for hepatic cryosurgery of non colorectal/non neuroendocrine metastases can be well established. In the meantime, certain patients can benefit from local therapies including cryosurgery and resection but these patients must be chosen judiciously and in combination with an extensive search for extrahepatic disease.

References

1. Healey WV, Priebe CJ, Jr., Farrer SM, Phillips LL. Hepatic cryosurgery. Acute and long-term effects. Arch Surg 1971; 103(3): 384–392.
2. Dutta P, Montes M, Gage AA. Experimental hepatic cryosurgery. Cryobiology 1977; 14(5): 598–608.

Table 9.2.7. Results of cryosurgery for neuroendocrine liver metastases

Study	Total no. of patients	Symptom free survival	Symptom relief			Overall survival	Morbidity & mortality
			Number of patients symptomatic prior to cryosurgery	Complete response	Partial Response		
Seifert et al. (35)	13	N/A	7	5	2	12/13 patients alive at median F/U = 13.5 months	4/13 morbidity
Bilchik et al. (6)	19	10 months	19	19 (2 patients required a second cryosurgery)	N/A	>49 months	morbidity N/A 0% mortality
Crews et al. (39)	2	NA	NA	NA	NA	NA–all died of disease – time not mentioned	NA
Cozzi et al. (16)	6	repeated data from Seifert series	—	—	—	—	—
Dale et al. (43)	1	NA	NA	NA	NA	NA	NA
Ravikumar et al. (44)	2	NA	NA	NA	NA	NA	NA

3. Dutta P, Montes M, Gage AA. Large volume freezing in experimental hepatic cryosurgery. Avoidance of bleeding in hepatic freezing by an improvement in the technique. Cryobiology 1979; 16(1): 50–55.
4. Ravikumar TS, Steele G, Jr., Kane R, King V. Experimental and clinical observations on hepatic cryosurgery for colorectal metastases. Cancer Res 1991; 51(23 Pt 1): 6323–6327.
5. Sarantou T, Bilchik A, Ramming KP. Complications of hepatic cryosurgery. Semin Surg Oncol 1998; 14(2): 156–162.
6. Bilchik AJ, Sarantou T, Foshag LJ, Giuliano AE, Ramming KP. Cryosurgical palliation of metastatic neuroendocrine tumors resistant to conventional therapy. Surgery 1997; 122(6): 1040–1047.
7. Seifert JK, Morris DL. Prognostic factors after cryotherapy for hepatic metastases from colorectal cancer. Ann Surg 1998; 228(2): 201–208.
8. Onik GM, Chambers N, Chernus SA, Zemel R, Atkinson D, Weaver ML. Hepatic cryosurgery with and without the Bair Hugger. J Surg Oncol 1993; 52(3): 185–187.
9. Cady B, Jenkins RL, Steele GD, Jr., Lewis WD, Stone MD, McDermott WV et al. Surgical margin in hepatic resection for colorectal metastasis: a critical and improvable determinant of outcome. Ann Surg 1998; 227(4): 566–571.
10. Seifert JK, Morris DL. World survey on the complications of hepatic and prostate cryotherapy. World J Surg 1999; 23(2):109–113.
11. Yeh KA, Fortunato L, Hoffman JP, Eisenberg BL. Cryosurgical ablation of hepatic metastases from colorectal carcinomas. Am Surg 1997; 63(1): 63–68.
12. Berney T, Mentha G, Roth AD, Morel P. Results of surgical resection of liver metastases from non-colorectal primaries. Br J Surg 1998; 85(10): 1423–1427.
13. Weaver ML, Ashton JG, Zemel R. Treatment of colorectal liver metastases by cryotherapy. Semin Surg Oncol 1998; 14(2): 163–170.
14. Silverstein JC, Staren E, Velasco J. Thermal bile duct protection during liver cryoablation. J Surg Oncol 1997; 64(2): 163–164.
15. Frank JL, Navab F, Ly K, Reed WP, Jr. Hemobilia complicating hepatic cryosurgery. J Surg Oncol 1998; 67(2): 130–133.
16. Cozzi PJ, Englund R, Morris DL. Cryotherapy treatment of patients with hepatic metastases from neuroendocrine tumors. Cancer 1995; 76(3): 501–509.
17. Stewart GJ, Preketes A, Horton M, Ross WB, Morris DL. Hepatic cryotherapy: double-freeze cycles achieve greater hepatocellular injury in man. Cryobiology 1995; 32(3): 215–219.
18. Blackwell TS, Debelak JP, Venkatakrishnan A, Schot DJ, Harley DH, Pinson CW et al. Acute lung injury after hepatic cryoablation: correlation with NF-kappa B activation and cytokine production. Surgery 1999; 126(3): 518–526.
19. Seifert JK, Junginger T, Morris DL. A collective review of the world literature on hepatic cryotherapy. J R Coll Surg Edinb 1998; 43(3): 141–154.
20. Tandan VR, Harmantas A, Gallinger S. Long-term survival after hepatic cryosurgery versus surgical resection for metastatic colorectal carcinoma: a critical review of the literature. Can J Surg 1997; 40(3): 175–181.
21. Parkin DM, Pisani P, Ferlay J. Estimates of the worldwide incidence of 25 major cancers in 1990. Int J Cancer 1999; 80(6): 827–841.
22. Zhou XD, Tang ZY. Cryotherapy for primary liver cancer. Semin Surg Oncol 1998; 14(2): 171–174.
23. Mazziotti A, Grazi GL, Cavallari A. Surgical treatment of hepatocellular carcinoma on cirrhosis: a Western experience. Hepatogastroenterology 1998; 45 Suppl 3: 1281–1287.
24. Wong WS, Patel SC, Cruz FS, Gala KV, Turner AF. Cryosurgery as a treatment for advanced stage hepatocellular carcinoma: results, complications, and alcohol ablation. Cancer 1998; 82(7): 1268–1278.
25. Korpan NN. Hepatic cryosurgery for liver metastases. Long-term follow-up. Ann Surg 1997; 225(2): 193–201.
26. Robertson JM, Lawrence TS, Walker S, Kessler ML, Andrews JC, Ensminger WD. The treatment of colorectal liver metastases with conformal radiation therapy and regional chemotherapy. Int J Radiat Oncol Biol Phys 1995; 32(2): 445–450.
27. Bertuccelli M, Falcone A, Campoccia S, Conti M, Brunetti I, Caramella D et al. Intrahepatic chemotherapy with floxuridine, leucovorin and dexamethasone in continuous infusion and mitomycin-C bolus in unresectable hepatic metastases from colorectal cancer: a phase II study. Tumori 1999; 85(6): 473–477.
28. Howell JD, Warren HW, Anderson JH, Kerr DJ, McArdle CS. Intraarterial 5-fluorouracil and intravenous folinic acid in the treatment of liver metastases from colorectal cancer. Eur J Surg 1999; 165(7): 652–658.
29. Kemeny N, Conti JA, Cohen A, Campana P, Huang Y, Shi WJ et al. Phase II study of hepatic arterial floxuridine, leucovorin, and dexamethasone for unresectable liver metastases from colorectal carcinoma. J Clin Oncol 1994; 12(11): 2288–2295.
30. Que FG, Nagorney DM, Batts KP, Linz LJ, Kvols LK. Hepatic resection for metastatic neuroendocrine carcinomas. Am J Surg 1995; 169(1): 36–42
31. McEntee GP, Nagorney DM, Kvols LK, Moertel CG, Grant CS. Cytoreductive hepatic surgery for neuroendocrine tumors. Surgery 1990; 108(6): 1091–1096.
32. Grazi GL, Cescon M, Pierangeli F, Ercolani G, Gardini A, Cavallari A et al. Highly aggressive policy of hepatic resections for neuroendocrine liver metastases [In Process Citation]. Hepatogastroenterology 2000; 47(32): 481–486.
33. Elias D, Cavalcanti dA, Eggenspieler P, Plaud B, Ducreux M, Spielmann M et al. Resection of liver metastases from a noncolorectal primary: indications and results based on 147 monocentric patients. J Am Coll Surg 1998; 187(5): 487–493.
34. Chamberlain RS, Canes D, Brown KT, Saltz L, Jarnagin W, Fong Y et al. Hepatic neuroendocrine metastases: does intervention alter outcomes? J Am Coll Surg 2000; 190(4): 432–445.
35. Seifert JK, Cozzi PJ, Morris DL. Cryotherapy for neuroendocrine liver metastases. Semin Surg Oncol 1998; 14(2): 175–183.
36. Maksan SM, Lehnert T, Bastert G, Herfarth C. Curative liver resection for metastatic breast cancer. Eur J Surg Oncol 2000; 26(3): 209–212.
37. Selzner M, Morse MA, Vredenburgh JJ, Meyers WC, Clavien PA. Liver metastases from breast cancer: long-term survival after curative resection. Surgery 2000; 127(4): 383–389.
38. Adam R, Akpinar E, Johann M, Kunstlinger F, Majno P, Bismuth H. Place of cryosurgery in the treatment of malignant liver tumors. Ann Surg 1997; 225(1): 39–8.
39. Crews KA, Kuhn JA, McCarty TM, Fisher TL, Goldstein RM, Preskitt JT. Cryosurgical ablation of hepatic tumors. Am J Surg 1997; 174(6): 614–617.
40. Wren SM, Coburn MM, Tan M, Daniels JR, Yassa N, Carpenter CL et al. Is cryosurgical ablation appropriate for treating hepatocellular cancer? Arch Surg 1997; 132(6): 599–603.
41. Bilchik AJ, Sarantou T, Wardlaw JC, Ramming KP. Cryosurgery causes a profound reduction in tumor markers in hepatoma and noncolorectal hepatic metastases. Am Surg 1997; 63(9): 796–800.
42. Lam CM, Yuen WK, Fan ST. Hepatic cryosurgery for recurrent hepatocellular carcinoma after hepatectomy: a preliminary report. J Surg Oncol 1998; 68(2): 104–106.
43. Dale PS, Souza JW, Brewer DA. Cryosurgical ablation of unresectable hepatic metastases. J Surg Oncol 1998; 68(4): 242–245.
44. Ravikumar TS, Kane R, Cady B, Jenkins R, Clouse M, Steele G, Jr. A 5-year study of cryosurgery in the treatment of liver tumors. Arch Surg 1991; 126(12): 1520–1523.

9.3 Cryoablation in the Treatment of Liver Lesions

Georgij G. Prokhorov with contributions by O. A. Litvinov and D. G. Prokhorov

9.3.0 Introduction

This report summarizes our 3-year experience with cryosurgery of liver tumors. In the period from 1997 through 2000, 8 patients (7 men and 1 woman) were entered into this study. The liver was exposed with laparotomy, and existing tumors were subjected to one or two freeze-thaw cycles using liquid nitrogen (temperature −196°C) delivered by five cryoneedles with a diameter of 3.85 mm. The cryoablation was monitored with intraoperative ultrasonography. The histologic characteristics of the tumors were as follows: colorectal cancer lesions, 6 patients; stomach cancer lesions, 2 patients. The follow-up period ranged from 71 to 446 days (median follow-up 233.7 ± 43.3 days). Six patients died in the period between 2 and 10 months after surgery. Two patients are alive, one of them has lived more than a year with signs of a relapse of disease in the liver. In this report we estimate the opportunities and efficiency of cryosurgery in the treatment of large liver lesions.

9.3.1 Material and Methods

The mean age of the patients was 57.5 years (46–65 years). The diagnosis of liver lesions was established on the basis of the results of ultrasonography and computed tomography. Cryodestruction was carried out in cases in which the liver tumors were unresectable (1,9): multiple lesions, tumor located in immediate proximity to major vessels, such as the portal vein and the vena cava, severe multimorbidity. Preoperative clinical and biochemical analyses of blood, liver function tests, coagulation test, abdominal computed tomography and liver ultrasonography were performed in all patients. Bilateral location of the liver lesions was detected in 5 cases, in 3 patients the lesion was located in one lobe. In 4 cases lesions were found in segment VIII, involving hepatic veins and a wall of the vena cava inferior. Synchronous lesions were found in 3 patients, metachronous in five. Computed tomography and ultrasonography were used in radiologic evaluation of tumor response and recurrence. We did not perform regional or systemic chemotherapy after cryodestruction.

9.3.2 Cryosurgical Engineering

Cryodestruction was carried out with a standard technique by laparotomy (1,5). Operative access to the liver was provided by a right subcostal incision. The liver was examined bimanually and the peritoneal cavity was explored to rule out extrahepatic disease. An intraoperative ultrasound unit (Aloca-630, Philips-360) was used to obtain real time images of the entire liver. 5 mHz linear-array transducers were used for this scanning. 3.85 mm trocar-type probes were used for hepatic cryoablation. Plate probes 40 mm in diameter were applied to freeze the liver's surface lesions. The probe was driven by a cryosurgical system, LCS 3000 Candela USA, which circulates the liquid nitrogen (temperature −196°C) through the probe. The placement of probes in the lesions, and also the freeze-thaw process were monitored with intraoperative ultrasonography. Cryosurgical ablation was performed with up to 5 cryoprobes placed simultaneously to expand the resulting ice ball over all the metastases. Intraoperative ultrasound monitored ice ball formation, the aim being to achieve a 1 cm frozen margin around the lesion. To achieve this purpose, it was necessary to carry out a change in position of the cryoneedles. The maximal size of a tumor that allows adequate cryodestruction of a lesion by simultaneous placement of probes with a diameter of 3.85 mm is 40 mm. The freeze portion of each freeze-thaw cycle took 15–20 minutes, and thawing took approximately 20–25 minutes. Spontaneous thawing extended the duration of the operation slightly, but allowed us to save stocks of nitrogen in the cryosystem, needed for adequate cryodestruction of large tumors. Single or double freeze–thaw cycles were carried out for each lesion. The choice of the mode of cryodestruction in each case depended on the number of lesions, their size, and their anatomic location, also the condition of the patient at the time of surgery, and whether cryodestruction was combined with conventional surgery. The probe was withdrawn after complete rewarming and the site was packed with an absorbable knitted fabric. A single freeze–thaw cycle was conducted in 7 patients, a double freeze-thaw cycle in 1 case.

9.3.3 Results

Eight patients were entered into this study in the period 1997–2000. Their mean age was 57.5 years (46–65 years). In all cases the liver tumors were metastatic. Histologically, tumors were metastases of colorectal cancer in 6 patients, metastases of stomach cancer in 2 patients. Metachronous lesions were found in 5 patients, synchronous in 3. In all cases these were adenocarcinomas. In all patients, cryodestruction was carried out 3–48 months after resection of a primary tumor. The basic clinical data on the patients are shown in Table 9.3.1.

Combined operations were carried out in 3 patients. Cryoablation of liver metastases was combined with cholecystectomy (1 patient), with nephrectomy (1 patient), and with cryodestruction of pelvic metastases (1 patient). The median hospital stay was 14 days (range 2–18 days). There were no intraoperative or postoperative complications. The duration of surgery was 5 h 42 min ± 39.1 min (3 h 45 min to 9 h 25 min). Average blood loss was 650 ± 197.3 ml (range: 400 to 1200 ml). The intraoperative bleeding from the postcryosurgical lesion was controlled by packing with an absorbable knitted fabric. Patients spent 2 to 3 days in the intensive care unit. Transient elevation of liver enzymes (to more than 7 times the preoperative level on the 2nd and 3rd postoperative days) and leukocytosis (up to 18 000) were observed. These levels normalized by the 10th postoperative day. The patients had a temperature as high as 38–39°C for 6–7 days after the operation, in 1 case for 20 days as a reaction to cryoablation, with negative cultures for systemic sepsis or purulent complications. Serum secretion for 14 days was seen in 1 patient who had undergone cryoablation of a large lesion (diameter 10.8 cm).

A perioperative complication occurred in 1 case when a double freeze-thaw cycle was carried out. One patient died 12 hours after the operation due to cryoshock. He had bilateral lesions and the percentage of hepatic replacement by the tumor was in the 25–50% range. It is known (2,3) that intraoperative coagulation disturbances can be exacerbated by general hypothermia, and, as is routine, a warming device surrounded the patient's body and warming fluid and plasma (300–600 ml) were administered. But long-term hypothermia (duration of surgery was 9 h 25 min, there were 12 freeze-thaw cycles, the patient's temperature at the end of the operation was 32°C) led to coagulopathy and multiple organ failure.

Table 9.3.1. Clinical patient data

Number of patients	8
Average age	57.5 years
Female	1
Male	7
Percentage hepatic replacement by tumors (PHR)	
<25%	2
25–50%	4
>50%	2
Liver disease only	6
Liver and extrahepatic disease	2
Number of lesions present (mean)	6,25 ± 2,4
Range	1–19
Average diameter of lesions	3,31 ± 0,48
Range	0,8–13
Follow-up in days	233,7 ± 43,3 days
Range	71–446 days

Our data indicate that within the first three hours of the operation the body temperature of the patient fell by 1.5°C. As the duration of surgery and of hypothermia increased, the patient's temperature was further reduced.

The follow-up period ranged from 71 to 446 days (not including the patient who expired), median follow-up: 233.7 ± 43.3 days. Two patients are alive to date, 6 patients died of recurrent tumors between 71 and 280 days after cryoablation.

The most important prognostic indicators were the size of tumors treated, expressed as percentage hepatic replacement (PHR) (3), anatomic location of the lesions and combination of liver disease with extrahepatic disease. For a PHR < 25% (n=2) the median survival was 323 ± 123 days. Two patients are still alive, one of whom has residual disease. He underwent bowel resection of colorectal cancer recurrence 8 months after the cryosurgical procedure. Tumor recurrence was found in the areas of cryodestruction as well as in other parts of the liver. The follow-up period of the second patient is 200 days, and at present there are no signs of progressive growth of metastases in the liver.

Of the 6 patients with colorectal metastases, one had evidence of residual disease (extrahepatic pelvic disease) documented at the time of cryosurgery. Two patients had PHR > 50%, two patients had PHR of 25–50% and had from 10 to 19 lesions. One of the patients with PHR > 50% had a large lesion in the pelvis (diameter 10 cm), and in his case cryodestruction of the liver metastases was performed in a single freeze-thaw cycle combined with cryoablation of the pelvic lesion. The patient lived for 9 months after surgery. The follow-up period for the second patient with PHR > 50% and central location of metastases was 71 days.

Of the 2 patients with stomach metastases one had evidence of residual disease (extrahepatic nodal disease). Both patients had PHR of 25–50%. Long-term disease control was not achieved in any of these cases.

We used 3.85 mm cryoprobes to increase safety in the passage of the probes through the liver and reduce blood loss. But we had to perform cryoablation with the probes in several positions to expand the ice ball to cover the metastases extending over a surface of more than 40 mm in diameter. In patients with PHR 25–50% and >50% only a single freeze-thaw cycle was performed. Our trying to do double freeze-thaw cycle cryoablation led to cryoshock in one patient. Median survival in patients with PHR > 25% was 198 ± 36.2 days, which correlated with median survival for untreated hepatic metastases (6,7,8).

Our data suggest that single freeze-thaw cryodestruction of large metastases in the liver have not essentially increased the survival rate. Our experience has shown that double freezing such large lesions can lead to cryoshock. The larger the diameter of the lesion, the greater their number, the closer they are located to major vessels, such as the vena cava inferior or the hepatic veins, the worse the results of cryoablation. Poor prognostic indicators also include a combination of liver disease with extrahepatic disease and the recurrence of a primary tumor. The performance of cryoablation of the liver lesions located close to hepatic veins and involving a wall of the vena cava inferior does not result in damage to the vein's wall because of the powerful bloodstream in the vessels.

Finally we surmise that a good clinical effect from cryodestruction may be expected in patients with liver lesions metastasized from colorectal cancer, with PHR by tumors less than 25% and with an absence of extrahepatic metastases at the time of performance of a double freeze-thaw cycle.

References

1. Littrup P, Lee F, Rajan D. Hepatic cryotherapy . State of the art techniques and future developments. Ultrasound Quarterly 1998; 14: 171–188.
2. Weaver Ml, Atkinson D, Zemel R. Hepatic cryosurgery in the treatment of unresectable metastases. Surg Oncol 1995; 4: 231–236.
3. Morris DL, Ross WB, Iqbal J. Cryoablation of hepatic malignancy: an evaluation of tumor marker data and survival in 110 patients. GL Cancer 1996; 1: 247–251.
4. Ravikumar TS, Kane R, Cady B. A 5 year study of cryosurgery in the treatment of liver tumors. Arch Surg 1991; 126: 1520–1524.
5. Korpan NN. Hepatic cryosurgery for liver metastases. Annals Surg 1997; 225: 193–201.
6. Bengmark S, Hafstrom L. The natural history of primary and secondary malignant tumors of the liver: the prognosis for patients with hepatic metastases from colonic carcinoma by laparotomy. Cancer 1969; 23: 198–202.
7. Wood CB, Gillis CR, Blumgart LH. A retrospective study of the natural history of patients with liver metastases from colorectal cancer. Clin Oncol 1976; 2: 285–288.
8. Bengtsson G, Caelsson G, Hafstrom L, Jonsson PE. Natural history of patients with untreated liver metastases from colorectal cancer. Am J Surg 1981; 141: 586–589.
9. Steele G Jr, Ravikumar TS. Resection of hepatic metastases from colorectal cancer: biologic perspectives. Ann Surg 1989; 210: 127–138.
10. Onik GM, Cooper C, Goldberg HI, Moss AA, Rubinsky B, Christianson M. Ultrasonic characteristics of frozen liver. Cryobiology 1984; 21: 321–328.
11. Onik G, Rubinsky B, Zemel R, et al. Ultrasound-guided hepatic cryosurgery in the treatment of colorectal metastatic colon carcinoma: preliminary results. Cancer 1991; 67: 901–907.
12. Ravikumar TS. The role of cryotherapy in the management of patients with liver tumors. Adv Surg 1996; 30: 281–291.

9.4 Minimally Invasive Hepatic Cryosurgery

Calvin H. L. Law with a contribution by Véd R. Tandan

9.4.0 Introduction

Hepatic cryosurgery provides a method with which indications for surgical intervention for hepatocellular carcinoma or hepatic metastases can be expanded. The advantages of cryosurgery include: (1) the ability to ablate targeted tissue; (2) minimal and controlled destruction of surrounding normal parenchyma; (3) possible increase in immune stimulation. However, for many years, hepatic cryosurgery has been limited by the need for a subcostal laparotomy to allow for hepatic exposure and subsequent placement of cryosurgical probes.

A minimally invasive technique would expand the advantages of hepatic cryosurgery even more by eliminating the morbid, large subcostal incision. Laparoscopic techniques have revolutionized surgery, allowing surgeons access to the abdominal cavity using very small incisions that minimize morbidity and maximize cosmesis. Hepatic cryosurgery is ideally suited to this approach since it uses small probes that can be passed through trocars and it does not necessitate the removal of any specimen. Several experiments have shown its feasibility, and limited clinical studies are reporting success with the technique.

9.4.1 Experimental Basis for Minimally Invasive Hepatic Cryosurgery

Minimally invasive hepatic cryosurgery requires that the lesion can be accessed via limited exposure, and that there are cryoprobes that are small enough to be introduced via limited incisions. In addition, it requires the use of a modified intraoperative ultrasound transducer probe capable of being placed through a limited incision.

Two techniques of minimally invasive hepatic cryosurgery have been tested in pig models. The more common technique has been the laparoscopic approach and there is one report studying the use of a "mini-laparotomy".

The mini-laparotomy technique was described by Lee et al. (1). In this study, a percutaneous creation of "agar" lesions was carried out in 17 pigs followed by a 2 cm subcostal incision and intraoperative imaging using an end-fire multiple array ultrasound transducer. Cryoprobes were then placed directly into the lesions and a 15 minute freeze cycle was initiated. The pigs were then sacrificed and their livers were to be studied. Problems with the technique included: (1) the lesions created were 0.7 cm in size and there was still a positive "agar" margin in one pig; (2) imaging in the same line of sight as the cryoprobe made it difficult to accurately monitor the developing ice ball; (3) the "agar" lesions were made in the inferior portion of the liver whereas the typical liver metastasis is often in the superior portion of the liver where it is made unresectable by virtue of its anatomic location; and (4) lack of an easy ability to visualize the rest of the abdominal cavity to rule out extra-hepatic metastases. Potential advantages of this technique as advocated by the authors include (a) the ability to use this despite dense adhesions that precluded laparoscopy; and (b) the relative ease of this technique compared to laparoscopy.

There are several experimental studies for the laparoscopic approach (2–4). The study from Tandan et al. helped to establish (in a pig model) (a) the ability to maintain pneumoperitoneum while using the cryoprobes; (b) the lack of skin destruction at the port site using a cryoprobe through the Teflon laparoscopic port and (c) the ability to identify, target, and completely ablate a lesion via laparoscopic ultrasound and cryosurgery was confirmed. McCall et al. found that none of their rabbit models of laparoscopic hepatic cryosurgery suffered a potentially fatal gas embolus.

Limitations to treating high right lobe lesions was noted by Tandan et al. and transpleural placement of cryoprobes was suggested but with the warning of the need for a chest tube and double lumen endotracheal intubation to allow for a right sided lung collapse prior to transpleural port placement.

9.4.2 Technique of Laparoscopic Hepatic Cryosurgery

General anesthesia is used in all patients. Positioning is the next step and can be critical. Good knowledge of the lesion location is needed to determine whether the procedure can be performed supine or left decubitus. The left decubitus position allows for laparoscopic treatment of segment VI or VII by allowing posterior access as well (5). Pneumoperitoneum was established via Veress needle (2,6) or open Hasson trocar (5). Ianitti et al. argued for an open approach since most patients may have had a previous surgery (primary lesion) and thus postoperative scarring may be an issue. The laparoscope is placed into the abdomen. Using an angled scope allows for better visualization (30 to 45 degrees), and keeping all ports 10 mm or greater allows any camera to be moved to any port. The first step here is to rule out the presence of carcinomatosis or distant or recurrent disease that would terminate the procedure. Once this is ruled out, the other ports should be placed under direct vision. Adhesions are taken down where needed and the liver can be mobilized along the falciform and triangular ligaments where necessary. The port to be used for the laparoscopic ultrasound transducer must be kept lateral and level with the surface of the liver to allow better optimization of ultrasound imaging. In addition, we have found that a plastic trocar without a trumpet valve is required here, since the metal trocars with trumpet valves had the propensity to strip the plastic lining off the laparoscopic ultrasound resulting in major transducer damage. The appropriate site for the Teflon port is then chosen and the liver capsule scored with an L-hook prior to the placement of the cryoprobe under directed ultrasound guidance. Temperatures, core and intra-abdominal, should be monitored. Fluid bolus should be started if a larger amount of lesion is to be cryoablated. Two cycles of freeze/thaw are used and the probe is removed once the temperature rises above −20°C. The tract can then be packed with hemostatic agents using narrower 5 mm laparoscopic forceps. As in the open technique, drains should be left inside and can be brought out through the laparoscopic port sites.

Pistorius (7) emphasized the critical steps to laparoscopic hepatic cryosurgery: (a) targeting the lesion; (b) visualizing the ice ball; (c) successfully approaching deep lesions; (d) appropriately monitoring blood loss.

9.4.3 Patient Selection for Minimally Invasive Hepatic Cryosurgery

Several clinical studies looking at laparoscopic hepatic cryosurgery have been published (2, 5, 6, 8, 9). There were a variety of reasons to choose laparoscopy. First, the general guidelines for open hepatic cryosurgery are applicable. Additional indications specific to the laparoscopic approach include: poor risk candidate for major laparotomy; unresectable disease in easily accessible range of a laparoscopic approach; and in one study (5) patient preference.

Table 9.4.1. Clinical results of laparoscopic hepatic cryosurgery

Study	Number	Extrahepatic disease	OR time (min)	Blood loss (cc)	No. of lesions and size (cm)	Complication	Postoperative stay (days)
Heniford et al. (8) Ianitti et al. (5)	9	2	210	235	3/3.4	1 – hemorrhage 1 – biliary leak	4.5
Lezoche et al. (9)	18	0	131.2	N/A	1.5/N/A	2 – hemorrhage 8 – pleural effusion 3 – subphrenic collection 1 – worsening of liver function 1 – wound infection	6.4
Tandan et al. (2)	1	0	N/A	N/A	1/2	0	4
Wallis et al. (6)	5	0	N/A Freeze time 32 minutes	100	N/A	1 – parenchymal fracture 2 – pleural effusion	N/A

9.4.4 Clinical Results of Minimally Invasive Hepatic Cryosurgery

The results of the limited series of laparoscopic hepatic cryosurgery are presented in Table 9.4.1 as well. With very limited numbers it is difficult to draw firm conclusions. However, it appears that laparoscopic hepatic cryosurgery may result in a shorter hospital stay, consistent with the results of other laparoscopic procedures. However, the usual complications of hepatic cryosurgery were not spared including the development of pleural effusion, the possibility of parenchymal fracture with significant blood loss requiring a conversion to an open approach for hemorrhage control, biliary leak and critical destruction of normal parenchyma resulting in an exacerbation of liver failure. These are important considerations for the anesthetist as well and it is critical not to be lulled into a sense of security because the laparoscope is being used. No incidents of cryoshock were noted but this may be related to the limited size and number of lesions treated with cryosurgery.

References

1. Lee FT, Jr., Chosy SG, Weber SM, Littrup PJ, Warner TF, Mahvi DM. Hepatic cryosurgery via minilaparotomy in a porcine model: an alternative to open cryosurgery. Surg Endosc 1999; 13(3): 253–259.
2. Tandan VR, Litwin D, Asch M, Margolis M, Gallinger S. Laparoscopic cryosurgery for hepatic tumors. Experimental observations and a case report. Surg Endosc 1997; 11(11): 1115–1117.
3. Cuschieri A, Crosthwaite G, Shimi S, Pietrabissa A, Joypaul V, Tair I. Hepatic cryotherapy for liver tumors. Development and clinical evaluation of a high-efficiency insulated multineedle probe system for open and laparoscopic use. Surg Endosc 1995; 9(5): 483–489.
4. McCall JL, Jorgensen JO, Morris DL. Laparoscopic hepatic cryotherapy: a study of safety in rabbits. Surg Laparosc Endosc 1996; 6(1): 29–31.
5. Iannitti DA, Heniford T, Hale J, Grundfest-Broniatowski S, Gagner M. Laparoscopic cryoablation of hepatic metastases. Arch Surg 1998; 133(9): 1011–1015.
6. Wallis CB, Coventry DM. Anaesthetic experience with laparoscopic cryotherapy. A new technique for treating liver metastases. Surg Endosc 1997; 11(10): 979–981.
7. Pistorius G, Menger MD, Feifel G. Minilaparotomy vs the percutaneous approach for minimally invasive hepatic cryosurgery [letter]. Surg Endosc 2000; 14(2): 207–209.
8. Heniford BT, Arca MJ, Iannitti DA, Walsh RM, Gagner M. Laparoscopic cryoablation of hepatic metastases. Semin Surg Oncol 1998; 15(3): 194–201.
9. Lezoche E, Paganini AM, Feliciotti F, Guerrieri M, Lugnani F, Tamburini A. Ultrasound-guided laparoscopic cryoablation of hepatic tumors: preliminary report. World J Surg 1998; 22(8): 829–835.

9.5 Cryosurgery for Liver Alveococcosis

Boris I. Alperovich

Alveococcosis results from the invasion of an organism by Echinococcus multilocularis in its larval stage and its further development (Leuckart 1863). The parasitic nature of the disease was first established by R. Virchow (1856). The real nature of the disease and the biological cycle of the development of alveococcus were investigated only in the last decades by Rausch (USA), Vogel (Germany), Lucashenko (Russia). Morphological peculiarities of parasitic lesions of the liver have been investigated by Posselt, Melnikov-Razvedenkov, Mirolyubov and Konstantinov.

The disease is found in northeastern Tirol (Austria) and in the neighboring districts of Bavaria (Germany), southern France, in Alaska (USA), on Hokkaido Island (Japan), in Russia and in other countries of the former USSR (Kirghistan, Armenia, Azerbaijan). In Russia the largest epidemic regions for alveococcosis are Bashkiria, Western Siberia, Yakutia, Kamchatka, Chukotka, and the Kirov Region.

In fact the disease invades only the liver, in which a parasitic tumor develops. Because of its peculiar biological structure and its clinical manifestations, the parasitic tumor is similar to the malignant liver tumor. The Alveococcus node in the liver has infiltrating growth as have malignant tumors, and in the process of growth it can invade the porta hepatis (Fig. 9.5.1), neighboring tissues and organs–pancreas, diaphragm, pericardium and even the myocardium (Figs. 9.5.2–9.5.3). Invasion of blood and lymphatic vessels leads to the development of metastatic lesions of regional lymphatic nodes (Fig. 9.5.4), of the lung (Fig. 9.5.5), and the brain (Fig. 9.5.6). The alveococcosis node (parasitic cavern) can rupture and the contents flow into the abdominal and pleural cavities and even into the pericardiac cavity, resulting, respectively, in peritonitis, pleurisy, and pericarditis. All these complications lead inevitably to death. Therefore, optimal methods of treating the disease should be elaborated.

In 1890 Langenbuch stated that "for long this sad and awful form of the disease will induce doctors to look for some specific means" and the Russian scientist N.F. Melnikov-Razvedenkov stated in 1902: "The danger of mortality resulting from infection by alveolar echinococcosis stimulates the doctor's interest in studying the etiology of infection and the peculiarities of the parasite's development in the human body. The opportunity of surgical treatment makes alveolar echinococcosis interesting both for internists and surgeons". In the past century the etiology, epidemiology and morphology of alveococcosis were investigated in

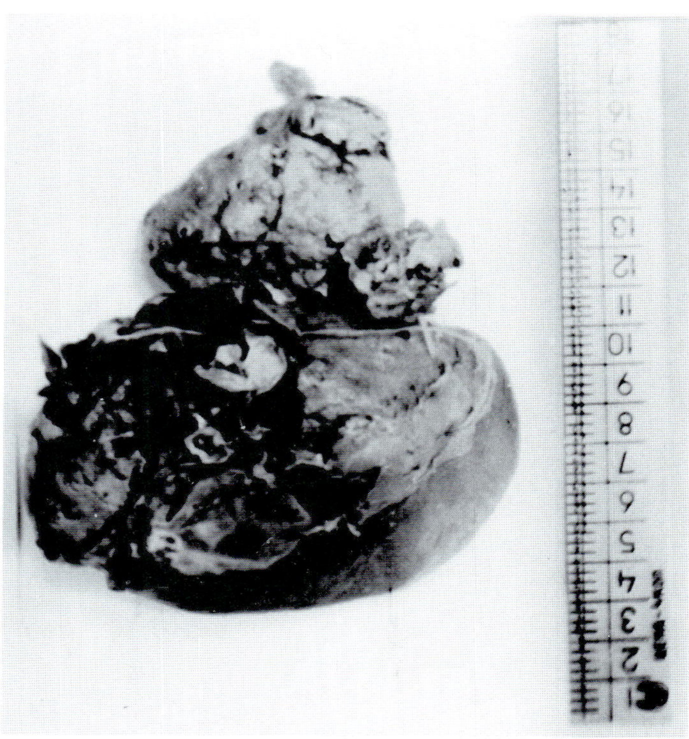

Fig. 9.5.2. Alveococcosis of the liver. Invasion of the parasite into the pericardium

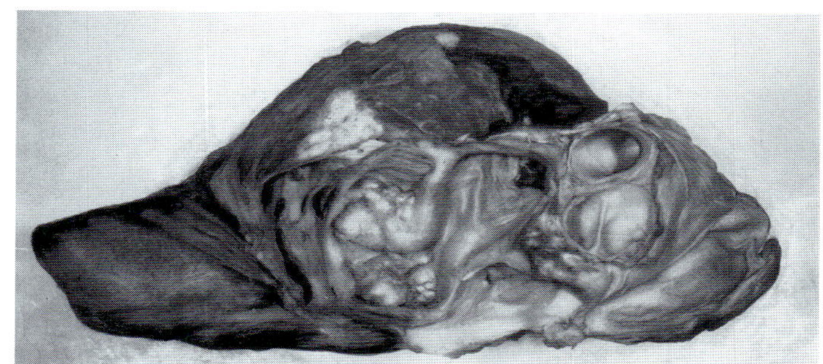

Fig. 9.5.3. Alveococcosis of the liver. Invasion of the parasite into the myocardium

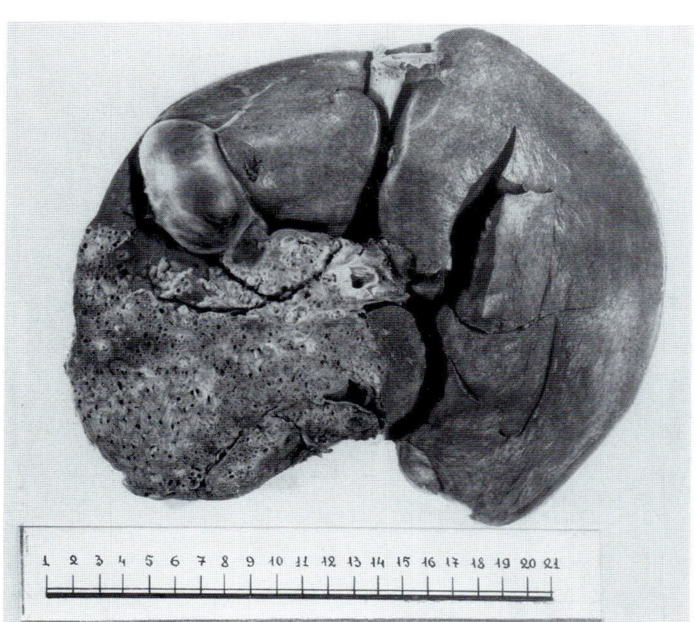

Fig. 9.5.1. Alveococcosis of the liver. Invasion of the porta hepatis

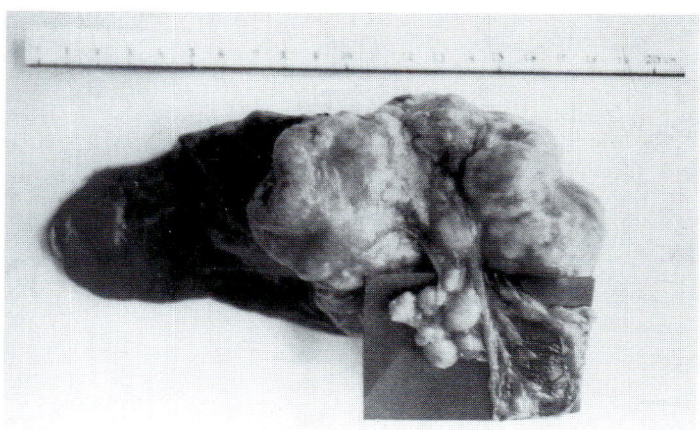

Fig. 9.5.4. Alveococcosis of the liver. Metastasis in lymph node

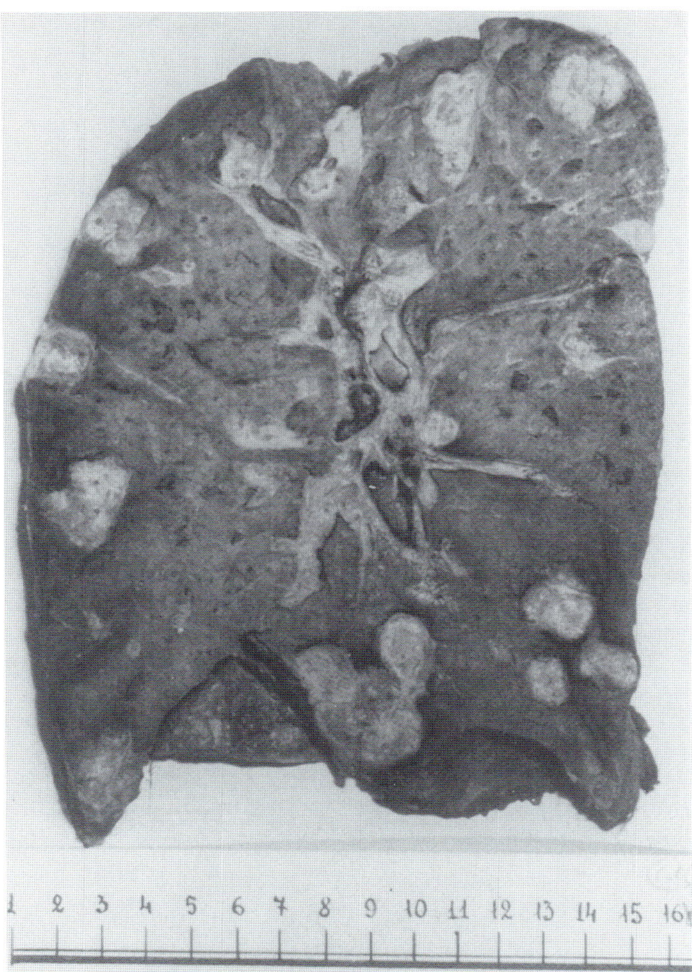

Fig. 9.5.5. Alveococcosis of the liver. Metastasis to the lungs

detail. Unfortunately, surgical treatment is the only chance of saving the patient's life.

Worldwide, surgeons have performed about 1000 resections of the liver for alveococcosis since the first resection performed by Bruns in 1896 and Mysh in 1912 (Alperovitch 1967, Bregadze 1963, Dederer 1975, Reifferscheid 1960, and Stucke 1963).

Although advances have been made, only 25%–30% of advanced cases can be radically operated, according to the data of the majority of the investigators. Unfortunately most cases are advanced on presentation, because of the long symptom-free larval period of the disease. Palliative operations do not prevent the growth of a parasitic "tumor", which characteristically grows on the periphery of the parasitic lesion in the liver.

During the last 45 years the authors have seen about 1000 patients with alveococcosis. About 500 of them have been operated, including 234 resections of the liver, 154 of them were radical and 84 operations were palliative.

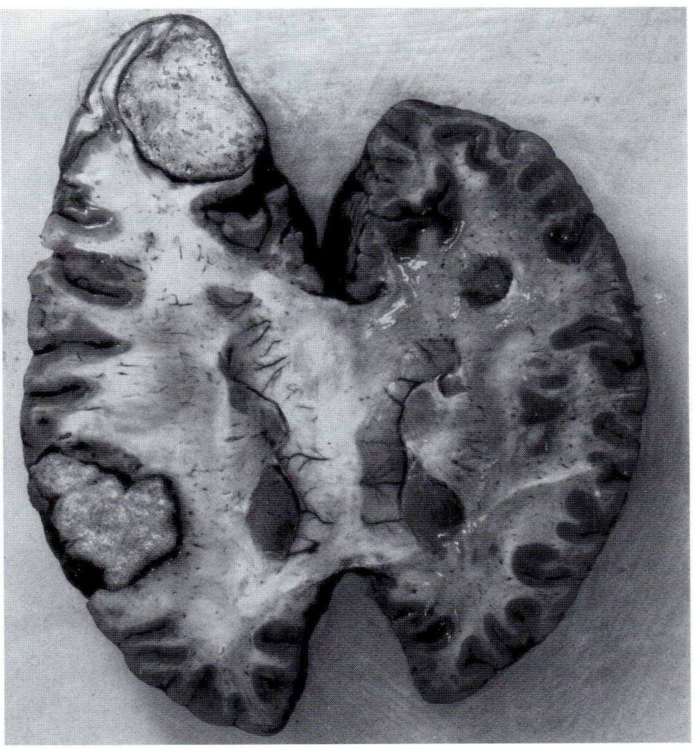

Fig. 9.5.6. Alveococcosis of the liver. Metastasis to the brain

Experimental research carried out by Milonov and colleagues proved in experiments on cotton rats that the parasitic tissue and embryonal elements of alveococcus die at temperatures below −80°C. These experimental data and our experimental investigations and clinical observations have given us grounds to use cryosurgery for alveococcosis. Our clinical observations showed that cryosurgical treatment kills embryonal elements of alveococcus and destroys the parasitic tissue (Figs. 9.5.7–9.5.8).

We developed and carried out the following cryosurgical operations for alveococcosis:

1. Cryoresection of the liver
   - 1.1. Cryoresection of the liver by cryoscalpel and cryoultrasonic scalpel
   - 1.2. Resection of the liver with cryodestruction in its stump.
2. Palliative resections of the liver with cryodestruction of the remaining parasitic tissue.
3. Drainage operation of parasitic caverns with cryodestruction of their walls.
4. Cryodestruction of parasitic "tumor" of a liver as an independent operation.

The above-listed operations are here described:

1. The resection of the liver for alveococcosis is the main operation ensuring complete and long-lasting recovery. But operability remains low. The resection of a liver, especially an extensive one, is a complicated operation. Its main complication is massive intraoperative hemorrhage, especially parenchymal hemorrhage, which is especially difficult to stop during the operation. The use of a cryoscalpel during resection of the liver makes it possible to reduce hemorrhage considerably during the operation. The cryoscalpel developed by us reduces blood loss by 40–50% and makes large tubular liver structures (vessels and bile ducts) more visible during the operation. According to our clinical research the large reduction in operational blood loss during cryoresection results from stopping parenchymal hemorrhage and hemorrhage from vessels up to 2 mm in diameter (Figs. 9.5.9–9.5.11). The size of the cryoresected parts of the liver can be considerable (hemihepatectomy, extended hemihepatectomy) (Fig. 9.5.12).

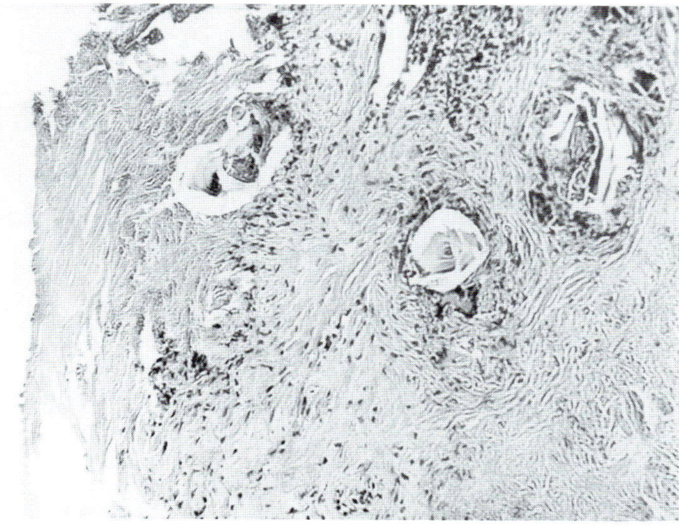

Fig. 9.5.7. Alveococosis of man. Microscopic image. Hematoxylin-eosin stain, magnification ×200

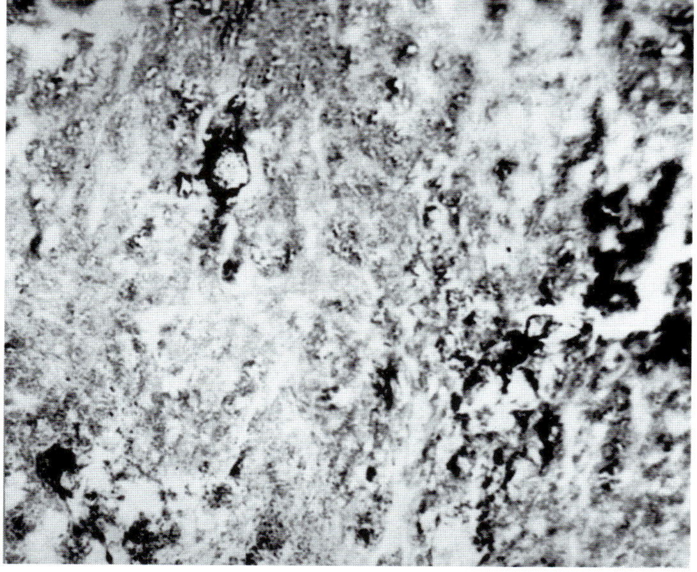

Fig. 9.5.8. The liver of the same patient 21 days after cryodestruction. Microscopic image. There are no elements of alveococcus in the preparation. Hematoxylin-eosin stain, magnification ×200

1.2. The usual liver resection for alveococcosis can be supplemented by cryodestruction of the stump of the organ after the resection, which is sufficient to prevent recurrence of alveococcosis (Fig. 9.5.13).

Cryoresection of a liver is technically analogous to conventional resection. After the liver is exposed by cutting its ligaments, block-like sutures are applied on the resection line, or vascular secretory elements (arteries, veins, ducts) of part or as much as half of the liver are ligated. The affected part of the liver can be excised thereafter with almost no blood loss with the help of the cryoscalpel of our design. If the application of hemostatic sutures is too difficult, and vasoligation of the hepatic vessels is undesirable, cryoresection can be performed with a cryoscalpel. In this case after the incision of the liver tissue, it is necessary to clamp the vessels on the resected line, followed by vasoligation in the plane of incision (Fig. 9.5.14).

When a parasitic "tumor" invades the porta hepatis or the area of the vena cava inferior, palliative resection of the liver, followed by cryodestruction of the remaining parasitic tissue in these anatomically dangerous zones can be performed (Fig. 9.5.15). These operations can be carried out according to the principles of conventional liver

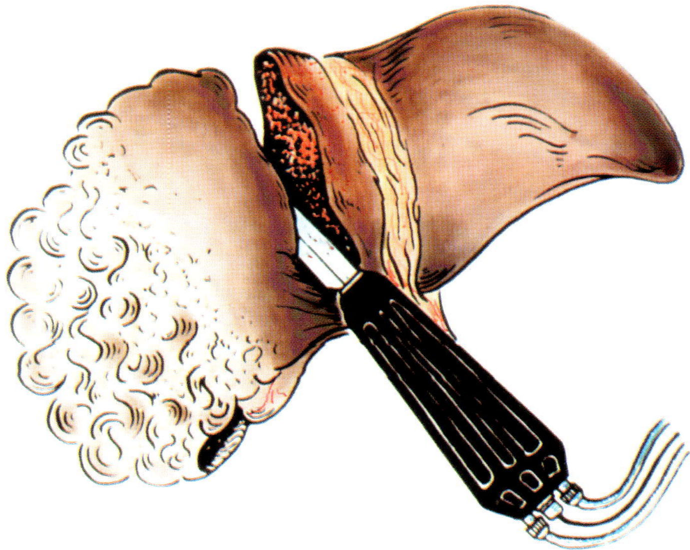

Fig. 9.5.9. Liver cryoresection. Schematic representation

resection. The surgeon leaves a thin layer of parasitic tissue 0.5 cm thick on the vessels in this zone of risk. The area of the remaining parasitic tissue is subjected to cryodestruction by a cryosurgical probe. These operations are, practically speaking, radical operations by virtue of their immediate and late results, although they are defined as "palliative" resections, because subzero temperatures destroy the remaining parasitic tissue. At the same time there is no need to fear the destruction of the walls of large blood vessels, as Cooper proved in numerous experiments that even complete freezing of large vessels does not destroy them.

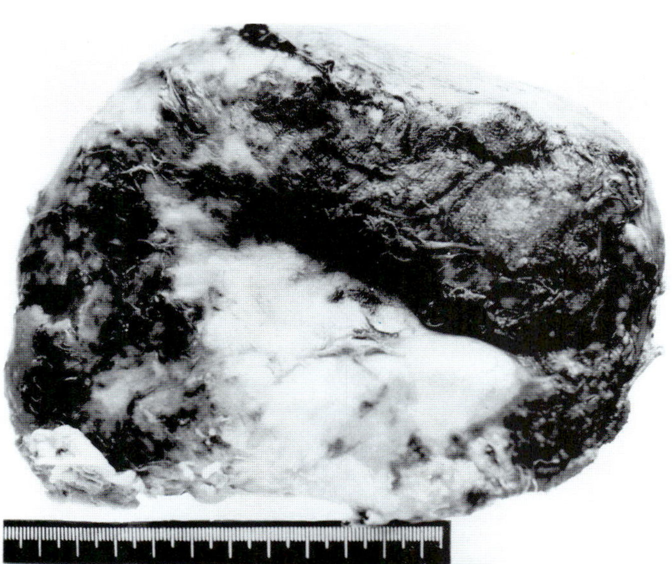

Fig. 9.5.10. Preparation, liver cryoresection

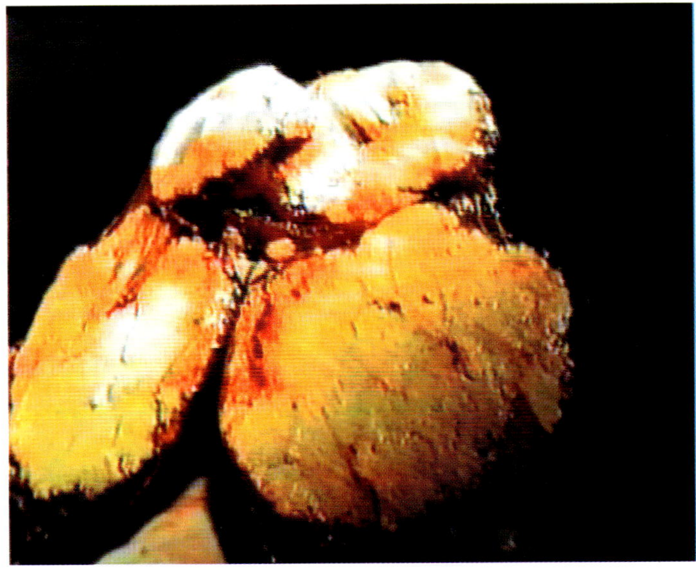

Fig. 9.5.11. Preparation, liver cryoresection. Right hemihepatectomy

2. We have carried out 18 resections of the liver and 35 palliative resections followed by cryodestruction of the remaining elements of alveococcus without lethal exit and with good direct and late results over many years.

The first liver cryoresection, performed by us in 1977, has set a record for recurrence-free follow-up. In 22 years following the operation, the patient

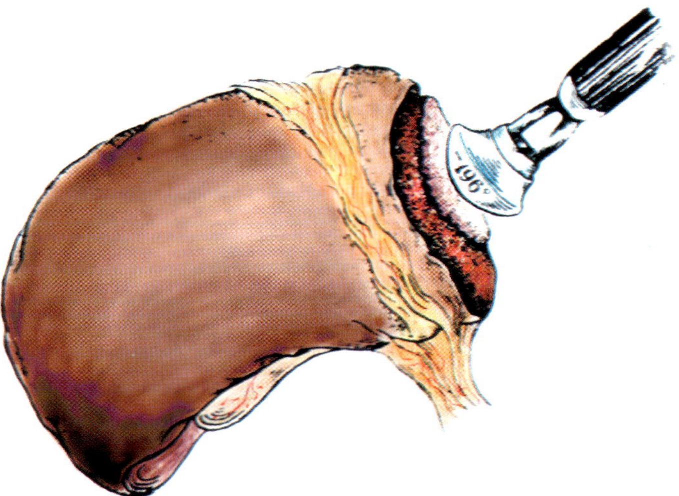

Fig. 9.5.12. Cryodestruction of the liver stump after resection. Schematic representation

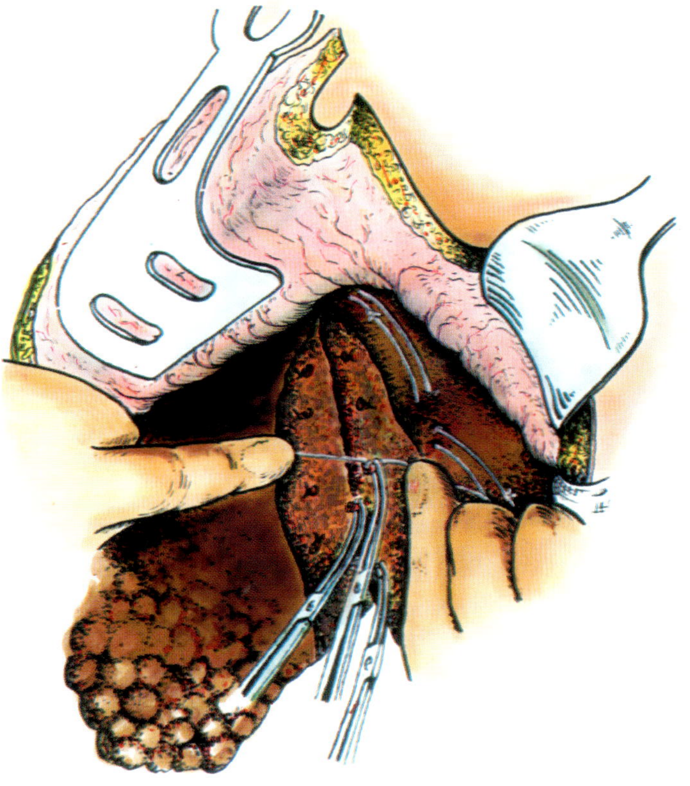

Fig. 9.5.13. Vasoligation at the site of incision. Schematic drawing

has no symptoms of alveococcosis, and she is disease-free after postoperative herniotomy.

Case 1: A 31-year-old patient presented at the clinic of the Siberian Medical University on November 14, 1977 with a suppurating fistula in the epigastrium, general weakness and poor appetite. She had been ill for 12 years. She had been previously operated three times in other clinics to excise fistulas in the hypochondriac region.

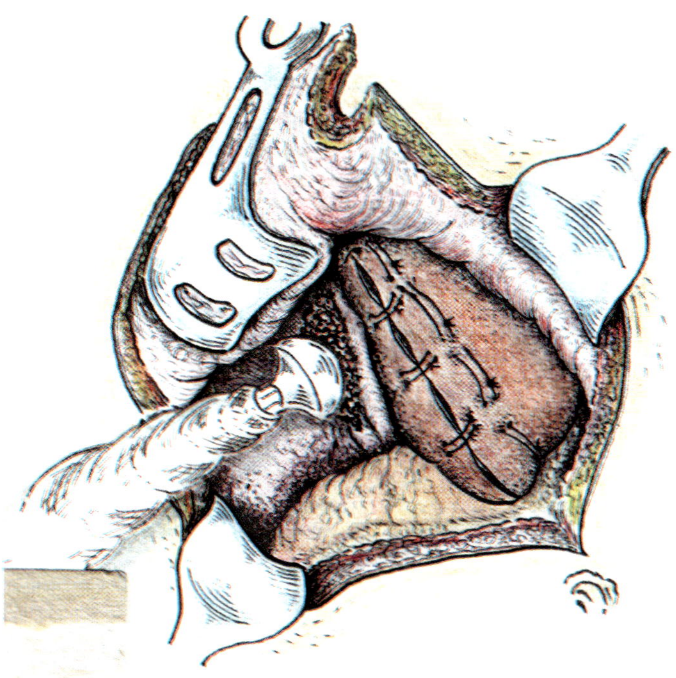

Fig. 9.5.14. Palliative liver resection with cryodestruction. Schematic representation

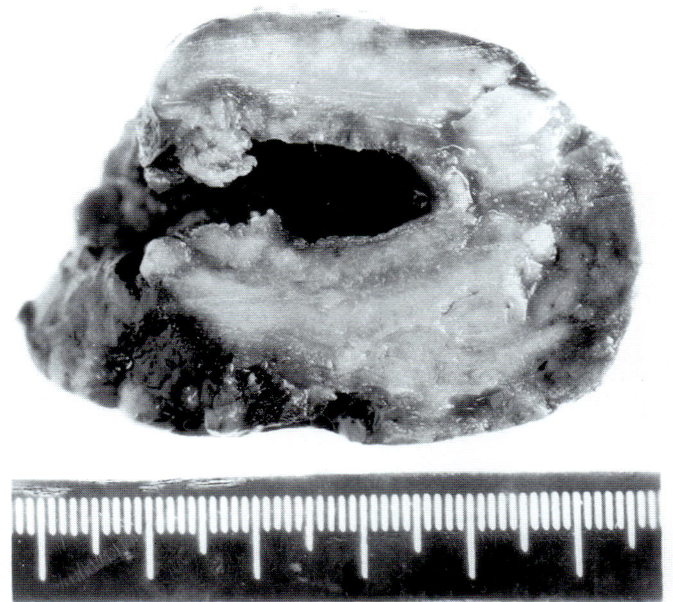

Fig. 9.5.15. Preparation, liver cryoresection

The general condition of the patient was satisfactory. The organs of the thoracic cavity were free of pathology. The abdomen was symmetric. In the epigastrium area there was a transverse postoperative cicatrix, in the center of which a purulent fistula opened. Around the fistula was an infiltrate up to 3 cm in diameter, slightly painful at palpation. The liver did not extend beyond the edge of the costal arch. Blood analysis and urinalysis were unremarkable, except for an increase in the erythrocyte sedimentation rate (to 18 mm/h) and the serum level of bilirubin (to 100 mcmol/l).

On the fistulogram the fistula duct was thin, was connected to the liver in the sagittal fissure, where there was a cavity of 6 × 6 cm.

The operation was performed on December 16, 1977. The upper intermediate laparotomy preceded excision of the fistula duct which reached the border of liver segments II–IV. In this zone there was a dense site of infiltrate 5 × 5 cm, which consisted of thick adhesions. Cryoresection of the part of the liver including the fistula and parasitic tumor was performed (Fig. 9.5.16). The patient recovered well.

Histological diagnosis: alveococcosis of the liver (Fig. 9.5.17).

22 years after the operation there is no evidence of recurrence of alveococcosis in the liver. The patient is in good health.

During cryoresection the volume of the resected part of the liver can be rather significant up to hemihepatectomy and extended hemihepatectomy. An example follows:

Case 2: A 35-year-old patient came to the clinic complaining of weakness, suppuration from a fistula in the upper part of the post-operative cicatrix, on May 4, 1982. The patient had been ill since 1978, when a dense tumor-like formation was determined in the epigastrium. The patient was operated in another city in 1979, when an alveococcus node in the left lobe of the liver was found during laparotomy. The operating surgeon considered the process inoperable and only drained the cavity. The purulent fistula did not heal after this operation, and the patient next presented in our clinic.

The general condition of the patient was satisfactory. The thorax was unremarkable. The abdomen was symmetric. There was a postoperative cicatrix along the median line of the epigastrium. In the upper third of the cicatrix there was a fistula with suppuration. The liver extended 3.5–4 cm from under the costal arch. Blood analysis and urinalysis were unremarkable.

Fistulography revealed that the fistula duct was twisted with different branches and ducts reminiscent of a bunch of grapes in the left lobe of the liver.

On the rheohepatogram changes in blood circulation could be seen in the middle and left part of the liver.

The operation was carried out on May 11, 1982. The abdominal cavity was opened by a staple-like incision in the Alperovich technique and the fistula excised. The parasitic cavity in the remaining part of the left lobe of the liver, 10 × 10 cm in size, had grown into the diaphragm and the forward wall of the stomach in the zone of lesser curvature. The right lobe of the liver was hypertrophic. The elements of the porta hepatis were free. Left hemihepatectomy followed by cryodestruction of the liver stump was performed (Fig. 9.5.18).

Histological diagnosis: alveococcosis (Fig. 9.5.19).

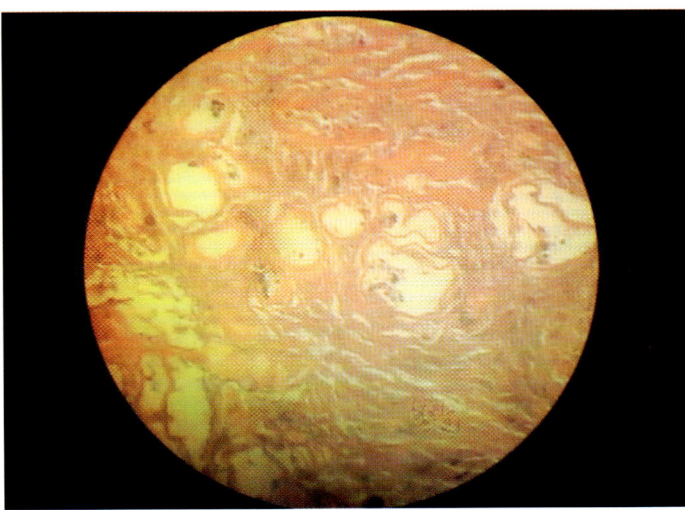

Fig. 9.5.16. Preparation from the same patient. Hematoxylin-eosin stain, magnification ×200

Case 3: An example of palliative resection of the liver with cryodestruction of the remaining parasitic tissue.

A 52-year-old patient came in November 1981 to the clinic from one of the Siberian regions complaining of a feeling of fullness in the epigastrium and in the right hypochondriac region, anorexia, and progressive weight loss. She had felt ill since April 1981.

Clinical examination revealed no ascites, ruling out a malignant liver tumor.

At laparoscopy a yellow–white calculus-like dense formation (alveococcus) was seen in the right lobe of the liver.

On scintigram of the liver, a "cold focus" was seen in the right half of the organ.

On the rheohepatogram there was a change in the blood flow in the right lobe of the liver, with a change in blood circulation in the area of the porta hepatis.

The operation was performed on November 19, 1981. The abdominal cavity was opened layer-by-layer with a staple-like incision (the Alperovitch technique). An enormous node of alveococcus 20 × 20 × 15 cm with the degradation cavity

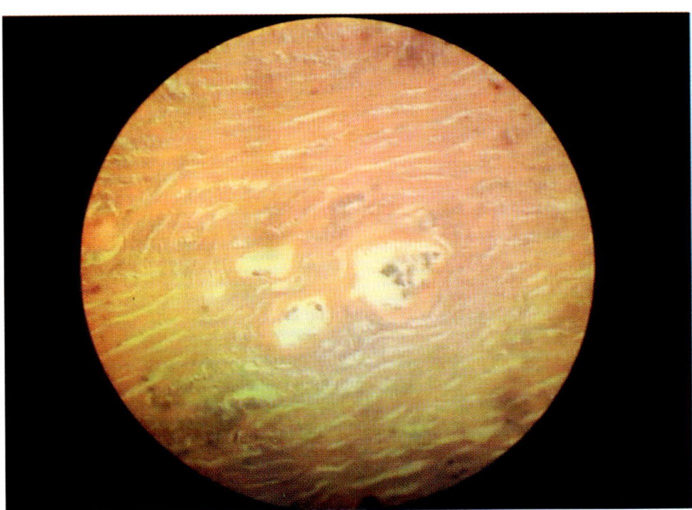

Fig. 9.5.17. Preparation from the same patient 22 years after cryoresection. Hematoxylin-eosin stain, magnification ×200

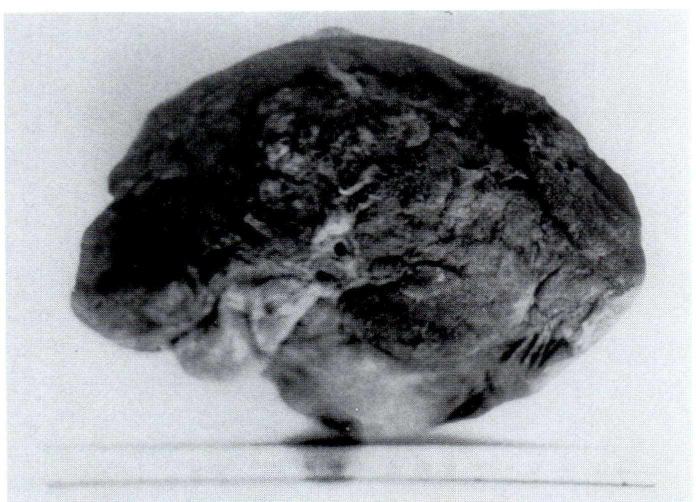

Fig. 9.5.18. Alveococcosis of the liver. Left hemihepatectomy with cryodestruction of the liver stump. Preparation

(300 ml) occupied the entire right lobe of the liver, was fixed to the porta hepatis and vena cava inferior, and infiltrated the diaphragm and the wall of the abdominal cavity. After exposing the liver by cutting the ligaments, a right extended hemihepatectomy was performed. The removed pathological liver tissue weighed approximately 1500 g. Parasitic tissue, 3 × 2 × 0.3 cm in size, was left on the vena cava inferior. It was subjected to cryodestruction at −195°C for 5 minutes (Fig. 9.5.20).

The patient recovered.

Histological findings: alveococcosis (Fig. 9.5.21).

The patient was examined 12 years after the operation. She is in good health and works around the house.

In some cases, when there are great technical difficulties (extremely large size of the parasitic node, atypical topographic anatomic conditions), it is possible to remove a parasitic node in the dangerous zones of the porta hepatis or in the area of the vena cava inferior only partially. The remaining parasitic tissue is subjected to cryodestruction.

3. Drainage operation of parasitic caverns with cryodestruction of their walls (Fig. 9.5.22).

This operation can be performed if the palliative resection of the liver is impossible because of the extent of the pathological process. This operation ranks below the previously described operations in effectiveness but it can be used if a more radical operation is not possible. The remaining parasitic tissue has to be fully destroyed by the cryosurgical approach. The thickness and the size of the parasitic cavity are always different and are of particular significance for postoperative results. The thinner the walls of the parasitic cavern are, the more effective cryodestruction is. A secondary infection always follows the operation and the parasitic tissue sloughs off through the wound in the abdominal wall. Eight patients were operated similarly in the clinic.

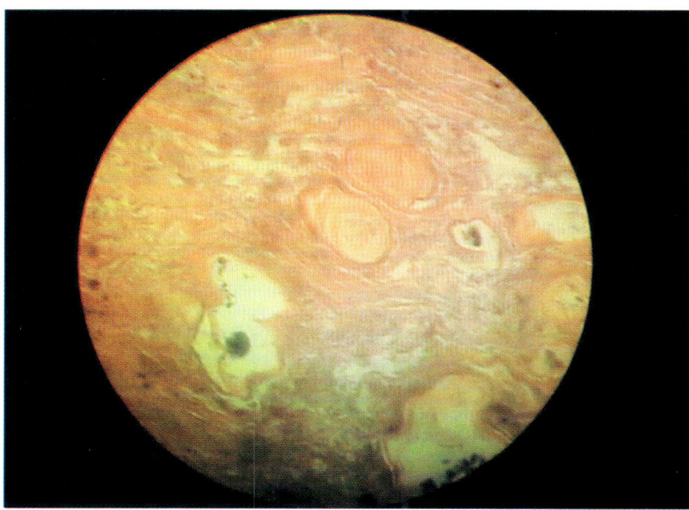

Fig. 9.5.19. Micropreparation from the same patient. Hematoxylin-eosin stain, magnification ×200

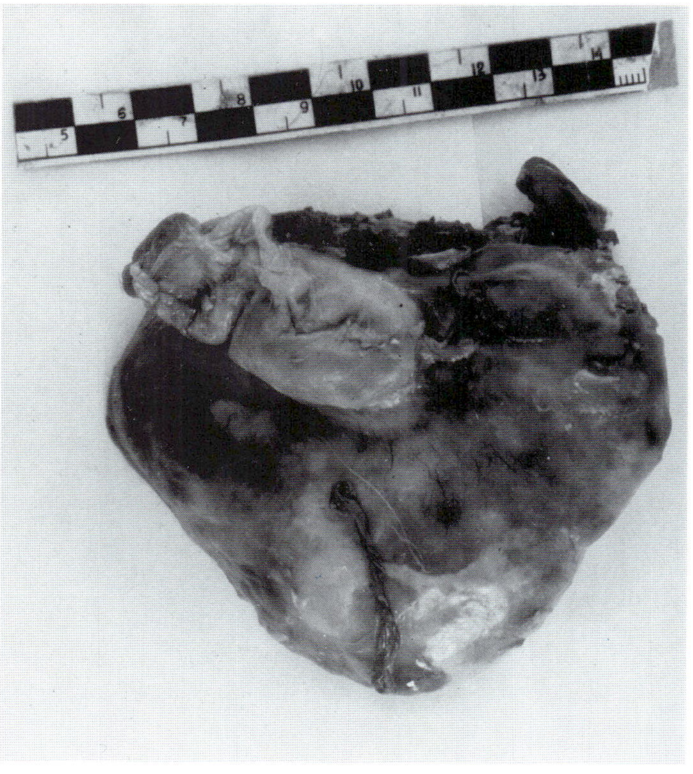

Fig. 9.5.20. Palliative liver resection for alveococcosis. Extended right hemihepatectomy. Preparation (weight 1500 g)

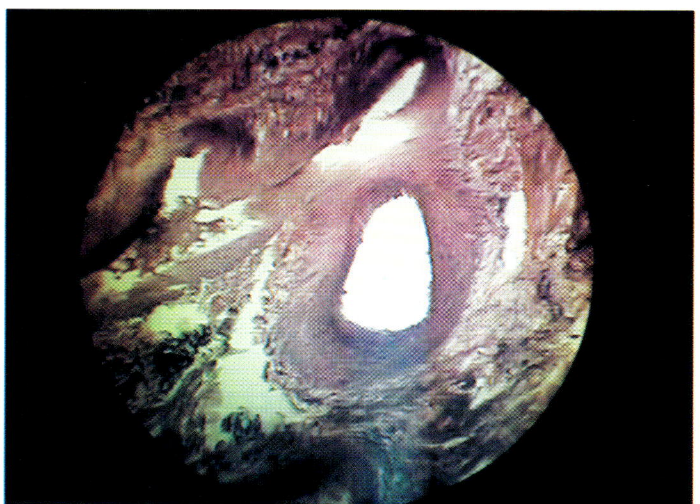

Fig. 9.5.21. Micropreparation from the same patient. Hematoxylin-eosin stain, magnification ×200

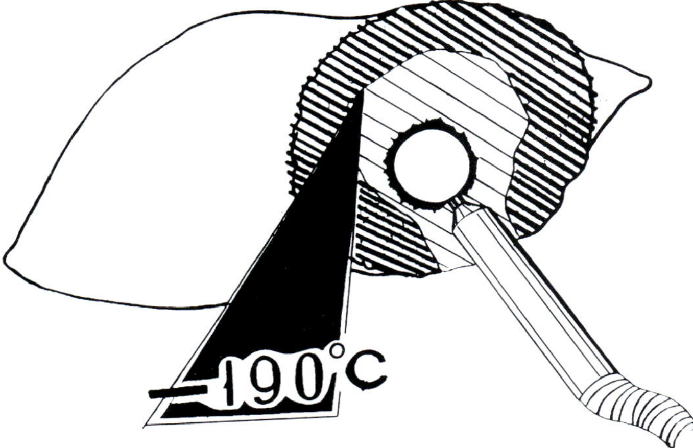

Fig. 9.5.22. Surgery of the parasitic (alveococcus) node with drainage of the parasitic cavern and cryodestruction of its walls. Schematic representation

It is difficult to judge the efficiency of these operations, but the undoubted clinical effect is diminution in toxemia, improvement of general health and prolongation of life.

The technique of the operation is as follows. After laparotomy and examination of the organs of the abdominal cavity, the surgeon must assess the size of the parasitic tumor. The larger the size of the parasitic cavity is, the more effective and less traumatic the operation is. The very evacuation itself leads to diminution of toxemia and less mechanical pressure on the surrounding organs and vessels of the porta hepatis. Thereafter, a part of the walls of the parasitic cavern is excised, and its edges are sutured to the abdominal wall (marsupialization). After marsupialization of the walls of the parasitic cavity, parasitic sequestra are evacuated out of it (Fig. 9.5.23). Its walls are subjected to cryodestruction from within the cavity from several points. The thinner the walls of the parasitic cavern are, the more effective cryodestruction is (Fig. 9.5.24). As a result of postoperative aseptic necrosis, the parasitic tissue dies and subsequently it sloughs off into the wound. Generally, after this operation, the wound heals by secondary intention or the formed bilious-purulent fistula can be operated to empty into the intestine.

Case 4: A 30-year-old patient presented at the clinic on August 22, 1978 complaining of pains in the right hypochondriac region and epigastrium. He had felt ill since 1974, when hepatomegaly was revealed during a prophylactic examination. The patient was repeatedly treated in various hospitals with the diagnosis of cirrhosis hepatis.

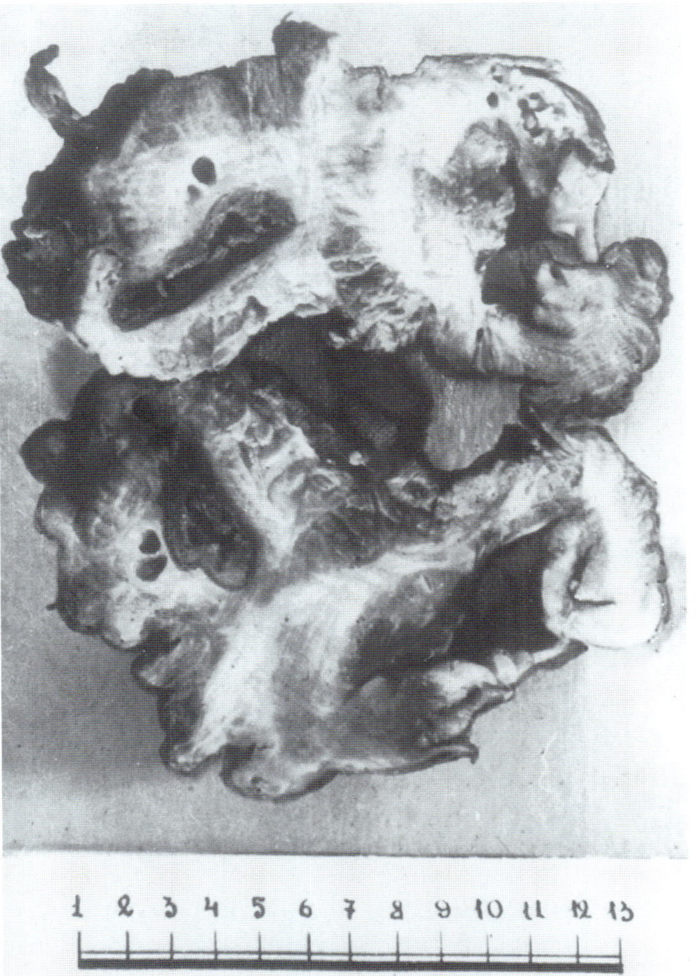

Fig. 9.5.23. Alveococcosis of the liver. Sequestrum

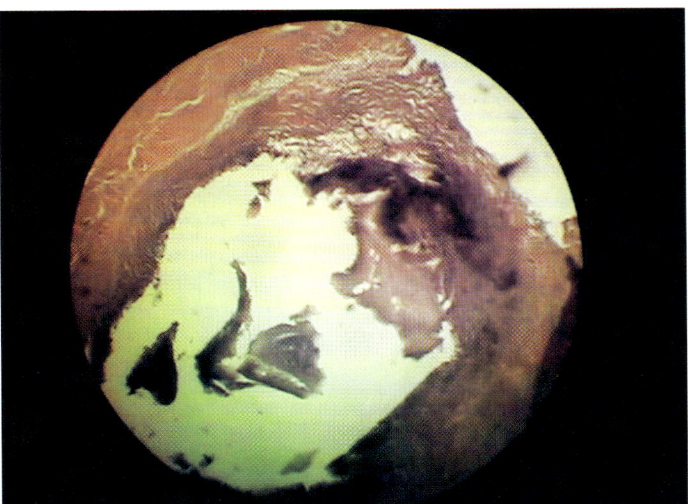

Fig. 9.5.24. Intraoperative biopsy, preparation from the same patient. Hematoxylin-eosin stain, magnification ×200

The patient's general condition was satisfactory. Skin color was normal. There were no remarkable findings.

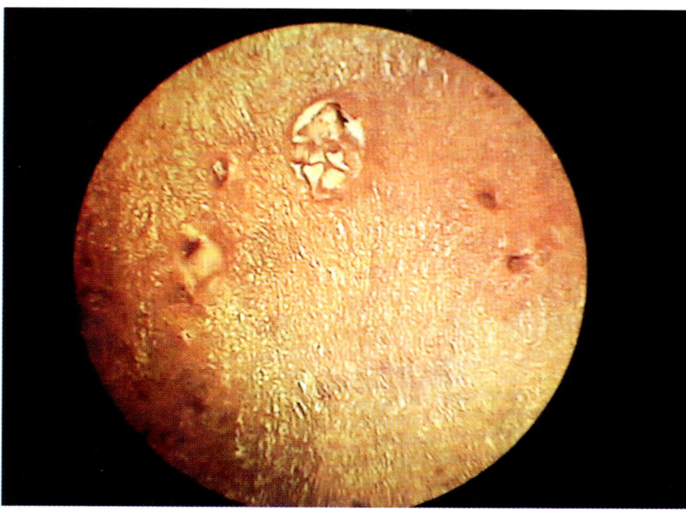

Fig. 9.5.25. Preparation from the same patient 8 days after cryodestruction. There are no elements of alveococcus in the preparation. Hematoxylin-eosin stain, magnification ×200

Two small contrast shadows were seen in the left lobe on the survey hepatogram.

The operation was carried out on September 13, 1978. An enormous node of alveococcus was found on inspection. The node spread over the area of the porta hepatis and was attached to the vena cava inferior. The size of the parasitic node was 30 × 30 × 25 cm. The front wall of the decay cavity, measuring 10 × 8 cm, was excised. The decay cavity was evacuated. The walls of the cavity were sutured to an abdominal wall (marsupialization) and subjected to cryodestruction for 30 minutes. The depth of freezing was up to 1.5 cm, and the area of freezing in the area of the porta hepatis was 10 × 8 cm. In the first postoperative month, the parasitic node sloughed off through the wound. The last part of the parasitic tissue was evacuated on November 11, 1978, after which the wound healed by secondary intention.

During the operation and on the 8th and the 21st postoperative days, a biopsy was taken from the parasitic node.

Histological diagnosis: alveococcosis (Fig. 9.5.25).

In the biopsy material no elements of alveococcus were found three weeks after cryodestruction (Figs. 9.5.25–9.5.26).

Examination of biopsy specimens of the liver, taken out of the parasitic node after cryodestruction showed the effectiveness of this method in treating alveococcus in the human.

It will be possible to judge the efficiency of similar operations only after analysis of long-term results.

4. Cryodestruction of the parasitic node as an independent operation.

Such an operation should be reserved for patients with very wide distribution of parasitic nodes in the liver, multiple nodes with invasion of the porta hepatis, considerable invasion of the node into the diaphragm over a considerable length, when other, more radical operations are impossible. In the clinic 8 patients have been operated similarly.

The technique of the operation is simple enough. The operation is made after laparotomy and inspection of the abdominal cavity, at which point the surgeon decides about the need for cryodestruction.

It is necessary to note that the entire node must be frozen to kill the parasite. There are two conditions for this. First, a high-technology cryoprobe should be used, secondly, sufficient exposure is necessary, which depends on the size and topography of the parasitic tissue. In the clinic, exposure was increased to 30 minutes at every locus of cryodestruction.

An example of such an operation.

Case 5: A 26-year-old patient came to the clinic on November 25, 1976 complaining of dull constant pains and the feeling of fullness in the right hypochondriac region, weakness, and anorexia. She had been ill for 3 years.

Her general state was satisfactory. The clinical findings were unremarkable.

The hepatogram showed multiple calcifications in the right lobe of the liver under the diaphragm.

An occlusion of the main portal vein was seen on the portohepatogram.

A hepatic scan showed that the form of the liver was changed, its size increased. In the upper part of the right lobe there was an extensive area in which there was no accumulation of colloidal gold. In the lower part of the right lobe, there was a zone with low accumulation of a radiopharmaceutical.

The operation was carried out on October 1, 1976. A huge stagnant liver is determined on examination. An alveococcus node, 10 × 12 cm in size, without the degradation cavity, occupied almost the entire right lobe of the liver. The node spread over the first segment of the liver, the area of the porta hepatis and the area of the vena cava inferior. Over a large surface, there was growth into the diaphragm. Cryodestruction of the parasitic node was performed at a temperature of the cryoprobe of −196°C. The focus of freezing was 8 cm in diameter. The exposure was 20 minutes. We took a biopsy and performed omentohepatopexia. A suture closed the abdominal wall without a drain.

In the postoperative period, the patient had some fever without any special changes in the blood during the month after surgery. The patient was discharged from the clinic in a satisfactory state.

Histological examination: alveococcosis of the liver.

Half a year after the operation, the patient experienced a sudden rise in temperature. Hyperthermia remained for a week. Then the patient had defecation with pus up to 1000 ml. The temperature became normal after this.

The patient was examined in the clinic a year later. Her condition was satisfactory. All clinical tests were unremarkable. The patient felt well and was back at work. The period of observation was 3.5 years. Then contact with the patient was lost.

In summary, it is possible to conclude that the application of cryosurgery has opened a new door in surgery of alveococcosis and has expanded the surgeon's possibilities. The problem, however, demands further scientific investigation and improvement of the cryosurgical equipment.

References

1. Alperovich BI. Alveococcosis. Yacutsk, Russia, 1967.
2. Alperovich BI. Alveococcosis and its treatment. Medicine, Moscow, 1972.
3. Alperovich BI, Paramonova LM, Merzlikin NV. Cryosurgery of the liver and pancreas. Tomsk, Tomsk State University Press, 1985.
4. Alperovich BI. Surgery of the liver. Tomsk, Tomsk State University Press, 1985.
5. Alperovich BI. Liver and biliary tract surgery. Tomsk, Siberian Medical University, 1997.
6. Bregadze IL, Konstantinov VM. Alveolar echinococcosis. Medgis, USSR, 1963.
7. Dederer YM, Krylova NP. Atlas of operations on the liver. Medicine, Moscow, 1975.
8. Bruns P. Leberresection bei multilokulaerem Echinococcosis. Beitr.f.klin.Chir., 1896; 50(7): 1353.
9. Cooper IS. Cryogenic Surgery. Engineering in the Practice of Medicine. Baltimore, 1967.
10. Reifferscheid M. Chirurgie der Leber. Stuttgart, 1957.
11. Stucke K. Zur chirurgischen Therapie der Echinococcus alveolaris. Der Chirurg, 1963; 34: 165.

9.6 Cryosurgery for Liver Echinococcosis

Boris I. Alperovich

Echinococcosis of the liver results from the invasion into the liver of the larval stage of the tape worm (Echinococcus granulosus) and its further development (Batsch 1786). The disease has been known since ancient times. Hippocrates wrote about ''jecur aqua repletum''. In 1681 Redi described the worm and in 1833 Sibold reproduced a development cycle of the parasite in an experiment.

The epidemiology, morphology and spread of echinococcosis have been investigated in detail. The disease is usually found in countries with highly developed agriculture, since domestic animals, especially dogs, play the main role in the development cycle of the parasite. The echinococcosis frequency varies greatly from country to country. Echinococcosis is found in Chile, Argentina, Uruguay, Brazil, Australia, New Zealand, Northern Africa, Greece, Yugoslavia, Bulgaria, Armenia, Azerbaijan, Kirghizia, Kazakhstan. In Russia the sites of origin for echinococcosis are on the middle and lower Volga River, in western Siberia, Dagestan, Yakutia, Chukotka, and the Kamchatka regions.

Man is an intermediate host of echinococcus, he falls ill by chance, and is the biological end station for the parasite. The morphology of echinococcus of man was investigated in detail by Deve in 1937.

Irrespective of the size of the cyst, echinococcus consists of three layers and is filled with a transparent opalescent liquid with little salt content or amber acid. The internal wall of a parent cyst represents a germinative layer. Outside of it is a white shell, similar in appearance to mother of pearl, with a chitin shell (the result of the parasites' vital functions). The cyst is surrounded by a dense fibrous capsule, the product of vital functions of the host, who attempts to separate from the parasite. The parasite is characterized by oppositional growth – it grows moving apart and compresses neighboring structures.

When a parasitic cyst has been in the liver for many years, the thickness of the fibrous capsule can be as much as 5–7 mm.

In due course an echinococcus cyst can partially or completely degrade, undergo aseptic necrosis or suppuration. If the cyst is located on the periphery of the liver, otherwise insignificant trauma can perforate the cyst, whose content can flow into the abdominal or pleural cavities. In this case scoleces from echinococcus sand are spread into the peritoneum and pleura, where cysts similar to the parent begin to develop.

Surgical treatment of echinococcosis of a liver was begun by Volkmann (1874), Thornton (1883), and Koenig (1890).

Major developments were made by the Russian scientists Bobrov (1894) and Spasokukotsky (1926). Loretta was the first to perform a resection of a liver for echinococcosis in 1888. In 1956 Melnikov published data collected from the Russian literature on 159 liver resections performed by Soviet surgeons. At the same time, there are a number of controversial questions and unsolved problems in the surgery of echinococcosis. Despite the achievements of modern surgery the recurrence rate of the disease after radical operations is still high. The majority of researchers are of the opinion that recurrence depends on the invasion of the abdominal cavity by scoleces of echinococcus during the operation. There are also other reasons for recurrences, for example, small cysts deep in the liver, unrecognized during the operation, and insufficiently radical treatment.

An operation for liver echinococcosis aims at removing echinococcus cysts and their contents out of the organism and in so doing not to leave scoleces or hydatids of echinococcus in the liver or elsewhere in the abdominal cavity.

The effectiveness of surgical treatment of echinococcosis depends on absolute removal of mother cysts and their contents and prevention of embryonal elements (hydatids and scoleces) from entering the wound.

The modern surgical treatment of liver echinococcosis can be classified as follows:

1) Closed echinococcotomy performed in one operation on uncomplicated or suppurated echinococcus (Bobrov 1897; Spasocucotsky 1926).
2) Open echinococcotomy performed in one operation (Volkmann 1874).
3) Enucleation of the parasite together with the fibrous capsule (Melnikov 1955).
4) Resection of the liver (Loretta 1888).

Two-phase operations are not performed nowadays. Enucleation of the parasite with the fibrous capsule is a very traumatic and sanguineous operation, even more so than liver resection. Basically most authors perform resections of the liver or closed echinococotomy in one operation. In case the echinococcus cyst is suppurating, the open echinococcotomy is indicated.

The greatest drawback to the resection of the liver is its traumatic effect and hemorrhage during the operation, and after closed echinococcotomy the rate of recurrence is as high as 10–20%.

The recurrences are more often observed in the more complicated forms of the disease.

Recurrences of echinococcosis are possible in the following cases:

1) When the operating surgeon does not notice a number of small cysts in the depths of the liver, lying separately from the main cyst. In this case special methods of examination (intraoperative ultrasonography) makes it possible to avoid this mistake.
2) Recurrence may occur during a puncture or the exposure of the mother cyst when scoleces of echinococcus flow into parts of the abdominal cavity or remain in the liver wound. It is possible to avoid this by using special vacuum aspirators to evacuate the contents of the echinococcus cyst (Babur 1976).
3) Finally, scoleces of echinococcus that remain in the walls of the fibrous capsule are the most frequent reason for local recurrences of echinococcosis of the liver. Fissures can emerge in the walls of the chitin capsule of the mother cyst and the walls of the fibrous capsule in complicated forms of echinococcosis. The embryonal elements of the parasite (scoleces) can flow into these fissures (Fig. 9.6.1). After resection of the contents of the cyst and its capsules these scoleces can become the reason for the development of recurrent echinococcosis.

In this connection many scientists attach great significance to processing the walls of the fibrous capsule of the parasitic cyst during echinococcotomy. The walls of the capsule are worked with a formalin solution or with an iodine tincture. But these measures do not always appear to be effective.

The use of subzero temperatures in the treatment of echinococcosis has been shown to be very promising in several ways.

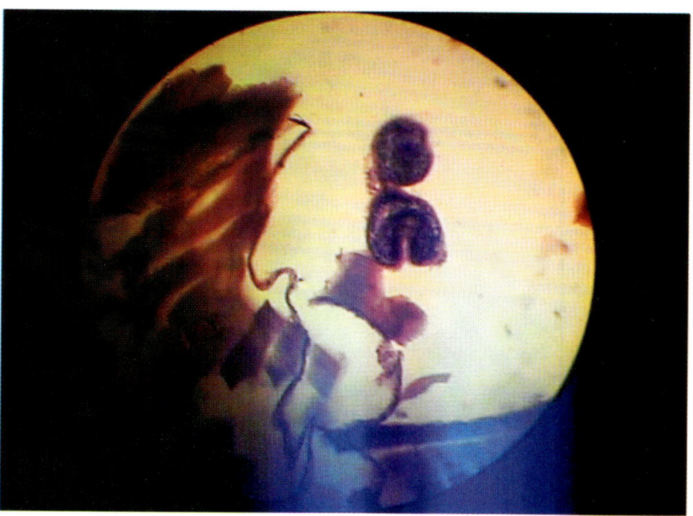

Fig. 9.6.1. Embryonal elements (scoleces) of echinococcus deep in the fibrous capsule. Hematoxylin-eosin stain, magnification ×400

The resection of the liver is effectively carried out with the help of a cryoscalpel when there are multiple echinococcus cysts, occupying a lobe of the liver, or when there are single cysts located on the periphery of the organ.

The resection of the liver is made close to the surface of the cyst. Preliminary suture application prevents bleeding, but is not necessary (Fig. 9.6.2). After resection of the liver tissue, large tubular structures of the organ (vessels and bile ducts) are grasped by hemostatic clamps and separately ligated (Fig. 9.6.3). After resection, the stump of the liver should be subjected to cryodestruction to destroy embryonal elements of the parasite in the wound (Fig. 9.6.4).

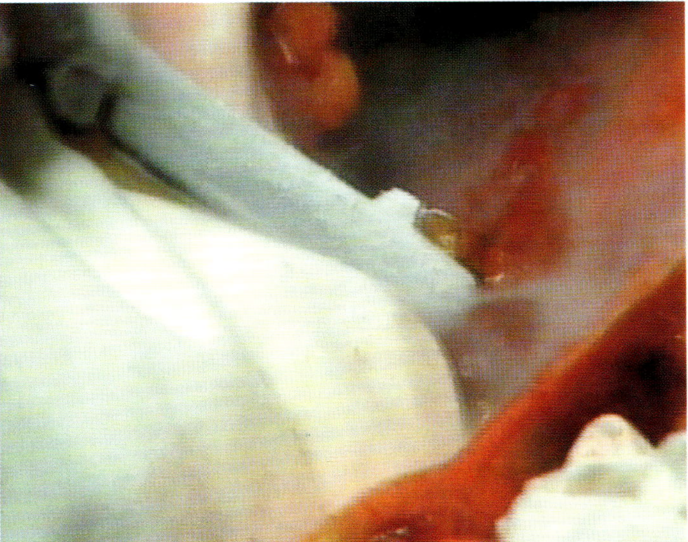

Fig. 9.6.2. Liver cryoresection for echinococcosis

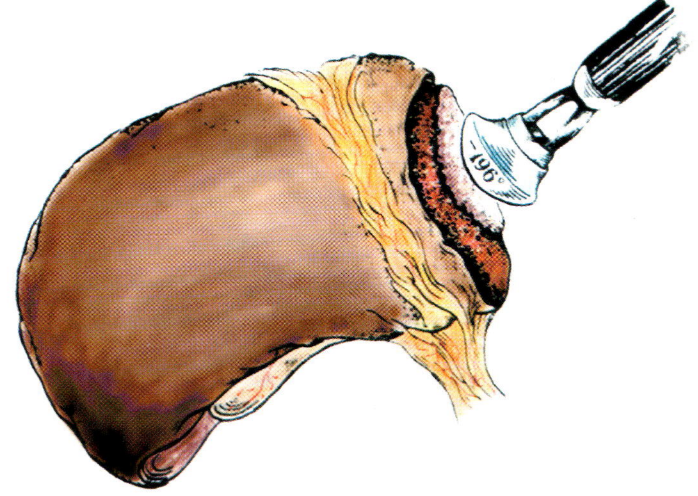

Fig. 9.6.4. Cryodestruction of the stump of the liver after resection. Schematic representation

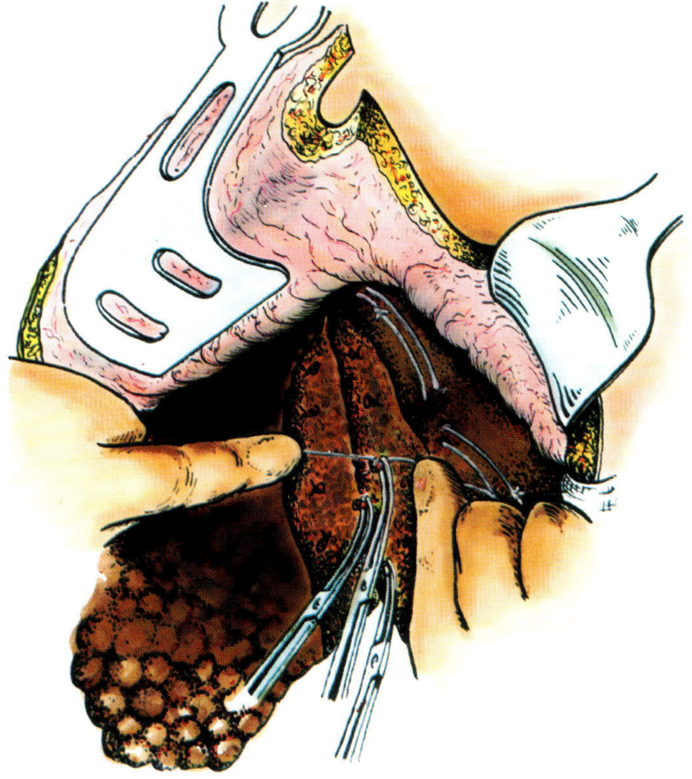

Fig. 9.6.3. Ligation of tubular structures in the plane of the incision in cryoresection of the liver. Schematic representation

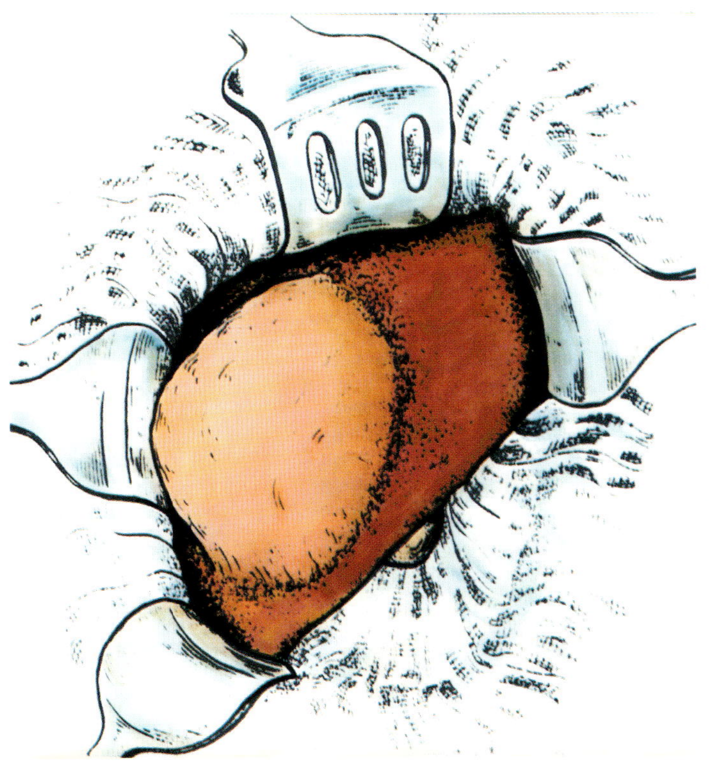

Fig. 9.6.5. View of echinococcus cyst during the operation. Schematic representation

The advantages of the method are:

1. Essential reduction of hemorrhage during resection by stopping parenchymal bleeding and hemorrhage from vessels up to 2 mm in diameter. Parenchymal bleeding can be reduced from 40–60%, according to our clinical data.
2. The use of the cryoscalpel also makes it possible to prevent the recurrence of the disease, and cryodestruction of the stump of the liver after resection strengthens this effect.

A closed echinococcotomy in one operation is more usually performed. The technique of the operation using cryosurgery has been developed in the clinic.

The location of the echinococcus cyst is determined after laparotomy (Figs. 9.6.5–9.6.6). After the puncture of the cyst it is opened and its contents and especially mother and daughter parasitic chitin capsules are removed (Fig. 9.6.7). At this moment of the operation, special care must be taken to avoid disseminating scoleces and hydatids into the abdominal cavity.

Then parts of the fibrous capsule are resected wherever possible (Fig. 9.6.8). After that the remaining parts of the fibrous capsule are subjected to cryodestruction with the purpose of destroying scoleces that are in the cystic cavity and in the walls of the fibrous capsule (Figs. 9.6.9–9.6.10). This step of the operation promotes prevention of recurrence of the disease and also promotes prompt healing of the wound of the liver, as the superficial destruction of the fibrous capsule leads to rapid appearance of granular tissue and prompt cicatrization. The remaining parts of the walls of the cavity should be sewn with block sutures (Fig.9.6.11).

When the remaining cavity is large, it can be tamponed by the epiploon in the flap technique (Kourias 1951; Askerhanov 1976) (Fig. 9.6.12).

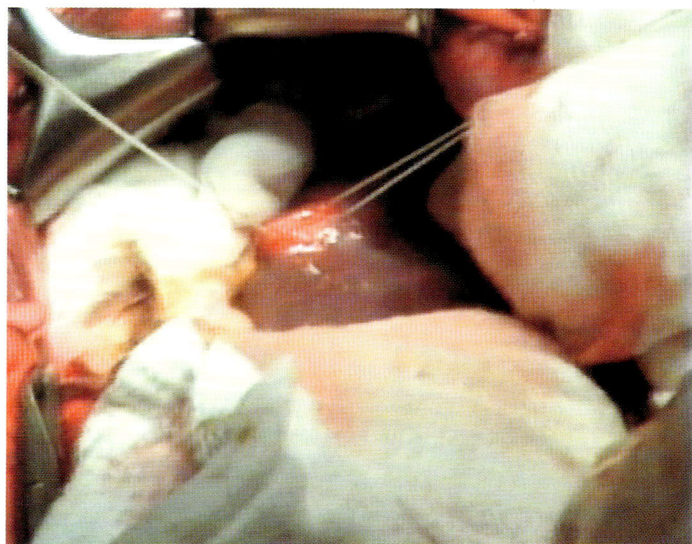

Fig. 9.6.6. View of echinococcus liver cyst

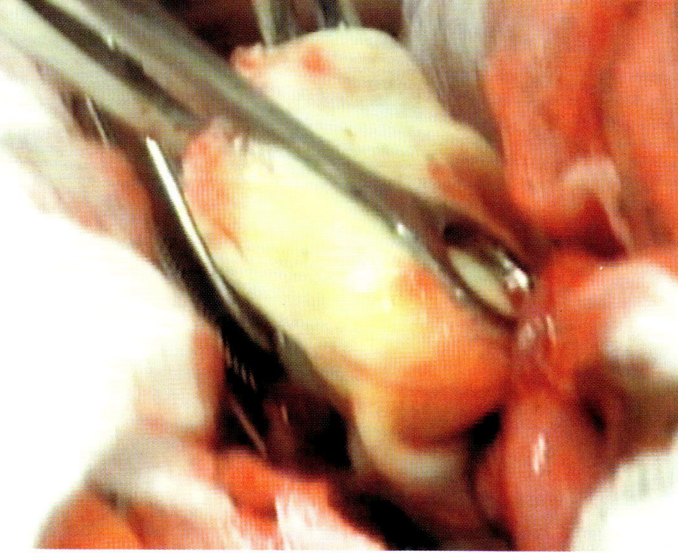

Fig. 9.6.7. Echinococcotomy. Resection of chitin capsules of echinococcus

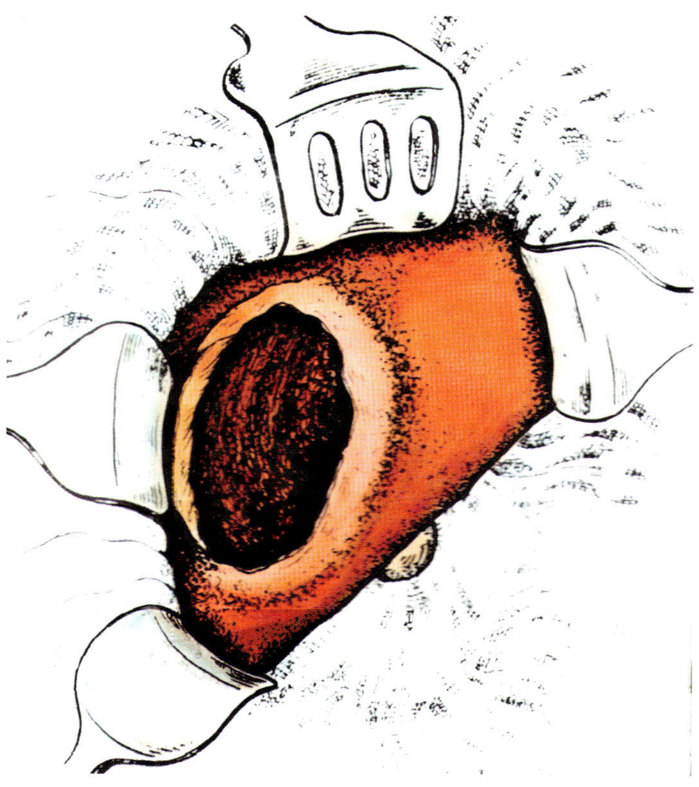

Fig. 9.6.8. Echinococcotomy. Excision of part of the fibrous capsule

In the clinic 22 similar operations have been carried out without mortality and with good immediate and late results.

Optimum modes of cryotreatment in closed echinococcotomy are: the temperature of the cryoprobe should be (−160°C) – (−190°C). The frequency of vibrations of cryovibroprobe should be 400 KHz. The exposure time of each cryocycle should be 5–8 minutes. In a large area exposed to cryodestruction, cryotreatment is carried out at several points of the area involved.

A 31-year-old patient came to the clinic on September 13, 1995, complaining of dull pains in the right hypochondriac region and moderate

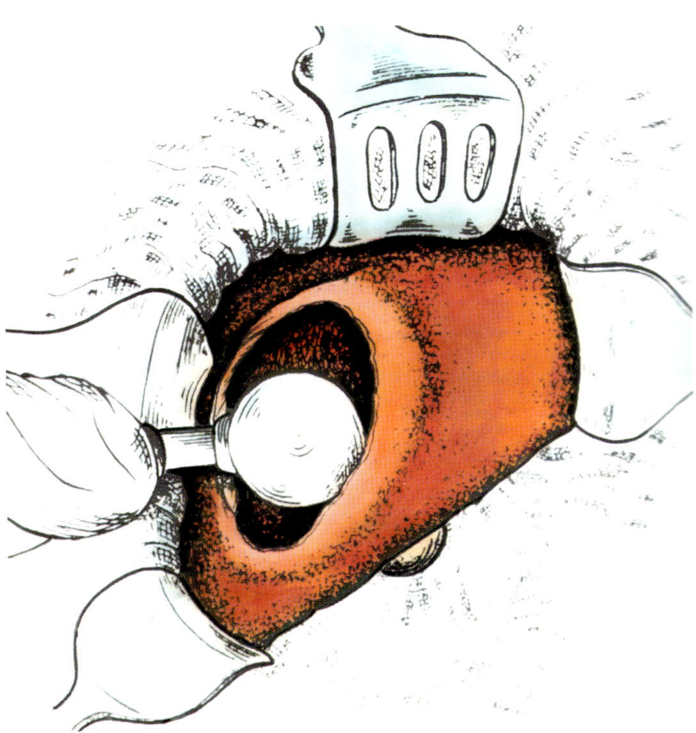

Fig. 9.6.9. Echinococcotomy. Cryodestruction of part of the fibrous capsule. Schematic representation

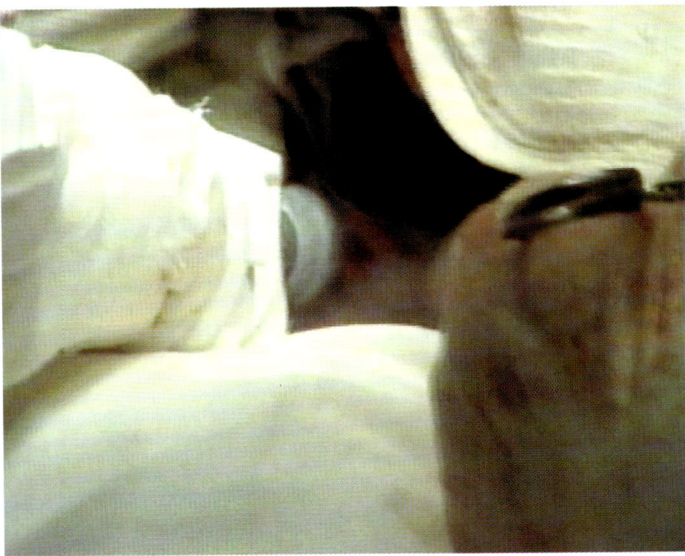

Fig. 9.6.10. Echinococcotomy. Cryodestruction of a fibrous capsule

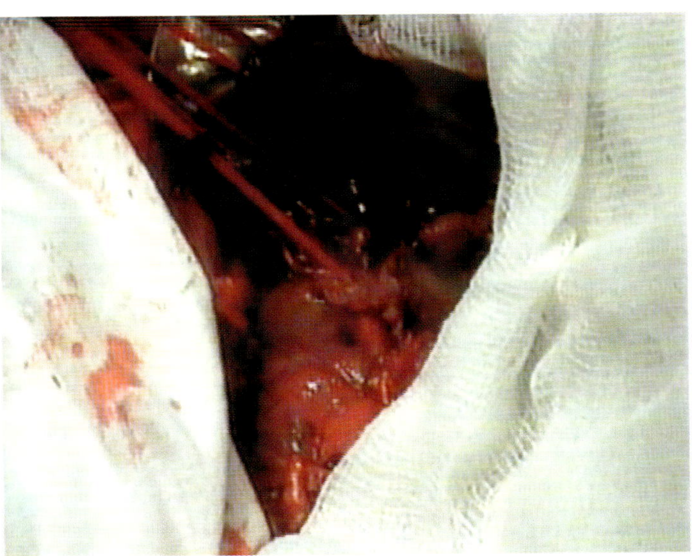

Fig. 9.6.11. View of the walls of the cavity of echinococcus after cryodestruction

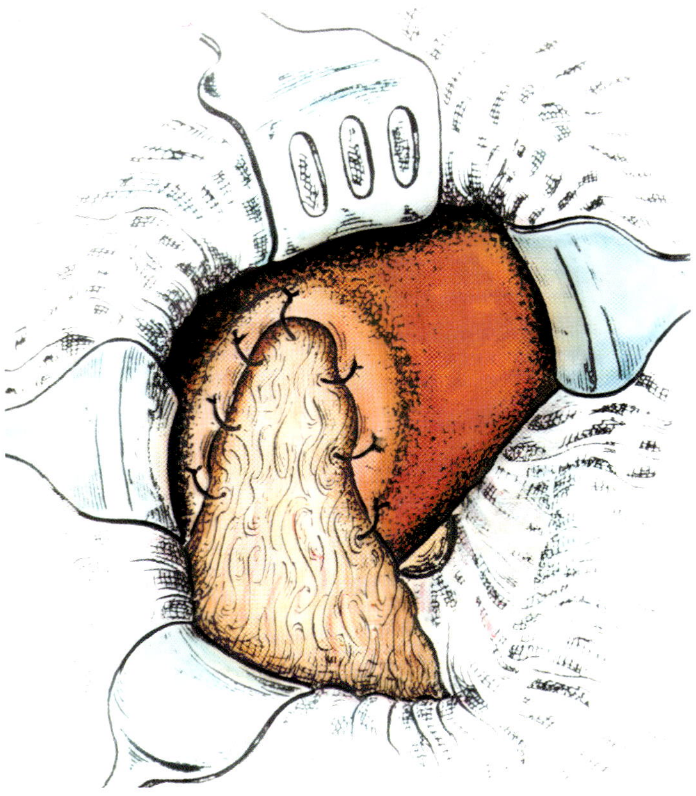

Fig. 9.6.12. Echinococcotomy. Tamponade of the cyst cavity with epiploon. Schematic representation

weakness. It was established from anamnesis that the patient has been ill since 1978 when an ultrasonic investigation revealed echinococcosis of the liver and of the right lung. The patient was operated in another clinic, where a resection of the lung was made, and the patient was sent to our clinic for further treatment.

At presentation the patient's general condition was satisfactory. The organs of the thorax were without pathology. The abdomen was symmetric. There was pain at palpation in the epigastrium and in the right hypochondriac region. The liver extended 3 cm beyond the costal arch, its edges were elastic but not very movable. There was increased serum ALT – 2.96 mmol/l. The Casoni test with echinococcus antigens was positive. The ultrasonic investigation revealed hepatomegaly, with a smooth liver surface, and the left lobe reduced in size. In segments I–III, there was a mass consisting of 3 spherical cysts, their overall size was 10–11 cm. In the back of the right lobe in segment VII, there was a similar formation of a rounded shape measuring 10 cm with an alveolar structure and a dense capsule. These formations were not connected with the large vessels of porta hepatis. Intrahepatic bile ducts of the left lobe were moderately dilated.

The operation was performed on September 19, 1995. The abdominal cavity was opened by bilateral subcostal access. Inspection yielded the following: the entire left lobe was occupied by three cysts of echinococcus, grown together, with dense walls, and a number of hydatids. In the right lobe of the liver, on its subdiaphragmatic surface, there was a large dense cyst measuring 10 cm in diameter.

Resection of the left lobe of the liver was made in the method of the clinic. The liver stump was subjected to cryosurgery. The cyst in the right lobe was evacuated. Most of the wall of the cyst was excised. The remaining parts were subjected to cryosurgery. The resected surface was tamponed with epiploon and sutured. The abdominal cavity was closed without a drain.

The patient recovered well.

Histological findings: echinococcosis of the liver

The use of the cryotechnique in operations for echinococcosis makes the execution of the operation easier, reduces hemorrhage during cryosurgical resection of the liver and improves the results of closed echinococcotomy in one operation. Cryosurgical operations prevent the recurrence of the disease to a large degree, since subzero temperatures kill embryonal elements of echinococcus.

References

1. Alperovich BI. Surgery of liver and bile ducts. Tomsk, Siberian State Medical University, 1997.
2. Alperovich BI, Paramonova LM, Merslikin NV. Cryosurgery of the liver and pancreas. Tomsk, Tomsk State University, 1985.
3. Askerhanov RP. Surgery of echinococcosis. Makhachkala, Dagestan Publishing House, 1976.
4. Petrovsky BV, Milonov OB, Deyenichin PG. Surgery of echinococcosis. Moscow, Medicina, 1985.

10. Pancreas Cryosurgery

10.1 Pancreatic Cancer

Nikolai N. Korpan with contributions by Jaroslav V. Zharkov, Iwan S. Tchekman, Gerhard Hochwarter, Franz Beer, and Franz Sellner

10.1.0 Introduction

The incidence of pancreatic cancer is increasing nationally as well as worldwide. The linear trend shows an increase of 3% to 15.1 per 100,000 (WHO standard 7.9 per 100,000). In contrast to other malignancies, in about 42% of all cases of pancreatic cancer the patient presents in a disseminated stage at the time of first diagnosis. Early diagnosis is difficult, because pancreas cancers develop relatively slowly and without clinical signs until the tumor has grown to a large size. Unfortunately the results of curative as well as of palliative treatment are not satisfactory to date.

Alarming disease symptoms unfortunately first appear much too late and form the basis for a poor prognosis. At present only between 10% and 20% of all pancreatic tumors can be radically excised. Only a very small proportion of 5% of all patients profit from such interventions. At present the survival time after surgical resection of pancreatic cancer is just 5 years. 70–80% of the patients die within the first year after diagnosis. The survival time for patients in advanced stages of the disease is just 6 to 10 months.

The detailed reports from the WHO as well as from the Japanese Pancreatic Society on pancreatic cancer for the first time provided surgeons with scientifically based statistics on the postoperative prognosis of pancreatic cancer in different stages. The results showed unfortunately that only a very small percentage of patients have a real chance of survival after an extensive resection.

The majority of patients may anticipate interventional or minimally invasive, palliative therapy, which will provide them a good quality of life and short hospitalization during their remaining life span.

New scientific insights gained in basic research in biology and experimental surgery as well as modern technical developments provide an important and fascinating look at the treatment strategies in advanced stages of pancreatic cancer. In patients with pancreatic tumors that can no longer be treated curatively, cryosurgical interventions are motivating and promising of success.

10.1.1 Experimental Studies

Our own experiments on dogs as well as other theoretical and experimental tests have been carried out to determine how low temperatures produce their effect on tissue.

Most important are the ice crystallization processes, in which two important mechanisms were identified: first, intra- and extracellular ice formation, by which the cell structure and the tissue are destroyed (damaged). Second, cell and tissue dehydration develop along with protein denaturation, which lead to rupture of the cell membrane.

Experiments on 28 dogs (Figs. 10.1.1–10.1.4) showed that at first there is a mild hyperemia with the formation of a cryozone as a result of the ice formation. The cryodestruction zone of the pancreatic parenchyma was clearly defined with a sharp demarcation line with good visual contours. Particularly noticeable after thawing was a considerable discoloration (reddening) with mild swelling and a clear border between the intact and the cryodestroyed tissue (see Fig. 10.1.3). The tissue very seldom retains it original color and consistency.

In the following hours, the focus exposed to cold become edematous (swollen) and reddened, i.e., an aseptic necrosis with thrombus formation developed.

After four weeks, it could be seen how loose connective tissue with numerous blood vessels had developed, after 9–10 weeks tight connective tissue developed, and after 12 weeks, the transformation

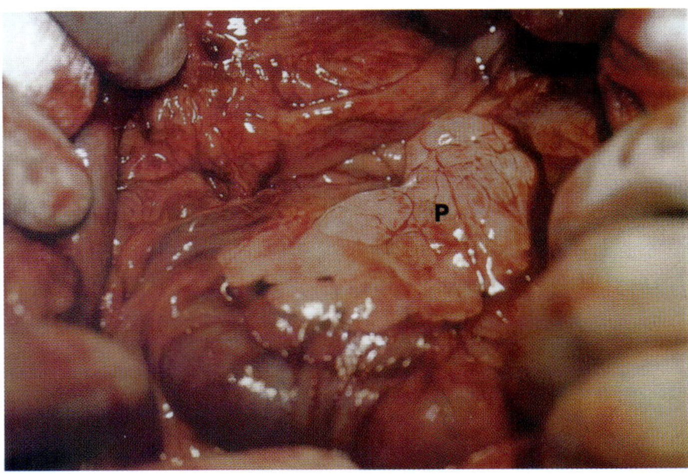

Fig. 10.1.1. Appearance of a dog pancreas before cryosurgery. The picture shows normal parenchyma. *P* Pancreas

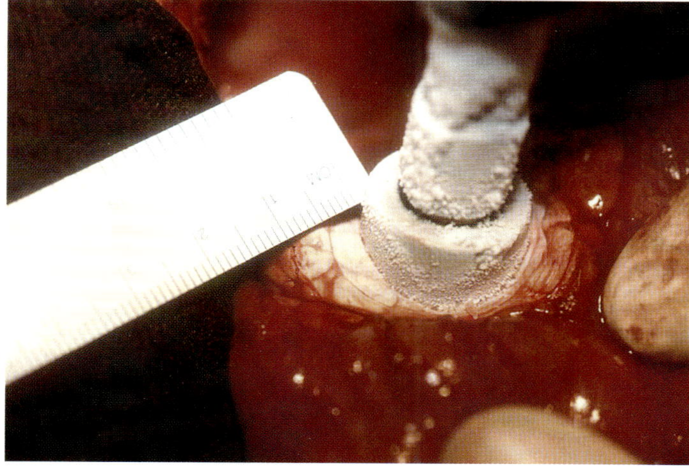

Fig. 10.1.2. The technique of cryosurgery. The disc probe with a diameter of 20 mm is placed on the pancreas at a temperature of −180°C for 9 min in a single freeze-thaw cycle to induce aseptic cryonecrosis (tissue destruction). Formation of an ice ball around the cryoprobe and line of demarcation of the cryozone. The cryosurgical margin measures 12 mm in diameter

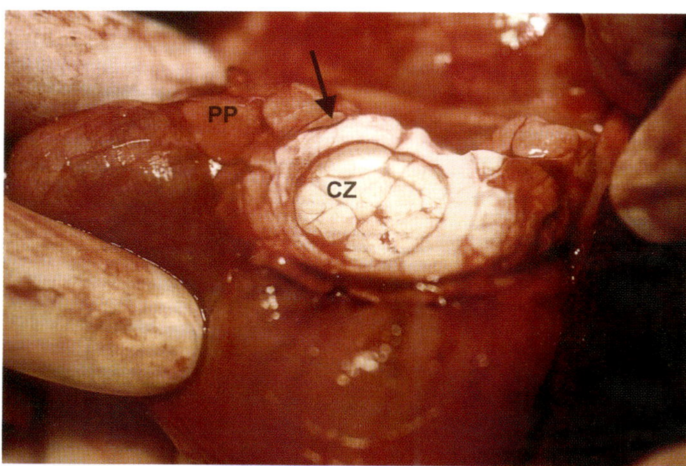

Fig. 10.1.3. Post-cryosurgical view. Appearance of the cryozone with ice crater in the center and visible ice margin with line of demarcation immediately after the cryosurgical procedure. *PP* Pancreas parenchyma, *CZ* cryosurgical zone

of the cryozone of the pancreatic parenchyma was complete.

Based on these experimental results, the following optimal cryoparameters for cryosurgical interventions in patients with pancreatic carcinomas was determined:

- Freeze temperature between −170°C and −190°C
- Freeze speed 300°C/min
- Spontaneous thawing
- Duration of application

Crash treatment:	10 sec
Short treatment:	1 min
Medium-duration treatment:	3 min
Long treatment:	5–7 min, in special cases longer

- Number of sessions: 1–3
- Volume of the cryozone: 1–180 cm^3
- Constancy of temperature at the tip of the probe
- The freeze process should be pre-programmed and proceed automatically in line with the established values

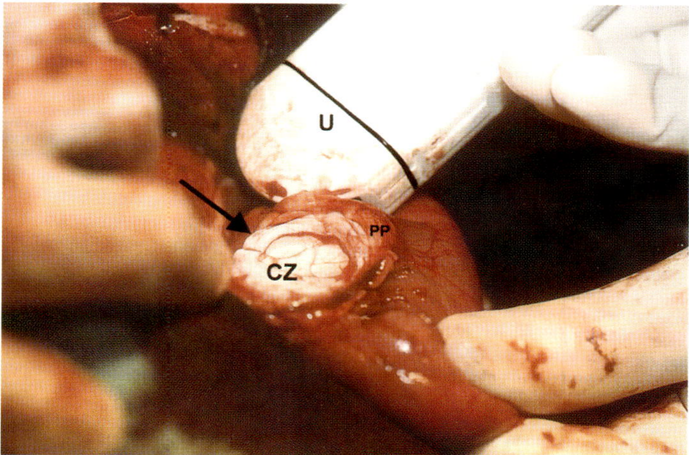

Fig. 10.1.4. Intraoperative monitoring of pancreas cryosurgery: Intraoperative ultrasound of the pancreas after single freeze-thaw cycle. *CZ* Cryosurgical zone, *U* ultrasound

10.1.2 Clinical Experience

Many years of international experience with the use of cryosurgery in advanced stages of pancreatic cancer have demonstrated the possibilities and limits of this surgical method. Cryosurgical pro-

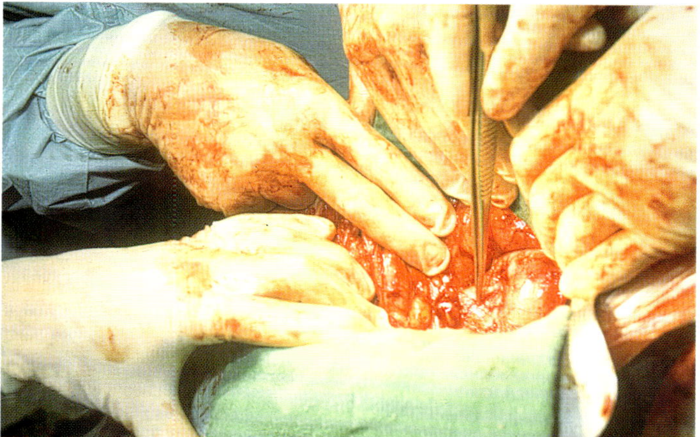

Fig. 10.1.5. Primary pancreas head carcinoma in a 53-year-old male. Intraoperative view

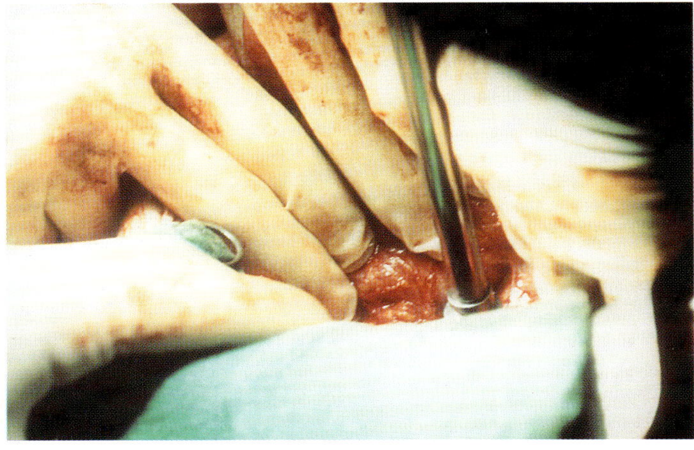

Fig. 10.1.6. The same patient. A single cryosurgical freeze-thaw cycle; the 20-mm-diameter disc cryoprobe is placed on the tumor lesion at a temperature of −180°C. The disc is very briefly applied to the lesion

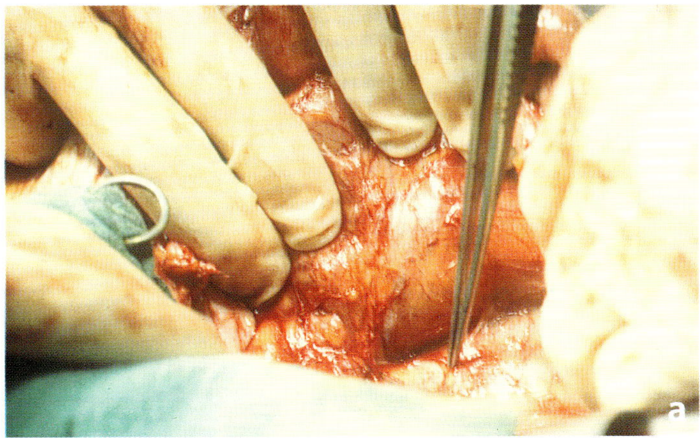

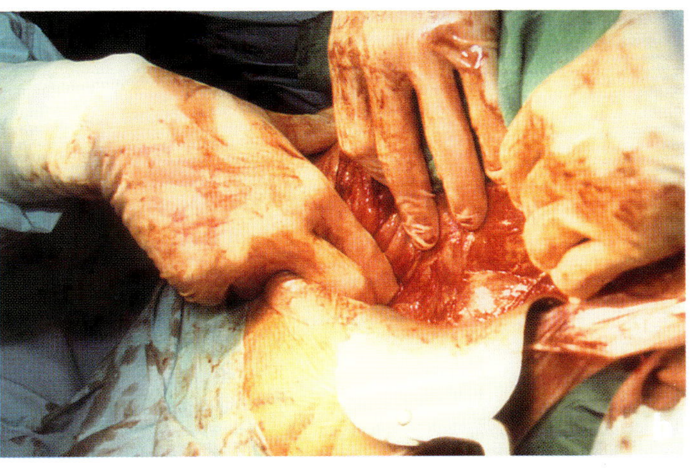

Fig. 10.1.7. In the same patient, the tumor lesion after cryosurgical session: immediately after freezing (**a**) and thawing (**b**) of the pancreas parenchyma

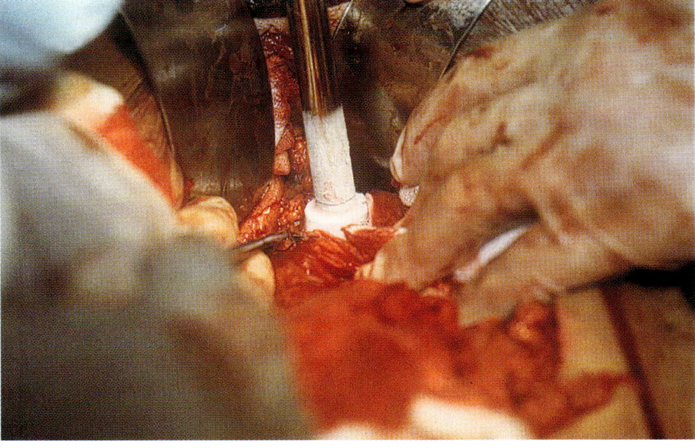

Fig. 10.1.8. Primary pancreas head carcinoma in a 46-year-old male. Intraoperative view: Cryosurgical treatment with a 30-mm-diameter disc cryoprobe, placed on the pancreas lesion at a temperature of −180°C. The disc is very briefly applied to the lesion

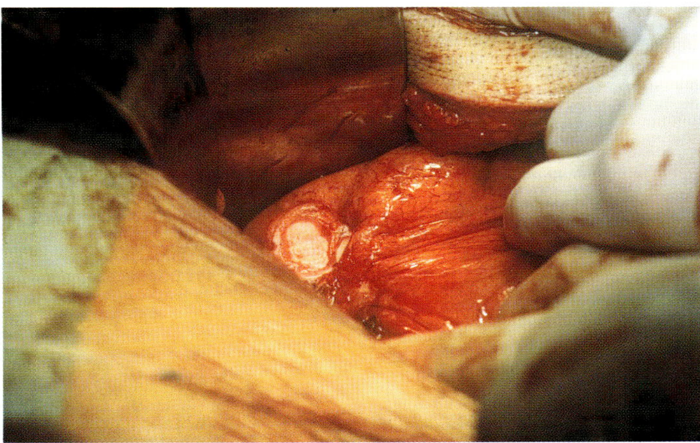

Fig. 10.1.9. Post-cryosurgical view in the same patient. Ice block formation. Appearance of a cryozone with the ice crater in the center, and of the ice margin with the visible line of demarcation, immediately after the cryosurgical session

cedure en bloc of the inoperable pancreas carcinoma (Fig. 10.1.5) is carried out by application of the round tip to the tumorous pancreas parenchyma (Fig. 10.1.6). The cold shock destroys the cancerous tissue at a temperature of −190°C (Fig. 10.1.7a, b), but healthy tissue is spared, because the effect of the cold can be exactly regulated with regard to depth and extent. The length of application and the number of treatment cycles must be individually determined, depending on the clinical picture.

10.1.3 Cryosurgical Procedure

The pathological focus should be removed with some healthy tissue, i.e., the macroscopically observed cryozone should always be a few centimeters wider than the focus (Figs. 10.1.8–10.1.9). The depth and extent of the cryozone is dependent

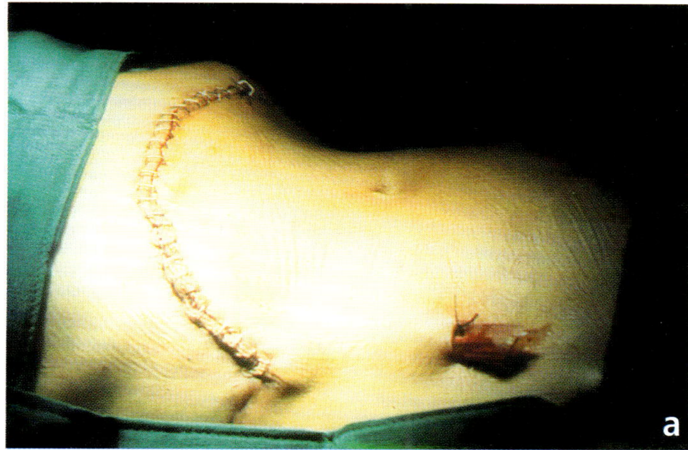

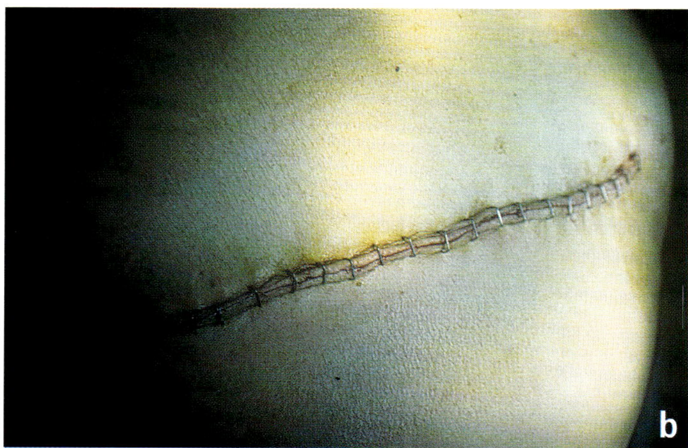

Fig. 10.1.10. After the pancreas cryosurgery the abdominal cavity can be closed with drainage (**a**) or without drain (**b**)

on the freeze temperature and on the length of exposure. The lower the temperature, the deeper and wider the cryozone. Of course, other factors, such as the size or the location of the tumor, play a not unimportant role.

The operation is normally ended with a drain (Fig. 10.1.10a) but the abdominal cavity can also be closed without a drain (Fig. 10.1.10b). Intraoperative sonography is usually carried out to monitor the cryosurgical procedure.

All patients with pancreatic carcinoma have responded well to cryosurgery. There were no surgical complications or mortality directly associated with the cryosurgery. Nor were intra- or postoperative bleeding, fistulas or sepsis determined. The postoperative course was unproblematic and free of complications. In-hospital stays are normally no longer than 5–7 days. At present there are no known contraindications.

Thus, since the cryosurgical method is far less invasive than conventional pancreas resection, the rate of complications and postoperative mortality are very low.

References

1. Cooper IS. Cryogenic surgery: a new method of destruction or extirpation of benign or malignant tissues. N Engl J Med 1963; 268: 743–749.
2. Gage AA, Baust J. Mechanisms of tissue injury in cryosurgery. Cryobiology 1998; 37(3): 171–186.
3. Korpan NN, Zemskov VS, Skiba VV. Cryomethods in General Surgery. Medizinskii Referativnii Zhurnal 1984; Kiev/Moscow, 77: 93–98.
4. Korpan NN. Möglichkeiten und Grenzen der modernen Kryochirurgie. In: Neugebauer H. (Ed.) Was gibt es Neues in der Medizin. 1996; Medizinisches Jahrbuch, Dr. Peter Müller Verlag-Wien, 207–213
5. Korpan NN. Hepatic Cryosurgery for Liver Metastases. Long-Term Follow-Up. Ann. Surg 1997; 225(2): 193–201.
6. Korpan NN. Pancreas Cryosurgery. An Animal Study. 2000; 1st European Congress of Cryosurgery (San Sebastian, Spain, March 29-April 2, 2000), Abstract Book, 7.
7. Korpan NN, Hochwarter G. Pancreatic cryosurgery – a new surgical procedure for pancreatic cancer. Europ J Clin Invest 1997; 27 (Suppl 1): A33.
8. Korpan NN, Hochwarter G, Sellner F, Zharkov JV. Pancreatic cryosurgery- a new surgical strategy for pancreatic cancer. 1997; 37th World Congress of Surgery, International Surgical Week ISW97 (Acapulco, Mexico, August 24–30, 1997), Abstract Book, 156.
9. Korpan NN, Muskin JN, Zemskov VS, Skiba VV. Abdomen Cryosurgery. Vestnik Surg 1985; 9: 141–145.
10. Korpan NN, Zharkov JV, Sacher R. A morphological study of cooling rate response in normal animal liver tissue: Cryosurgical Implications. Eur J Clin Invest 1999; 29 (Suppl 1): 22.
11. Rabin Y, Steif PS, Taylor MJ, Julian TB, Wolmark N. An experimental study of the mechanical response of frozen biological tissues at cryogenic temperatures. Cryobiology, 1996; 33(4): 472–482.

10.2 Acute Destructive Pancreatitis

Tatjana Komkova

Acute destructive pancreatitis is a serious disease, the cause of which are necrobiotic processes of pancreatic cells and enzyme autoaggression, with subsequent development of necrosis, degeneration of the pancreas and later infection. The choice of the method of surgery for acute pancreatitis depends on a number of factors, including etiology, depth and extent of destructive processes in the pancreas, as well as hypertension in the extrahepatic bile ducts. The majority of authors recommend the application of extracorporeal methods of detoxication in combination with conservative and surgical treatment. The degree of enzyme toxemia is of great importance for the course of the disease (Aldrete et al. 1980; Lasson et al. 1985; Shabalin 1989). Clinical experience shows that the treatment of acute destructive pancreatitis should not be limited to only one approach. The choice of therapy, including surgical treatment, depends on the patient's general condition, the serum level of pancreatic enzymes, and the intensity of peritoneal symptoms. Despite an active surgical approach to destructive pancreatitis, mortality in this disease remains high, regardless of the type of operation (Ronson 1990; Savelev 1983).

Analysis of the results showed that after operations on early-stage disease mortality is up to 54.5%, and after surgery on late-stage disease mortality is up to 70%. Surgery for acute destructive pancreatitis ranges from the drainage of the epiploon bag to resection (Miller et al. 1993; Shalimov et al. 1993). However, even this variety of operations has not improved the results of treating this disease and has led surgeons to develop new methods of operative treatment of acute destructive pancreatitis.

Merslikin's experimental work, carried out at the Tomsk Regional Hepatological Center (Tomsk, Russia) has proved the efficiency of application of subzero temperatures for acute destructive pancreatitis. In animal experiments (on female dogs), acute destructive pancreatitis was modelled by injection of bile taken from the same dog's gall bladder into the pancreas. As a result fat pancreonecrosis developed in the majority of the cases. Then relaparotomy and cryodestruction in the pancreas was performed at a temperature of (−180)–(−196)°C. Cryodestruction was performed at several points across the surface of the pancreas at an exposure of 30–40 sec. The effectiveness was judged on the basis of the clinical outcome and biochemical data (serum level of activity of the pancreatic enzymes, serum glucose).

A day after the operation the serum level of the pancreatic enzymes was reduced considerably in comparison with the initial level.

The serum level of pancreatic enzymes remained within the normal range during the next 30 days after the operation. The general condition of the animals was improved. Morphological investigations were performed at different times after the operation. They showed that the pancreatic tissue was replaced by a fibrous cicatrix in the zone of cryodestruction by the 45th–90th day after the operation. Pancreonecrosis foci were not evident.

The analysis of the experimental results allowed us to draw conclusions about the efficiency of the cryosurgical method of treatment of acute destructive pancreatitis. Subzero temperatures cause "functional" pancreatectomy. In comparison with conventional pancreatectomy, which is a very traumatic and disabling operation, cryodestruction in the pancreas is performed quickly and easily and does not cause such complications as hemorrhage, formation of cysts and fistulas. Furthermore, in those patients with pancreonecrosis who have symptoms of pancreas lysis, it is not always possible to undertake a resection of the organ or pancreatectomy, and crysurgery is indicated and is technically easy to perform. The operation is short and can be performed in 30–40 min, which is of great importance for the treatment of patients with severe toxemia, when the time factor can play the decisive role in a patient's successful recovery.

Cryodestruction preserves the anatomic integrity of the pancreas and stops the processes of autolysis. The islets of Langerhans remain functionally intact despite suppression of normal carbohydrate metabolism. The short term increase in serum glucose self-corrects and does not require additional injections of insulin. A sharp decrease in enzyme activity makes it possible to prevent the development of a number of complications in vital organs (pleuritis, pericarditis, etc.). In the postoperative period the zones of cryonecrosis are replaced by a fibrous cicatrix, which prevents the development of acute destructive pancreatitis in the late postoperative period (Fig. 10.2.1). Furthermore, subzero temperatures cause degenerative and destructive changes in nerve conductors and intramural nerve endings, which reduces pain considerably (Fig. 10.2.2).

Experimental research has proved the hemostatic effect of the influence of subzero temperatures: the tissue at biopsy bleeds moderately, the walls of large vessels are not destroyed during cryodestruction, and the entire volume of blood circulation is preserved (Fig. 10.2.3). The position of the organs is preserved and no deformation of the duodenum and extrahepatic bile ducts takes place after cryosurgery. However, it is necessary to remember that the minimal distance of cryodestruction from the duodenum wall should be not less than 1.5–2.0 cm.

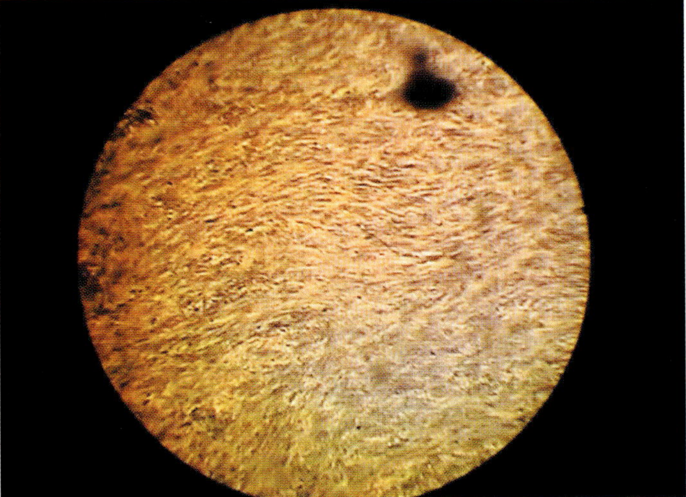

Fig. 10.2.1. Formation of the fibrous cicatrix after cryodestruction in acute destructive pancreatitis. Hematoxilin-eosin stain. Magnification ×200

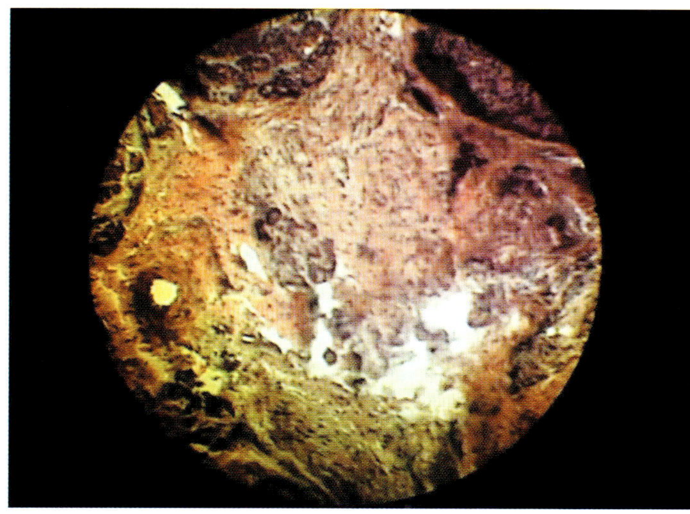

Fig. 10.2.2. Nerve conductors of the pancreas after cryodestruction. Impregnation by nitrogen oxide silver by Bilshovsky-Gros. Magnification ×500

These good experimental results made it possible to apply the methods in clinical practice. The indications for the cryosurgical approach in the pancreas in acute destructive pancreatitis were defined as follows:

1. Absence of effect of the conservative treatment within the first few days
2. Increase of symptoms of peritonitis during infusion therapy
3. Increase of activity of pancreatic enzymes or their stabilization at high levels
4. No effect of application of cytostatics and anti-enzyme medications

The contraindications are an increase in signs of nephro-hepatic insufficiency, cardiac weakness, elderly age (older than 70).

Upper medial laparotomy is the most convenient access for cryosurgical treatment of acute destructive pancreatitis. It is expedient to expose the pancreas before beginning cryosurgery. Moving the organ into the wound improves the conditions for freezing the adjacent large vessels without the danger of damage to the vessels. Cryosurgery is performed with a cryoprobe whose freezing surface is 30–40 mm in diameter and at a temperature of (−180)–(−196)°C. Cryoexposure is applied in 3 or 4 of the most morphologically altered areas of the pancreas, with exposure up to 120 sec at each treated point in separate cryocycles (Fig. 10.2.4). Duration of exposure is determined by the size of the pancreas, as it can increase in acute pancreatitis because of an increase in interstitial edema.

Freezing is carried out at each point in several cryocycles (2–3 cycles in each point) to amplify the effect of cryodestruction. The tissue of the pancreas should be allowed to thaw after each cryocycle. It is necessary to maintain sufficient distance between the cryoprobe and the wall of the duodenum to avoid freezing of the latter. Omentopancreatopexy and drainage of the epiploon bag end the operation.

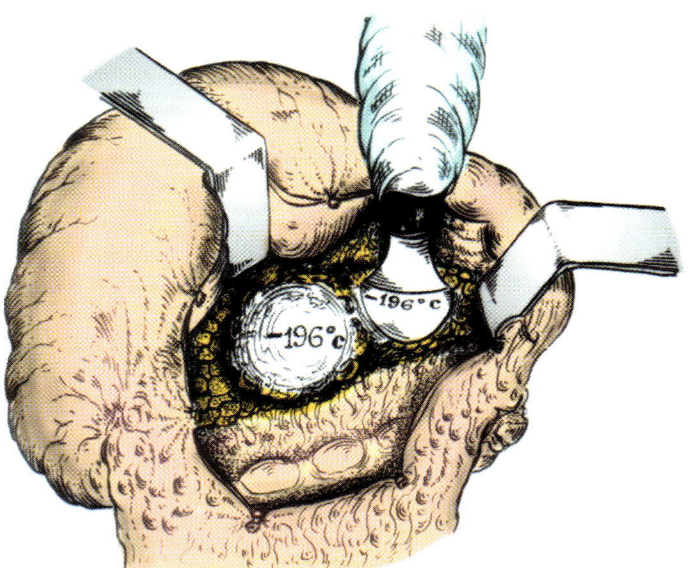

Fig. 10.2.3. Cryodestruction in the pancreas in acute destructive pancreatitis

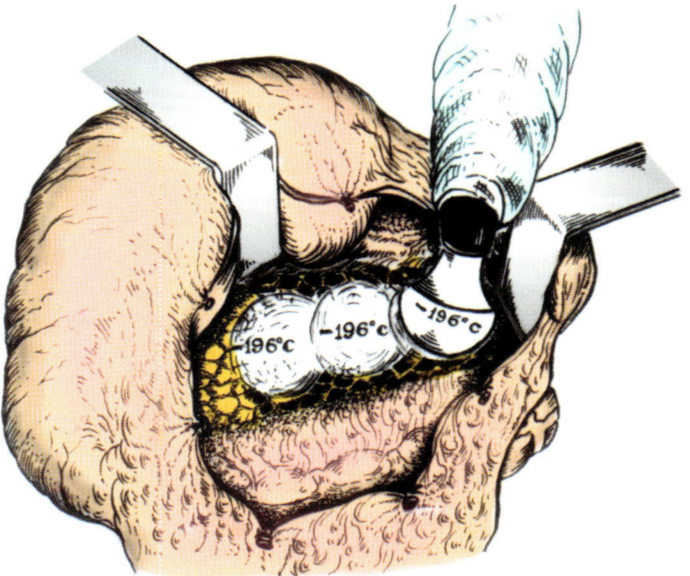

Fig. 10.2.4. Additional points of cryodestruction in the pancreas in acute destructive pancreatitis

Cryodestruction in the pancreas was applied in clinical practice alongside the conventional methods. It is necessary to point out that acute destructive pancreatitis often develops on the basis of chronic Opistorchosus invasion and cholelithiasis, and it also may be accompanied by the development of enzymatic cholecystitis and mechanical icterus. In these cases, the cryosurgical approach should be combined with cholecystectomy and drainage of the main bile duct according to one of the conventional methods. Preoperative examination of the patient includes ultrasonography, which reveals any increase in the size of the pancreas, which develops basically through edema and destruction of the parenchyma. It is also possible to see changes in echodensity in the pancreas parenchyma and irregular intensity of echosignals (the location of the foci of necrosis and their intensity, the presence of the zones of normal pancreatic tissue, etc.).

The key clinical symptom indicating surgery is an increase in peritoneal irritation and signs of toxemia during conservative treatment. Mortality is high after conventional methods of surgical treatment, being 73.6% and 29.6% after abdominization and omentopancreatopexy, respectively. After cryosurgery in the pancreas in acute destructive pancreatitis, mortality was much lower at 18%.

Case report: Patient I, 35 years old, was brought by ambulance to the surgical department of the Tomsk city hospital on February 3, 1987. The patient complained of pains in the epigastrium and the right hypochondriac region, nausea, and xerostomia. Anamnesis showed that the patient had been treated conservatively for chronic pancreatitis for a year and a half. The patient's symptoms had appeared two days earlier. The objective examination showed that the patient's general condition was satisfactory, the tongue was dry, the skin was icteric. At palpation there was pain in the epigastrium and the right hypochondriac region. Musset's sign, Ortner's sign, Mayo-Robson's sign were positive, serum bilirubin was 83 mmol/l, amilase of urine was 1066 g/l. Ultrasonography revealed concrements in the gall bladder. Symptoms of acute pancreatitis increased. On February 11 laparotomy, cholecystectomy, main bile duct drainage, with abdominization and cryodestruction at three different points in the pancreas at −196°C at exposure of 60 sec in each point were performed. Interoperatively the pancreas was inspected and showed signs of fat pancreonecrosis, a gall bladder with phlegmonous inflammation. There were no stones in the main bile duct. Postoperatively, symptomatic conservative therapy was administered. On the second postoperative day, urine amylase was 100 g/l and the course of the postoperative period was unremarkable. The patient was discharged to ambulatory treatment on the 20th day after the operation in satisfactory general condition.

In this case the choice of the surgical method depended on morphological changes in the pancreas, on pathological processes in the extrahepatic bile ducts, as well as on any complications.

Regardless of the morphological form of pancreonecrosis, cryosurgery is performed according to the suggested scheme: the temperature is (−180)–(−196)°C, exposure is 30–40 sec in separate cryocycles depending on the size of the pancreas. The pancreas must be frozen across its entire width to achieve a positive result. Combining cryosurgery in the pancreas with abdominization can be considered to be a very effective method, which considerably simplifies cryodestruction and improves the results of the operation.

The results achieved by clinical application of cryodestruction in the pancreas in pancreonecrosis are good, postoperative mortality being a low 18.6%. The suggested method is quite simple to perform, has few complications, provides good results in the late postoperative period, and prevents the formation of pancreatic fistulas and cysts. The replacement of acinous tissue by a fibrous cicatrix makes it possible to prevent the development of acute destructive pancreatitis in the late postoperative period.

The normalization of the activity of pancreatic enzymes by the second or third day after the operation is of great importance, which influences positively the patient's general condition, and reduces enzyme toxemia. At the same time, the endocrine function of the pancreas remains normal, and serum glucose in patients with diabetes mellitus reaches preoperative levels by the third or fourth day. For all these reasons, the cryosurgical approach can be recommended for the treatment of acute destructive pancreatitis.

References

1. Aldrette JS, Jimens H, Halpern N. Evaluation and treatment of acute and chronic pancreatitis. A review of 380 Cases. Ann Surg 1980; 191(6): 664–671.
2. Lasson A, Laurel AB, Ohlsoon K. Correlation Among Complement Activation Protease Inhibitors and Clinical Course in Acute Pancreatitis in Man. Scand J Gastroenterol 1988; 20(3): 335–345.
3. Miller BJ, Henderson A. Necrotizing Pancreatitis: Operating to Life. International Surgery Week. Hong-Kong 1993; 239.

4. Ronson JH. The Role of Surgery in the Management of Acute Pancreatitis. Ann Surg 1990; 4: 382–392.
5. Savelev VS. Late results of conservative and surgical treatment of pancreonecrosis. Surgery 1983; 7: 11–12.
6. Shalimov AA, Lifshits HZ, Kozhara SP. New approach to surgical treatment of patients with necrotic pancreatitic abscesses. International Surgery Week.Hong-Kong 1993; 245.
7. Shabalin VN. Immune therapy for destructive pancreatitis complicated by hepatic insufficiency. Surgery 1989; 7: 76–79.

10.3 Chronic Pancreatitis

Tatijana Komkova

Cryosurgery is one of the most progressive trends in modern medicine. Achievements in physics and cryobiology have made it possible to develop and introduce into clinical practice a relatively simple surgical method, with good therapeutic effects and a low level of postoperative complications. J. Cooper was the first to use freezing to treat a brain tumor in 1961. There is practically no bleeding in cryosurgical operations, the zone of operation may be extended, duration of exposure and the temperature applied in the operation can be well controlled, different diameters of the working part of the cryoprobe make it possible to use subzero temperatures in otorhinolaryngology, oncology and other areas of surgery.

The wider introduction of cryomethods has required the development of special equipment designed to freeze tissues and organs having different degrees of vascularization. The blood circulation in the organ being subjected to cryodestruction determines the speed of heat exchange. Thus, the basic characteristics of the freezing agent were determined and the specifications of cryosurgical apparatuses were suggested as a result of experimental and clinical research (Afanasjev et al. 1987; Tchireshkin 1972; Bellows 1967).

Liquid nitrogen, with a boiling point of −196°C, is in widespread use nowadays. The pancreas being a highly vascularized organ, high-powered cryoequipment is required for operations on this organ to keep the temperature of the working surface not higher than −180°C for 30–40 seconds during the contact time. Only such a low temperature makes it possible to achieve optimum freezing of pancreatic tissue even with substantial inflammatory growth. Experimental investigations have shown that freezing should be carried out in several cryocycles to expand the zone of cryonecrosis. The structure of blood vessels and pancreatic ductules is preserved, but glandular tissue is subjected to aseptic necrosis, and degenerative and destructive changes develop in nerve conductors and intramural nerve endings.

Besides traditional methods, the application of a cryoultrasonic scalpel is possible in pancreas resection, in which the cryogenic method is combined with ultrasound and increases the speed of formation of the ice ball, intensifies cryodestruction and simultaneously reduces adhesion of organ tissue to the cutting surface of the instrument. The application of a powerful cryoprobe and ultrasonic scalpel makes it possible to freeze pathological foci to a considerable depth, to resect the organ with minimum bleeding, and also to prevent the development of a number of postoperative complications common in traditional methods of surgical treatment of pancreatic disease.

The first reports on cryosurgery of the pancreas came from A. Carraro (1910), who froze the pancreas of goats and rabbits with a jet of chlorethyl. The author proved as a result of his experiments that the focus of necrosis is substituted by fibrous tissue of the pancreas parenchyma.

In 1970, J. Myers and co-authors published the results of research on morphological changes in pancreas tissue of rhesus monkeys under cryoinfluence. Cryodestruction was elicited by a device in which liquid nitrogen was the freezing agent and the temperature of the working part was −180°C. In all these experiments neither edema nor bleeding was observed in the part of the pancreas that was subject to cryodestruction. It was also seen that a general inflammatory reaction in the form of pancreatitis did not develop. The authors pointed out the danger of carrying out cryodestruction too close to the duodenum, as the danger of necrosis of the wall of the latter arises. The same authors determined that the structure of vascular walls in contact with the subzero temperatures is preserved, which is extremely important for prevention of bleeding during the operation and in the postoperative period.

The creation of the original cryosurgical equipment required its testing under experimental conditions as well as detailed study of morphological changes brought about by different levels of subzero temperatures in different organ areas.

Experiments were carried out on male and female dogs of different ages weighing from 7 to 16 kg. It was necessary to make preparations at different times after the operation with application of special methods of fixing and coloring for more detailed research of morphological processes arising in nervous conductors, vessels and acinic tissue of the pancreas. The area in which the vascular nerve fascicle passes into the pancreas contains a great number of intramural nerve endings and was determined to be a basic zone of cryodestruction. The temperature for cryodestruction was −180 to −196°C with exposure of 30–120 seconds in separate cryocycles. The macroscopic view of the cryodestruction focus after freezing resembled a white ball, which became dark crimson with moderate perifocal edema after thawing.

Extensive foci of necrosis of glandular tissue, acini are not differentiated precisely in the early period after cryodestruction (1–2 days). Isolated granulo- and agranulocytes are found between acini and the layers of fibrous tissue. Blood vessels of different diameter are seen along deferent ductules and between the lobules. The wall of the vessels preserves its structure despite perivascular edema (Fig. 10.3.1).

The study of histological preparations later showed that isolated fibroblasts appear with signs of aseptic necrosis of acinic tissue from the 14th day, which points to the primary stages of the formation of the fibrous cicatrix (Fig. 10.3.2). The foci of necrosis of acinic tissue, the cells of glandular epithelium of acini after cryodestruction, have homologous cytoplasm in the apex and the base of the acini. The zones of necrosis are gradually replaced by friable, shapeless fibrous tissue (Fig. 10.3.3).

The changes arising under the influence of subzero temperatures in deferent ductules and the vascular wall are of great importance for clinical practice. Deferent ductules and blood vessels accompanying them are seen clearly against the necrotic background immediately after cryodestruction. Pancreatic ductules preserve their structure, the epithelium of the ductules is clearly seen. The majority of blood vessels of different diameter are filled with blood corpuscles, and the vascular wall, whose structure has been preserved, has moderate perivascular edema (Fig. 10.3.4). The fact that deferent ductules are dilated when fibrous cicatrices develop following cryodestruction is significant (Fig. 10.3.5). Stasis and thrombosis are seen in blood vessels; however, dilated vessels with moderate perivascular edema are more frequently seen later in the observation period after cryodestruction. The morphological picture described above has formed the basis for developing the technique of cryosurgery, which does not cause lesions of pancreatic ducts even with the

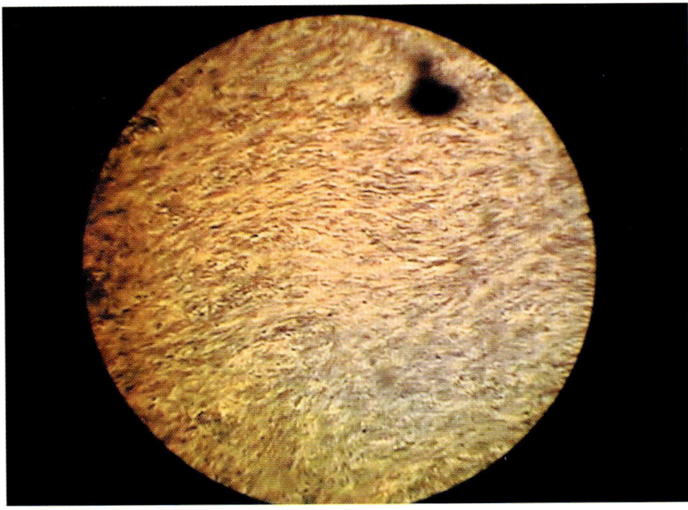

Fig. 10.3.2. Formation of the fibrous cicatrix replacing acinous tissue after cryodestruction in the pancreas. Day 14. Hematoxylin-eosin stain, magnification ×200

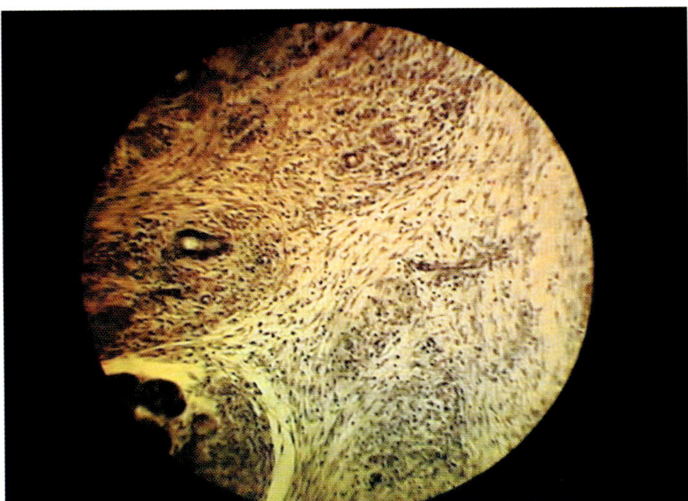

Fig. 10.3.3. Formation of the fibrous cicatrix replacing acinous tissue after cryodestruction in the pancreas. Day 21. Hematoxylin-eosin stain, magnification ×200

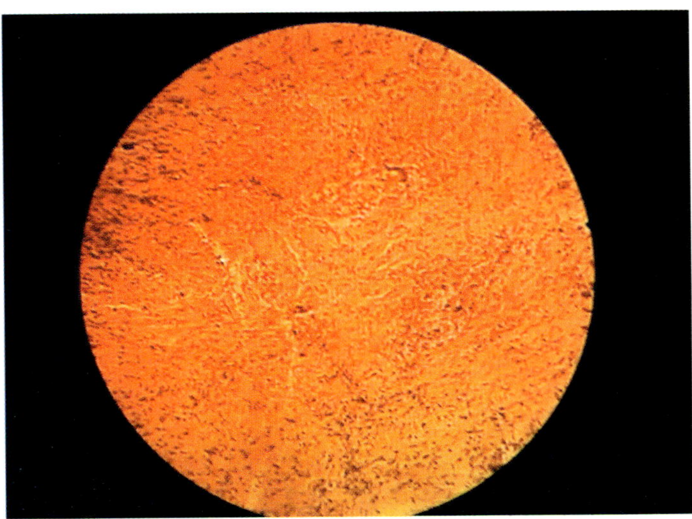

Fig. 10.3.1. The tissue of the pancreas on the first day after cryooperation. Hematoxylin-eosin stain, magnification ×200

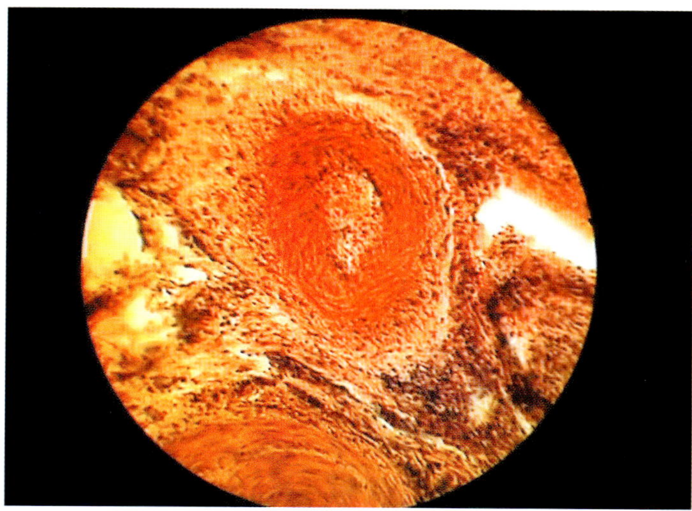

Fig. 10.3.4. The vessels of the pancreas after cryodestruction. Day 21. Hematoxylin-eosin stain, magnification ×200

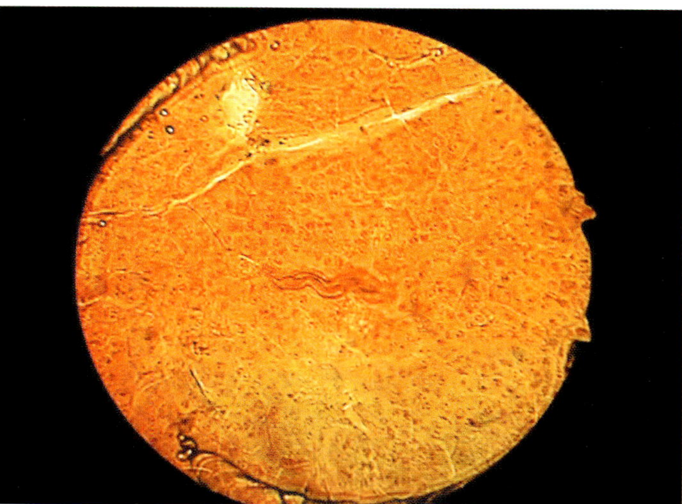

Fig. 10.3.6. Nerve conductors of the pancreas after cryodestruction. Day 14. Nitrogen oxidic silver, magnification ×500

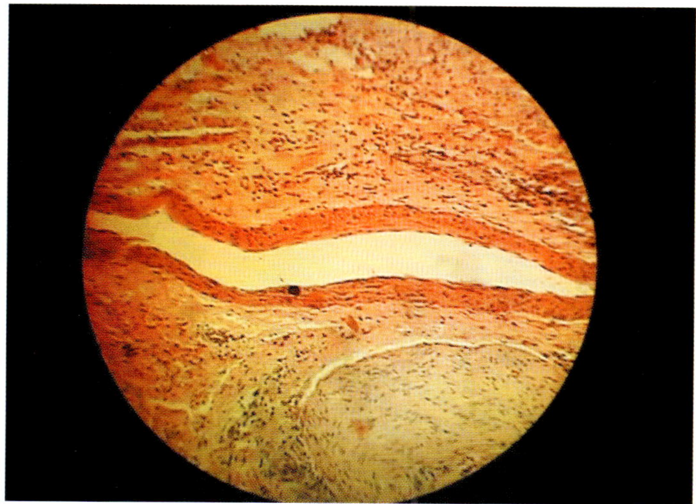

Fig. 10.3.5. Deferent ductules of the pancreas after cryodestruction. Day 21. Hematoxylin-eosin stain, magnification ×200

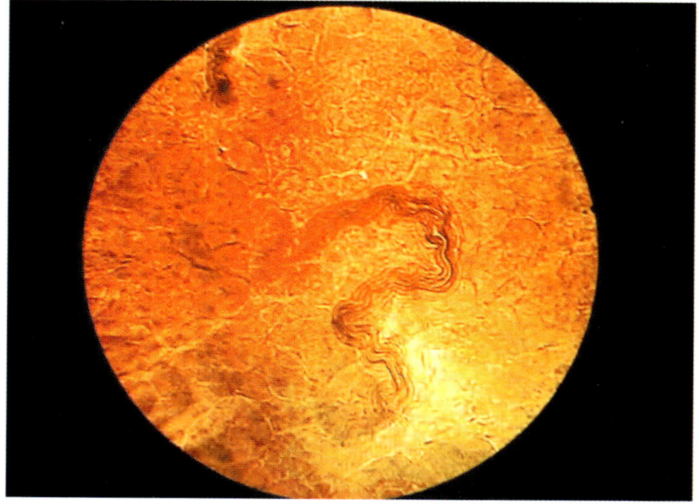

Fig. 10.3.7. Nerve trunks of the pancreas after cryodestruction. Day 21. Nitrogen oxidic silver stain, magnification ×500

development of fibrous cicatrices. The resistance of the vascular wall to subzero temperatures makes it possible to carry out cryodestruction close to major vessels and also to prevent hemorrhage during the operation.

In spite of the achievements of cryosurgery, the morphological changes in intramural nerve endings and nerve conductors resulting from cryodestruction have not been investigated up to now. Nerve conductors of different diameters of myelin and non-myelin type and nerve trunks of unequal diameter are normally found between the lobules in the layers of friable shapeless fibrous tissue.

In this case axons in the majority of myelin and non-myelin filaments are of equal diameter with single small varicose intumescences over the entire length (Fig. 10.3.7). In parallel with it, a small number of oligodendroglia cells are found, when their nuclei are moderately or weakly impregnated with nitrogen silver. Small ganglions of different forms consisting of one or two neurons are seen on closer study.

Nerve trunks of different diameter and isolated nerve filaments are noticeable in the layers of friable, shapeless fibrous tissue and accompanying blood vessels on the background of the deviations in the exocrinic part of the pancreas shortly after cryodestruction. Nerve filaments are particularly noticeable in the area of maximal cold influence. Nerve filaments with axons revealing dischromia can sometimes be seen among the nerve filaments that no longer take up the nitrogen silver stain. In this case the sites are already intensively impregnated with silver compared to the structures which have lost affinity to silver. As a result, fragmentation of the filament can be seen (Fig. 10.3.8). Nerve filaments do not differ in their structure from the control sites in the pancreas that are distant from the area of maximal cold influence.

In addition, the few varicose intumescences and disfilamentations of the neurofibrillar apparatus can be seen in axons of filaments of the nerve trunks and in isolated nerve conductors. The glial cells in the majority of objects are not easily discernible.

The results of our experiments showed that a temperature higher than –100°C is not cold enough to freeze all the morphological structures of the pancreas. The temperature of the working part of the instrument should be −180 to −196°C to achieve a maximal clinical effect.

The morphological changes arising in the tissue, vessels, ducts and nervous conductors of the pancreas as well as anatomophysiological peculiarities of the organ innervation, the location of nerve plexuses, intramural nerve endings and ganglions were all taken into consideration in the process of elaborating the technique of cryodestruction. The majority of these formations accompany the arteries and concentrate mainly in the head of the pancreas.

Thus, the "key" point for cryodestruction in chronic pancreatitis was determined on the basis of the experimental research data with regard to the anatomic structure of nervous conductors and structure of the pancreas. The "key" point is the transit zone where the head of the pancreas joins the body. The maximal number of the nerve conductors and intramural nerve endings undergoing degenerative and destructive changes are subjected to subzero temperatures during cryodestruction in this area. Cryodestruction causes partial cold denervation of the organ with preservation of nervous conductors and plexuses innervating the duodenum, the stomach and the extrahepatic bile ductules.

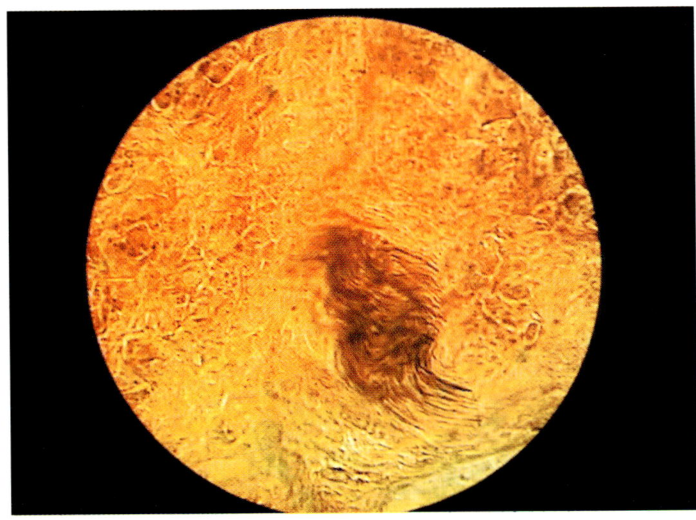

Fig. 10.3.8. Nerve conductors of the pancreas after cryosurgery. Day 21. Nitrogen oxidic silver stain, magnification ×500

Cold denervation of the pancreas in chronic pancreatitis is in principle different from the techniques of the mechanical denervation of the organ suggested earlier. All the operations on the vegetative nervous system described earlier interrupted the innervation of only one or two plexuses. These types of surgical correction do not completely interrupt the innervation of any of them because of the arborescent structure of the plexuses. Nervous formations located near the vessels and intramural nerve endings remain unchanged at the intersection of large nerve trunks.

These nervous conductors coming from several nerve plexuses are subjected to subzero temperatures during the operation on the pancreas in the transit zone between the head and the body. This zone contains the largest number of nerve conductors and intramural nerve endings, with arborescent innervation. In addition, the transit zone of the pancreas head into its body is the entrance zone of arteries into the pancreas tissue. The arteries have three nerve plexuses, so that periarterial nerve endings located directly in the tissue of the pancreas are subjected to subzero temperatures when cryodestruction takes place in this zone.

Consideration of indications and contraindications in each individual case and the choice of the adequate method of surgical treatment are of great importance in achieving an effective therapeutic result in cryosurgical operations. The following indications for cryodestruction in the pancreas in chronic pancreatitis have been formulated on the basis of analysis of the experimental and clinical data gathered:

1. Presence of a strong pain syndrome
2. Absence of therapeutic effect of conservative treatment
3. Frequent exacerbations of chronic pancreatitis
4. Strong pain in posttraumatic pancreatitis
5. Pseudotumorous pancreatitis with pain syndrome
6. Pseudotumorous pancreatitis with suspicion of malignant transformation.

The basic indication for an operation is the pain syndrome, whose etiology can include, *inter alia*, alcohol abuse, Opisthorchis invasion, preceding trauma. It is expedient to combine cryosurgery of the pancreas with cholecystectomy when chronic pancreatitis is accompanied by cholelithiasis.

The contraindications for the operation are:

1. Presence of multiple foci of calcifications in pancreas parenchyma
2. Concretions in pancreatic ductules
3. Active opisthorchiasis
4. An elderly or senile age with existing somatic pathology
5. Young patients with existing somatic pathology accompanying chronic pancreatitis
6. Obstruction of the main pancreatic duct

Chronic pancreatitis is a long-term disease with exacerbations of different intensity. Simultaneously, inflammatory processes in pancreatic tissue progress gradually, and tears in small ductules and enzymes diffusing into the parenchyma lead to "self-digestion" of the pancreas (Becker 1981; Saveljev 1983). The choice of the method of surgical correction is determined by the location of the pathological focus (head, body, tail), the character of the changes in the parenchyma, the state of the duct system, and changes in the incretory and excretory function of the organ. Traditional methods of surgical treatment of chronic pancreatitis have a number of essential drawbacks. Depending on the volume of the resected pancreatic tissue, the procedure can be technically quite complex, with the possible development of different postoperative complications, such as pancreatic fistulas and diabetes mellitus, as well as decreased motor function of the extrahepatic bile ductules, of the duodenum, and of the jejunum.

Developing original methods of cryosurgery for chronic pancreatitis, the authors aimed to achieve a good therapeutic effect and to prevent most intra- and postoperative complications. Cryosurgical operations in chronic pancreatitis do not require special preoperative preparation of the patient. Required are general clinical methods of examination, ultrasonography, computed tomography of the pancreas, and retrograde cholangiopancreatography to verify the diagnosis.

The technique of the operation is as follows. The size, the form and the consistency of the pancreas are estimated at inspection after laparotomy to define the points and the regime of cryodestruction. The authors consider it to be expedient to take biopsy material before cryodestruction to verify the diagnosis, to exclude malignancy, and to define postoperative therapy. The incision in the peritoneum along the inferior edge of the pancreas and removal of the pancreas into the wound site facilitate cryodestruction. It is important to remember during cryodestruction that the distance between the working part of the instrument and the wall of the duodenum should be not less than 15–20 mm to avoid freezing the wall of the duodenum, which can be a potentially fatal complication. Furthermore, it is not recommended to use cryosurgery on the tail of the pancreas, as this part of the organ contains incretory apparatus – islets of Langerhans. Their lesion can cause the development of postoperative diabetes mellitus. Besides, morphological changes rarely develop in the tail of the pancreas in chronic pancreatitis.

During cryodestruction it is not necessary to fear freezing the wall of large vessels (aorta) located behind the pancreas: after laparotomy the pancreas is easily removed into the wound site, where it can be held away from the vessels; further, the correctly chosen cryodestructive exposure makes it possible to restrict freezing to the pancreas.

Cryodestruction is carried out with the use of a cryoprobe, the diameter of the working part being 30–40 mm. The temperature is −180 to −196°C, the exposure time is 2–3 min, depending on the size of the pancreas. Cryodestruction should provide freezing of the tissue of the pancreas in the optimal area and at an optimal depth to achieve positive results. The maximal number of nerve formations will be subjected to cryodestruction only under this condition. The duration of cryodestruction can increase or decrease depending on the extent of chronic inflammation. The cryosurgical exposure also depends on the temperature and the diameter of the working part of the cryoprobe: the higher the temperature and the smaller the diameter, the longer the duration of application should be to achieve a desirable result (Figs. 10.3.9–10.3.10).

Thus, assuming a width of the pancreatic tissue to be destroyed of 30–40 mm, the optimal extent of freezing of the pancreatic tissue is achieved by an exposure of 2–3 minutes in separate cryocycles, a temperature of the working part of −180 to −196°C, and a diameter of the cryoprobe of 30–40 mm.

Besides treatment to the basic ("key") point during the operation, two or three other sites in the pancreas should be subjected to cryodestruction

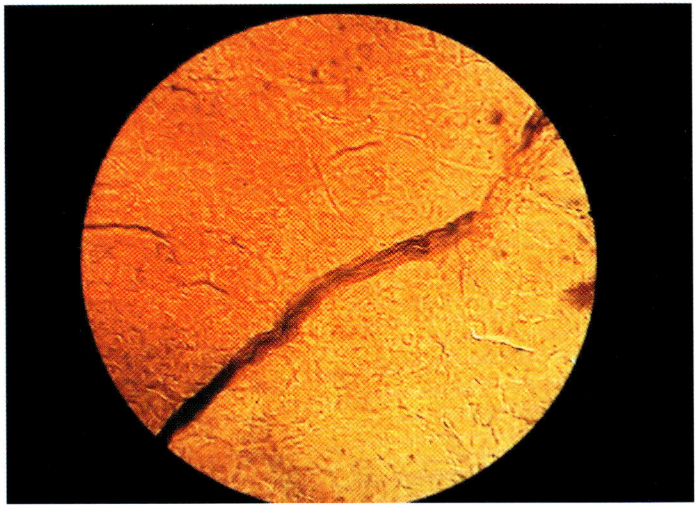

Fig. 10.3.9. Nerve conductors of the pancreas after cryodestruction. Day 40. Nitrogen oxidic silver stain, magnification ×500

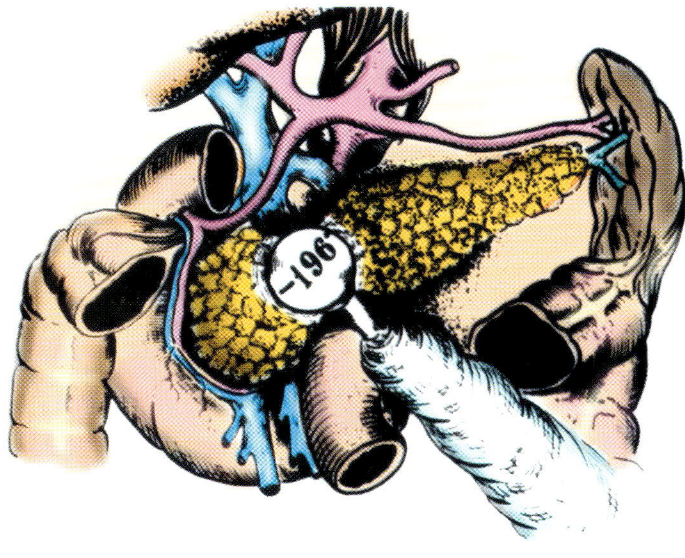

Fig. 10.3.10. The "key" point for cryodestruction in the pancreas for chronic pancreatitis

(Fig. 10.3.11). The aim of this operation is to create a zone of aseptic necrosis in the affected parts of the pancreas with the subsequent formation of fibrous cicatrices in place of acinic tissue, which makes it possible to prevent the development of acute destructive pancreatitis in the postoperative period. Pancreatic excretion is suppressed in consequence of the development of sclerosis.The operation ends with the drainage of the epiploon bag.

Cryodestruction in chronic pancreatitis has a number of advantages over the traditional methods of surgical treatment of this pathology.

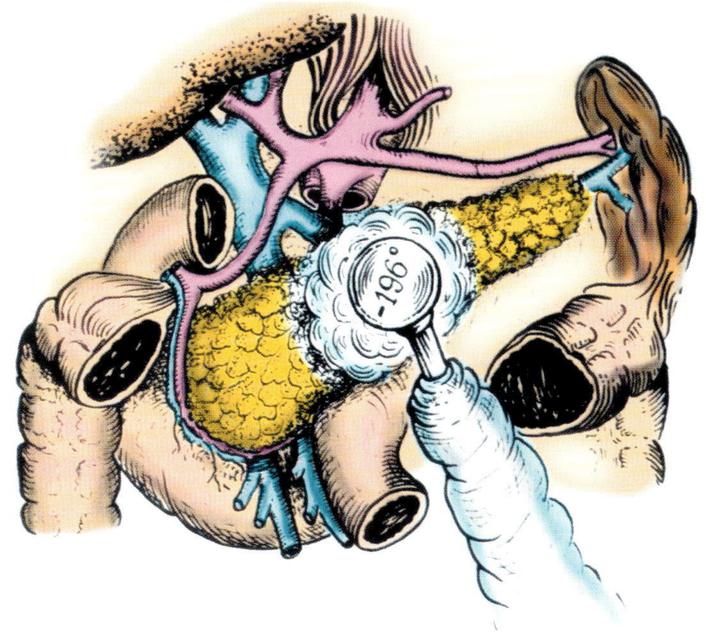

Fig. 10.3.11. Cryodestruction in the pancreas for pseudotumor pancreatitis

1. The operation is relatively simple, but its efficiency is high
2. It does not give rise to potentially fatal complications as compared with traditional methods (shock, hemorrhage)
3. The operation is quite short, its duration is 40–60 min

In addition, the cryodestruction of the pancreas can be combined with cholecystectomy for calculous cholecistitis, and the excision of pancreatic fistulas after previous operations.

The analysis of early and late results after cryodestruction has shown that the pain syndrome of the majority of the patients ceased completely or almost completely, exacerbations of the chronic pancreatitis that occurred were rather mild and did not require stationary treatment, and that serum glucose remained within the normal range.

Thus, patient Z, 33 years old, presented at the surgical department of the Tomsk Regional Hepatological Center (Russia) as scheduled in September 1987 complaining of pains of belt-like character in the epigastrium and in the right hypochondriac region, and with periodic vomiting. The patient was repeatedly treated conservatively for chronic pancreatitis. He had been treated surgically for pancreonecrosis (the form is not known) in 1977. The patient had been suffering from diabetes mellitus type II since 1986. At presentation the general state of the patient was satisfactory, the abdomen was soft, with pain in the epigastrium, and the Mayo-Robson sign was positive. At ultrasonography there were moderately expressed signs of chronic cholecystitis, the pancreas had a heterogeneous echostructure, with foci of increased echodensity. Clinical diagnosis: chronic painful pancreatitis, medium-grade diabetes mellitus. Pancreatic cryodestruction following laparotomy was performed under general anesthesia in October 1987. During the inspection of the abdominal cavity, a commissure process was revealed, the pancreas was deformed and hardened to a calculous density, with even harder foci in both the head and body. A puncture biopsy was performed, and cryodestruction was carried out at three points at a temperature of −196°C and with an exposure of 2 minutes at each point in separate cryocycles. The patient was discharged from the hospital to the care of his primary physician in satisfactory condition. The result of the histological investigation was chronic pancreatitis (Fig. 10.3.12). The patient experienced no pain for five years after the operation and felt generally well.

In the postoperative period, special attention should be paid to changes in biochemical findings. It was established that all the patients operated according to the suggested methods had a postoperative serum glucose level at the preoperative level. Two patients suffering from diabetes mellitus had hyperglycemia. The determination of enzyme levels was made pre- and postoperatively to estimate excretory function of the pancreas and to choose treatment accordingly. The development of reactive edema of the pancreas in the first days after the operation resulted in a moderate increase in the activity of pancreatic enzymes in all the patients. It did not require active correction and ceased by the 5th–6th day after the operation.

Thus, the analysis of the immediate and subsequent results showed that pancreatic cryodestruction in chronic pancreatitis makes it possible to achieve an absence of pain with minimum mortality (2.8%). The operation is rather simple, does not cause dyspeptic symptoms, and allows a good therapeutic outcome.

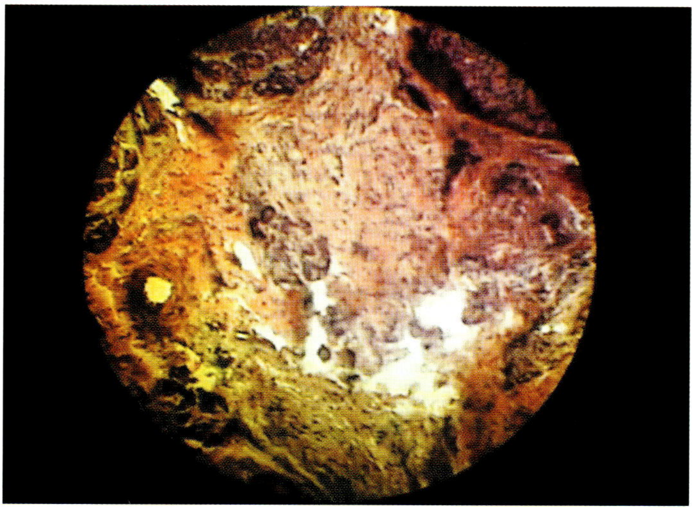

Fig. 10.3.13. Histological examination (intraoperative biopsy) of the pancreas of 44-year-old patient with chronic pancreatitis. Hematoxylin-eosin stain, magnification ×200

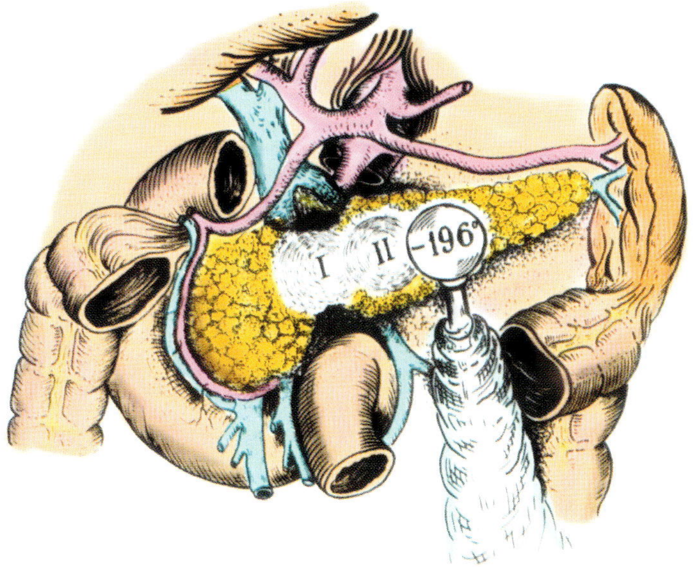

Fig. 10.3.12. Additional points of cryodestruction in the pancreas for chronic pancreatitis

References

1. Becker V. Pathological Anatomy and Pathogenesis of Acute Pancreatitis. World J Surg 1981; 5(3): 303–309.
2. Bellows JG. Cryosurgical Instruments. Theoretical and clinical consideration. Surgery 1967; 47(5): 416–424.
3. Cooper J. Principles and rationale of cryogenic Surgery. Med Bull 1962; 1(5): 10.
4. Cooper J. Cryogenic Surgery for Cancer. Fed Proc 1965; 24: 237–240.
5. Fay T, Henney GC. Correlation of body segmental temperature and its relation to the location of carcinomatous metastasis. Surg Gynecol Obstet 1938; 5: 512–524.
6. Hess W. Partielle and totale Pancreatektomien bei chronischer Pankreatitis. Helv Chir Acta 1967; 34 (1–2): 99–102.
7. Hiraoka T, Watanabe E, Katch T. A new surgical approach for control of pain in chronic pancreatitis complete denervation of the pancreas. Am J Surg 1986; 152 (5): 549–551.
8. Mallet-Guy P. Surgical treatment of chronic relapsing pancreatitis. Arch Surg 1955; 70 (4): 609–610.
9. Myers RS, Hammond WC, Kemcham AS. Cryosurgical necrosis of the head of the pancreas. Ann Surg 1970; 171(3): 413–418.
10. Puchalski L, Ladny JR, Piotrowski Z, Rog I. Surgical management of chronic pancreatitis: indication and procedures. Int Surg Week. Hong-Kong. 1993; 820.

10.4 Pancreas Cysts

Tatjana Komkova

Cysts of the pancreas are a rare pathology. Acquired cysts or pseudocysts having no capsule of their own are more common. Acute pancreatitis, trauma of the organ, Opistorchosus invasion can cause pancreatic cysts to develop (Lankisch et al. 1993; Swiklus et al. 1993). The disease is usually accompanied by a pain syndrome regardless of the primary reason for the development of the cyst. Suppuration, hemorrhage and other potentially fatal complications are also possible. The factors mentioned above are the basic indications for an operation.

Surgical options for the treatment of pancreatic cysts include different types of outside drainage, pancreas resection of different volume, creation of cystogastro- and cystoenteroanastomosis, and filling the cyst with self-hardening plastics (Nevel et al. 1990; Galeev et al. 1992; Anderson et al. 1993). The operations of outside drainage can be performed as a temporary matter, if there are technical problems or contraindications for a more complicated and more extensive operation. Such patients need secondary surgical treatment later.

If the pathological process is located in the tail of the pancreas, the clinical picture is more scanty, the pain syndrome is less severe. However the development of splenomegaly and disturbances in carbohydrate metabolism are possible. Distal resections of the pancreas are often complicated by the development of destructive pancreatitis of the stump and the formation of pancreatic fistulas (Sulkowski et al. 1990; Fedorov 1993). Unfortunately, mortality after pancreas resection remains at 4.5%, and it is even higher, 16%, after extended operations. Pancreatoduodenal resection is indicated for a cyst located in the head of the pancreas, which is also a very complex and traumatic operation.

Cysts caused by Opistorchosus occupy a special place in this group of diseases, being a complication of chronic Opistorchosus pancreatitis. In this case the disease proceeds with a strongly expressed clinical symptom, which is caused by Opictorchosus cholangitis and the expressed inflammatory process in the pancreatic ducts. As a result, strictures develop along with deformation of the duct, leading to hypertension of the pancreatic ducts. Hindrance of the outflow of the pancreatic secretion causes intensification of the pain syndrome and of the inflammatory process in the parenchyma and contributes to the development of recurrence of pancreatic cysts (Brazhnikova 1989).

The achievements of cryosurgery have made it possible to elaborate the methods of combined operations on pancreas cysts. The aim of the operation is the resection of a pathological focus (cyst) and prevention of disease recurrence. One group of operations consists of the excision of the external wall of the cyst within the limits of probably healthy tissue, the resection of the cyst contents and cryodestruction of the cyst bed. The influence of subzero temperatures causes replacement of acinic tissue by a fibrous cicatrix. Degenerative and destructive changes develop in nerve endings, which makes it possible to stop the pain syndrome and to prevent disease recurrence (both cyst formation and acute destructive pancreatitis) in the remote postoperative period. These operations are organ preserving, as no part of the organ is resected, and it does not interfere with carbohydrate metabolism or digestion. The preservation of the structure of the main pancreatic duct is of great importance to prevent the formation of fistulas in the postoperative period. Multiple cysts of the body and tail of the pancreas, isolated cysts with external pancreatic fistulas are the indication for left-sided resection of the pancreas. In these cases the combination of the resection or cryoresection of the pancreas and the cryodestruction of the remaining part is expedient. The resection is carried out according to one of the conventional methods with suturing and ligation of the main pancreatic duct. The remaining part of the pancreas is subjected to cryodestruction at a temperature of −196°C, which makes it possible to prevent the development of acute destructive pancreatitis of the remaining part in the postoperative period. The replacement of the acinic tissue by a fibrous cicatrix makes it possible to decrease the activity of pancreatic secretion, which is also important to achieving a good therapeutic effect. In some cases we use a cryoultrasonic scalpel which makes it possible to influence the remaining tissue of the pancreas. The advantages of the suggested methods of operations create conditions to reduce the number of postoperative complications after surgery for pancreatic cysts.

The basic indication for combined operations are:

1. Pancreatic cysts of Opistorchosus etiology in different parts of the organ
2. Pancreatic pseudocysts which have developed after trauma or acute destructive pancreatitis

3. Pancreatic cysts which have developed as a result of strictures of pancreatic ductules
4. Recurrent cysts of the pancreas
5. Multiple congenital or parasitic cysts
6. Direct or indirect signs of cyst malignancy or signs of malignant transformation of the cysts

The contraindications for such operations are limited. They are cyst suppuration, somatic pathology accompanying the basic disease, advanced age of the patient.

The combined operations can be divided into two groups. They are:

1. Resection and cryoresection of the pancreas with additional cryodestruction of the remaining part of the organ
2. Excision of the cyst wall including some apparently healthy tissue with additional cryodestruction of the cyst bed

It is expedient to apply the first variant of the operation when the cyst is located deep in the parenchyma of the organ (body, tail), when the external wall, consisting of glandular tissue, is comparatively thick and its excision can cause complications (hemorrhage, damage to pancreatic ductules). Resection of the pancreas is the operation of choice for deep multiple cysts, and also for pancreatic fistulas which have formed after previous surgery. Resection of the tail or body with subsequent conventional procedures depends on the location of the cyst. The remaining part of the pancreas is subjected to cryodestruction at a temperature of (−180)–(−196)°C and a diameter of 30–40 mm of the working surface of the cryoinstrument. The duration of cryoexposure depends on the volume of the remaining part of the pancreas, the intensity of the pathological process, and the condition of the duct system (Figs. 10.4.1–10.4.2).

The influence of subzero temperatures causes aseptic necrosis with subsequent formation of the fibrous cicatrix, which prevents the development of postoperative pancreatitis, promotes the smooth course of the postoperative period and achievement of a good therapeutic effect.

The creation and introduction into clinical practice of cryoequipment made it possible to replace the conventional resection of the pancreas with cryoresection. The application of a cryoscalpel or cryovibroscalpel in operations on the pancreas makes it possible to prevent the development of parenchymal hemorrage from the incision line during the operation. The freezing zone which then forms is subjected to transformation in the postoperative period: a fibrous tissue develops over the entire plane of cryoresection, which serves to prevent the development of postoperative fistulas. Thus, cryoresection of the pancreas combined with cryodestruction in the remaining part makes it possible to prevent the development of immediate postoperative complications in the

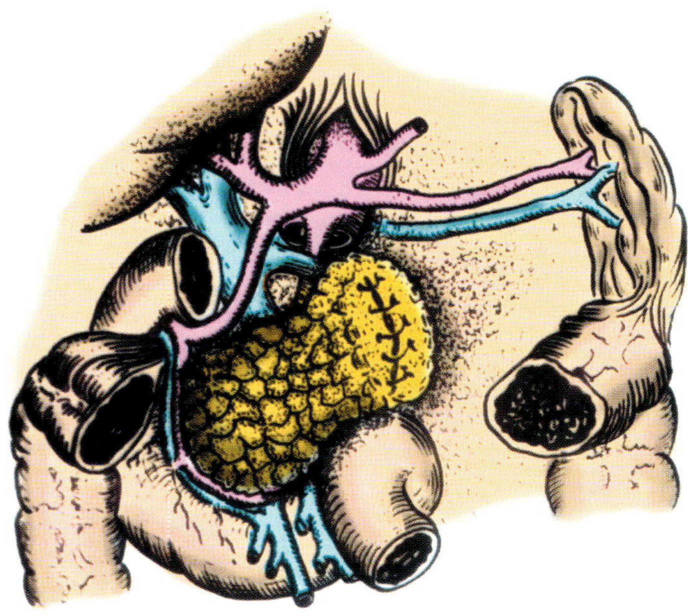

Fig. 10.4.1. The stump of the pancreas after resection (cryoresection) of the cyst

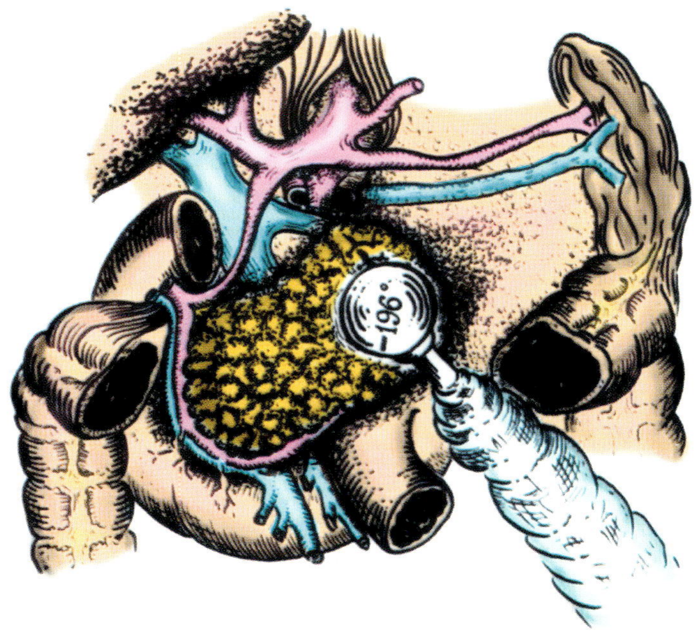

Fig. 10.4.2. Cryodestruction in the stump of the pancreas after resection (cryoresection)

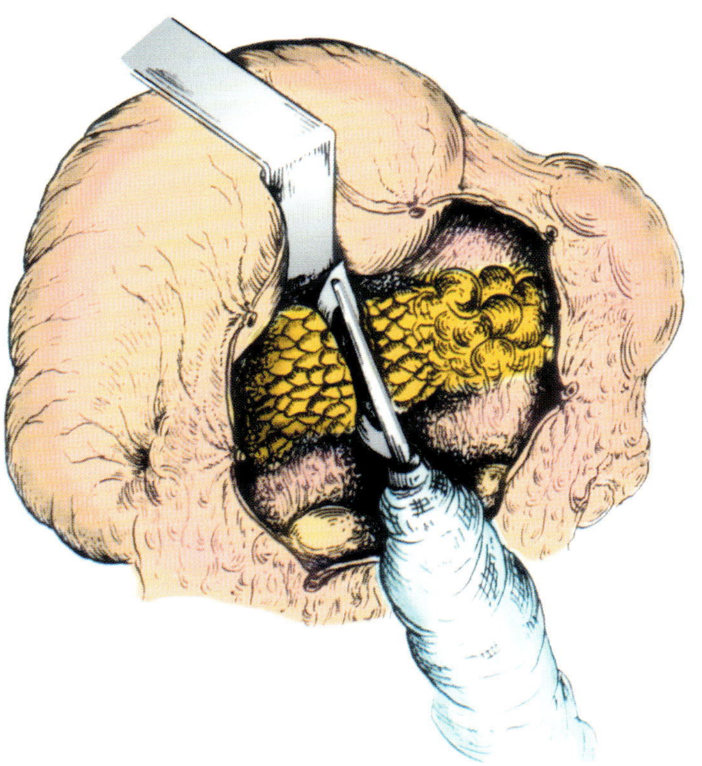

Fig. 10.4.3. Cryoresection of the pancreas

stump as well as over the plane of resection (Fig. 10.4.3).

The second group of combined operations consists of the excision of the cyst wall and cryodestruction of the area around the location of the cyst (Figs. 10.4.4–10.4.5). Special attention is required when the cyst is located in the pancreas head, for which the operation of choice is a pancreatoduodenal resection, which leads to invalidism of the patient. The excision of the cyst wall up to the parenchyma of the pancreas is possible if the location of the cyst is rather superficial. The cyst cavity is previously cleared of its contents.

Cryodestruction of the immediate area of the cyst is made at a temperature of −196°C after the excision of the cyst wall. It might be necessary for two or three points of the most pathologically affected parts of the pancreas body to be subjected to additional cryodestruction. The exposure is determined by the size of the pancreas. It is expedient to carry out cryodestruction in separate cryocycles of 20–30 sec each, in order to achieve the maximal freezing effect and to control the depth and extent of the cryoinfluence. In the case of an existing cyst this variant of combined surgery prevents its malignant transformation.

Thus, the suggested variants of operations on pancreatic cysts make it possible to prevent postoperative complications that can develop after

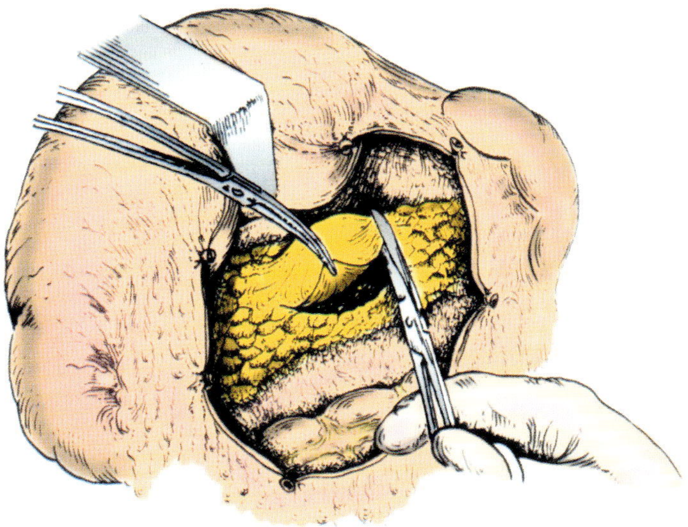

Fig. 10.4.4. Excision of the cyst wall of the pancreas

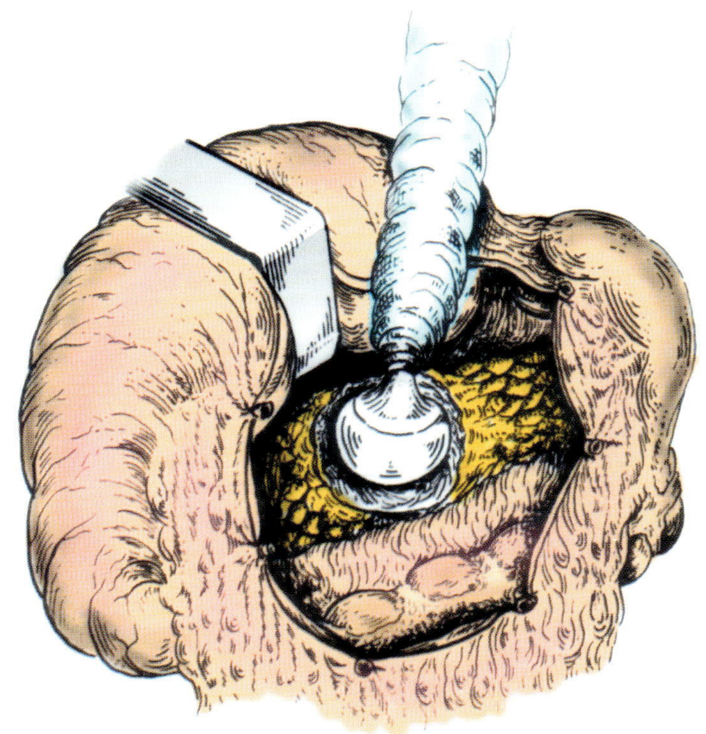

Fig. 10.4.5. Cryodestruction of the bed of the pancreatic cyst

conventional operations, including acute destructive postoperative pancreatitis, pancreatic fistulas, hormone and enzyme insufficiency, and cyst recurrences. This type of organ-preserving surgery makes it possible to expand the number of indications for cryosurgical treatment of this pathology.

Preoperatively, besides general clinical investigations, ultrasonography, computed tomography of the pancreas, retrograde cholangiopancreatography should be carried out to prepare the patient for the operation. Single and multiple formations with a liquid component in the centre can be seen in addition to signs of chronic pancreatitis as a result of the perifocal inflammation. Flakes and calcinates can sometimes be seen in the liquid component of pseudo-cysts (Figs. 10.4.6–10.4.7). Retrograde cholangiopancreatography makes it possible to estimate the condition of the duct system, to find strictures, concrements, or changes in the extrahepatic bile ducts. These findings will determine the choice of the method and the extent of the operation. Because of the small number of contraindications for the cryosurgical treatment of pancreatic cysts and the good therapeutic effect, this modern method of treatment can be recommended for wider use in surgical practice.

A case report follows. Patient B, 44 years old, came to the surgical department of the Tomsk Regional Hepatological Centre in November 1991, complaining of intense pain in the epigastrium radiating into the left hypochondriac region, increasing after fatty meals and alcohol consumption. The patient considered herself to be ill since 1990, when she felt pressure pains in the epigastrium. The patient was never previously examined or treated. The general condition of the patient was satisfactory, the abdomen was soft at palpation, and painful in the epigastrium, where a mass of dense elastic consistency was palpated. Multifocal cyst formation was seen in an ultrasonic investigation of the pancreas. The laparotomy, resection of the pancreas, and cryodestruction in the pancreatic stump, were made under general anesthesia in December 1991. The cyst, measuring 6 × 5 × 5 cm, was found in the body of the pancreas. After the pancreas was exposed, the cyst wall with some pancreatic parenchyma was0 resected. Cryodestruction in the stump was performed at a temperature of −196°C and an exposure of 1 min. After omentopancreatopexy and drainage, the abdominal cavity was closed. The postoperative course was unremarkable. The serum glucose level remained within the normal range, the activity of pancreatic enzymes was normalized after a moderate rise by the seventh day. The patient was discharged from the hospital in satisfactory condition. After a three-year follow-up period, the patient's condition was judged to be satisfactory, the cyst did not recur.

Thus, these operations on pancreatic cysts show good results, are a simple surgical method,

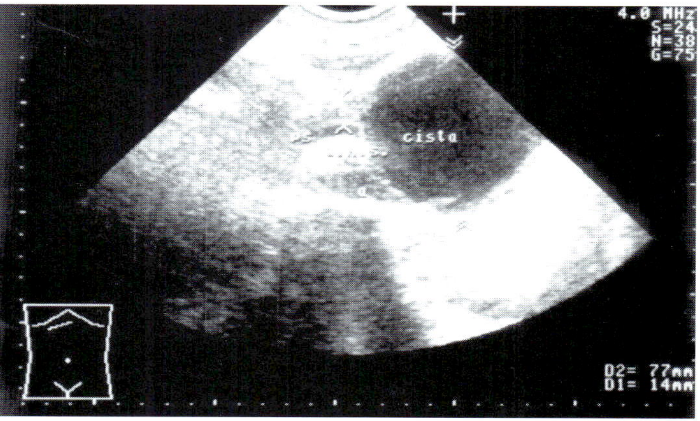

Fig. 10.4.7. Ultrasonography: the cyst in the pancreas body (patient K, 39 years old)

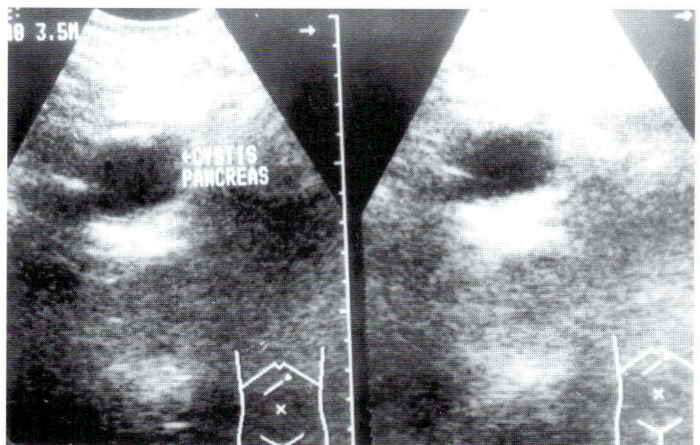

Fig. 10.4.8. Ultrasonography: cyst in the body of the pancreas (patient S, 40 years old)

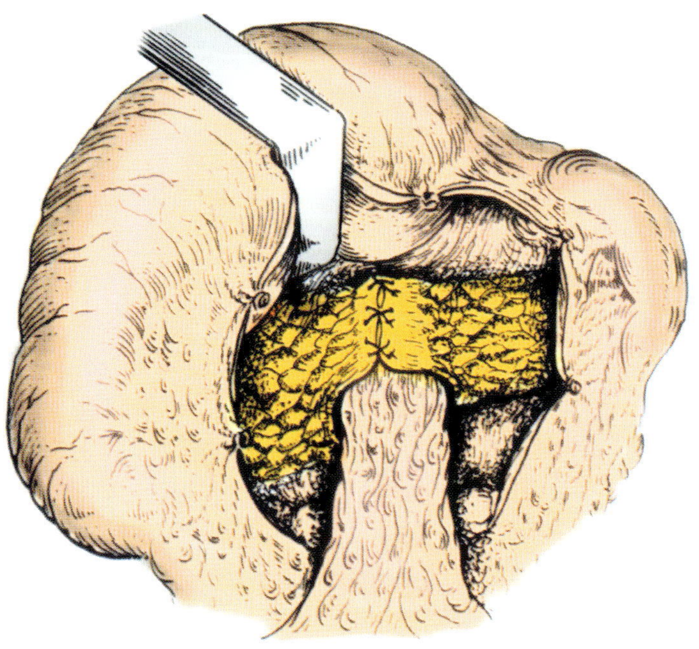

Fig. 10.4.6. Omentopancreatopexy of the stump after cryosurgical and conventional resection in the pancreas

which make it possible to preserve the organ with normal internal and external secretion intact.

Extension of the indications for cryosurgical treatment, development and improvement of cryosurgical equipment, and the use of combined surgery have made it necessary create a more detailed classification of the types of cryosurgical and combined conventional/cryosurgical operations. This classification is proposed by the author. Besides the type of the operation it also specifies the nosological form, which simplifies the choice of the optimal operative procedure.

Classification

1. Cryooperations
   a) cryodestruction in the pancreas in acute destructive pancreatitis
   b) cryodestruction in the pancreas in chronic pancreatitis at the "key point"
   c) cryodestruction in the pancreas in chronic pancreatitis at additional points
   d) cryodestruction of pancreatic tumors
   e) cryoresection in the pancreas + cryodestruction in the stump
2. Combined operations
   a) excision of the pancreatic cyst wall + cryodestruction of the area of its location
   b) resection of the pancreas + cryodestruction in the stump
   c) operations on extrahepatic bile ducts and on the gall bladder + cryodestruction in the pancreas

The results of experimental research and clinical application of subzero temperatures, reviews of the data in the literature, comparison of the results of conventional and cryosurgical methods of treatment of pancreatic diseases make it possible to point out some advantages of cryosurgery, namely:

1. Cryosurgical operations are relatively simple to perform
2. The duration of surgery is short
3. They have few contraindications
4. They stop the pain and enzyme toxemia in patients with pancreonecrosis, as a result of formation of a fibrous cicatrix in the cryosurgical zone
5. They stop the pain syndrome as a result of freezing denervation in the pancreas
6. They make it possible to stabilize the development of the tumor process and to improve the general condition of the patient with oncological disease
7. They prevent the development of such complications as hemorrhage and pancreatic fistulas in the postoperative period

Based on our own experimental and clinical experience as well as that of other authors, cryosurgery can be recommended for treatment of pancreatic disease in combination with conventional surgery.

References

1. Andersson R. Acute pancreatitis – management of complicating pseudocysts. International Surgery Week. Hong-Kong 1993; 814.
2. Brazhnikova NA. Clinics of Opistorchosus pancreatitis. In: Abstract book: Diagnostics and treatment of hepatic and pancreatic diseases, Russia, 1990; 251–253.
3. Fedorov VD. Pancreatic cysts. International conference, Moscow, Russia, 1993; 37–38.
4. Galeev MA. Diagnostics and surgical treatment of pancreatic cysts. Scientific conference, Novosibirsk, Russia, 1992; 201.
5. Lanckich P, Happe-Lohr A, Peiper M. Operative treatment of pancreatic pseudocysts in chronic pancreatitis. International Surgery Week. Hong-Kong 1993; 808.
6. Nevell KA, Aranka GV, Prinz RA. Are Cystgastrostomy and Cystjejunostomy Equivalent Operations for Pancreatic Pseudocysts? Surgery 1990; 108(4): 635–640.
7. Sulkowsky U, Meyer J, Kauts G, Bunte H. Argumente für ein abgewandeltes Konzept in der Therapie der akuten Pankreatitis zur Indikation konservativer und chirurgischer Verfahren. Chirurg 1989; 60(4): 246–250.
8. Svikluc AV. Surgical treatment for pancreatic tumors. International scientific conference, Kiev, Ukraine, 1988; 130–131.

11. Cryosurgery in Pulmonology

11.1 Cryosurgery in Respiratory Disorders

Omar Maiwand

11.1.0 Introduction

The anti-inflammatory properties of low temperature have been known for centuries, however its application for tissue destruction dates from the work of James Arnott in the period 1845 to 1851 (1). Arnott used direct application of salt and crushed ice to achieve local temperatures of around −20°C and was thus able to treat advanced uterine tumors. This resulted in a reduction of pain, regression of the tumor and control of symptoms. Significant progress in the use of cryo surgery, the controlled application of extreme cold, was made possible by the availability of liquefied gases. These were used successfully in the treatment of skin cancer in 1889 (2). Further advances were facilitated by the development of a number of different types of cryoprobe in the early 1960's. The first of these was developed by Cooper and Lee in 1961 (3) for neurological applications and used liquid nitrogen (−196°C) circulated through an insulated probe. In 1964 Amoils and Walker (4) developed an improved probe in which cooling was achieved by the Joule-Thomson effect (5), adiabatic expansion of a compressed gas (nitrous oxide), for the treatment of opthalmological conditions.

Cryosurgery for endobronchial disease, however, was delayed due to the anatomical inaccessibility of the bronchi and concern over the healing of endobronchial mucosa. These problems were overcome by experimental work on animals (6–11) and by the development of long probes, which were narrow enough to pass through a rigid bronchoscope. A limited amount of experimental work was carried out in the USA from about 1975 with the first study at the Mayo Clinic, with 28 patients with malignant and benign lesions treated with a rigid probe with liquid nitrogen as the cryogen, achieving probe tip temperatures of −160°C (12). A further study by Rodgers used a nitrous oxide cooled probe with a tip temperature of −80°C to treat a group of 27 patients (13). Endobronchial work in the USA was discontinued in favor of the newly developed laser treatment.

The first large scale study in Europe involved treating bronchial carcinoma with a specially designed rigid probe (Fig. 11.1.1) and was published by Maiwand in July 1986 (14), followed by a paper by Homasson in August of the same year (15) and Astesiano in November (16). All three authors used nitrous oxide cooled cryoprobes for palliation or treatment of malignant and benign endobronchial lesions. Cryosurgery is currently used widely around the world for endobronchial treatment.

11.1.1 Biophysical Aspects of Cryosurgery

Cooling cells to a temperature of about −10°C causes little damage as the cell is protected for a period of time from the effects of low temperature by the cell contents, mainly the cell cytoplasm. Once the temperature reaches −30°C, however, cell death is almost certain. This protective effect

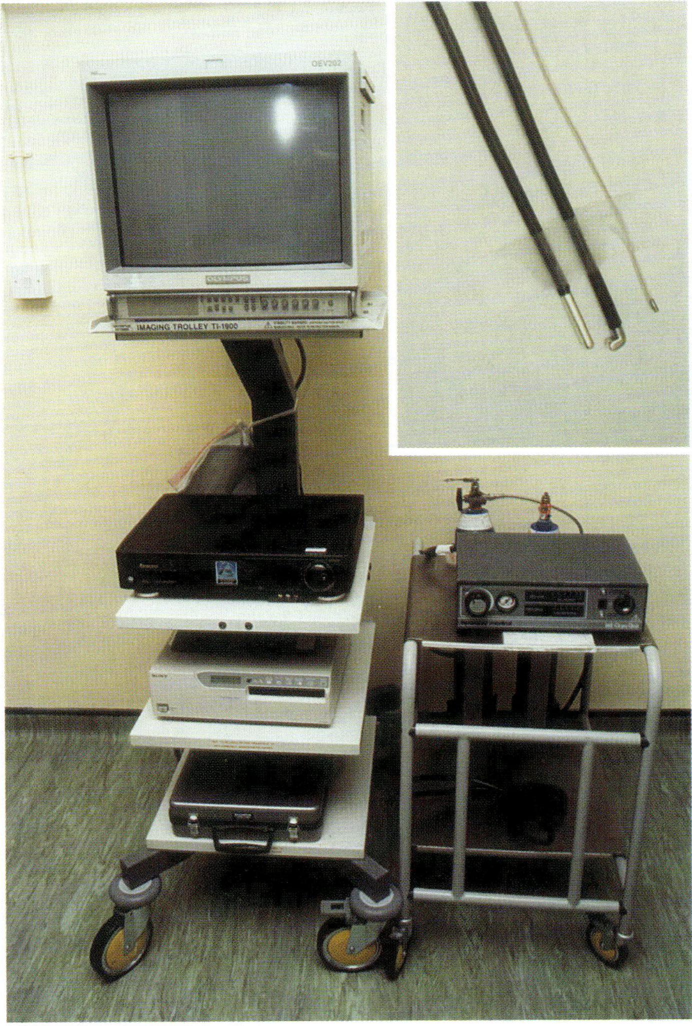

Fig. 11.1.1. Cryomachine and probes, straight, right angled and flexible

varies with different types of tissue. In general tissues can be divided into two types, cryoresistant and cryosensitive. The cryosensitivity of tissues is directly related to their free water content. Mucous membrane, skin, nerve fibres and granulation tissue are cryosensitive whereas connective tissue, fibrous tissue, fat and bone are cryoresistant and can withstand much colder and longer freeze applications.

The extent and permanence of a freeze injury is determined by the lowest temperature achieved (17), the rate of cooling (which should be as rapid as possible), the rate of thawing (as slow as possible) (18–20), the number of freeze thaw cycles performed (21–23) and the type of tissue being frozen. There are some differences of opinion over the optimal temperature delivered to the tissue that is required for cell destruction. It is generally agreed that a temperature of −30°C or below, delivered to the whole of the abnormal mass, is required to ensure cell destruction.

The destructive effects of freezing tissue are due to two major mechanisms, one immediate, the other delayed. The immediate cause of injury is the damaging effect of freezing and thawing on cells. The delayed cause of the injury is the progressive failure of microcirculation; ultimately, vascular stasis becomes operative as an important cause of tissue injury.

11.1.2 Immediate Biochemical Effects

The damaging effects of low temperature on cells begin as temperature falls into the hypothermic range. Local hypothermia is present for a time before and after the freezing temperature is reached and if it is continued for a prolonged time, cell metabolism progressively fails and cell death may occur.

Once the temperature falls into the freezing range, water is crystallized, which has more serious consequences than the earlier cooling. The effect of freezing on cells is based on ice crystal formation, the size and effect of which are related to the temperature achieved and to the rate of freezing, and the number of freeze thaw cycles. At around −15°C, ice crystals begin to form, initially in the extracellular spaces. As ice crystals form from pure water the extracellular spaces become hypertonic relative to the cell interior, a net movement of water from the intracellular to the extracellular space occurs, causing intracellular shrinkage and increasing intracellular solute concentration.

This osmotic gradient also precipitates a diffusion gradient between the extracellular and intracellular spaces, which can influence the ionic concentration within the cell due to the net movement of H^+ ions out of the cell, and the migration of solute ions into the cell. It is generally believed that saline concentrations greater than 2 moles per liter are damaging to most cellular proteins. A reduction of the intracellular pH to a value of 4 or below will cause further damage impairing enzyme systems and affect the lipoprotein components of the plasma membrane containing the cell and its organelles. This biochemical effect possibly has more destructive consequences than the physical effects.

11.1.3 Immediate Physical Effects

With further cooling, ice crystals may form within the cells. The cell membrane has been considered a barrier to ice nucleation, but ice crystals may enter the cell through membrane injury or perhaps micropores. Once ice crystals form within the cell, cell death is almost certain.

Slow freezing leads to large, stable crystals, forming principally in the extracellular spaces. Rapid freezing leads to smaller and thermodynamically unstable crystals. Continuous intracellular cooling eventually reaches the eutectic temperature immediately below which the remaining solvent and solute crystallize simultaneously. The resulting crystalline complex causes irreversible physical damage. Further physical damage ensues as the cryolesion is allowed to thaw. Slow thawing leads to recrystallization with larger, stable crystals, which are highly destructive over the longer time period.

11.1.4 Delayed Effects

The delayed effects of freezing are caused by vascular changes, in particular platelet aggregation and deposition of microthrombi on the vessel wall resulting in narrowing and obstruction of the vascular lumen. This phenomenon is more obvious in the venules than arterioles as the blood flow in the arterioles is about three times faster and heat exchange of blood flow protects the vessels. This process increases permeability of the vessel wall and edema of the tissues. The loss of blood supply deprives the cell of any possibility of survival. These changes explain the therapeutic value of cryosurgery for the control of surface bleeding.

11.1.5 Immunological Aspects of Cryosurgery

For a number of years now, it has been suggested that cryodestruction of a tumor can evoke an immune response and that this response may possess specific anti-tumor properties. In studies in tumor bearing animals, the natural immune responses to tumor infiltration can locally limit the spread of the disease, and can cause regression of non-local disease. Cryosurgery applied to prostatic carcinoma has been observed to cause remission of metastatic lesions (24, 25). Ablation of lung metastases using cryosurgery may control the growth of metastatic lesions (26) and similar observations have been made with metastatic liver tumors (27). Changes in immune responses have also been demonstrated following cryosurgery for rectal carcinoma (28) and malignant melanoma (29). Cryosurgery may therefore be utilized not only for local ablation of tumors but also as a possible means of engendering anti-tumor immune responses. The mechanisms underlying these responses remain largely unknown but may possibly be triggered by the release of cryonecrotized tumor antigens.

The experience of the author in treating a large number of patients with endobronchial tumors with cryosurgery, has shown an incidence of supraclavicular node enlargement of only 4% during the progression of the disease. Figures of more than 20% of patients with supraclavicular node enlargement for large groups of patients are commonly seen in the literature, suggesting that the treatment may also be inducing potentially beneficial immunological effects. Cryosurgery may cause regression of systemic disease through immunomodulation but the exact mechanism has yet to be elucidated.

11.1.6 Cryosurgical Equipment

The equipment required for endobronchial cryosurgery consists of a cryosurgical console, a selection of probes and source of cryogen. Cryomachines or consoles are manufactured by several companies, including Spembly Medical in the UK, Endocare and Cryomedical Sciences in the USA, Erbe in Germany, DATE in France and MST in the Czech Republic. The main differences among them are the method of temperature control and the cryogen used. Most consoles regulate the supply of cryogen by means of a foot controlled pedal and monitor cryogen cylinder pressure, time of application and probe tip temperature (Fig. 11.1.1).

Two types of bronchoscope can be used for cryosurgical procedures, rigid and flexible. Rigid bronchoscopes have the advantage that they can accommodate a fine suction catheter, which can be used to remove secretions and debris so that they do not accumulate and insulate the target area. The rigid bronchoscope also allows for larger biopsies, bleeding control and oxygen provision. The model of rigid bronchoscope is not critical so long as it has sufficient diameter to allow the insertion of the cryoprobe. The flexible bronchoscope has the advantage that it can be used under local or general anesthesia, but it is less robust and there is a possibility that the cryoprobe may cause it to become blocked or damaged by ice crystals forming in the return channel.

Cryoprobes for endobronchial use have been specially designed to fit the internal anatomy of the trachea, main bronchi and of the lobar and segmental divisions of the bronchial tree and must fit within the bronchoscope. The cryoprobe may be a rigid or flexible one, and rigid probes may be straight or have a right-angled tip. A probe with an angled tip is used for lesions of the trachea, main bronchi, and basal segments of the lower lobe, and a probe with a right angled tip for lesions in the upper lobes and apical segments of the lower lobes. Probe diameter is an important factor in the effectiveness of cryosurgery and while smaller diameter probes (2.2 mm) cool more rapidly, their area of treatment is limited and so can only be used for small to moderately sized lesions. Smaller probes also take a longer time to thaw. Larger diameter probes (5.5 mm) are most effective for larger tumor masses. The rigid probe has a number of advantages over the flexible probe in that it is more robust and can be used to treat a much larger area and allows for more rapid thawing (Fig. 11.1.1).

11.1.7 Cryogens

Cryogen is a term used for materials used specifically for the purpose of generating low temperatures. The choice of cryogen in cryosurgery is very important, as the result of the procedure is directly related to the lowest temperature delivered to the whole of the abnormal tissue. Several studies have shown that the temperature needed for a lesion to be destroyed is around −30°C. Freezing to −30°C or below at the rate of 100°C per minute will cause over 90% cell death. Therefore it is clear that the cooling agent used should have the capability to produce a local temperature of −30°C or less. Most cryogens used are in the liquid phase and remove

Table 11.1.1. Properties of cryogens

	CO_2	N_2O	N_2	Ar
Boiling point (1 atmosphere) (°C)	−78	−88	−196	−186
Heat of vaporization at boiling point (Kjmole^{-1})	15.8	16.5	2.9	6.5
Vapour pressure at 298K (kPa)	5984	4973	–	–
Critical temperature (°C)	31	36	−147	−122
Critical pressure (Mpa)	7.38	7.26	3.39	4.90

heat (via heat of vaporization) while maintaining a constant temperature, during the transition to the gaseous state. There are a number of cryogens, which have been used in cryosurgery including nitrous oxide, liquid nitrogen, carbon dioxide and argon (Table 11.1.1).

Carbon dioxide is easily available and can produce temperatures down to −79°C and has a high heat of vaporization but it can only be used with very large probes, as the solid phase would block finer ones.

Liquid nitrogen is also easily available and has a low saturation temperature of −196°C. It has the disadvantage of requiring vacuum insulated storage and that probe cooling is relatively slow.

Nitrous oxide is a readily available and inexpensive cryogen and can be stored in the liquid phase, at room temperature, in high-pressure cylinders. It is transferred to the cryoprobe via capillary tubes surrounded by either a metal or plastic sheath, but which do not require thermal insulation. Cooling occurs by means of the Joule-Thomson effect (adiabatic expansion of a compressed gas). When the gas reaches the tip of the probe, it passes through a small nozzle and expands, forming a vapor haze and causing an extremely rapid drop in temperature for up to 20 mm from the expansion nozzle. Nitrous oxide can reach −89°C, and this method of cooling causes the probe to cool and thaw extremely rapidly.

Argon has also been used as a cryogen in recent years and can achieve very low temperatures (−186°C) and also provides extremely rapid cooling.

11.1.8 Temperature Monitoring

As the destructive effect of cryosurgery is directly related to the lowest temperature delivered to the abnormal tissue, it is therefore essential to monitor the temperature at the tumoral level. An experienced operator may be able to judge the degree of freezing empirically by means of the ice ball formation, consistency of the frozen tissue and a knowledge of the time of probe application, although this cannot be regarded as accurate (24).

Some models of cryoprobe incorporate a thermocouple into the probe tip but this does not give a measure of tissue temperature. Although it is very important to monitor temperature at the application site, this would require a further probe to be placed in the tissue close to the cryoprobe. The anatomical size of the tracheobronchial tree limits the accessibility of an additional probe to be placed for temperature monitoring. Modern cryomachines do give a measure of probe tip temperature, however the temperature rises significantly when measured away from the probe tip. In our study of 100 patients, the mean temperature at a point 2 mm from probe tip was found to be −30°C (standard deviation ± 5.6) where the probe tip temperature was −70°C ± 3.8 (25).

The freezing process can also be monitored by the impedance method (26), which measures changes in resistance during freezing and thawing. The probe itself acts as one electrode and a further electrode, usually in the form of a metal pad, is placed on the skin of the patient. As cooling occurs, the impedance measured between the two electrodes rises rapidly from around 10 to 50 kÙ as pure water ice crystals form and the electrolyte becomes more concentrated. Once the eutectic point is reached and the electrolyte freezes, impedance rises even more rapidly to around 500 to 1000 kÙ. This technique allows the area of eutectic freezing to be monitored and controlled.

11.1.9 Cryosurgical Technique

Anatomical knowledge and the practical ability to perform rigid and flexible bronchoscopy are essential requirements for performing tracheobronchial cryosurgery. Tracheobronchial cryosurgery is performed under direct vision via the bronchoscope, using a rigid or flexible cryoprobe. The flexible cryoprobe is designed to be used through a fibreoptic bronchoscope under local or general anesthesia. The much larger rigid cryoprobe (5.5 mm diameter) requires the use of a rigid bronchoscope under general anesthesia. General anesthesia has the advantage that it provides complete relaxation of the patient giving maximum mobility to the neck. This facilitates the accurate positioning of the long cryoprobes to the trachea, main bronchus or lower lobes (Fig. 11.1.2). An additional advantage of the use of a rigid bronchoscope is that it allows for positioning a 3 mm catheter close to the lesion, which facilitates

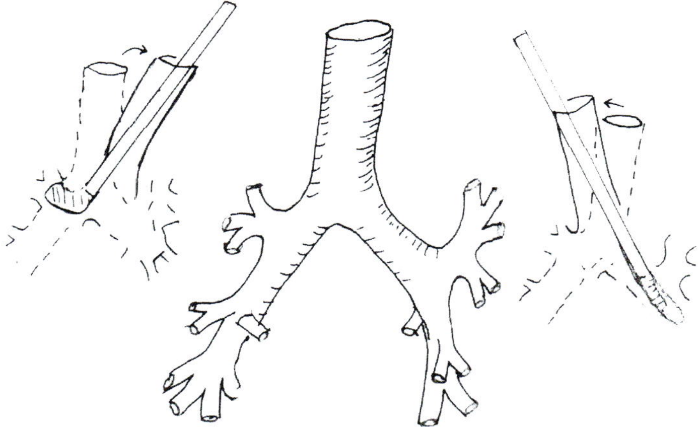

Fig. 11.1.2. Mobility of the airways achieved under general anesthesia. Full mobility of the neck facilitates effective insertion of the rigid probes

continuous suction of blood and secretions and provides better probe to tumor contact.

Before general anesthesia an intravenous access site is established with a plastic cannula typically 21 g or similar size. Monitoring includes a three-lead ECG to monitor lead V5 non-invasive blood pressure recording and arterial oxygen saturation using a pulse oximeter.

Following a period of preoxygenation, anesthesia is induced with propofol (0.75 to 1.8 mg/kg) administered over a 30–120 second period. Following the loss of the eyelash reflex, relaxation is provided with succinylcholine (0.5 to 1.0 mg/kg) or mivacurium (150 μg/kg). The airway is controlled and intermittent positive pressure ventilation is provided with 100% oxygen by means of a Sander's injector. Eye protection is applied at this point.

The patient is placed in the supine position with the head fully extended so that the chin points vertically upwards in a mid line position. The upper jaw should be protected from trauma with a swab or sponge. The rigid bronchoscope should be supported by the left forefinger and thumb to protect the teeth and gums. The operator should perform an initial visual assessment of the lesion, as site and macroscopic characteristics of the tumor can affect the choice of cryoprobe. The distal tip of the rigid bronchoscope should be placed about 5 mm above the lesion. With the lesion in direct vision, the appropriate probe is inserted on or into the tumor mass. It is important to excise any necrotic tissue or slough to prevent insulation of the target tumor.

Cryogen is supplied to the probe by the compression of the foot operated pedal and cooling is initiated for a period of 3 minutes after which thawing is allowed until the probe separates from the tissue. A second freeze-thaw cycle may then be carried out. If the lesion covers a large area of the bronchial tree, multiple applications may be necessary during the session. It is essential that the whole area affected by the tumor is frozen in order to achieve maximum tumor destruction. If the trachea or bronchi are blocked by a tumor mass, then as much of the tumor as possible is removed with forceps and the area refrozen for 3 minutes. At the end of the procedure the lumen frequently opens satisfactorily. Excessive bleeding from the tumor surface can be controlled by the application of adrenaline solution 1:1000. The procedure generally takes about 20 minutes and patients can usually be discharged home on the same day. A repeat treatment is carried out after 2 weeks and also where indicated after 6 weeks. Tissue samples for histological examination are taken before each cryosurgical treatment.

The following should be considered when treating tracheobronchial lesions.

- Histologically proven carcinoma of the trachea and bronchi.
- Inoperability based on the position of the tumor, performance status or poor respiratory function. Predominantly intraluminal tumors.
- Extraluminal elements of tumors should not cause occlusion by external pressure of more than 75% of the normal diameter.
- Tumor recurrence following radiotherapy, chemotherapy or lung resection.
- Benign lesions and carcinoid tumors.
- Granulation tissue following transplantation.

11.1.10 Cryosurgery for Malignant Tracheobronchial Lesions

Primary lung cancer is the commonest cancer and affects 900,000 people yearly and is also the most common cause of death from malignant disease in the world (27). It is rapidly disabling and has a very poor survival rate of only 10–13% over 5 years (27). Overall survival rates around the world have improved little over the years. Surgical resection is the only curative treatment and offers the best possibility of a cure, particularly for patients with stage I and II disease, but unfortunately most patients (over 80%) at the time of presentation are at such an advanced stage that symptomatic palliation is the only course of treatment. Since survival rates are so poor, the issue of quality of life for these patients becomes paramount. Around 30% of patients with lung cancer present with central airway obstruction, which itself causes significant morbidity and mortality (28) and causes distressing symptoms of cough, breathlessness, hemoptysis and recurrent infection which in extreme cases may lead to gradual asphyxiation where central airways are obstructed. The standard method of treatment of obstruction caused by lung cancer has been radiotherapy or chemotherapy. These treatments have limited effectiveness in reopening blocked lumina and may have a damaging effect on surrounding healthy tissue (29). They also have the disadvantage that patients may not be able to tolerate repeated courses of treatment. Cryosurgery is one of a number of techniques that can be used to reopen obstructed tracheobronchial lumina in patients with inoperable tumors. The alternatives include laser treatment, diathermy and stent placement.

A number of studies have shown that endobronchial cryosurgery is a safe and effective palliation for malignant obstructive lesions (14, 30–33). In a recent study in this hospital, we have found significant improvements in symptom quantification, performance status and respiratory function tests in patients treated with cryosurgery. These patients were referred for cryosurgery because they were considered inoperable on the basis of the position of their tumor, poor performance status or poor respiratory function. The study consisted of 305 consecutive patients with histologically proven carcinoma, treated between January 1995 and December 1999 (Table 11.1.2). Patients received an average of 2.51 cryotreatments. This was an elderly and late stage group of patients, with 80% of patients 70 or older and over 90% at stage III or IV. Results (Table 11.1.3) showed that cryosurgery effectively reopened blocked endobronchial lumina (Figs. 11.1.3–11.1.5) and provided improvements in performance status, respiratory function and symptom quantification.

Table 11.1.2. Patients, histology and TNM staging

Patients	
Mean Age (range)	68.4 (36–87)
Male: Female	1.88:1
Histology	
Squamous	67.3
Adenocarcinoma	15.3
Other NSC	6.4
Small cell	11.0
TNM staging (NSC)	
Stage IV	44.9
Stage IIIb	23.8
Stage IIIa	24.6
Stage II	6.7

11.1.11 Cryosurgery for Benign and Low Malignancy Lesions

Cryosurgery has been used in the treatment of a number of benign and low malignancy conditions including carcinoid tumors, granulation tissue

Table 11.1.3. Symptom, performance status and respiratory function improvement after cryosurgery and Kaplan Meier survival

Symptoms	Symptomatic %	Improved %	
Dyspnea	89.9	64.1	
Cough	81.8	69.9	
Hemoptysis	34.2	83.8	
Chest Pain	28.7	59.7	
Performance status	**Pre Cryo**	**Post Cryo**	**P value**
Karnofsky	67.5	74.6	
WHO	2.52	2.16	
Respiratory function			
FEV1/liter	1.39	1.52	<0.001
FVC/liter	2.00	2.23	0.003
Survival (Kaplar-Meier) (95%CL)	12.9 months (9.8–15.1)		

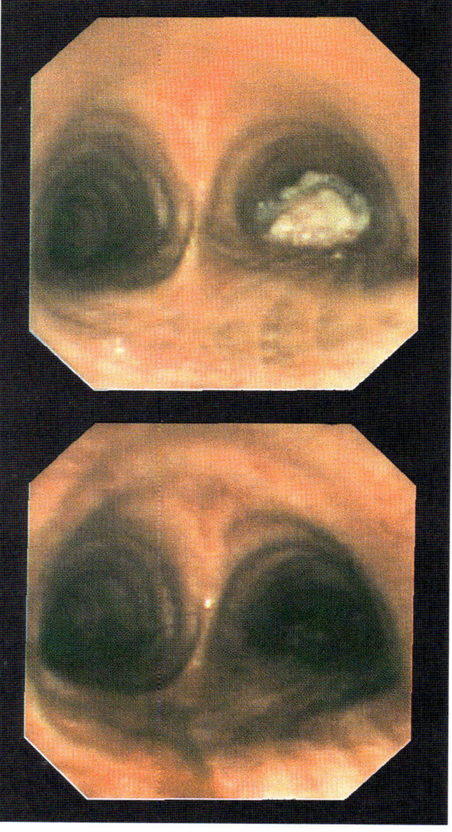

Fig. 11.1.3. Right main bronchus carcinoma before and after cryosurgery

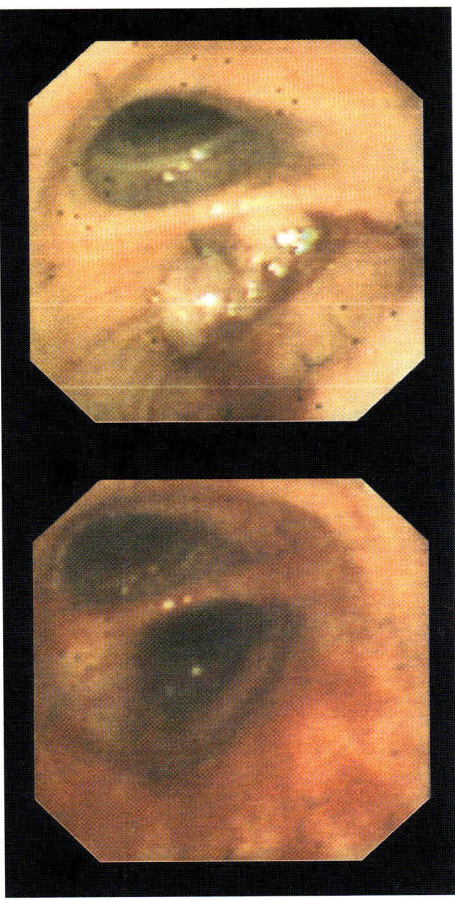

Fig. 11.1.4. Right lower lobe carcinoma before and after cryosurgery

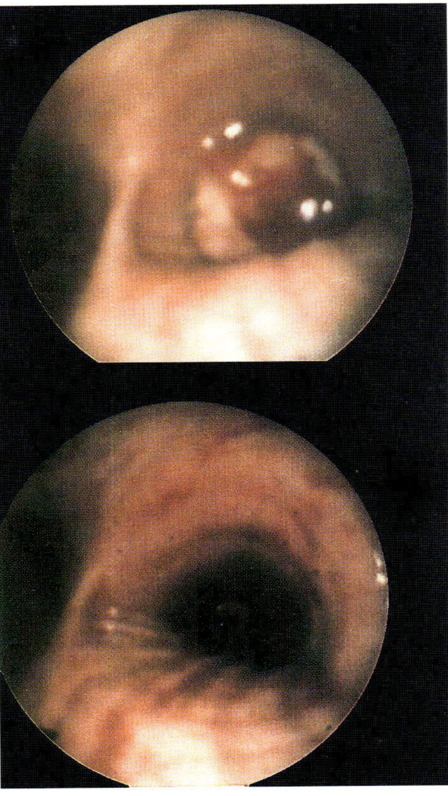

Fig. 11.1.5. Right main bronchus before and after cryosurgery

following heart/lung transplant (34), amyloidosis (35), tracheobronchopathia osteochondroplastica (TBOCP), sarcoid, lipoma, polyps, post-intubation tubal stenosis, leiomyoma, hemangioma and Wegener's granulomatosis.

In a study carried out at this hospital, fifteen patients with histologically proven endobronchial carcinoid tumors (12 typical, 3 atypical) were treated with cryosurgery between 1992 and 1998. Of the 12 patients with typical carcinoid tumor, all but one, who died accidentally, are still alive with a mean follow-up of 49.4 months. Nine of these, treated with cryosurgery only (mean 3.4 treatments), showed no tumor present on histological and radiological examination at follow-up. For the patient who died accidentally, post-mortem examination reported no residual tumor. For the other three patients, cryosurgery downstaged the tumor from the main bronchus to lobar bronchus, allowing resection by lobectomy rather than pneumonectomy. There was a significant improvement in respiratory function tests and performance status after treatment.

Two of the three patients with atypical carcinoid tumors had good endobronchial palliation with cryosurgery but subsequently died due to metastasis. The third is still alive and well after 49 months. The results suggest that cryosurgery is an effective palliative and potentially curative treatment for carcinoid tumors deemed inoperable because of the extent of their disease or co-morbid conditions. Cryosurgery can also be considered as a treatment for downstaging endobronchial carcinoid tumors to allow for less radical resection.

Cryosurgery has also been used successfully in this hospital for the treatment of a case of primary localized tracheobronchial amyloidosis of the respiratory tract, which caused narrowing of the intermediate bronchus and almost complete blockage of the lower lobe. Repeated sessions of cryosurgery to the lesions, over a follow-up period of eleven years, have been found to be an effective treatment for this progressive disease (35).

Cryosurgery has been used in this hospital as a first line treatment for airways compromised by granulation tissue after heart/lung transplantation. In a study of 21 patients (34), results were judged as good in 15 patients and fair in 6 patients. There were no cryosurgery related complications and 8 patients also received endobronchial stents and dilation. Respiratory function tests were shown to increase significantly after treatment. The use of cryosurgery markedly reduced the percentage of patients requiring stents compared to other series.

Tracheobronchopathia-osteochondroplastica (TBOCP) is a rare benign condition that affects large airways, which become narrowed by ossified or cartilaginous nodules in the submucosa with normal overlying mucosa. In this hospital, three patients with TBOCP have been treated with cryosurgery. Patients received between 3 and 7 sessions of cryosurgery which in all cases resulted in symptom improvement for cough and hemoptysis, although hemoptysis did return at a later date.

Extraction of foreign bodies has also been achieved with cryosurgery and the technique is particularly useful with friable matter, which could disintegrate with forceps (36).

11.1.12 Cryosurgery and Radiotherapy

A number of studies have suggested a possible synergistic effect between cryosurgery and external radiotherapy based on modification of tumor blood flow. The peripheral part of the cryonecrosis is inhomogeneous, sparing perivascular cells. These residual cells around the cryolesion exhibit a high mitotic index.

Vergnon et al. (37) carried out a study to assess the efficiency of cryosurgery followed by irradiation compared to irradiation alone in a study of 38 patients with inoperable lung cancer. Patients were treated with cryosurgery followed by a bronchoscopy in which the effectiveness of the procedure was assessed. After 15–21 days, radiotherapy with curative intent was started (40 Gy in 16 fractions to anterior-posterior fields and 10 days later an additional 15 Gy by tangential field). For the group for whom cryosurgery had been seen to be efficient (>50% of tumor destroyed), local control of the disease was achieved in 65% of patients. This compares to figures of 35% local control achieved by radiotherapy alone.

11.1.13 Cryosurgery and Chemotherapy

A study on the treatment of oral cancer indicated that chemotherapy might be more effective following cryosurgery (38). Ikekawa (45) using a murine tumoral system subsequently confirmed this accumulation of anti-cancer drugs at the tumor site following cryosurgery. Homasson et al. (40) have published a prospective study demonstrating that chemotherapy may be more effective after the application of cryosurgery. Twelve patients with inoperable, obstructive bronchial tumors were treated with intravenous bleomycin labelled with cobalt 57 before and after cryosurgery. The redistribution and elimination half-lives of the labelled bleomycin were determined with the use of a gamma camera. Tumor to normal tissue ratios were also calculated. A significant difference was found between tumoral uptake before and after cryosurgery, with a mean increase in tumor to normal tissue ratio of 30% where bleomycin was administered 2–6 hours after cryosurgery. This is thought to be caused by vascular destruction preventing clearance of the bleomycin. Further work with a larger group of patients is required to confirm these findings.

11.1.14 Cryoanalgesia

The pain after thoracotomy can be very intense and may cause severe postoperative complications. A number of methods are currently employed to provide relief of this post-thoracotomy pain, though each is associated with specific disadvantages and side effects. Conventional analgesia usually focuses on parenteral opiate administration, which is not always effective and can be associated with a number of side effects including respiratory depression, nausea and vomiting, constipation and peripheral vasodilatation. Intercostal infiltration is time consuming and often requires repeated blocks. It also carries the risk of the systemic effects of local anesthetics. Continuous intercostal infusion, although avoiding the need for repeated blocks, increases the risk of toxicity. Epidural analgesia requires skilled anesthetic technique and can induce hypotension, urinary retention and motor loss.

A number of studies have shown that cryoanalgezia, the localized freezing of intercostal nerves, is simple, well controlled and provides effective and prolonged analgesia in the majority of patients. The procedure involves the freezing of intercostal nerves by means of a cryoprobe, which induces changes consistent with a second-degree nerve lesion (axonotmesis). The parietal pleura is peeled back locally in order to locate the intercostal nerves, though with increased experience this may not be necessary for patients with a thin pleura. The probe is positioned, under direct vision, on the intercostal nerve close to the intercostal foramen proximal to the collateral branch. Freezing is applied for 30 seconds producing an ice ball approximately 2–3 mm in diameter that completely covers the nerve. The probe is left to defrost in situ to avoid damage to the nerve caused by its adhesion to the frozen probe. The intercostal nerve at the thoracotomy space (sixth or seventh), one nerve below and two above, are frozen and the probe is then allowed to thaw. To obtain the maximum benefit from the cryoanalgesia the chest drain is placed within the cryotreated area. This may mean placing the drain one or two spaces higher than normal.

Results obtained by Maiwand et al. (47) have shown a mean duration of analgesia of 27 days and numbness extending from the anterior chest wall and epigastric area for an average of 38 days. In a study of 600 patients only 7% reported severe postoperative pain. For female patients, freezing of the fifth and higher intercostal nerves should be avoided because of the temporary loss of sensation in the nipple area.

Indications for the use of cryoanalgesia are:

- Elderly patients, for whom early mobility is of the utmost importance for an early recovery.
- Patients with poor respiratory function tests, to assist in lung re-expansion and prevent further complications.
- Patients where early removal of the chest drain is required.
- Where a tumor is infiltrating the chest wall and mediastinal structures.
- Left thoraco-laparotomy incisions.

A number of studies have compared the use of cryoanalgesia against other forms of post-thoracotomy analgesia, with varying results. Orr (48) and Pastor (49) demonstrated a significant improvement in respiratory function and pain relief in comparison to parenteral opiates, using a 60 s application of the cryoprobe. Brichon (50) and Miguel (51), however, showed that epidural analgesia provided faster and more effective pain relief and better restoration of pulmonary function.

Cryoanalgesia is able to provide a therapy that reduces the postoperative analgesic requirement and facilitates control of post-thoracotomy pain. This improves respiratory function and hence reduces the incidence of any postoperative complications. This study suggests that cryoanalgesia of the intercostal nerves be considered as an economical, safe and easy to use technique for the long-term control of post-thoracotomy pain. By providing adequate analgesia it is possible to improve respiratory function, allow for a return to the patient's preoperative mobility and compliance with intensive physiotherapy and so prevent complications such as sputum retention, pneumonia or deep vein thrombosis, particularly important for patients with poor respiratory function (52, 53).

A study carried out at the China-Japan Friendship Hospital, Beijing, China in conjunction with this hospital, exposed intercostal nerves of dogs to varying periods of freezing (30–120 seconds) using a probe temperature of −50°C (carbon dioxide). Nerves were biopsied at various intervals over the following 6 months and the neural tissue examined histologically, using routine hemoxylin & eosin stains and immunohistochemical techniques, which specifically identified the axons and myelin sheaths. Following a one-minute cryo-application, the individual axons showed degeneration with accumulation of edema fluid. The endoneurium itself was intact and capillary stasis was also evident. Clumping of neural substance, indicating the beginning of axonal fragmentation was present. After one week axonal swelling had disappeared. There was Schwann cell proliferation, and a lymphocytic and histiocytic inflammatory infiltrate with phagocytosis was present. Axonal segments had appeared in some neurons, indicating partial nerve recovery. This neuronal recovery was progressive and was complete by one month. For longer periods of cryo-application, the immediate changes in the intercostal nerves were the same. However the time taken to complete recovery was increased, in particular by a delay in entering the recovery phase. After a two-minute cryo-application there was a 2-week delay before axonal swelling resolved and regeneration began.

11.1.15 Future Developments

The future success of cryosurgery depends on the development of suitable probes, improved temperature monitoring techniques and, more importantly, the use of new cryogens to provide practicable units delivering controllable lower temperatures. Advances in scanning technology would facilitate accurate location of tumors and allow them to be treated by minimally invasive techniques.

Therefore, further laboratory and clinical research is required in the uses of different cryogens and standardization of local temperature without damaging the surrounding tissues. Detailed study of the cryosensitivity of various tissues must be undertaken. Examination of the immunological effects of freezing may lead to improvements in tumoricidal responses of the host. Further research into the effects of cryosurgery combined with other techniques such as radiotherapy and chemotherapy may also provide more effective palliation and possibly improved survival for patients with advanced stage, inoperable lung cancer.

11.1.16 Conclusions

The use of extreme cold in the pulmonary area has been well established. Cryosurgery offers an effective and rapid method to restore the patency of blocked tracheobronchial lumina immediately and therefore improve symptoms and quality of life. The technique is easy to perform, economical, has minimal complications and is well tolerated by the patient. Cryotherapy often improves the patient tolerance to the stage that a further treatment such as radiotherapy or chemotherapy can be tolerated, providing a better outcome and improved quality of life and survival.

References

1. Arnott J. On the treatment of cancer by regulated application of anaesthetic temperature London: J Churchill 1851.
2. Campbell-White A. Possibilities of liquid air to the physician. JAMA 1901; 36: 426.
3. Cooper IS, Lee A. Cryothalamectomy-hypothermic congelation: A technical advance in basal ganglia surgery. J Am Geriatric Soc 1961; 9: 714–718.
4. Amoils SP, Walker AJ. The thermal and mechanical factors involved in ocular cryosurgery. Proc R Soc Med 1966; 59: 1056–1064.
5. Meldrum SJ. Some aspects of cryosurgery. Biomed Eng 1970; 5: 120–124.
6. Grana L, Kidd J, Swenson O. Cryogenic techniques within tracheobronchial tree. J Cryosurg 1969; 2: 62–67.
7. Thomford NR, Wilson WH, Blackburn ED, Pace WG. Morphological changes in canine trachea after freezing. Cryobiology 1970; 7: 19–28.
8. Neel HG, Farrell KH, Payne WS, De Santo LW, Sanderson DR. Cryosurgery of respiratory structures 1. Cryonecrosis of trachea and bronchus. Laryngoscope 1973; 83: 1062–1071.
9. Neel HB, Farrell KH, Payne WS, De Santo LW. Cryosurgery of respiratory structures 2. Cryonecrosis of the lung. Laryngoscope 1974; 84: 417–426.
10. Gorenstein A, Neel HB, Sanderson DR. Trans-bronchoscopic cryosurgery of respiratory structures. Experimental and clinical studies. Ann Otol Rhinol Laryngol 1976; 85: 670–678.
11. Carpenter RJ, Neel HB, Sanderson DR. Cryosurgery of bronchopulmonary structures. An approach to lesions inaccessible to the rigid bronchoscope. Chest 1977; 72: 279–284.
12. Sanderson DR, Neel HB, Fontana RS. Bronchoscopic Cryotherapy. Ann Otol 1981; 90: 354–358.
13. Rodgers BM, Moazam F, Talbert JL. Endotracheal Cryotherapy in the treatment of refractory airway strictures. Annal Thorac Surg 1983; 35: 52–57.
14. Maiwand MO Cryotherapy for advanced carcinoma of the trachea and bronchi. BMJ 1986; 293: 181–182.
15. Homasson JP, Renault P, Angebault M, Bonniot JP, Bell NJ. Bronchoscopic cryotherapy for airway strictures caused by tumors. Chest 1986; 90: 159–164.
16. Astesiano A, Aversa S, Ciotta D, Galietti F, Gandolfi G, Giorgis GE, Doliaro A, Scappaticci E, Pepino E. Distruzione crioterapica dei tumori invasvi tracheobronchiali. Casistica personale. Min Med 1986; 77: 2159–2163.
17. Miller RH, Mazur P. Survival of frozen-thawed human red cells as a function of cooling and warming velocities. Cryobiology 1976; 13: 404–414.
18. Fahy GM, Saur J, Williams RJ; Physical problems with the vitrification of large biological systems. Cryobiology 1990; 27: 492–510.
19. Gage AA, Guest K, Montes M, Caruana JA, Whalen DR. Effect of varying freezing and thawing rates in experimental cryosurgery. Cryobiology 1985; 22: 175–182.
20. Smith JJ, Fraser J. An estimation of tissue damage and thermal history in cryolesion. Cryobiology 1974; 11: 39–47.
21. Gage AA; Critical temperature for skin necrosis in experimental cryosurgery. Cryobiology 1982; 19: 273–282.
22. Rand RW, Rand RP, Eggerding FA, Field M, Denbesten L, King W, Camici S. Cryolumpectomy for breast cancer: an experimental study. Cryobiology 1985; 22: 307–318.
23. Gage AA, Baust J. Mechanisms of tissue injury in cryosurgery. Cryobiology 1998; 37: 11–86.
24. Soanes WA, Ablin RJ, Gonder MJ. Remission of metastatic lesions following cryosurgery in prostatic cancer: immunological considerations. J Urol. 1970; 104: 154–159.
25. Fukagai T, Tazawa K, Higaki Y, Imamura K. Changes in immunoparameters following cryosurgery in prostate cancer. Hinyokika Kiyo Acta Urologica Japonica 1990; 36: 307–317.
26. Largiader F, Uhlschim G, Gattiker HH. Kryochirurgie von Lungenmetastasen (cryosurgery of lung metastases). Thoraxchir Vask Chir 1975; 23: 515–522.
27. Preketes AP, King J, Caplehorn JR, Clingan PR, Ross WB, Morris DL. CEA reduction after cryotherapy for liver metastases from colon cancer predicts survival. Aust NZ J Surg 1994; 64: 612–614.
28. Wang ZS. Cryosurgery in rectal carcinoma-report of 41 cases. Chung Hua Chung Liu Tsa Chih 1989; 11: 226–227.
29. Weyer U, Petersen I, Ehrke C, Carstensen A, Nussgen A, Russ C et al. Immunomodulation durch Kryochirurgie beim malignem Melanom. (Immunomodulation by cryosurgery in malignant melanoma). Onkologie 1989; 12: 291–296.
30. Gage AA, Caruana JA, Garamy G. A comparison of instrument methods of monitoring freezing in cryosurgery. J Dermatol Surg Oncol 1983; 9: 209–214.
31. Maiwand MO, Homasson JP. Cryotherapy for tracheobronchial disorders. Interventional Pulmonology 1995; 16: 427–443.
32. Use of bioelectric impedance measurements as a control in the cryodestruction of normal or pathological tissue in vivo. C R Acad Sci Paris 1975; 281: 1191–1194.
33. Baue A, Geha AS, Hammond GL, Laks H, Naunheim KS. Glenn's Thoracic and Cardiovascular Surgery. Appleton and Lange, Stamford, Connecticut 1996.
34. Bolliger CT, Solèr M, Tamm M, Perruchoud AP. Kombinierte endobronchiale und konventionelle Therapiemöglichkeiten bei inoperablen zentralen Lungentumoren. Schweiz Med Wochenschr 1995; 125: 1052–1059.
35. Murren JR, Buzaid AC. Chemotherapy and radiation for the treatment of non-small cell lung cancer. Lung Cancer 1993; 14: 161–171.
36. Walsh DA, Maiwand OM, Nath AR, Lockwood P, Lloyd MH, Saab M. Bronchoscopic cryotherapy for advanced bronchial carcinoma. Thorax 1990; 45: 509–513.
37. Homasson JP, Renault P, Angebault M, Bonniot JP, Bell NJ. Bronchoscopic cryotherapy for airway strictures caused by tumors Chest 1986; 90: 159–164.
38. Morasso A, Gallo E, Massaglia GM, Onoscuri M, Bernardi V. Cryosurgery in bronchoscopic treatment of tracheobronchial stenosis. Chest 1993; 103: 472–474.
39. Maiwand MO. The role of cryosurgery in the palliation of tracheobronchial carcinoma. Eur J Cardio-Thoracic Surg 1999; 15: 764–768.
40. Maiwand MO, Zehr KJ, Dyke CM, Peralta M, Tadjkarimi S, Khagani A, Yacoub M. The role of cryotherapy for airway complications after lung and heart-lung transplantation. Eur J Cardio-Thoracic Surg 1997; 12: 549–554.
41. Maiwand MO, Nath AR. Kamath BSK. Cryosurgery in the Treatment of Tracheobronchial Amyloidosis. J Bronchology (in press).
42. Roden S, Homasson JP. Une nouvelle indication de la cryotherapie endobronchique: l'extraction de corps étrangers. Presse Med 1989; 18: 897.
43. Vergnon JM, Schmidt T, Alamartine E, Barthelemy JC, Fournel P, Emonot A. Initial combined cryotherapy and irradiation for unre-

sectable non-small cell lung cancer. Preliminary results. Chest 1992; 102: 1436–1440.
44. Benson JW. Combined chemotherapy and cryosurgery for oral cancer. Am J Surg 1975; 13: 596–600.
45 Ikekawa S, Ishihara K, Tanaka S, Ikeda S. Basic studies of cryochemotherapy in a murine tumor system. Cryobiology 1985; 22: 477–483.
46 Homasson JP, Pecking A, Roden S, Angelbaut M, Bonniot JP. Tumour fixation of bleomycine labeled with 57-cobalt before and after cryotherapy of bronchial carcinoma Cryobiology 1992; 29: 543–548.
47. Maiwand MO, Makey AR, Rees A. Cryoanalgesia after thoracotomy. J Thorac Cardiovasc Surg 1986; 92: 291–295.
48. Orr IA, Keenan DJM, Dundee JW. Improved pain relief after thoracotomy: use of cryoprobe and morphine infusion. BMJ Clinical Res Ed 1981; 283: 945–948.
49. Pastor J, Morales P, Cases E, Cordero P, Piqueras A, Galàn G, Paris F. Evaluation of intercostal cryoanalgesia versus conventional analgesia in post-thoracotomy pain. Respiration 1996; 63: 241–245.
50. Brichon PY, Pison C, Chaffanjon P, Fayot P, Burchberger, Neron L, Verdier J, Sarrazin R. Comparison of epidural analgesia and cryoanalgesia in thoracic surgery. Eur J Cardio-Thorac Surg 1994; 8: 482–486.
51. Miguel R, Hubbell D. Pain management and spirometry following thoracotomy: A prospective randomised study of four techniques. J Cardiothoracic Vascular Anaesthesia. 1993; 7: 529–534.
52. Katz J. Cryoanalgesia for post-thoracotomy pain. Ann Thorac Surg 1989; 48: 5.
53. Maiwand O, Makey AR, Sanmuganathan S. Increased effectiveness of physiotherapy after cryoanalgesia following thoracotomy. Physiotherapy 1982; 68: 288–290.

11.2 Indications of Cryosurgery in Pulmonology

Jean-Paul Homasson with a contribution by M. Angebault

11.2.0 Introduction

The rapidly developing field of interventional bronchoscopy with both the rigid as well as the flexible fiberoptic bronchoscope (FOB) offers a large variety of different endoscopic treatment modalities which have shown their utility in controlling different bronchial disorders or tumor progression. The key factor for successful tracheobronchial cryosurgery is not only the technique but more importantly the indications.

An initial endoscopy with a FOB permitting a diagnosis of endobronchial obstruction is generally performed; biopsies should be done in order to confirm the benign or malignant characteristics of the lesions.

If the patient has impending respiratory failure due to an obstructing tracheal tumor or stenosis, cryosurgery which has a delayed effect in relieving obstruction is not indicated; this clearly remains the domain of a different technique allowing an immediate debulking effect, such as laser or electrocautery. The lesion must be accessible to the cryoprobe through the endoscope. Rigid bronchoscopy can be carried out under neuroleptic or general anesthesia but endoscopic therapy may be performed under local anesthesia using a flexible cryoprobe which is inserted through the working channel of a FOB.

11.2.1 Indications

Symptom control indications: Cyrosurgery may be justified for treating troublesome syndromes such as cough, dyspnea, or hemoptysis of either malignant or benign lesions.

The major symptom amenable to cryosurgery is hemoptysis caused by a visible lesion. The hemostatic effect of cold causing vasoconstriction, capillary occlusion and rapid slowing of the circulation is well known (1). However, this effect is not immediate, and electrocautery is certainly more appropriate even if both techniques should be consecutively used during the same endoscopic session. All those who have tried cryosurgery alone have obtained a significant improvement or disappearance of hemoptysis. In our series (2) hemoptysis stopped in 80% of cases and similar good results are generally reported.

Dyspnea is also a frequent symptom due to an obstructing lesion. We have already stated that cryosurgery is not indicated in case of acute respiratory distress. However an overall improvement of dyspnea (37%–66%) is reported in different series (2–4).

Following cryosurgery the patients have less cough (64%) and stridor (70%) (5–7). Disappearance of wheeze and thoracic pain is sometimes reported.

Objective improvement of pulmonary function was seen in 58% of patients, and the changes in lung function correlated with symptoms (3–8).

Indications according to the type of lesion

Malignant tumors: Most lesions treated with cryosurgery are malignant tumors, either primary bronchial carcinomas or secondary deposits (Fig. 11.2.1). Cryosurgery will destroy the visible endobronchial portion, and therefore the results are difficult to assess, as they depend on various criteria, namely endoscopic appearance, tumor histology or symptoms. Cryosurgery is a palliative treatment. Overall, the results have been favorable in 70 to 80% of patients treated, regardless of the criteria used to measure performance (9,10), and cryosurgery provided excellent symptom relief and improved quality of life (11).

Tumors of intermediate malignancy: These tumors are much rarer. Cryosurgery may be indicated when conventional surgery is contraindicated.

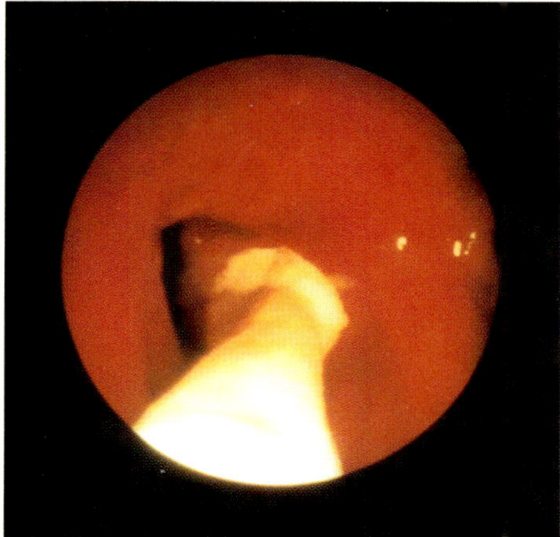

Fig. 11.2.1. Squamous cell carcinoma of the left main bronchus being treated with cryosurgery

Carcinoids, cylindromas, papillomatosis, muco-squamous (12) and other tumors of low malignancy have been successfully treated.

Benign lesions: These lesions constitute a small percentage of pathology seen in the tracheo-bronchial tree. Granulation tissue is very sensitive to the effect of cold. Cryosurgery has also been successful in treating tumors or granulation tissue regrowth around both silicone or wire mesh stents without the loss of the integrity of the stent. Cryosurgery is an effective therapeutic option to deal with bronchial stenosis secondary to excess granulation tissue following lung transplantation (4). Good results have been obtained when treating myomas, including leiomyomas, although several sessions may be needed. Less vascularized lesions, such as amyloidosis, fibromas, lipomas, hamartochondromas or fibrous stenosis, are rarely influenced by cryosurgery (7–13), but there is no risk in attempting treatment.

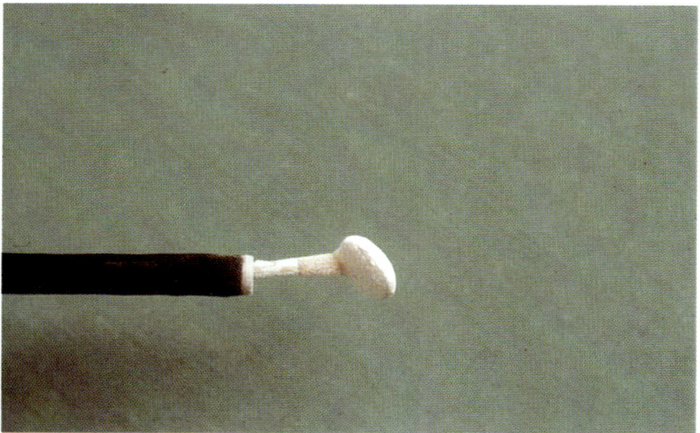

Fig. 11.2.2. Retrieval of foreign body (tablet)

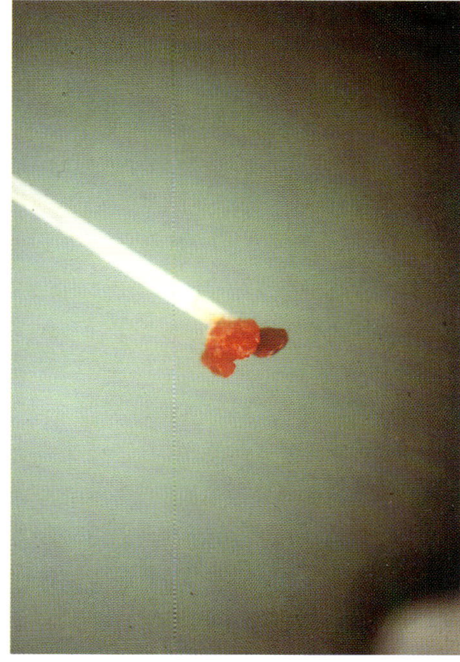

Fig. 11.2.3. Removal of slough using cryoadherence

Foreign bodies: Cryosurgery may be used to remove foreign bodies, including pills (Fig. 11.2.2), slough caused by previous treatment (Fig. 11.2.3), blood clots, peanuts, teeth, chicken bones, glass fragments. (7, 13–15).

11.2.2 Cryosurgery Associated with Chemotherapy or Radiotherapy. Experimental and Clinical Studies

Application in Pulmonology

The process of freezing and the mechanism of damage during cryosurgery have been widely described in previous reports (13, 16, 17).

Two factors contribute to cell death: a physical effect with cellular dehydration and extracellular followed by intracellular crystallization; and a vascular effect of microthrombosis. The result is a slough which occurs several days later. At the edge of the frozen area the hypothermia causes a heterogeneous destructive effect, and it is in this area that chemotherapy or radiotherapy has a complementary destructive effect. For this reason we have called this area the combined therapeutic area (Fig. 11.2.4). Very little is written concerning these combined treatments, but experimental studies confirm clinical results and merit further studies: the combination of cryosurgery and chemotherapy or radiotherapy is more effective than either therapy alone.

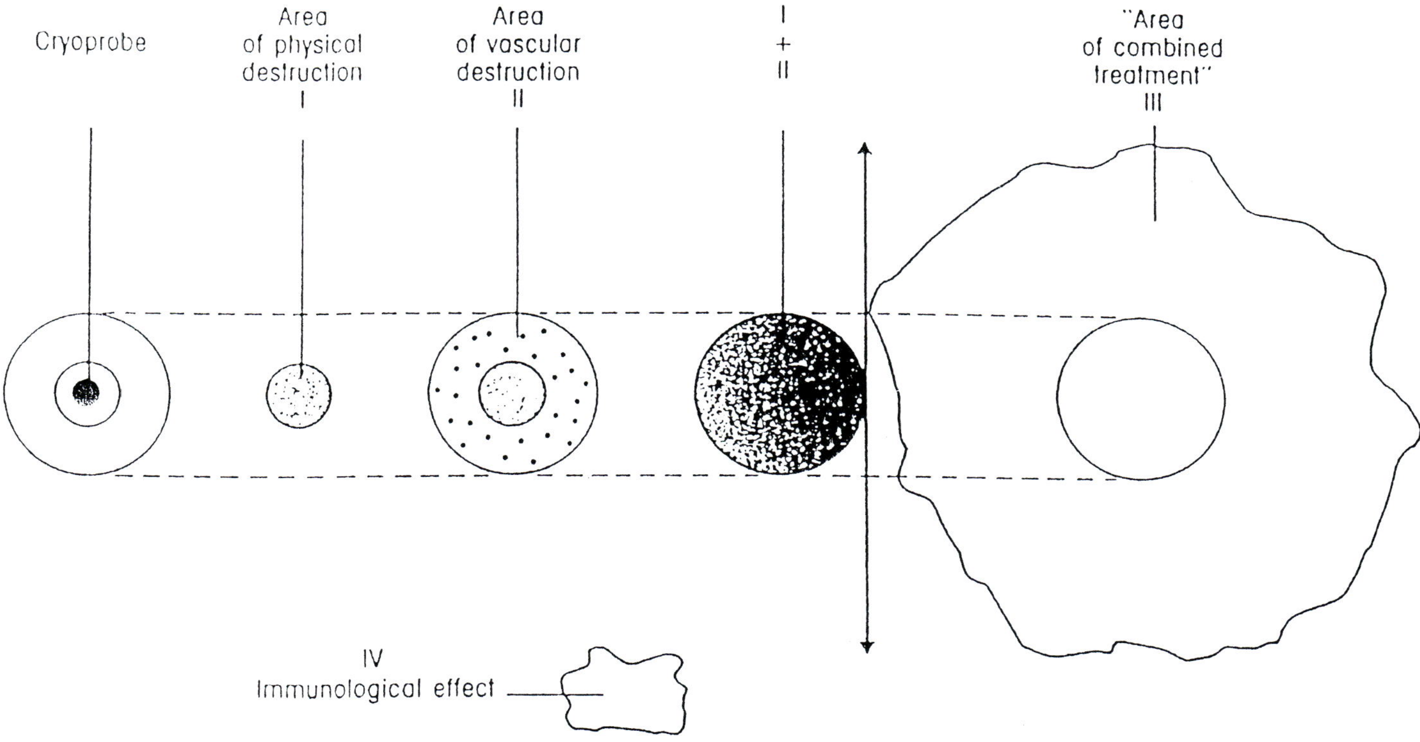

Fig. 11.2.4. Schematic illustration of a cryolesion

Cryosurgery – Chemotherapy

Experimental studies: The combined effect of cryosurgery and anticancer drugs was studied by Ikekawa et al. in an experimental B16 melanoma murine tumor system (18). The anticancer drugs pepleomycin and adriamycin were administered intraperitoneally in combination with cryosurgery. When the drugs were given 1 hour before cryosurgery, there was no significant difference between the frozen tumor and untreated tumor. However, when administered 5 min, 1 h or 3 h after cryosurgery, the drug concentration in the frozen tumor was significantly higher than in the control tumor. The authors conclude that in cryochemotherapy, it is necessary to administer the drug at the appropriate time. The trapping of the anticancer drug results in a higher concentration and lasts for a long time, so that cryochemotherapy is expected to be a new mode of cancer therapy.

Clarke et al. developed several model cell culture systems and evaluated the effects of 5-Fluorouracil alone or combined with cryosurgery (19). Cells exposed to 5-FU resulted in a minimal loss of viability. Cells exposed to freezing temperatures resulted in an approximate 30% loss of viability. Those cells subjected to the combination resulted in a greater loss of viability than either of the other treatments.

Using a N_2O driven cryoprobe that is currently used in bronchial endoscopy (Fig. 11.2.5) we studied together for the first time cryotoxicity and the effect of cryolesions on cells, in different layers of an ice ball formed around the cryoprobe tip, which was immersed in a tumor cell suspension (rat ascitic hepatoma). The diameter of the probe was 3 mm, and its length was reduced from 60 to 25 cm for convenience; this shortening did not alter its performance. We confirmed previous studies: cryotoxicity is greatest nearest to the cryoprobe. In contrast, at the ice ball periphery, discrete

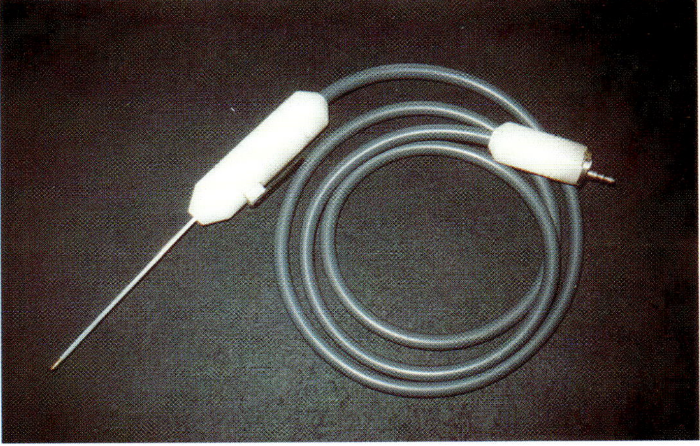

Fig. 11.2.5. N_2O-driven cryoprobe (DATE). Length = 25 cm. Diameter = 3 mm

lesions were visible (20). However, the conclusions thus obtained in our experimental model cannot be directly applied to solid tumors in situ. In these tissues, other factors play a role: in particular, the histological structure, the specific cryosensitivity of various tissues, and the vasculature. With the idea of improving the therapeutic efficacy of cryosurgery in the regions of low cryotoxicity (ice ball periphery and surrounding areas), we have combined intraperitoneal chemotherapy with cisplatin in the treatment of rat transplantable fibrosarcoma. The tumor (approximately 30 mm^3) was grafted into the back of a Sprague-Dawley strain rat. This tumor grows rapidly, and we used cisplatin (single dose 1 mg/kg), as this drug is generally part of anti-lung-cancer protocols. We treated 10 rats with cisplatin alone, ten with cryotherapy alone, and 10 with combined cryosurgery and chemotherapy and compared the results with the evolution of the tumor grafted in 6 control rats. The anticancer drug was administered 1 hour after cryosurgery. The tumor volume and body weight were measured daily. Poor results were obtained when the treatments were applied separately whereas their combined use significantly reduced the tumor growth (Figs. 11.2.6–11.2.8). The body weight increases as the tumor size rapidly reaches the size and weight of the rat itself. This experimental study also confirms the efficacy of combined treatments.

Clinical studies: Benson (21) combined chemotherapy and cryosurgery for advanced oral carcinomas. The majority of the patients had recurrent disease after other therapy. All treatments were performed using liquid nitrogen and a flexible copper mesh cryoprobe. A two-day post-cryosurgical infusion (intra-arterial) of 5-FU was administered. Electrosurgical subtotal tumor reduction was performed at the time of initial cryosurgery to reduce swelling and magnitude of *in situ* tissue slough. Among the 30 patients reported, 20 remain alive from six months to six years, only 2 of whom have clinically evident recurrent disease. This non-randomized study establishes a suprisingly favorable outcome of several cases treated with this combination of therapies, which merits further studies before decisive revision of traditional standards of practice.

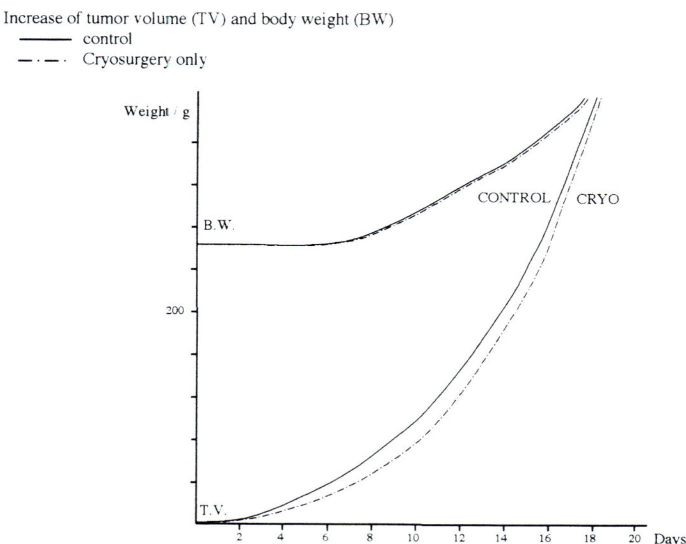

Fig. 11.2.7. Treatment: cryosurgery alone

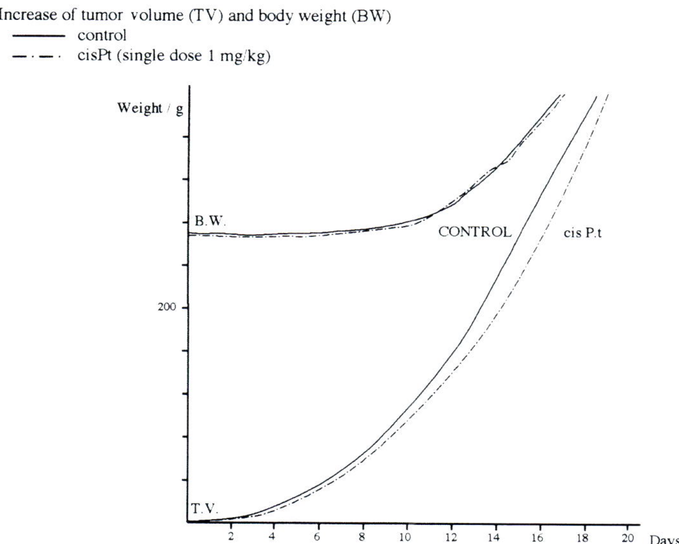

Fig. 11.2.6. Treatment: cisplatin alone

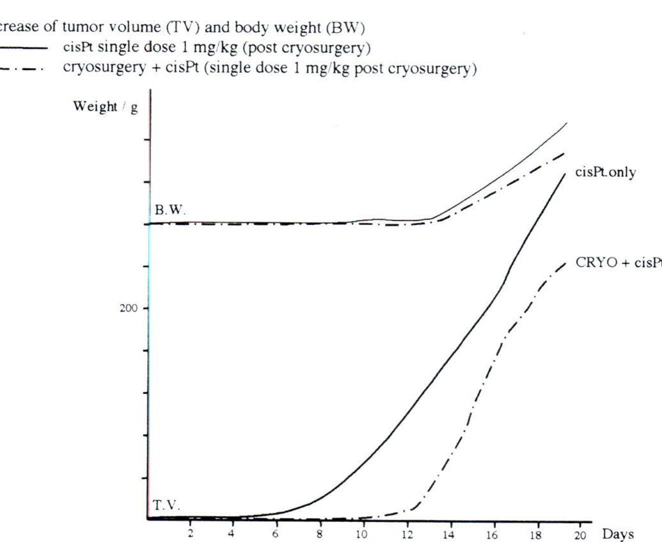

Fig. 11.2.8. Treatment: cryosurgery + chemotherapy (Cis Pt.)

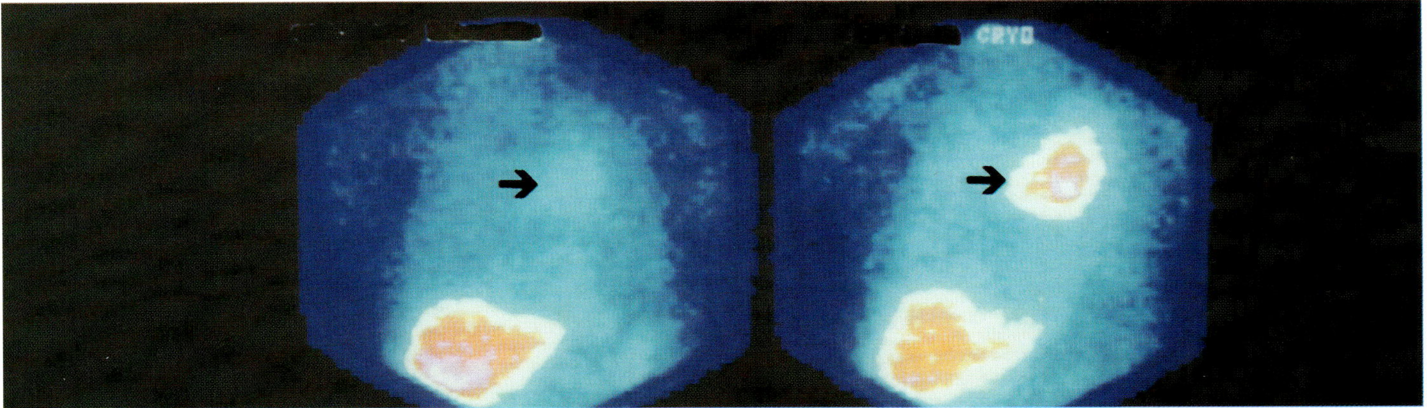

Fig. 11.2.9. Tumor uptake of radiolabelled bleomycin before cryosurgery and 15 days later (arrows) immediately after the cryosurgery procedure (bottom left = liver bleomycin concentration)

To confirm the experimental data, we carried out a prospective study on twelve patients (22). All presented with bronchogenic cancer at an advanced stage of illness. Surgical resection was not possible. The endoscopy in all cases revealed an endobronchial tumor obstructing one main bronchus, and cryosurgery was indicated as a palliative therapy. The patients received 15 mg bleomycin i.v. labelled with cobalt 57. Each patient was then placed under a gamma camera and a region of interest was drawn over the left ventricle in order to plot a time activity curve corresponding to the disappearance of the radiolabelled bleomycin from the blood. The redistribution and elimination half-lives of the labelled bleomycin were calculated from this curve. Further regions of interest were drawn to calculate uptake by both the tumor and normal tissue. A tumor to normal tissue ratio was then calculated. As the wash-out time of radiolabelled bleomycin was about 10 days, the same protocol was performed 15 days later, one hour after the cryosurgery procedure. The endoscopic treatment was carried out using either rigid or flexible probes, and nitrous oxide was the cooling agent. A significant difference was found in the tumoral uptake of radiolabelled bleomycin before and after cryosurgery with a mean increase in uptake of 30% following cryosurgery. The pharmacokinetic parameters demonstrate that after cryotherapy there was accelerated plasma clearance and it can be postulated that bleomycin is trapped in the tumor as a consequence of the vascular disruption caused by freezing (Fig. 11.2.9). Predictably, the endoscopic findings after 15 days, just before cryosurgery, were not modified by the single injection of 15 mg bleomycin, because the dose was clearly not high enough to have a therapeutic effect. The study thus confirms the experimental findings of Ikekawa in the mouse and offers an explanation for the initial clinical findings reported by Benson in ENT tumors. These clinical results confirm that the concentration of the anticancer drug was higher in the frozen zone and adjoining hypothermic area compared to untreated surrounding tissue, and tumor destruction is superior to that normally found with chemotherapy alone. The histology of the tumor did not influence the nuclear medicine measurements. More experimental and randomized clinical studies are needed to draw firm conclusions. Nevertheless, when surgical resection is not feasible, cryochemotherapy could be a new regimen for the treatment of bronchial (or other) carcinomas.

Cryosurgery – radiotherapy: In localized inoperable bronchial carcinomas, radiotherapy is an accepted treatment, but the mean survival of patients treated in this way is only 10 months and local eradication of tumor is only obtained in approximately 35% of cases. In obstructive tumors the regression of atelectasis is achieved after irradiation in only 21% of cases without local treatment of the disease. Treatment of these obstructive tumors with Nd-YAG laser has been suggested prior to irradiation. This protocol gives better survival and quality of life. Like laser therapy, cryosurgery will relieve bronchial obstructions and prevent local complications which are the cause of the majority of deaths. Certain studies have suggested a possible synergy between the effect of cryosurgery and external irradiation based on modification of tumor blood flow (23). In a study of the cryo-lesion of a rabbit esophagus studied under microangiography, Le Pivert (24) demonstrated the appearance of marked neovascularization 15

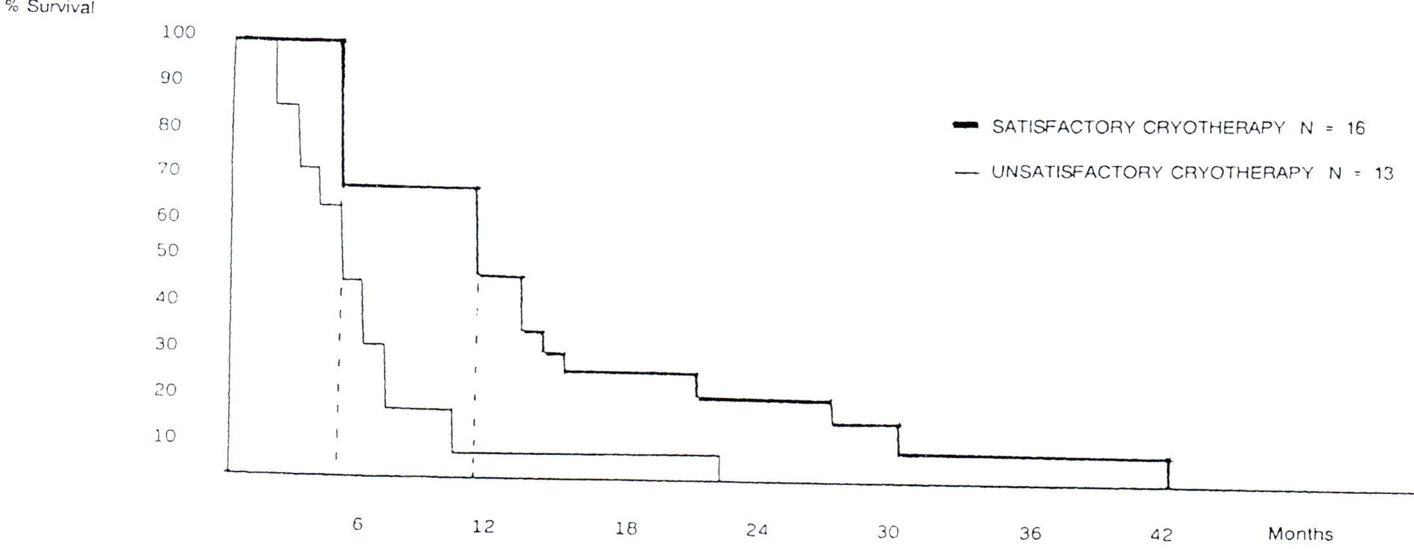

Fig. 11.2.10. Kaplan-Meier survival curves. Benefit in terms of survival determined by effective cryosurgical treatment

days after cryosurgery. This hypervascularization may increase the radio-sensitivity of well vascularized tissues.

In a prospective but not randomized series we enrolled patients in a protocol of cryosurgery associated with radiotherapy (25). These patients with non small cell carcinoma were classified according to their response to cryosurgery. Satisfactory outcome was defined as more than 50% tumor destruction. Two weeks after cryosurgery, radiotherapy was performed. The study group consisted of 29 inoperable patients. One or two sessions of cryosurgery were performed; cryosurgery was considered satisfactory in 16 cases, and unsatisfactory in 13 cases with persistent tumor lesions. 21 patients received 65 Gy and 8 patients with a poor general condition received 45 Gy. The results of this association were evaluated with FOB and biopsy two months after the end of irradiation. All patients survived more than 3 months after radiotherapy. Nevertheless, in the unsatisfactory cryosurgery group, patients died quickly of local complications, with a median survival of 5 months. In the satisfactory group, the median survival was 11 months and a significant improvement in survival was obtained (Fig. 11.2.10). This study does not prove the potentiating effect of cryosurgery on radiotherapy. However, it underlines several significant points:

I. Tumor debulking prior to irradiation helps improve survival and avert local complications.

II. The survival curves obtained correspond closely to those obtained with laser resection of endobronchial lesions.

III. The presence of local obstruction appears to be an important prognostic criterion, survival being more dependent on this factor than on TNM stage.

IV. This "curative" local efficacy raises the possibility of an increased tumor radiosensitivity, induced by the vascular effects of the cryosurgery.

References

1. Gage A, Maiwand MO. Cryosurgery and haemostasis. Cryosurgery 2000; 3: 4–6.
2. Homasson JP, Renault P, Angebault M, Bonniot JP, Bell NJ. Bronchoscopic cryotherapy for airway strictures caused by tumors. Chest 1986; 90: 159–164.
3. Walsh DA, Maiwand MO, Nath AR, Lockwood P, Llloyd MH, Saab M. Bronchoscopic cryotherapy for advanced bronchial carcinoma. Thorax 1990; 45: 509–513.
4. Maiwand MO, Homasson JP. Cryotherapy for tracheobronchial disorders. In: Mathur PN, Beamis JF. (eds): Clinics in Chest Medicine. Saunders, Philadelphia, 1995; 16: 427–443.
5. Homasson JP. Cryotherapy in pulmology today and tomorrow. Eur Resp J 1989; 2: 799–801.
6. Maiwand MO. Cryotherapy for advanced carcinoma of bronchi and trachea. Cryotherapy 1987; 9: 22–24.
7. Sheski FD, Mathur PN. Endobronchial cryotherapy for benign tracheobronchial lesions. Chest 1998; 114: 261–262.
8. Pesek M, Simecek C, Bruha F. Kryokoagulation in der Behandlung von Bronchialtumoren. Z Erkrank Atm Org 1990; 175: 126–131.
9. Homasson JP, Mathur PN. Cryotherapy in endobronchial disorders. In: Beamis JF, Mathur PN (eds): Interventional pulmonology. Mc Graw Hill, New York, 1999; 69–81.
10. Thommi G, Mc Leay M. Cryotherapy in the management of tracheobronchial obstruction by lung tumors. Chest 1998; 114: 262.
11. Maiwand MO. The role of cryosurgery in palliation of tracheobronchial carcinoma. Eur J Cardio Thor Surg 1999; 15: 764–768.

12. Debieuvre D, Gury JP, Kuntz P, Ory JP, Polio JC. Carcinome muco-épidermo bronchique après greffe de moelle traité par cryothérapie. Rev Mal Resp 2000; 17: 1- 103.
13. Homasson JP, Bell NJ. Cryotherapy in chest medicine. Springer, Paris. 1992.
14. Thommi G, Leay M. Cryobronchoscopy in the management of foreign body in the tracheobronchial tree. Chest 1998; 114: 303.
15. Marasso A, Gai R, Prota R. An unusual case of foreign bodies in the bronchial tree. Journal of Bronchol 1995; 2: 339–340.
16. Baust JG. Underlying mechanisms of damage and new concepts in cryosurgical instrumentation in cryosurgery. Mechanism and applications. International Institute of Refrigeration. Paris 1995; 2: 21–36.
17. Gage AA, Baust J. Mechanisms of tissue injury in cryosurgery. Cryobiology 1998; 37: 171–186.
18. Ikekawa S, Ishihara K, Tanaka S, Ikeda S. Basic studies of cryochemotherapy in a murine tumor system. Cryobiology. 1985; 22: 477–483.
19. Clarke DM, Van Buskirk RG, Baust JG. Timing dependency in cryochemo combination therapy: model cell systems. Cryobiology 1999; 39: 320.
20. Homasson JP, Thiery JP, Angebault M, Ovtracht L, Maiwand MO. The operation and efficacy of cryosurgical, nitrous oxide-driven cryoprobe. Cryoprobe physical characteristics: their effects on cell cryodestruction. Cryobiology 1994; 31: 290–304.
21. Benson JW. Combined chemotherapy and cryosurgery for oral cancer. Am J Surg 1975; 130: 596–600.
22. Homasson JP, Pecking A, Roden S, Angebault M, Bonniot JP. Tumor fixation of Bleomycin labeled with 57 cobalt before and after cryotherapy of bronchial carcinoma. Cryobiology 1992; 29: 543–548.
23. Vergnon JM, Schmitt T, Alamartine E, Barthelemy JC, Fournel P, Emonot A. Initial combined cryotherapy and irradiation for unresectable non small cell lung cancer. Chest 1992; 102: 1436–1440.
24. Le Pivert PJ. Basic considerations of the cryolesion. In: Handbook of Cryosurgery. Richard J. Ablin (Eds). Marcel Dekker, New York Basel 1980; 15–68.
25. Benis M. Association cryothérapie- radiothérapie dans le traitement des cancers bronchiques non à petites cellules inopérables. Etude de 29 cas. Thèse Paris V, Universite René Descartes, 1991.

11.3 Bronchoscopic Cryosurgery

Daniel Luna Sabaté

To the results obtained through methods deemed classic, such as the clamp resection or electrocauterization or the Yag-Laser, we have to add the results obtained in recent years through cryotherapy, photodynamic, intraluminal radiotherapy and high frequency thermocoagulation.

Cryosurgery is a form of cryotherapy based on the therapeutic use of the destructive effect of cold.

There is evidence for the use of cold in medicine as long ago as 3500 BC for treatment of infected wounds of the chest, fractures of the skull, and various battle injuries. Hippocrates (460–377 BC) described the use of cold to relieve the swelling and pain of trauma and other diseases affecting the bones and joints. Avicenne, in the 11th century, produced a study of the anesthetic properties of cold. The same properties were observed by Severino (1580–1656). Its anesthetizing properties were valued years later by D.J. Larrey, Napoleon's surgeon, in limb amputations, without pain or hemorrhage, following the application of snow and ice during the Russian campaign of 1812.

The destructive effect of cold was used for the first time by John Hunter (1777). Later, James Arnott at the Middlesex Hospital in 1841 was the first physician to use this destructive effect in the treatment of tumors.

Its applications in the field of modern medicine were initiated in 1959 by Lee Cooper using liquid nitrogen as the cooling agent and a cryoprobe with a metal tip, where temperatures reach −196°C. Later, this method was used extensively in other specialties such dermatology, general surgery, gynecology, proctology, and urology.

The history of cryotherapy for tracheo-bronchial lesions has been relatively short due to the difficulty of anatomic accessibility. It was only in 1977 that the first applications in pneumology appeared with Carpenter and later with Sanderson in 1981 and Rogers in 1983. In 1985, thanks to the work of J.P. Homasson in France and O. Maiwand in England the peak of this treatment was reached due to the perfecting of probes of small caliber – rigid, semi-rigid, and flexible (Le Pivert 1980). In France, there are over 100 units actively using this method.

The goal of cryotherapy in pneumology is based on the freezing of tissues of specific areas of the trachea or bronchi through a probe, with optical control and through impedance (Le Pivert 1977), reaching temperatures of at least −40°C, in order to obtain a specific cellular destruction (cryodestruction).

The choice of effective coolant for cryodestruction is important. Several studies have shown that the core temperature needed for a lesion to be destroyed is between –20°C and –40°C. There are several cooling agents that can be used as cryogens: chlorofluorocarbons (domestic and industrial refrigeration), rarely used in cryotherapy; carbon dioxide; liquid nitrogen and nitrous oxide.

The cooling agent most commonly used in cryotherapy is nitrous oxide (N_2O) stored at very high pressure (50−60 atmospheres). When transported through the very fine channel of the probe, it reaches a low pressure chamber, placed at the distal end of the probe, providing temperatures as low as −80°C, thus forming an important expansion of low temperatures (Joule-Thomson effect).

The cryodestruction is due mainly to two mechanisms: A direct physical effect, immediate

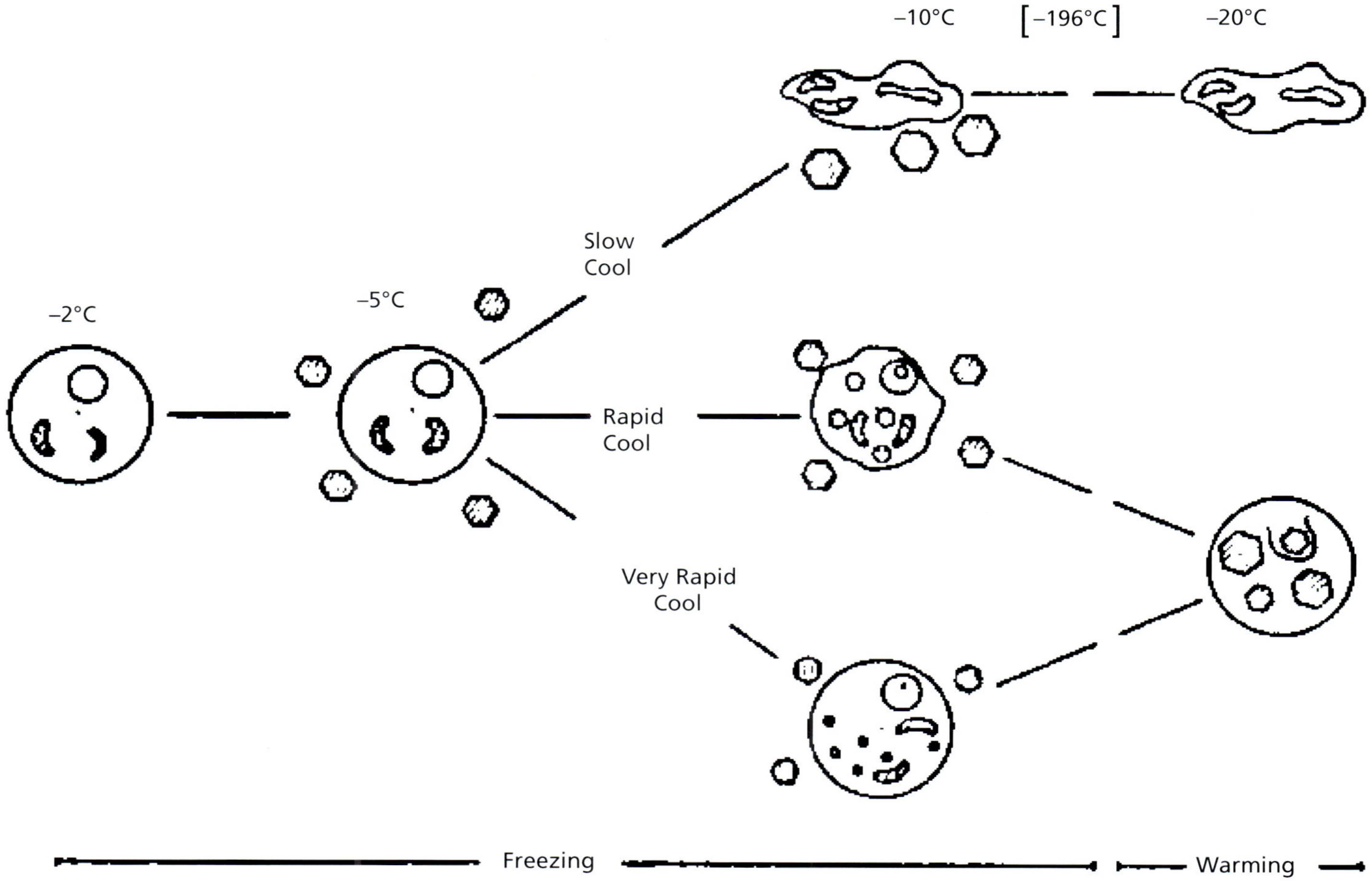

Fig. 11.3.1. Schematic representation. Extra- and intracellular crystallization by Mazur (1977)

and predominant (crystallization) and an indirect vascular effect, delayed due to thrombosis. Rapid freezing and, thereafter, slow thawing cause maximum cell death (Mazur 1977): extracellular and intracellular crystallization and thereafter migratory intracellular recrystallization, which are very toxic to the intracellular organelles (mitochondria, endoplasmic reticulum), causing cell death (Fig. 11.3.1). Ischemic and infarcted aspects of cryolesions appear from a few minutes to several hours after cryoapplication. We should point out an important effect, namely vasoconstriction, which appears at the moment of freezing, quickly giving a hemostatic effect, which allows biopsies to be performed on highly vascularized masses, which bleed easily, thus permitting histology to be performed without the risks of bleeding. We also point out a third mechanism, immunologic effect, which is still under investigation.

Further to the freezing effects (crystallization – thrombosis), a slough develops, which is expelled through expectoration, even though in some few cases the slough will have to be extracted with the biopsy clip during the control examination 8–12 days later.

Once the slough has detached from the area of the treated wall, there is no bleeding, it repairs itself spontaneously, and a non-retractile, non-fibrous scar develops.

Since 1987 we have used semi-rigid cryotherapy probes, which we introduce through a rigid bronchoscope at the same time as the optic tube, generally under total anesthesia. The area to be treated is then frozen, performing several applications at different points until the freezing of the involved area is obtained (Fig. 11.3.2). All of this takes place under optic and impedance control (Le Pivert 2000). We have also been using since 1992 flexible probes through the fiberoptic bronchoscope under local anesthesia.

In our hospital we have treated: 39 reactive granulomas at the tracheal tree; 3 subglottic stenosis; 2 papillomatosis; 1 subglottic carcinoid tu-

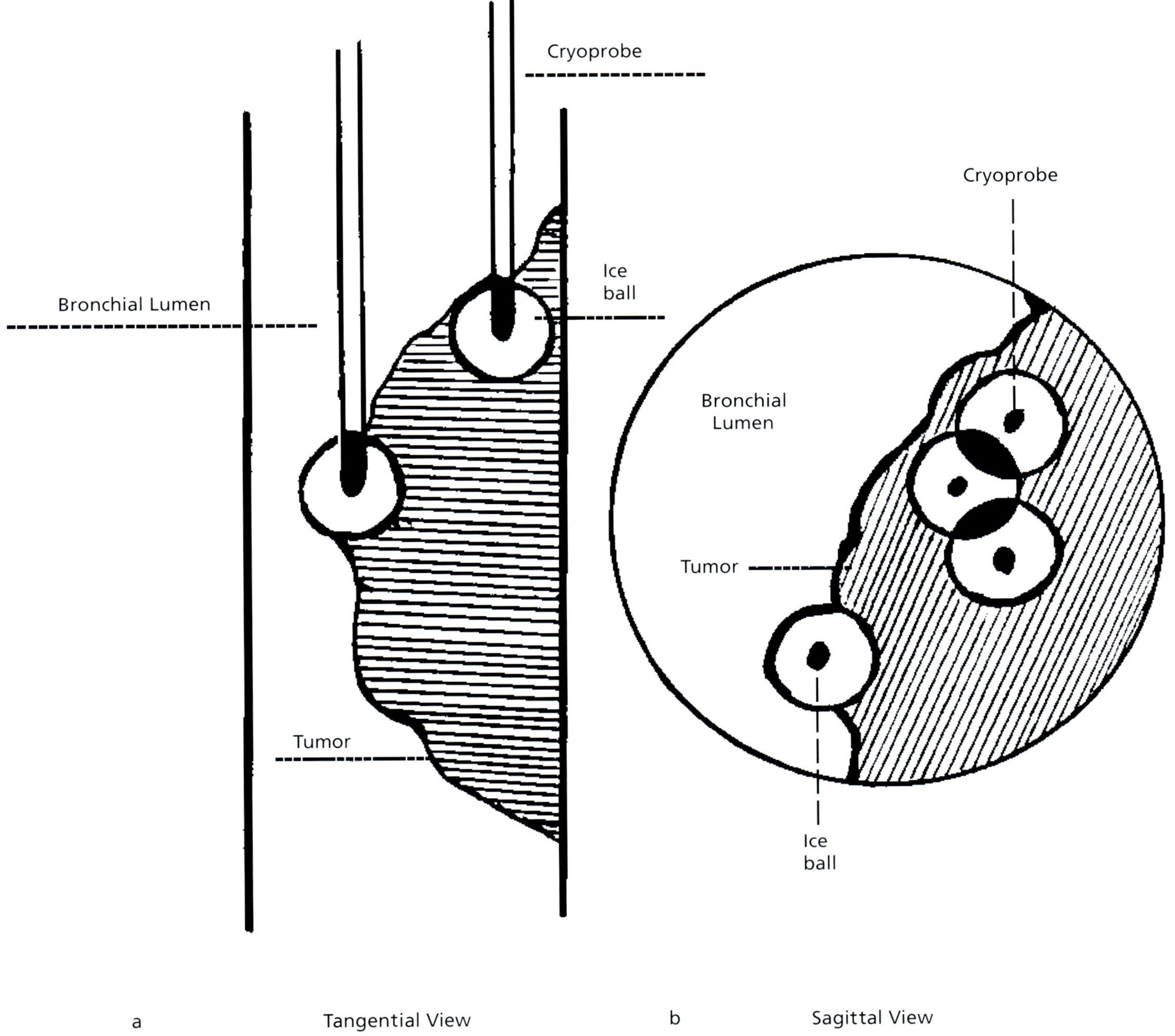

Fig. 11.3.2. Schematic representation. Freezing technique: Three freeze-thaw cycles are carried out at each site under direct vision and impedance

mor (relapsed after Yag-Laser); 1 subglottic cystic adenoid carcinoma of Laser treatment); 13 malignant tumors. In the bronchial tree: 4 tuberculous granulomas; 3 unspecified granulomatose masses; 1 granuloma due to actinomycosis; 5 typical carcinoid tumors; 31 malignant tumors (one case: mucous-epidermoid tumor treated later with intraluminal radiotherapy); 5 moderate to severe dysplasias (one case "in situ") and 6 post-lobectomy or post-pneumonectomy local recurrences treated later with intraluminal radiotherapy–brachytherapy). Most malignant tumors of the trachea and bronchi are treated with local irradiation.

The results obtained lead us to conclude that endoscopic cryotherapy is the treatment of choice in reactive granulomas, as well as in benign, or low malignancy, tumors. Very similar results have been attained in the treatment of precancerous lesions, according both with our personal experience and with the literature (Ozenne 1990; Vergnon 1992) (Fig. 11.3.3).

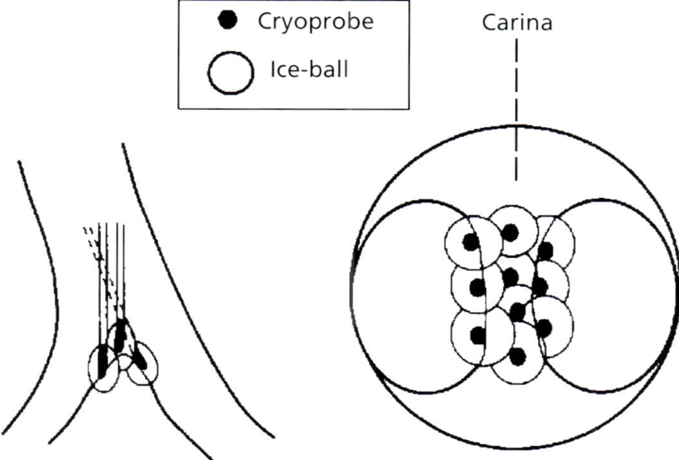

Fig. 11.3.3. Schematic representation. Technique of cryotherapy for the tumor *in situ*. 1. The probe is applied laterally on each side of the carina. 2. The tip of the probe is applied along the crest of the carina

We consider that this treatment is an excellent palliative method in malignant non-operative tumors with favorable outcomes in 80% of the cases, especially when combined with radiotherapy after about 15 days of the freezing of the tumor (Vergnon 1999).

We wish to point out the possibility of performing biopsies on highly vascularized masses with a decrease of the possibility of bleeding, and even of death, due to the precocious vasconstriction effect, without histological changes which may interfere with the anatomopathological interpretation, at least, in optical microscopy. We also wish to point out the beneficial effect of the combination of cryotherapy with chemotherapy (Homasson 1995).

The complementary, fundamental effect of cryotherapy should be considered whenever another endoscopic treatment is started with a different technique (Yag-laser, thermocoagulation, etc.). In our experience, various tumors that have been treated previously with the techniques just mentioned, in order to reduce tumor volume, to reduce signs of asphyxia, etc, need thereafter to be treated with cryotherapy as a complement to avoid rapid recurrence (Fig. 11.3.4).

In conclusion, we believe endoscopic cryotherapy to be an inexpensive, easy to use, effective and safe therapy. It is the treatment of choice in benign pathology (reactive granulomas, benign tumors, central typical carcinoid tumors, precancerous lesions, etc.) and it is very important in vascularized masses with the possibility of biopsies free of risk of bleeding. It is very effective in patients with endobronchial carcinoma and airway obstruction (inoperable malignant tumors), especially when subsequently combined with radiotherapy and/or chemotherapy.

References

1. Amoils SP, Walker AJ. The thermal and mechanical factors involved in ocular cryosurgery. Proc R Soc Med 1966; 59: 1056.
2. Arnott J. On the present state of therapeutic enquiry. London, 1845.
3. Breasted JH. The Edwin Smith Surgical papyrus, vol. 3. Chicago, University of Chicago Oriental Institute, 1930.
4. Carpenter RJ, Neel HB, Sanderson DR. Cryosurgery of the bronchopulmonary structures. An approach to lesions inaccesible to the rigid bronchoscope. Chest 1977; 72: 279–284.
5. Cooper IS, Lee A: Cryothalectomy-hypothermic coagulation: a technical advance in basal ganglia surgery. Preliminary report. J Am Geratr 1962; 9: 714.
6. Gage AA: Cryotherapy for cancer. In: Rand R, Rinfret A, Von Leden H. Eds. Cryosurgery. Springfield, IL: Charles C. Thomas, 1968; 376–387.
7. Homasson JP, Renault P, Angebault M, Bonniot JP, Bell N: Bronchoscopic cryotherapy for airway strictures caused by tumors. Chest 1986; 90: 159–164.
8. Homasson JP, Angebault M, Boniot JP, Baud D, Roden S, François-Coudray S: Cryotherapy of benign and malignant tracheo-bronchial tumors. Report of 250 cases. Chest 1990; 98 (Suppl 2); 131.
9. Homasson JP, Pecking A, Roden S, Angebault M, Bonniot JP: Tumor fixation of bleomycin labeled with 57 cobalt before and after cryotherapy of bronchial carcinoma. Cryobiology 1992; 29: 543–548.
10. Homasson JP and Bell NJ: Cryotherapy in Chest Medicine. Paris: Springer 1993.
11. Homasson JP: Bronchoscopic Cryotherapy J Bronchol. 1995; 2: 145–153.
12. Homasson JP, Jean-François R, Maiwand O, Vergnon JM: Abstracts of the area of endobronchial cryotherapy in the 1st European Congress of Cryosurgery in San Sebastian (Spain): 30 March–2 April, 2000.
13. Larrey DJ: Memoires de chirurgie militaire et campagne. Paris: F. Buisson, 1812.
14. Le Pivert P: Cryochirurgie en cancerologie: Contribution experimentale à l'ètude de la cryodestruction des cellules tumorales in vivo. Thèse de Doctorat en Medicine. Lyon 1974; 350.
15. Le Pivert P, Binder P. Utilisation des mesures d'impedance biolectriques comme mèthode de contrôle de la cryodestruction "in vivo". CR Acad Sci Paris 1975; 285: 1191–1194.
16. Le Pivert P, Binder P, Ougier T. Measurement of intratissue bioelectrical low frequency impedance: A new method to predict peroperative the destruction effect of cryosurgery. Cryobiology 1977; 14: 245–250.
17. Le Pivert P. Basic considerations of the cryolesion. In: Handbook of cryosurgery. RJ. Ablin, M. Dekker, New York 1980, 2: 15–68.
18. Le Pivert P, Eckhoff G, Sramek M Bioelectrical Impedance Imaging for Monitoring Cryosurgery. Abstract of 1st European Congress of Cryosurgery in San Sebastian (Spain), 30 March–2 April, 2000.
19. Luna Sabaté D, Hernandez C, Aldama L, and cols: Crioterapia endoscópica en 5 carcinoides bronquiales intraluminales típicos. Abstracts of the V International Meeting on Respiratory Endoscopy (May 8–10th, 1977, Barcelona Spain), 1977.
20. Luna Sabaté D. Endoscopic treatment of the obstructive tracheobronchial tumors through cryotherapy. Abstract. The Third International Conference of the Arab Thoracic Association (7–10 November, 1999, Amman (Jordan), 1999
21. Maiwand MO. Cryotherapy for advanced carcinoma of the trachea and bronchi. Br Med J 1986; 293: 181–182.
22. Maiwand MO, Homasson JP. Cryotherapy for tracheobronchial disorders. Clin Chest Med 1995; 16(3): 427–443.
23. Mazur P. The role of intracellular freezing in the death of cells cooled at supraoptimal rates. Cryobiology 1977; 14: 251–252.

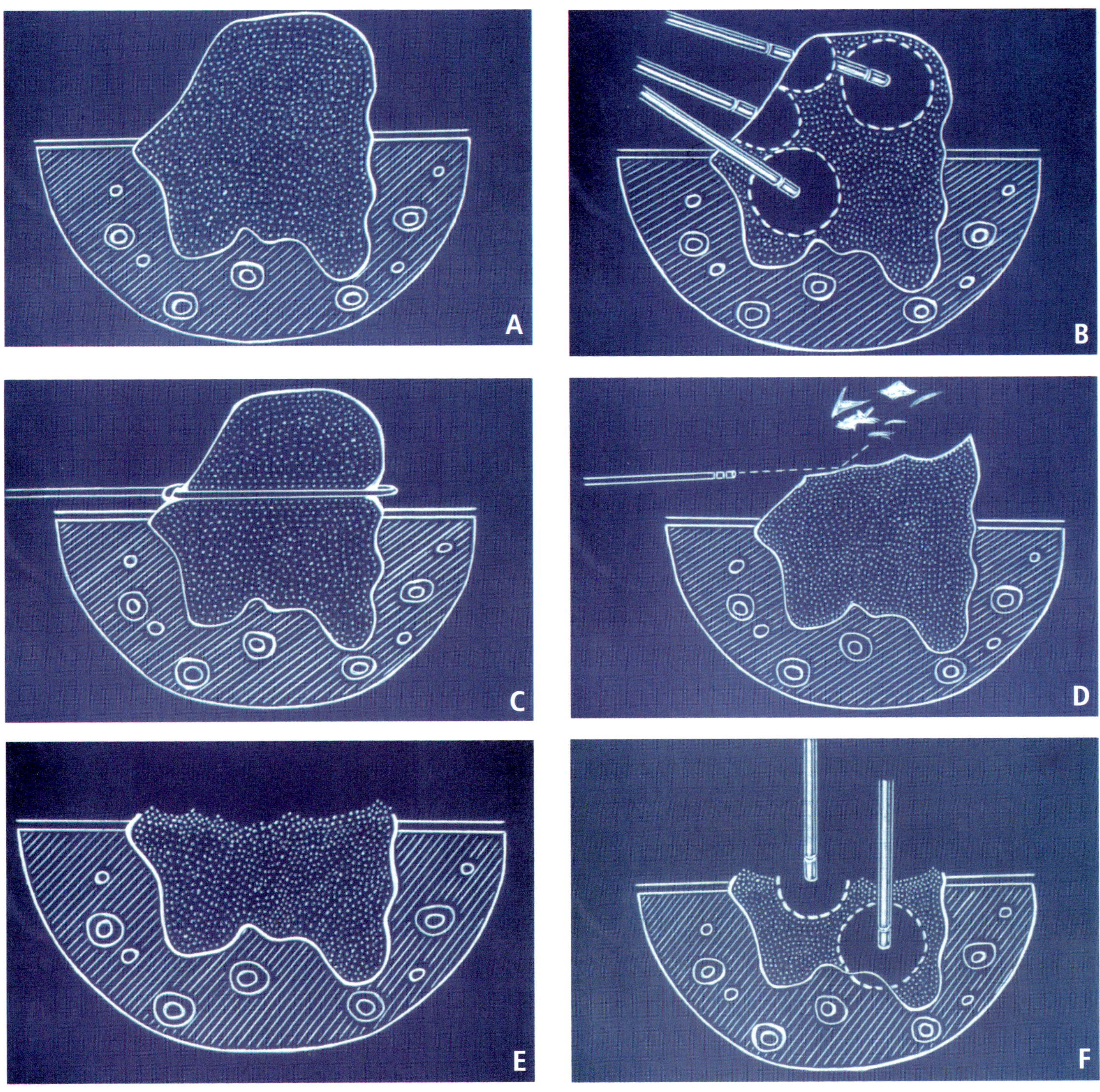

Fig. 11.3.4. Schematic illustration of endobronchial therapies: **A** Cryotherapy, **B** Endoluminar tumor cryosurgical treatment, **C** Clamp resection, **D** Laser or high frequency thermocoagulation treatment, **E** Remaining intramural tumor, **F** Freezing the remaining intramural tumor with the cryoprobe

24. Mazur P, Wolf KM, Busk MF. Fiberoptic bronchoscopic cryotherapy in the management of tracheobronchial obstruction. Chest 1996; 110: 718–723.
25. Ozenne G, Vergnon JM, Roullier A, Blanc-Jouvan F, Courty G: Cryotherapy of in situ or microinvasive bronchial carcinoma. Chest 1990; 98 (Suppl): 105.
26. Reuter HJ. Histoire de la cryochirurgie. Cryotherapy 1987; 9: 5–7.
27. Rodgers BM, Moazam F, Talbert JL. Endotracheal cryotherapy in the treatment of refractory airway strictures. Ann Thor Sur 1983; 35: 52–57.
28. Rubinsky B. The process of freezing and the mechanism of damage during cryosurgery. In: JP Homasson, NJ Bell, eds, Cryotherapy in Chest Medicine. Paris: Springer 1993; 7–18.
29. Sanderson DR, Neel HB, Fontana RS. Bronchoscopic Cryotherapy. Ann Otol 1981; 90: 354–358.

30. Vergnon JM, Boucheron S, Bonamour D, Fournel P, Emonot A. Destruction endobronchique des lesions tumorales: laser ou cryotherapie. Analyse préliminaire. Rev. Pneumol Clin 1987; 43: 19–25.
31. Vergnon JM. How I do it: Bronchoscopic cryotherapy. J Bronchol 1995, 2: 323–327.
32. Vergnon JM, Schmiitt T, Alamartine E, Barthelemy JC, Fournel P, Emonot A. Initial combined cryotherapy and irradiation for unresectable non small cell lung cancer. Chest 1992; 102: 1436–1440.
33. Vergnon JM Cryothérapie endobronchique: techniques et indications. In: Pneumologie Interventionelle. Rev Mal Respir 1999; 16: 619–623.

12. Cryosurgical Urology

12.1 Experimental Targeted Cryoablation for the Treatment of Symptomatic Benign Prostatic Hypertrophy (BPH)

Douglas Chinn

12.1.0 Introduction

One of the earliest roles of urologic cryosurgery was the treatment of BPH. A transurethral approach was utilized with liquid nitrogen. A single closed probe system, using liquid nitrogen, was placed transurethrally. Transrectal digital palpation and/or thermocouple monitoring were used to help monitor the freezing process. Suprapubic cystoscopy was used to monitor the bladder neck. This treatment was usually reserved for patients with very large glands and severe symptoms, but who were not good surgical candidates for conventional procedures (1). For unknown reasons, the focus of modern cryosurgery has since its advent been on malignant tissue. Perhaps this is due in part to the large number of excellent treatment choices available for BPH by the time a multiprobe liquid nitrogen system was developed (2). The extensive clinical experience in treating prostate cancer with cryosurgery has clearly demonstrated the efficacy of this method in decreasing prostate volume as measured by ultrasound in post cryosurgical biopsies. To date, there have been no published studies exploring the role of cryosurgery for the treatment of BPH using the current technique and technology.

In 1998, to investigate the role of cryotherapy as treatment for BPH, a three-patient pilot study was performed. The goals of the procedure were to decrease the volume of the transition zone while avoiding cryoinjury to the urethra, bladder neck, external sphincter, rectal wall, and neurovascular bundles.

12.1.1 Materials and Methods

After informed consent and IRB approval were received, three patients, ages 70–76 years, were treated for BPH utilizing the CRYOcare® cryosurgical unit (Endocare, Inc., Irvine, CA), and the Aloka 650 true biplane ultrasound unit (Aloka, Wallingford, CT). The indications for the procedure were a failure of medical therapy, and that cryosurgery represented the only other available alternative to simple open retropubic prostatectomy. All patients were screened to rule out prostate cancer, and the following parameters were measured pre- and post-operatively: PSA, prostate volume, postvoid residual, uroflow, and AUA symptom scores. Urinalysis, serum chemistry and CBC were also performed. All patients had previously received conservative daily medical therapy for their BPH symptoms. Two patients received an alpha-blocker and all 3 patients received Proscar™ (Merck & Co., Inc., Whitehouse Station, NJ). All medications were permanently discontinued prior to baseline studies and cryosurgery.

12.1.2 Technique

The technique was modified from the standard targeted approach for treating prostate cancer, such that all cryoprobes were placed equidistant between the urethra and the gland capsule (Fig. 12.1.1a and b). This allowed for symmetrical ice propagation between the surface of the gland and the urethra (Fig. 12.1.2), and reduced the chance of injuring either the urethra or the prostate capsule. The number of probes deployed was decided by the gland volume and dimensions. The transition zone of the prostate was targeted for freezing. Four cryoprobes were used in all cases

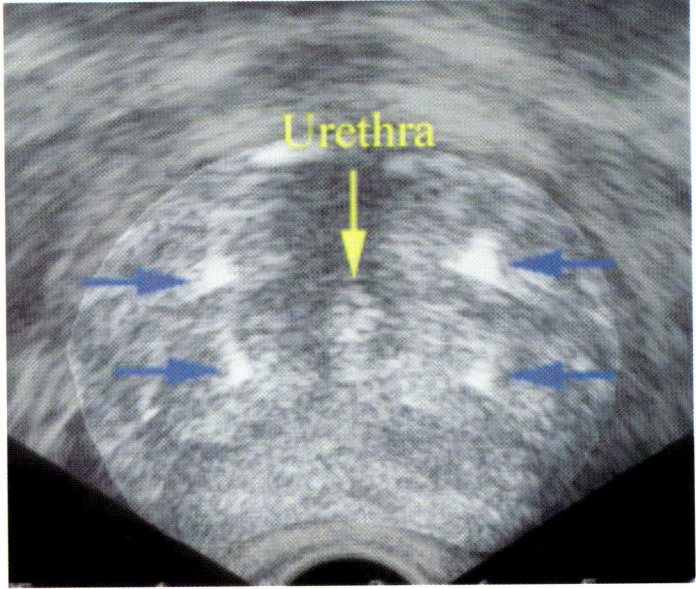

Fig. 12.1.1a. Cryoprobe placement methodology: Transrectal ultrasound permits visualization of the BPH cryoablation procedure in real time. This image was taken following cryoprobe placement. The four cryoprobes are depicted by the blue arrows

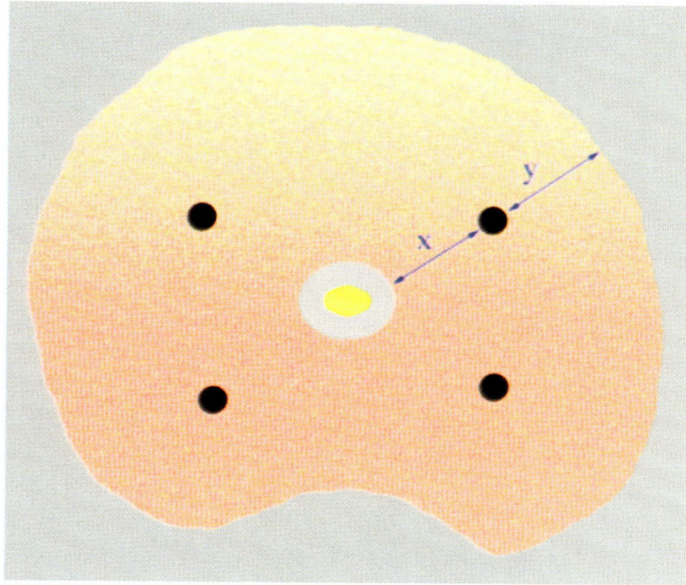

Fig. 12.1.1b. Schematic demonstrating cryoprobe placement, depicted in the ultrasound image above. The cryoprobes are advanced into the gland such that they are equidistant between the urethra and prostate capsule (distance x = distance y)

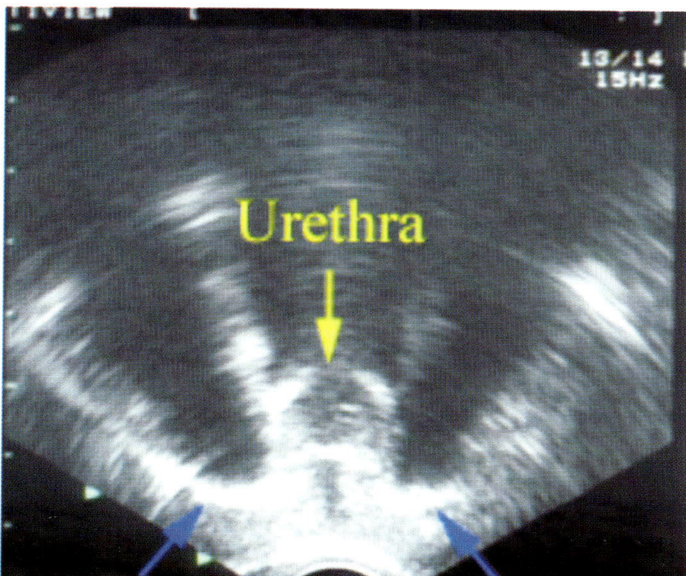

Fig. 12.1.2. Ultrasound image demonstrating ice ball growth (blue arrows) draping over the urethra, thus avoiding any chance of urethral injury

and all patients underwent a double freeze-thaw cycle. Thermocouples were placed in the right and left neurovascular bundles, between the rectal wall and posterior prostate capsule (Denonvillier's fascia), at the apex and at the external sphincter. The endpoint of the procedure was determined when a target temperature of 0°C was achieved at the apical, neurovascular, and Denonvillier's thermocouples. All procedures were performed on an outpatient basis.

12.1.3 Morbidity

As with standard prostate cryosurgery, there is scrotal edema, and perineal discomfort from the access sites, which resolves in 7–10 days. There is also urinary retention lasting from 6–8 weeks. A suprapubic catheter was placed in all cases, and the time of removal was determined when the postvoid residual was 50 cc or less. In two of the patients, the suprapubic tube remained for 6 weeks, while the tube remained in the third patient for 8 weeks. There was no urethral slough, urinary incontinence, pelvic pain, or impotence as a result of the procedure. Two patients were impotent preoperatively, and the one who was potent prior to surgery remains potent. Two patients developed epididymitis which was treated conservatively, and the condition resolved.

12.1.4 Results

Minimum follow-up time was 12 months for all 3 patients. Three months after the postoperative effects of cryosurgery resolved, the patients' symptoms measured by uroflow, postvoid residual, and symptom score, improved. The AUA symptom scores, peak uroflow rates (Fig. 12.1.3), and postvoid residuals all demonstrated marked improvement (Tables 12.1.1–12.1.3). Interestingly, the gland volumes did not change dramatically (Table 12.1.4). There were no changes in serum chemistries or blood count noted, but the PSA did decrease (Table 12.1.5). Much like microwave therapy, the improvement in symptoms took about 3 months and then was durable, for at least 12 months. The patients stated that the post cryosurgical improvements were greater than those with medical therapy alone. Patient satisfaction was 100%, and all 3 patients stated that they would have the procedure done again.

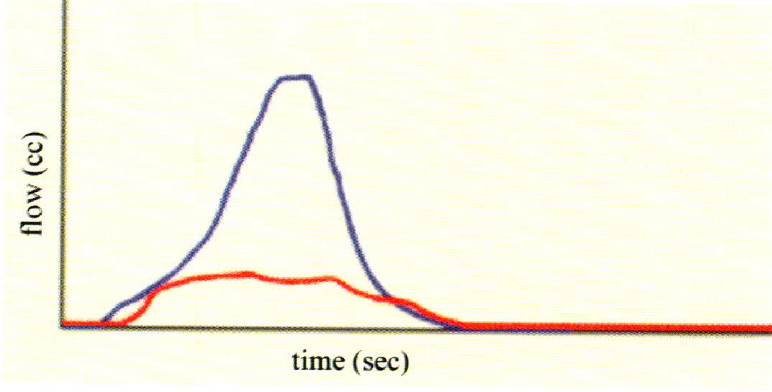

Fig. 12.1.3. Comparison of flow rates, pre-cryo (red line) and post-cryo (blue line). Patients in this limited series experienced increases in peak flow rates ranging from 56%–78%

Table 12.1.1. AUA scores before and after cryosurgery

Variable	Pt #1	Pt #2	Pt #3
PreOp AUA score	24	14	13
PostOp AUA score	5	3	3
% Change	84	79	77

Table 12.1.2. Peak uroflow rates before and after cryosurgery

Variable	Pt #1	Pt #2	Pt #3
PreOp peak flow (cc/sec)	14	8	11
PostOp Peak flow (cc/sec)	32	26	50
% Change	56	69	78

Table 12.1.3. Changes in postvoid residual volumes with cryosurgery

Variable	Pt #1	Pt #2	Pt #3
PreOp postvoid residual (cc)	122	460	260
PostOp Postvoid residual (cc)	32	26	50
% Change	74	94	96

Table 12.1.4. Gland volume changes with cryosurgery

Variable	Pt #1	Pt #2	Pt #3
PreOp Gland vol. (cc)	96	69	67
PostOp Gland vol. (cc)	44	52	44
% Change	54	25	34

Table 12.1.5. Effect of cryosurgery for BPH on PSA

Variable	Pt #1	Pt #2	Pt #3
PreOp PSA	5.6	7.9	1.9
PostOp PSA	1.9	2.6	0.8
% Change	66	67	58

12.1.5 Conclusion

The preliminary results indicate that cryoablation represents a viable mode of therapy for BPH, especially for glands >60 cc. Patient evaluation and selection is crucial, and this therapy is best suited for larger glands that would otherwise require an aggressive TURP, LAP or simple open prostatectomy. Smaller glands can be treated with any of the standard modalities including transurethral needle ablation (TUNA), transurethral resection (TURP), laser prostatectomy (LAP), transurethral microwave therapy (TUMT), or medical therapy. As with all minimally invasive treatment modalities, cryosurgery will not currently treat middle lobe disease. The procedure requires general or spinal anesthesia and there is still postoperative urinary retention. The ability to avoid urethral slough, bladder neck and neurovascular bundle injury, and to preserve urinary continence are all favorable parameters of this procedure. Because this was a pilot study, alpha-blockade was terminated after the procedure, but continuation after cryosurgery may help decrease the catheterization time. The gland volume changes are not as dramatic as with conventional cryosurgery, but the freezing is not as aggressive either. Since the relationship between gland size and degree of symptomatic BPH is not completely understood, it may be difficult to conclude exactly how cryosurgery improves symptoms. However, there is real volume change, and the improvement in measurable BPH symptoms are greater than those achieved by TUNA or TUMT. Whether the effects also include destruction of the periurethral alpha receptors aside from volume change remains to be further elucidated.

The safety profile of this procedure follows that of contemporary cryosurgery for prostate cancer. Because this therapy is minimally invasive, has minimal long term side effects, and is an outpatient procedure, cryosurgery represents an interesting alternative for symptomatic BPH. The continued use of Proscar™ and alpha blockers postoperatively may decrease the morbidity, and perhaps when a reliable temporary urethral stent becomes available, the morbidity will be further decreased. This short term experience has clearly demonstrated that cryosurgery is an effective treatment for symptomatic BPH, but more studies are required to ascertain the long term efficacy.

References

1. Gonder MJ, Soanes WA, Smith V. Chemical and morphologic changes in the prostate following extreme cooling. Ann. N.Y. Acad. Sci. 1965; 125: 716–729.
2. Wong WS, Chinn DO, Chinn M, Chinn J, Tom WL, Tom WL. Cryosurgery as a treatment for prostate carcinoma, results and complications. Cancer 1997; 79: 963–974.

12.2 Targeted Cryoablation for the Treatment of Localized Prostate Cancer

Douglas O. Chinn with contributions by Fred Lee, Duke K. Bahn, and Wilson S. Wong

12.2.0 Introduction

Cryoablation has long held promise for the treatment of prostate disease. There is ample evidence demonstrating the efficacy of freezing to ablate tissue. However, the search for an effective method for applying extreme cold to treat prostate adenoma has been arduous. The purpose of this chapter is to discuss briefly the history of prostate cryoablation, ending with contemporary instrumentation and technique. The specific pathophysiologic and physics theories informing the current approach will be described. Finally, the improved efficacy and advantages of contemporary methodology over previous techniques will be highlighted.

12.2.1 Pathophysiology of Prostate Cryosurgery

Cryosurgery is a thermal therapy, and like all such therapies, be it heat or cold, specific thermal parameters are required to increase the likelihood of cell death. In cryosurgery, there are many theories, based upon in vitro and in vivo experiments concerning the factors that contribute to cell death (15, 32, 33, 53, 54). Two types of ice formation occur during the freezing process, extracellular, and +intracellular. The factors that play a role in determining the lethality of intracellular versus extracellular ice are the following: (1) rate of freeze; (2) lowest temperature achieved; (3) length of time at lowest temperature; (4) number of freeze-thaw cycles; and (5) thaw rate (32–35, 53, 54, 57). Water tends to freeze more easily in a pure form (without solutes/electrolytes). Thus, ice outside of the cells (extracellular) forms more easily, drawing water out of the cells, dehydrating and shrinking them. Cooling also disrupts the cellular/biochemical functions as well. For intracellular ice formation, the cell must not be dehydrated, allowing ice crystals to actually form within the cell. Intracellular ice formation is felt to be uniformly more lethal to cells and tissue versus extracellular ice (32, 33, 53). It is hypothesized that intracellular ice relies primarily on mechanical shearing forces to disrupt the cell membrane, leading to cellular death. The intracellular volume increases with the conversion of water to ice, also contributing to cellular disruption and destruction. Extracellular ice relies on dehydration, denaturization and disruption of biochemical cycles and membrane structures to cause cell death (53, 54). A faster freeze rate traps the water in the cells, allowing intracellular ice formation, while a slow rate will encourage extracellular ice and cellular dehydration (32, 33, 53, 54).

However, these parameters may vary from organ to organ within a species, and animal models may not be directly correlative to human tissue. The only studies to date that have attempted to correlate the technique specifically to prostate cell death are the papers by Tatsutani et al. (50), Larson et al. (24), Bischof et al. (4), and Wong et al. (56). Tatsutani et al. (50) studied prostate cancer cell cultures, and compared freeze rates, number of freeze-thaw cycles, and minimal targeted temperature reached with cell death. With cultured human prostate cancer cells, they re-confirmed that a double freeze-thaw cycle to −40°C had a very high probability of cell kill, and they also demonstrated that a triple freeze-thaw to −20°C was equally effective in the laboratory setting, if a high enough freeze rate was achieved, indicating that freeze rates play a significant role.

Larson et al. did a study in which patients had focal cryosurgery followed by radical prostatectomy several weeks later. They compared the whole mount and microscopic pathology with the number of freeze cycles, temperature mapping and gadolinium MRI. They concluded that a double freeze to −40°C, was consistently lethal. Bischof et al. did *in vitro* and *in vivo* studies with Dunning AT-1 prostate tumor. They studied freeze rates, target temperatures and lethality. Their *in vitro* studies also reconfirmed that intracellular ice is uniformly lethal at −40°C and that freeze rate is less important than targeted end-temperatures. Their *in vivo* studies demonstrated that even sub-lethal *in vitro* parameters resulted in *in vivo* cell death, and suggested that other factors such as vascular thrombosis may play a role, and that further studies are necessary.

Thaw rates have also been felt to affect the lethal effect of cryosurgery (32–35). However, some of the data have been contradictory, but may also be related to other freezing parameters. It has been stated that a slow thaw is crucial. However, with the prostate, we cannot control the peripheral zone, where the thaw rate is most crucial. There is surrounding fat and muscle which will increase the thaw rate peripherally. The slowest rate is in the central gland with a passive thaw. Also, a passive thaw is very time consuming for impatient surgeons. Though research indicates otherwise, in the clinical setting, the rate of thaw does not appear to affect the successful outcomes of prostate cryosurgery.

In summary, the laboratory and clinical research studies have defined the lethal parameters required for successful prostate cryosurgery: a rapid double freeze-thaw cycle with a targeted lethal temperature of –40°C. The use of more frequent cycles at a warmer targeted temperature with longer hold times awaits clinical validation. However, the cryosurgeon must remember that achieving all of the targeted parameters safely and 100% of the time is not always possible.

12.2.2 Evolution of Modern Prostate Cryoablation

Early cryoablation methodologies applied cryoprobes to the gland surface, either transurethrally or in an open transperineal procedure (5, 16, 42). For the treatment of prostate diseases, this method met with limited efficacy and numerous complications. Direct application of the cryoprobe to the gland surface proved to be insufficient for treatment deep in the gland. The process was also impossible to visualize and difficult to control. Incontinence and retention, in addition to residual cancer, were usual outcomes of the treatment. The goal of modern cryoablation is to encompass the target tissue in addition to a ''surgical'' margin for thorough treatment. The periprostatic fascia is encompassed during the freeze to cover potential extracapsular involvement.

Because of the limitations of this application methodology, more sophisticated closed cryoprobe systems have been developed and represent a major step forward in the evolution of the technology. This technology involves multiple cryoprobes that are controlled using a computer microprocessor, allowing fine-tuned control of the freezing process. The long, thin cryoprobes can be inserted deep into the prostate gland for thorough coverage with percutaneous access. Multiple commercial instruments are currently available for the closed-system application. The most commonly utilized cryogens are pressurized, super-cooled liquid nitrogen, and argon gas. Both are efficacious for freezing. Liquid nitrogen systems super-cool the cryogen, then force it under pressure through the cryoprobes. In practice, this instrumentation can be slow, requiring several minutes to establish a baseline critical temperature. This is because the liquid nitrogen naturally boils as it moves through ambient-temperature cryoprobes, and the probes themselves must be cooled by continuous inflow of liquid nitrogen before nadir temperatures are achieved. In contrast, argon gas-based systems operate by supplying high-pressure gas to the cryoprobes through a Joule-Thompson port, resulting in ablative temperatures. An argon gas-driven system is known to be faster to operate due to the cryogen delivery methodology, reaching nadir temperatures in seconds (45).

The introduction of ultrasound in the early 1980's added a new option for procedural monitoring during cryoablation. Transrectal ultrasound (TRUS) was identified as an ideal imaging modality for the procedure (6). In the late 1980's and early 1990's, a percutaneous multiprobe cryoablation technique was developed using ultrasound to guide probe placement and to monitor the freeze (40). Transrectal ultrasound (TRUS) is an indispensable tool in modern cryoablation of the prostate gland. Ultrasound examinations detect and evaluate the extent of disease. The size and geometry of the gland is also evaluated with TRUS. During cryoablation, ultrasound is utilized to guide the precise placement of the cryoprobes and thermocouples. It is used to monitor the freezing process in real time, a critical process needed to confirm that gland coverage is thorough while at the same time insuring that surrounding structures are protected. The success or failure of the procedure is highly dependent upon the skill of the operator or operators who employ ultrasound. The following section will explain critical concepts concerning the physics of ultrasound and delineate its limitations.

12.2.3 Ultrasound and Cryoablation

Ultrasound is generated when an electrical signal is sent to the piezoelectric crystal of an ultrasound transducer. The sound waves are mechanical pressure waves similar to audible sounds. Diagnostic ultrasound frequencies generally fall in the range of 2 to 10 megahertz (MHz), or million-cycles/sec, and are called ultrasonic because they are higher than the human sound range of 20 to 16,000 hertz.

The ultrasound instrument creates images of organ structures when ultrasound waves are reflected back to the transducer. This is accomplished by measuring the time in which it takes sound to travel to and from the interface and by measuring the amplitude of the sound as well. The time delay for sound to travel to an interface and reflect back to the transducer provides information on depth of the tissue while the amplitude of the sound reflected back provides information concerning the type of tissue.

The speed of sound in a medium is determined by the characteristics of the medium itself. Sound will travel more quickly through frozen tissue than through unfrozen tissue. Thus, during cryoablation, ultrasound waves passing through unfrozen tissue will suddenly accelerate upon reaching the frozen tissue, or freeze front.

The amplitude of the reflected and transmitted waves at an interface between two media is dependent on the relative acoustic impedances of the two media. Impedance is the product of the density of a material and the speed of sound in that material. When an ultrasound beam is incident on an interface between two materials differing in acoustic impedance, a portion of the energy in the beam will be reflected and the remainder will be transmitted. The amplitude of the reflected wave depends on the severity of the acoustic impedance mismatch. When the acoustic properties of the two media are similar, very little of the sound is reflected at the interface, and the sound wave passes through without alteration. When there is significant mismatch in the acoustic impedance, most of the sound is reflected. The interface between frozen and unfrozen tissue represents an extreme impedance mismatch. Very little information can be obtained about an area behind a highly reflective interface. This phenomenon is known as acoustic shadowing (Fig. 12.2.1). Structures creating acoustic shadowing include gallstones, kidney stones, bones and air. Similarly, acoustic shadowing occurs behind the ice ball freeze front.

Refraction is the bending of sound beams at an interface. Refraction is dependent upon two factors: (1) the angle at which the incident sound beam strikes the interface and (2) the relative acoustic characteristics of the media comprising the interface. Refraction is important in cryoablation because the leading edge of the ice ball presents a convex, highly mismatched interface to encroaching sound waves. When sound strikes the ice front at 90 degrees, all of the sound is reflected back to the transducer. However, when the sound strikes the ice ball at an angle more than or less than 90 degrees, the beam is refracted. As the angle between incident sound waves and the frozen-unfrozen interface diverge increasingly from 90 degrees, refraction increases, and the apparent location of the ice edge becomes distorted. This phenomenon is known as critical angle shadowing (Fig. 12.2.2).

Due to this distortion, the ice ball may appear larger on the ultrasound display than it is in reality. It is of critical importance to recognize that ultrasound can only provide information concerning the leading edge of the ice ball. Reliable information cannot be obtained by ultrasound posterior to the ice ball because of acoustic shadowing from the effect of reflection. Likewise, the ultrasound image of the lateral edges of the ice ball is also not reliable due to the critical angle refraction shadowing. The overall area of shadowing is slightly larger than the true size of the ice ball. Modern cryoablative technique overcomes this limitation of ultrasound by deploying temperature sensors to the areas obscured under ultrasound. Temperature monitoring provides critical information about these hidden areas. This idea will be discussed in detail in the technique section.

Transducers: Modern ultrasound transducers can be divided into two types: (1) mechanically driven and (2) electronically driven, or phased-array transducers. Older generation transducers are mechanically driven, wherein a single piezoelectric crystal is rotated around an arc. The use of these transducers is not in favor at present because

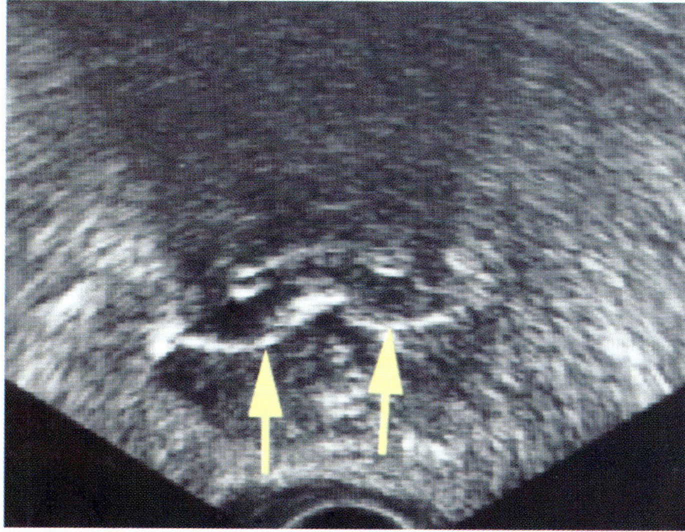

Fig. 12.2.1. Posterior acoustic shadowing. The frozen-unfrozen interface at the freeze front represents an extreme impedance mismatch. Incident ultrasound beams will be reflected from this interface (yellow arrows). As a result, the area behind the freeze front is masked from view

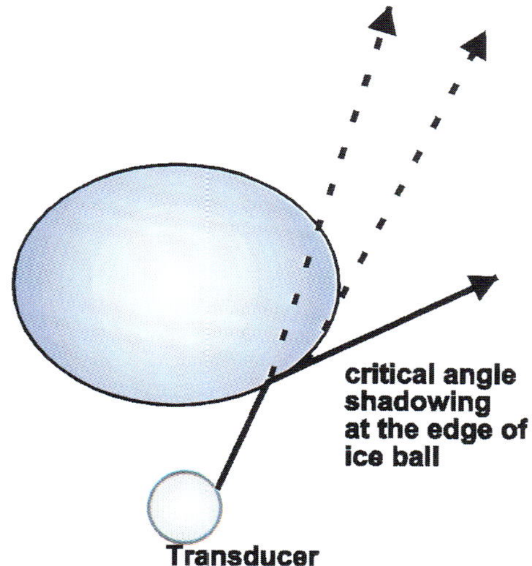

Fig. 12.2.2. Critical angle shadowing: Critical angle refraction, is seen at the curved edges of the ice ball. When the incident US beam strikes the convex ice interface at an angle greater or less than 90°, the beam is refracted or bent. This makes the ice ball appear to be larger than it truly is

mechanical problems are common and the available transducer resolutions are lower than contemporary, electronically driven transducers.

Electronically driven transducers are comprised of numerous crystals. The crystals may be aligned in linear fashion. This arrangement is classified as a linear array. The field of view of a linear array transducer is dependent on the number of crystals contained in the transducer. A linear transducer is typically 6 cm in length. The entire length is applied to the tissue of interest to maximize image size and quality. However, the crystal size, or footprint, can prove unwieldy and difficult to apply in anatomically constricted locations.

A linear array transducer is particularly useful in the precise placement of needles during the cryoablation procedure. The transducer can image the needle along its entire path. The needle is imaged when the needle is parallel to the surface of the transducer and perpendicular to the ultrasound beam, creating a highly accurate image free of distortion. Further, due to the large size of the crystal, the transducer can image the needle along its entire path, with minimal movement.

While the crystals in a linear transducer are fired constantly, crystals can be driven in a phased, rather than continuous, sequence. These types of transducers are classified as phased array. An advantage of the phased-array transducer is that it can be made to image in an arc by sequential firing of different groups of crystals. Such a transducer is classified as a sector scanner. A sector scanner has an important advantage over a linear array transducer in that it offers a wider field of view while having a relatively small footprint.

Biplane versus Endfire Transducers: Transrectal ultrasound transducers are available in sector, linear array, or endfire configurations. In order to image the prostate in the transverse plane, one must have a sector transducer because of the small cross-sectional area of the rectum. Since the prostate and the rectum are relatively long organs, a linear array transducer is useful to image these organs in the longitudinal plane. A biplane transducer combines a sector scanner and a linear array scanner in one transducer (Fig. 12.2.3). It allows precise imaging of both the transverse and longitudinal axis of the prostate without physically replacing the transducer.

An endfire transducer is a sector scanner in which the crystals are located at the tip of the instrument. It can be used to image the prostate in both transverse and longitudinal planes by rotating the transducer along its own axis (Fig. 12.2.4). This affords the endfire transducer great utility in biopsy guidance. However, it is critical that one be aware of a shortcoming of endfire transducers. Specifically, the two imaging planes for an endfire transducer are not truly orthogonal to each other. This makes placement of needles and cryogenic probes difficult and less precise. Therefore, endfire transducers should not be used in cryoablation. The physician's ultrasound instrumentation for cryoablation will typically include an endfire transducer for biopsy and staging of diseases, and a biplane transducer containing linear and sector crystals for the cryoablation procedure.

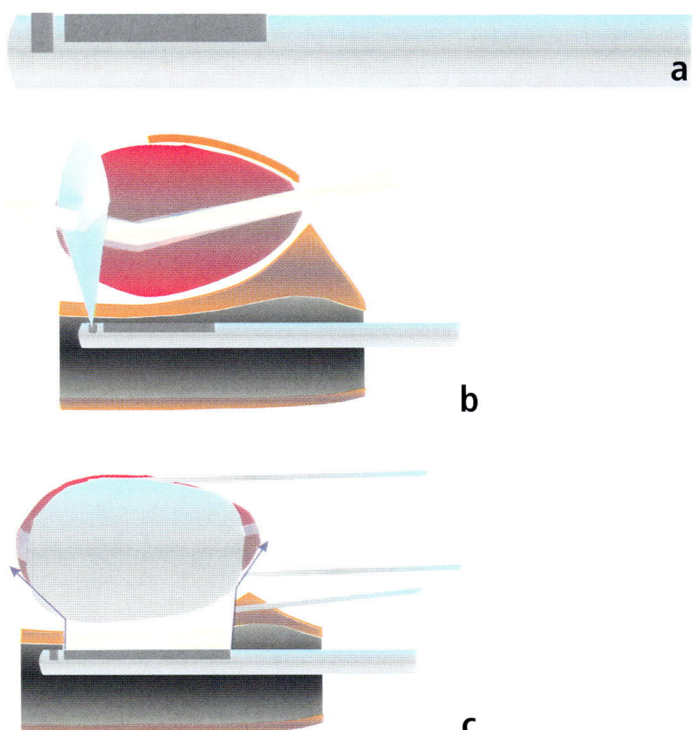

Fig. 12.2.3. **a** Biplane transrectal ultrasound transducer that incorporates both sector and linear arrays. The transverse sector (**b**) provides a transaxial view of the prostate gland. The prostate gland is examined by pushing the transducer in and out of the patient's rectum. Note that this crystal is not of the endfire configuration utilized in prostate biopsy. Reliable imaging of the gland in the axial plane during cryosurgery can only be achieved with a sector type crystal. The longitudinal component (**c**) is a linear array transducer. The gland is examined in the sagittal plane by rotating the transducer along its long axis

Transducer Frequency: Attenuation refers to the loss of strength of the acoustic waves as they travel through a medium. As ultrasound frequency increases, tissue attenuation increases. Thus, higher frequency transducers will permit higher resolution, and thus sharper images. However, increased resolution comes at the expense of depth of penetration. A higher-frequency transducer will create

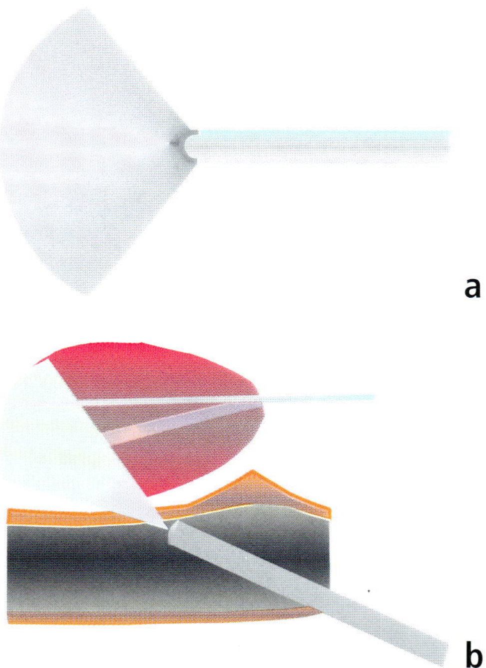

Fig. 12.2.4. a Endfire transducer. An endfire transducer is comprised of a sector type crystal located at the tip of the transducer. It can be used to image the prostate in both transverse and longitudinal planes (**b**) by rotating the transducer along its own axis. However, this instrumentation is prone to image distortion and does not enable the length of the gland to be visualized in a single image. This type of transducer is insufficient for prostate cryoablation

images that lose sharpness as depth increases. The desirable frequencies for cryoablation are 5 MHz in the sector transducer and 7.5 MHz in the linear transducer.

Color Doppler and Power Doppler: One of the major developments in the field of ultrasound is Doppler imaging. This modality has permitted the investigation of flow pattern in vascular systems in the human body. Unfortunately, Doppler imaging has not provided a useful addition to the cryoablation procedure to date. One suggested use of color Doppler imaging in cryoablation of the prostate is to identify blood flow in the rectal wall and thus allow for better monitoring of the freezing process. It is thought that this may prevent overfreezing the rectum during cryoablation. A second possible use of Doppler imaging is in the evaluation of neurovascular bundle areas. However, several critical technical factors prohibit Doppler from being of utility in this regard. First, the blood flow to and around the rectum and the neurovascular bundle areas tend to be perpendicular to the beams of the transducer, making Doppler less sensitive to flow of blood. Hence, Doppler is only able to detect blood flow around the rectum less than 50 to 60% of the time. The detection is not consistent and not uniform enough around the rectum to make this reliable. Second, shadowing by the ice ball (reflective and refractive) also blocks any ultrasound signals including Doppler signals. Like conventional gray-scale ultrasound, Doppler ultrasound cannot gather information beyond the freeze front. Third, any tissue movement or movement of the transducer will cause "flash" artifacts which may be confused with real blood flow, thereby leading to potentially serious inaccuracies. Finally, one must have an excellent command of the Doppler physics, i.e., pulse repetition frequency, phase, gate width, wall filtering, etc., in order to set the scanner properly to detect blood flow. These settings must be changed constantly in order to meet the changing condition of the freezing process.

12.2.4 Contemporary Cryoablation

Due to the shortcomings of ultrasound used alone, a combination of ultrasound and temperature monitoring was developed (9, 49). Briefly, clinical investigations of this revised technique revealed that the nadir temperatures within the ice ball, as reported by temperature sensors deployed to anatomic locations not visualized by ultrasound, as well as repeated freeze-thaw cycles, correlated to PSA and biopsy outcome data (9, 22, 23, 49). These studies strongly suggest that the use of ultrasound in combination with temperature monitoring to targeted lethal temperatures (−40°C), and a double freeze-thaw cycle represents an exciting and promising avenue of treatment in contemporary cryoablation (Figs. 12.2.5–12.2.7). Targeted cryoablation appears to be associated with promising outcomes, as well as minimal morbidity (Tables 12.2.1–12.2.2).

12.2.5 Indications and Patient Selection for Cryoablation

As a potentially curative therapy, cryoablation is offered primarily for patients with localized disease (stages T1-T3). Cryoablation is an option in patients considering radical prostatectomy, external beam therapy, or brachytherapy. As with all treatment options, the greater the stage of the disease, the higher the likelihood of failure. Patients with known seminal vesicle involvement (T3) have been treated with cryoablation, but may have higher failure rates. As with radical prostatectomy and brachytherapy, pelvic lymph node dissection is recommended in patients with a PSA of 15 ng/ml or higher before treatment. In general, cryo-

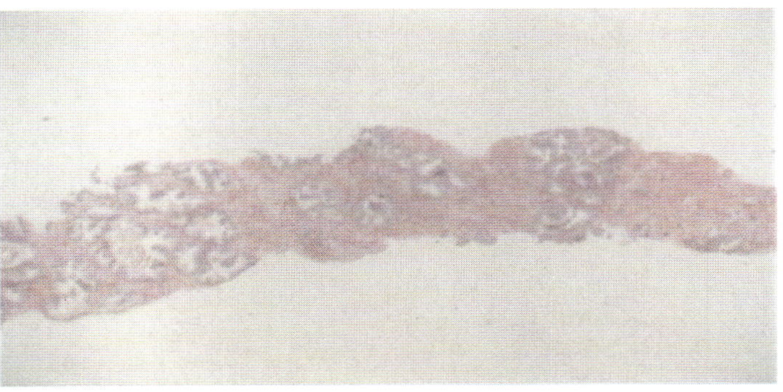

Fig. 12.2.5. Five year biopsy on a patient treated with cryoablation under TRUS guidance without temperature monitoring. The pathology shows normal prostate glandular tissue without cryosurgical effect

ablation is chosen by patients who do not desire, or who are not candidates for, radical prostatectomy. Patients usually choose cryoablation because it is a minimally invasive procedure with relatively quick recovery time, has a low incidence of incontinence, and can be repeated (2).

12.2.6 Targeted Cryoablation Technique

The goals of prostate cryoablation are the following: to freeze the entire prostate gland and beyond, to protect the prostatic urethra including the bladder neck and external sphincter, to avoid freezing through the rectal wall (fistula), and to preserve urinary continence. With these goals in mind, the technique required for successful targeted ablation have been refined (27).

12.2.7 Procedure Overview

The patient is placed in the dorsal lithotomy position, and the scrotum retracted away from the perineum, which defines the surgical field. Access to the prostate gland is achieved percutaneously, under transrectal ultrasound (TRUS) guidance. Cryoprobes are inserted percutaneously through small incisions in the perineum. The gland is examined using TRUS to determine the number and position of cryoprobes to be used. Detailed placement planning is described below. Prior to advancing the cryoprobes themselves, tracks must be created, and the thermocouples and urethral warmer are placed.

Using the Seldinger technique, tracks for the cryoprobes are created. The dedicated coaxial access kit includes an 18-gauge diamond-tipped needle and trocar, a j-wire, and an 11 French dilator/sheath combination. The initial track is created by advancing the needle and trocar under TRUS guidance. Once the track has been defined, the needle is removed, and the j-wire advanced down the channel. The flexible j-tip will anchor the wire firmly in the prostatic tissue. The trocar is then removed, leaving the wire in place. The sheath and dilator are then advanced over the wire. The dilator and guidewire are then removed, leaving

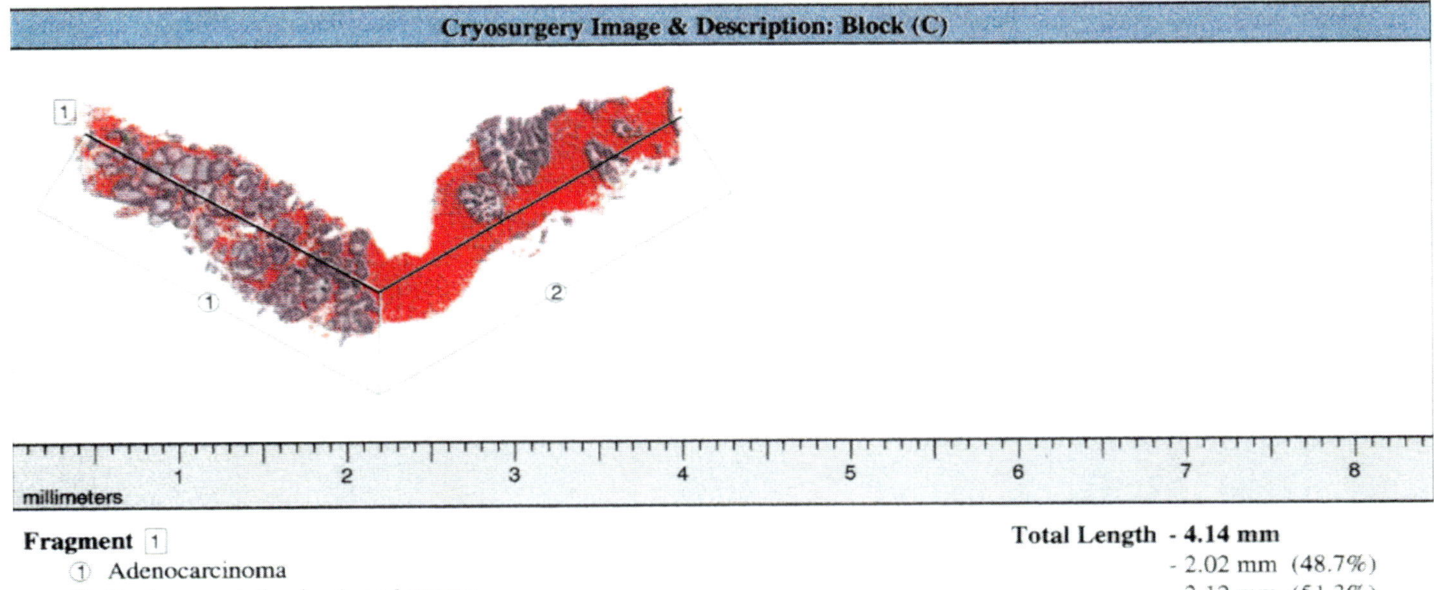

Fig. 12.2.6. Biopsy specimen for patient treated with a double freeze cycle to a target temperature higher than −40°C. Both residual prostate cancer and normal benign glandular tissue are identified in the biopsy

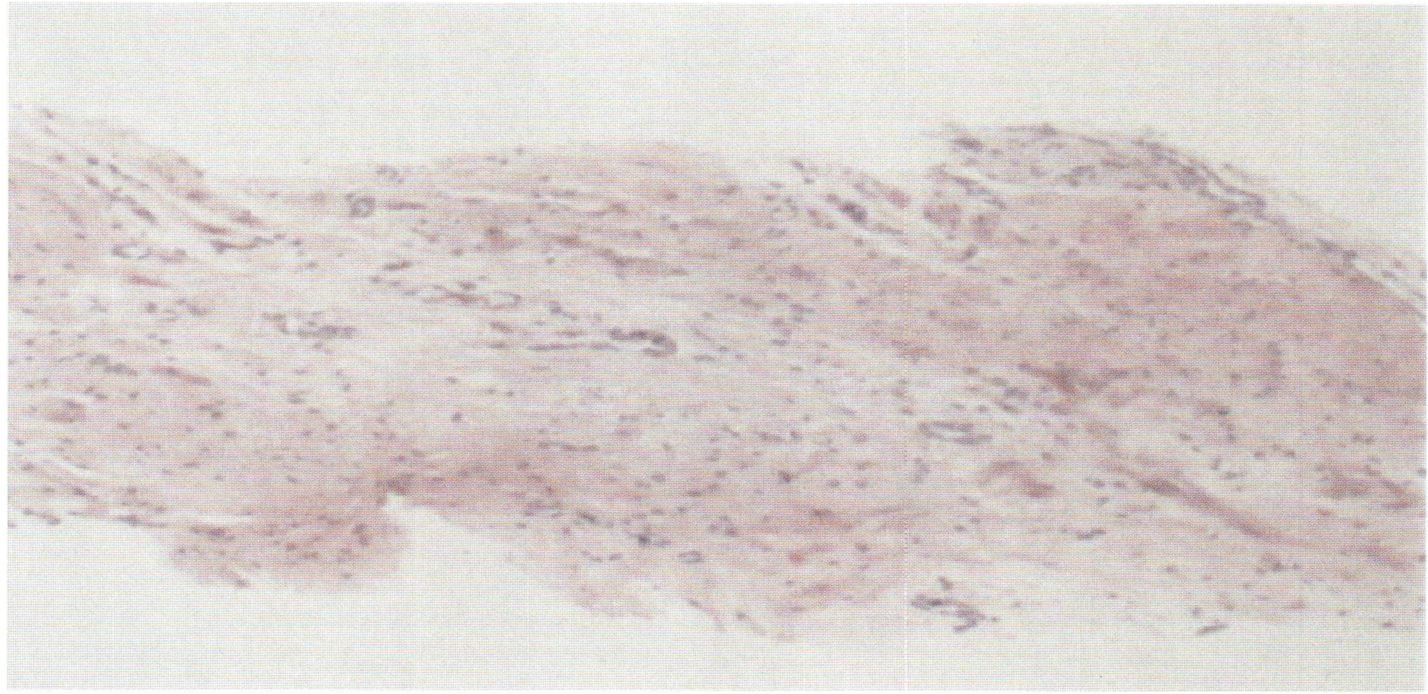

Fig. 12.2.7. Biopsy from a patient treated with cryoablation under combined TRUS and temperature monitoring. The treatment protocol included a double freeze with confirmation of target temperatures of −40°C. There is no evidence of residual adenocarcinoma, nor is there any residual normal prostate tissue present

the 11 French sheath in place to accept the cryoprobe.

Thermocouples are next placed in strategic locations surrounding the gland. These include right and left neurovascular bundles, Denonvillier's fascia, gland apex, and the external sphincter. Additional thermocouples may be placed at the physician's discretion.

A warming catheter is now advanced retrograde into the bladder via the urethra. This catheter is comprised of a closed system within which warmed saline is circulated to protect the bladder neck, prostatic urethra, and external sphincter.

Finally, the cryoprobes themselves are advanced down the sheaths. Cryoprobe placement planning is a critical step affecting the result of the procedure. The prostate gland volume should ideally be less than 35 cc in volume. Neoadjuvant hormone therapy is recommended to downsize larger glands. For glands within the recommended size, six cryoprobes are sufficient for treatment. For larger glands that do not respond to hormone therapy, or cases of seminal vesicle involvement, additional cryoprobes may be utilized [PG1]. The advanced technique required for treatment of such cases is beyond the scope of this chapter. The placement procedure for routine cryoablation is described below.

Table 12.2.1. Primary targeted cryoablation outcomes: PSA and biopsy

Authors	No.	% Negative biopsy	Mean PSA
Chinn (10)	93	94	0.30
Lee et al. (26)	163	96	0.12

12.2.8 Cryoprobe Placement

All cryoprobes enter at the apex of the gland. This ensures that the ice will encompass the apex without freezing the external sphincter. The pos-

Table 12.2.2. Complications following targeted cryoablation

Authors	No.	Incontinence (%)	Bladder outlet obstruction (%)	Rectal injury* (%)	Impotence (%)
Chinn (9)	93	2	3	0	100
Badalament et al. (2)	267	4.3	10	0	85
Lee et al. (25)	163	2	7	0.33	91

* Primary therapy

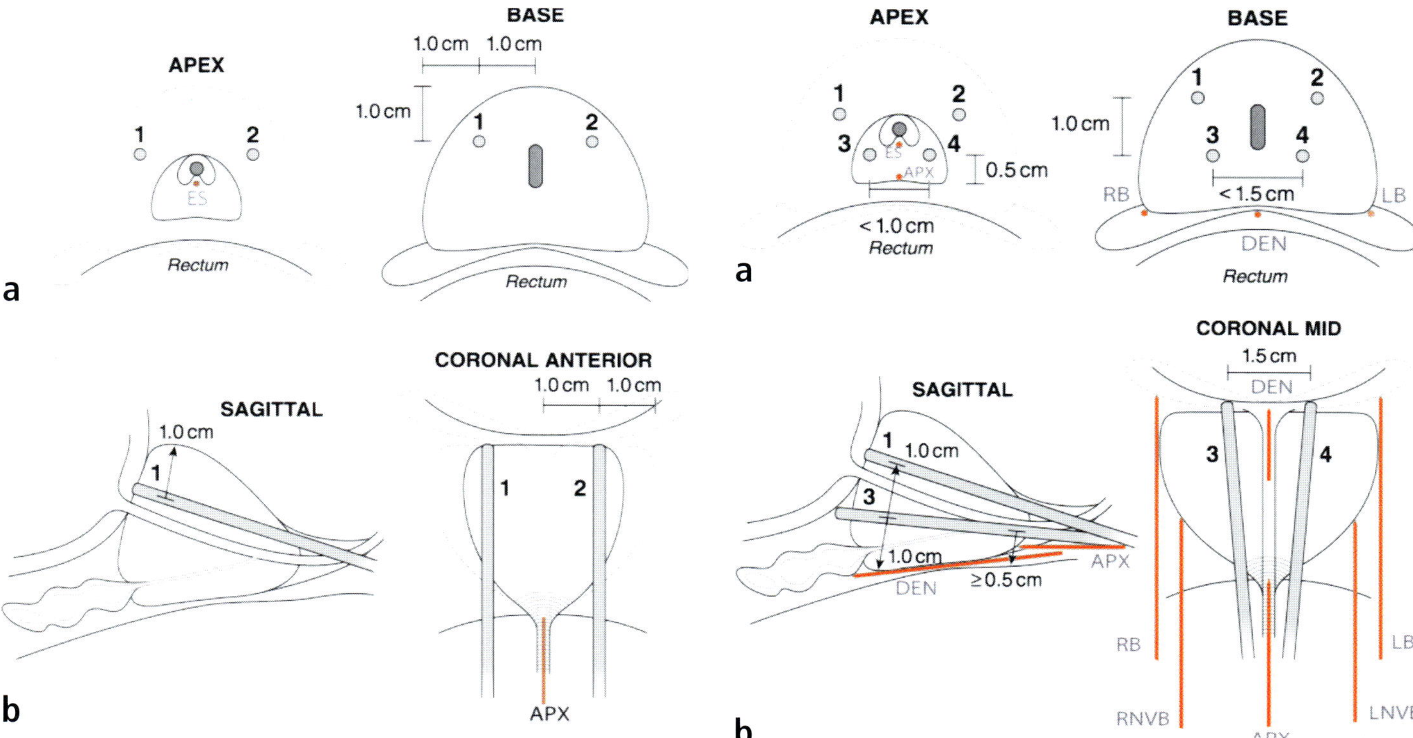

Fig. 12.2.8. a Insertion of the anterior-medial cryoprobes (1&2), axial projection. **b** Insertion of the anterior-medial cryoprobes (1&2), sagittal and coronal projection. Thermocouple placement (red line) is also demonstrated

Fig. 12.2.9. a Insertion of the posterior-medial cryoprobes (3&4), axial projection. Placement of the thermocouples (red dots) is also demonstrated. **b** Insertion of the posterior-medial cryoprobes (3&4), sagittal and coronal projection. Thermocouple placement (red lines) is also demonstrated

terior cryoprobes are flared laterally from apex to base, following the geometry of the gland.

Placement of Anterior Cryoprobes (1 and 2): Cryoprobes 1 and 2 are placed 1 cm lateral to and at the same level as the external sphincter (Fig. 12.2.8a). The cryoprobes are advanced until the tips reach the base of the prostatic capsule (Fig. 12.2.8b). They are flared as they are advanced to the base, so that they are separated by 2 cm. In this fashion, they will be lateral to the urethra by 1 cm at the base. This will assure glandular ablation of the transition zone while preserving the integrity of the urethra. The distance of the cryoprobes to the edge of the prostatic capsule should be no more than 1 cm. A gland larger than 4 cm in diameter will not accommodate this placement strategy, and placement of additional cryoprobes will be necessary.

Placement of Midline Posterior Cryoprobes (3 and 4): The cryoprobes enter the apex 0.5 cm posterolateral to the urethra, and separated by no more than 1 cm from each other (Fig. 12.2.9a). This assures a safe distance from the muscularis propria of the anal sphincter. The cryoprobes are advanced, again flaring laterally, so that the tips are separated by no more than 1.5 cm at the base. The tips of cryoprobes 3 and 4 are advanced until they project through the prostatic capsule by 0.5 cm (Fig. 12.2.9b).

Placement of Posterolateral Cryoprobes (5 and 6): These cryoprobes enter the prostate just posterolateral to cryoprobes 3 and 4 (Fig. 12.2.10a). The distance from the prostate capsule at the apex should be no more than 0.5 cm. The cryoprobes are advanced, flaring and following the contour of the prostate gland, while maintaining a distance from the capsule of 0.5 cm. The tips of cryoprobes 5 and 6 are advanced until they extend through the prostate capsule by 0.5 cm (Fig. 12.2.10b).

12.2.9 Thermocouple Placements (Figs. 12.2.8–12.2.10)

All patients have temperature monitoring. This allows confirmation of ablative temperatures (−40°C) at the site of the temperature sensor. Both the axial and the sagittal ultrasound projections are used to properly assure 3-dimensional placement of thermocouples. The real time depiction of the temperatures (Endocare software) governs the

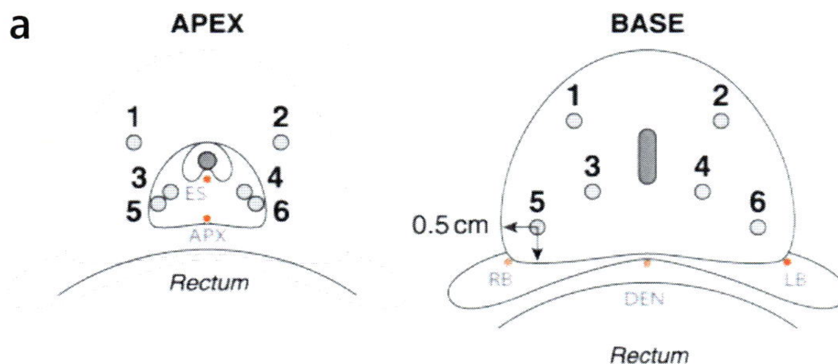

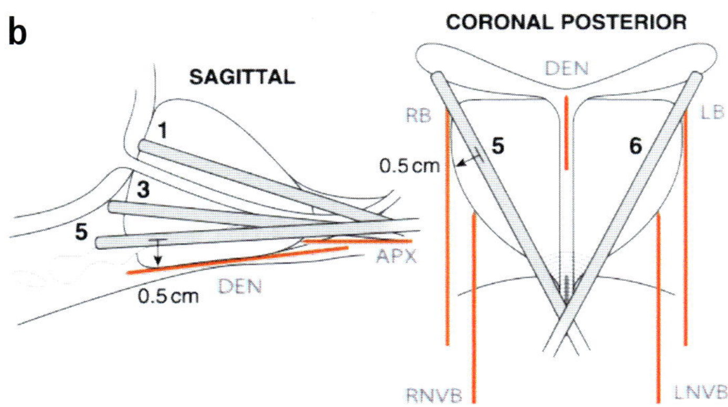

Fig. 12.2.10. a Insertion of the posterior-lateral cryoprobes (5&6), axial projection. Placement of the thermocouples (red dots) is also demonstrated. **b** Insertion of the posterior-lateral cryoprobes (5&6), sagittal and coronal projection. Thermocouple placement (red lines) is also demonstrated

cryoablation procedure. Thermocouples confirm the targeted temperature, and the slope of the temperatures curve delineates the velocity of ice ball growth.

1. External sphincter: The external sphincter thermocouple (ES) is placed in the midline of the posterior wall of the distal urethra at the level of urogenital diaphragm to monitor and prevent cryoinjury to the external sphincter (Figs. 12.2.8a, 12.2.9a).
2. Apex: Equidistant between cryoprobes 3 and 4, the apical thermocouple (APX) is positioned on the posterior prostatic capsule at the apex (Fig. 12.2.9a,b).
3. Denonvillier's fascia midline base: This thermocouple (DEN) is placed at midline base at the confluence of the seminal vesicles (Figs. 12.2.9 and 12.2.10).
4. Mid-gland neurovascular bundles: Mid-gland neurovascular bundle thermocouples (RNVB and LNVB) are placed at the midgland level, directly into the the neurovascular bundles on the lateral edge of the prostate (Figs. 12.2.9b, 12.2.10b).
5. Gland base: These thermocouples (RB and LB) are placed at the lateral edge of the gland, but all the way to the base, opposite the tips of cryoprobes 5–6 (Figs. 12.2.9b, 12.2.10b).

Cryoprobe Activation: The cryoprobes are activated in an anterior to posterior sequence, sculpting the ice to encompass the prostate gland and surrounding adventitia. The ice is sculpted to fit the geometry of the gland, and until the thermocouples outside of the gland (LB, LNVB, DEN, APX, RB and RNVB) reach −40°C. TRUS is utilized both to monitor ice growth and to prevent encroachment into the rectal wall. Temperature monitoring is used to confirm that lethal temperatures within the target area have been achieved, and also to confirm that the temperature at the external sphincter is maintained at or above 0°C throughout the procedure. The freeze protocol includes two freeze-thaw cycles.

Complete Glandular Thaw: After the first freeze cycle is completed, the cryoprobes are then placed into the "thaw" mode, utilized to thaw all of the ice that developed during the "freeze" mode. Before instituting the second freeze cycle, the positions of the cryoprobes and thermocouples are checked to make sure that they have not been accidentally displaced during the thaw mode.

Complications of Cryoablation: Patients recover remarkably well after cryoablation, with minimal pain medication requirements. The procedure can be performed either on an outpatient basis or as an overnight stay in the hospital. Most usual life activities can be resumed within seven to 10 days of the procedure. The most common complications associated with cryoablation are temporary urinary retention, impotence, mild urinary incontinence, and urethral slough (2,56).

Urinary Retention: The prostate swells dramatically after cryoablation creating outlet obstruction and transient urinary retention in virtually all patients. When the edema subsides, normal voiding will ensue. Retention may last from two to six weeks. A suprapubic catheter or a urethral Foley catheter may be placed in the patient, depending upon the surgeon's preference.

Impotence: The nerves responsible for creating erections are located in the neurovascular bundles, which course along the adventitia surrounding the prostate gland. Therefore, they will be engulfed when the ice ball is driven past the edge of the prostate and into the surrounding tissue. As a result, virtually all patients are impotent following the procedure. Many patients have had success with vacuum pump and injection therapies for impotence. This arena deserves further investigation. It is hoped that technique, technology, or concomitant medications may one day alleviate this complication. For now, as with any cancer treatment modality, each patient and physician must weigh the relative advantages and disadvantages of urological cryoablation.

Urinary Incontinence: Cryoablation is associated with low post-procedure urinary incontinence. A higher incidence of incontinence is reported in patients undergoing cryoablation following radiation failure. This will be discussed later in this chapter.

Bladder Outlet Obstruction: Bladder outlet obstruction can occur as a result of urethral slough. This complication occurs when the urethra is inadequately protected. The result is necrotic tissue of the prostatic urethra that occludes the urethra, causing various degrees of outlet obstruction.

Diagnosis and Treatment of Urethral Slough: A urethral slough typically manifests at four to six weeks post-procedure. Symptoms and degree of slough should be evaluated with cystoscopy. There are many treatment options available, depending upon the characteristics of the slough. Mild slough (Fig. 12.2.11) is treated expectantly and resolves spontaneously. Cases that do not resolve spontaneously may require Foley catheterization for two to four weeks until the slough passes. When catheterization does not suffice to alleviate the condition, more prolonged catheterization and/or a non-aggressive TURP (Fig. 12.2.12) may be required.

Rectal Injury: Careful technique and the use of thermocouples will minimize the possibility of rectal injury, and fortunately, this complication is rare. The entire prostate should be monitored using ultrasound as the freeze progresses towards the rectal wall. In addition, it is critical to observe the rectum carefully at the apex. At this area, the rectal wall is tented up and is thinner. Therefore, there is a smaller margin for freezing in this region and ultrasound is not as reliable, since the rectal wall is pulled away from the ultrasound probe. Patients must be instructed that they should not take any enemas or engage in any type of rectal manipulation after cryoablation.

Suspicion of rectal injury is raised by symptoms of watery stool, passing bubbles with urination, or fecal material in the urine. A Hypaque enema is the best conclusive test to diagnose rectal injury (Fig. 12.2.13). Small defects often will close spontaneously with a Foley catheter in place for 6 to 12 weeks. Large defects will require a temporary diverting colostomy, and probably transperineal closure.

12.2.10 Repeat Cryoablation

A distinct advantage held by cryoablation over other prostate cancer treatment options is that it can be repeated if necessary. Initial results are

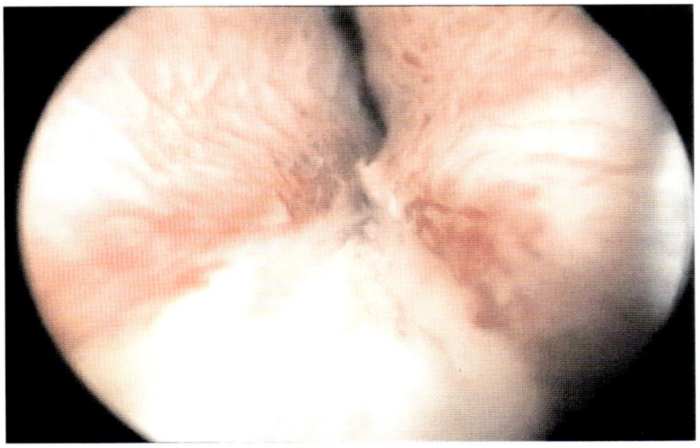

Fig. 12.2.11. Mild slough. Viable tissue is readily differentiated at cystoscopy from necrotic tissue injured by the freeze. The incomplete injury suggests that the slough will resolve spontaneosly. Treatment is expectant

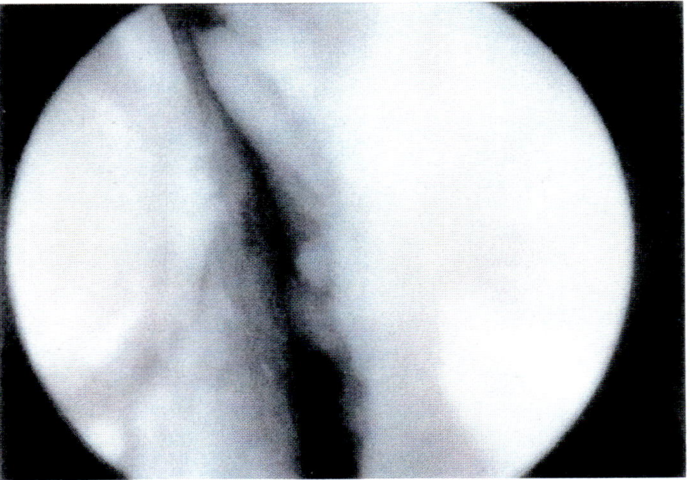

Fig. 12.2.12. Severe slough. The cystoscopy is characterized by circumferential necrosis. TURP will be required to resolve the obstruction

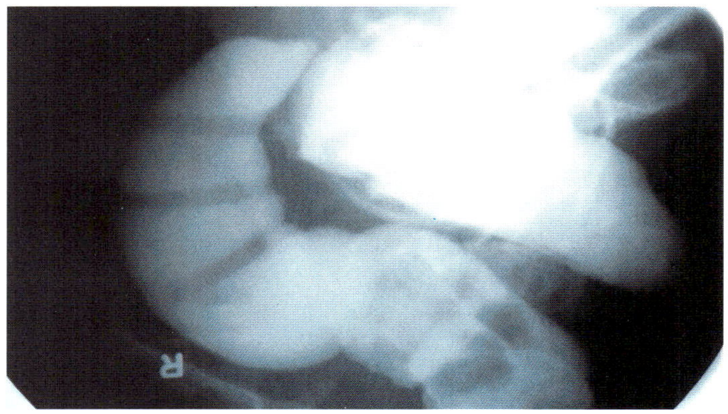

Fig. 12.2.13. Severe rectal injury. A Hypaque enema is the best method for diagnosis of urethrorectal fistula. This image demonstrates that contrast material has leaked into the bladder

excellent, and morbidity does not appear to increase with repeat procedures (31, 51, 56). Repeat cryoablation can be more difficult to perform due to dystrophic calcification of the gland, which creates acoustic shadows that impede ultrasound visualization. Fibrosis can also make access difficult. In repeat cryoablation, it is imperative for the surgeon to review the histopathology slides, because most of the gland is fibrotic. It is felt that only the areas of visibly viable prostatic tissue need to be treated.

12.2.11 Salvage Cryoablation

Cases of local recurrence following external beam or brachytherapy treatments have limited treatment options. The difficulty and high complication rate associated with salvage radical prostatectomy is well known (8,12,28,46). Salvage cryoablation following radiation failure offers patients an additional opportunity for potential cure. The morbidity rates associated with salvage cryoablation are lower than that with salvage radical prostatectomy (Table 12.2.3). As with salvage radical prostatectomy, cryoablation is most effective if performed on patients with early rising PSA's that are below 10 ng/ml (46). Proper staging and workup of these patients is critical to ensure selection of patients with localized disease. The procedure is more difficult to perform due to fibrosis caused by the radiation. The gland is smaller and more difficult to visualize. Biopsy outcomes for salvage cryoablation compare favorably to those for salvage radical prostatectomy (Table 12.2.3). Salvage cryoablation may provide a treatment advantage for patients failing radiation therapy, and desirous of intervention.

12.2.12 Conclusion

Cryoablation represents a vital treatment option for prostate cancer therapy. Patients who choose not to receive radical surgery or who are not good candidates for radical surgery, are appropriate candidates for this procedure. Morbidity is low compared to other treatment modalities, and continues to decrease with experience and equipment evolution. Although impotence remains a usual result of cryoablation, the ability of cryoablation to ablate cancerous tissue with fewer post-operative complications makes this procedure an appealing treatment option. For failed radiotherapy patients, cryoablation offers additional hope for cure. Disease-free survival rates are comparable to those with salvage radical prostatectomy, with lower associated morbidity and shorter hospital stays. Therefore, the minimal invasiveness, repeatability, low morbidity, and quick recovery time, coupled with excellent efficacy, all contribute to make cryoablation an attractive and viable therapeutic option in the battle against prostate cancer.

References

1. Ahlering TE, Lieskovsky G, Skinner DG. Salvage surgery plus androgen deprivation for radioresistant adenocarcinoma. J Urol 1992; 147: 900–902.
2. Badalament, R.A., Bahn, D.K., Kim, H., Kumar, A., Bahn, J.M., Lee, F. Patient-reported complications after cryoablation therapy for prostate cancer. Urology 1999; 54(2): 295–300.
3. Bahn, D.K., Lee, F., Solomon, M.H., Gontina, H., Klionsky, D.L., Lee, F.T. Jr., Prostate cancer, US-guided percutaneous cryoablation. Radiology 1994, 190(2): 551–556.
4. Bischof, J.C., Smith, D., Pazhayannur, P.V., Manivel, C., Hulbert, J., Roberts, K.P. Cryosurgery of dunning AT-1 rat prostate tumor:

Table 12.2.3. Outcomes and complications: salvage cryoablation *versus* salvage radical prostatectomy

Procedure	No. of patients	Mean incontinence rate (%)	Mean rectal injuries (%)	Bladder outer obstruction (%)	Negative margin on biopsy (%)
Salvage cryosurgery 8,9,12,13,26,36,43	379	24	3	15	73
Salvage radical prostatectomy 1,28,29,37,39,44,45,48,57	260	37	10	20	59

thermal, biophysical, and viability response at the cellular and tissue level. Cryobiology 1997; 34: 42–69.

5. Bonney, W.W., Fallon, B., Gerber, W.L., Hawtrey, C.E., Loening, S.A., Narayana A.S., Platz, C.E., Rose, E.F., Sall, J.C., Schmidt, J.D., Culp, D.A. Cryosurgery in prostatic cancer: survival. Urology 1982; 19: 37–42.
6. Brandt, B., Hibon, J. Lemaire, Ph., Domina, D., Lardennois, B. Ultrasonography and cryosurgery of the prostate. Cryotherapy 1985; 7.
7. Brenner, P.C., Russo, P., Wood, D.P. Salvage radical prostatectomy in the management of locally recurrent prostate cancer after 125-I implantation. Br J Urol 1994; 75: 44–47.
8. Cepedes, R.D., Pister, L.L., von Eschenbach, A.C., McGuire, E.J. Long-term follow-up of incontinence and obstruction after salvage cryosurgical ablation of the prostate: results in 143 patients. J Urol 1997; 157: 237–240.
9. Chin, J.L., Downey, D.B., Mulligan, M., Fenster, A. Three-dimensional transrectal ultrasound guided cryoablation for localized prostate cancer in nonsurgical candidates: a feasibility study an report of early results. J Urol 1998; 159: 910–914.
10. Chinn, D. Prostate cryosurgery: scientific and technical advancements. Urology News 1999; 3(4): 10–12.
11. Cohen, J.K., Miller, R.J., Rooker, G.M., Shuman, B.A. Cryosurgical ablation of the prostate: Two year prostatic specific antigen and biopsy results. J Urology 1996; 47: 395–401.
12. Corral, D.A., Pister, L.L., von Eschenbach, A.C. Treatment options for localized recurrence of prostate cancer following radiation therapy. Urol Clin North Am 1996; 23: 677–684.
13. De La Taille, A., Hayek, O., Benson, M.C., Bagiella, E., Olsson, C.A., Katz, A.E. Salvage therapy for recurrent prostate cancer after radiation therapy: the columbia experience. Urology 2000; 55(1): 79–84.
14. De La Taille, A., Benson, M.C., Bagiella, E., Burchardt, M., Shabsigh, A., Olsson, C.A., Katz, A.E. Cryoablation for clinically localized prostate cancer using an argon-based system: complication rates and biochemical recurrence. BJU International 2000; 85: 281–286.
15. Farrant, J., and Walter, C.A. The cryobiological basis for cryosurgery. J Dermatol Surg Oncol 1977; 3: 403–407.
16. Flocks, R.H. , Nelson, C.K., Boatman, D.L. Perineal cryosurgery for prostatic carcinoma. J Urol 1972; 108: 933–935.
17. Fowler, F.J., Barry M.J., Lu-Yao, Roman, A., Wasser, J., Wennberg, J.E. Patient-reported complications and follow-up treatment after radical prostatectomy. The national Medicare experience 1988–1990 (updated June 1993). Urology 1993; 42: 622–629.
18. Gondor, M.J., Soanes, W.A., Shulman, S. Cryosurgical treatment of the prostate. Investig Urol 1966; 3: 372–375.
19. Grampsas, S.A., Miller, G.J., Crawford, E.D. Salvage radical prostatectomy after failed transperineal cryotherapy: histologic findings from prostate whole-mount specimens correlated with intraoperative transrectal ultrasound images. Urology 1995; 45(6): 936–941.
20. Gursel, E., Roberts, M., Veenema, R.J. Regression of prostatic cancer following sequential cryotherapy to the prostate. J Urol 1972; 108: 928–932.
21. Jønler, M., Ritter, M.A., Brinkman, R., Messing, E.M., Rhodes, P.R., Bruskewi, R.C. Sequelae of definitive radiation therapy for prostate cancer localized to the pelvis. Urology 1994; 44: 876–882.
22. Jordan W.P., Walker D., Miller Jr., G.H., Drylie D.M. Cryotherapy of benign and neoplastic tumors of the prostate. Surg Gyn & Ob, 1967; 1265–1268.
23. Koppie, T.M., Shinohara, K., Grossfield, G.D., Presti Jr., J.C., Carroll, P.R. The efficacy of cryosurgical ablation of prostate cancer: The University of California, San Francisco experience. J Urol 1999; 162: 427–432.
24. Larson, T.R., Robertson, D.W., Corica, A., Bostwick, D.G. In vivo interstitial temperature mapping of the human prostate during cryosurgery with correlation to histopathologic outcomes. Urology 2000; 55(4): 547–552.
25. Lee, F., Bahn, D.K., McHugh, T.A., Onik, G.M., Lee, Jr., F.T. How I do it. US-guided percutaneous cryoablation. Radiology 1994; 192: 769–776.
26. Lee, F., Bahn, D.K., McHugh, T.A., Kumar, A.A., Badalament, R.A. Cryosurgery of prostate cancer: use of adjuvant hormonal therapy and temperature monitoring-a one year follow-up. Anticancer Res 1997; 17: 1511–1516.
27. Lee, F., Bahn, D., Badalament, R., Kumar, A., Klionsky, D., Onik, G., Chinn, D., Greene, C. Cryosurgery for prostate cancer: improved glandular ablation by use of 6–8 cryoprobes. Urology 1999; 54(1): 135–140.
28. Lerner, S.E., Blute, M.L., Zincke, H. Critical evaluation of salvage surgery for radio-recurrent/resistant prostate cancer. J Urol 1995; 154: 1103–1109.
29. Link, P., Freiha, F.S. Radical prostatectomy after definitive radiation therapy for prostate cancer. Urology 1991; 37: 189–192.
30. Loening, S., Lubraoff, D. Cryosurgery and immunotherapy for prostatic cancer. Urol Clin North Am 1984; 11: 327–336.
31. Long, J.P., Fallick, J.L., LaRock, D.R., Rand, W. Preliminary outcomes following cryosurgical ablation of the prostate in patients with clinically localized prostate carcinoma. J Urol 1998; 159: 477–484.
32. Mazur P. Causes of injury in frozen and thawed cells. Fed Proc 1965; 24 (2) part 3: S175–182.
33. Mazur, P. The role of intracellular freezing in the death of cells cooled at supraoptimal rates. Cryobiology, 1977; 14: 251–272.
34. McGrath, J.J., Cravalho, E.G. An experimental comparison of intracellular ice formation and freeze-thaw survival of Hela S-3 Cells. Cryobiology 1975; 12: 540–550.
35. Meryman, H. Mechanics of freezing in living cells and tissues. Science 1956; 124 (3221): 515–521.
36. Miller, Jr., R.J., Cohen, J.K., Shuman, B., Merlotti, L.A. Percutaneous, transperineal cryosurgery of the prostate as salvage therapy for post radiation recurrence of adenocarcinoma. Cancer 1996; 77: 1510–1514.
37. Moul, J.W., Paulson, D.F. The role of radical surgery in the management of radiation recurrent and large volume prostate cancer. Cancer 1991; 68: 1265–1271.
38. Neel III, H.B., Ketcham, A.S. Requisites for successful cryogenic surgery of cancer. Arch Surg 1971; 102: 45–48.
39. Neerhut, G.J., Wheeler, T., Cantini, M., Scardino, P.T. salvage radical prostatectomy for radiorecurent adenocarcinoma of the prostate. J Urol 1988; 140: 544–548.
40. Onik, G., Cobb, C., Cohen, J., Reyes, G.D., Rubinsky, B., Chang, Z., Baust, J. Transrectal ultrasound-guided percutaneous radical cryosurgical ablation of the prostate. Cancer 1993; 72(4): 1291–1298.
41. Patel, B.G., Parson, C.L., Bidair, J., Schmidt, J.D. Cryoablation for carcinoma of the prostate. J Surg Oncol 1996; 63: 256–264.
42. Petersen, D.S., Milleman, L.A., Rose, R.F., Bonney, W.W., Schmidt, J.D., Hawtrey, C.E., Culp, D.A. Biopsy and clinical course after cryosurgery for prostatic carcinoma. J Urol 1978; 120: 308–311.
43. Pisters, L.L., von Eschenbach, A.C., Scott, S.M., Swanson, D.C., Dinnery, C.P., Pettaway, C.R., Babaian, R.J. The efficacy and complications of salvage cryotherapy of the prostate. J Urol 1997; 157: 921–925
44. Pontes, J.E., Montie, J., Klein, E., Huben, R. Salvage surgery for radiation failure in prostate cancer. Cancer 1993; 71: 976–980.
45. Rewcastle JC, Sandison GA, Saliken JC, Donnelly BJ, McKinnon JG. Considerations during clinical operation of two commercially available cryomachines. J Surg Oncol 1999 Jun; 71(2): 106–11.
46. Rogers, E., Ohori, M., Kassabian, V.S., Wheeler, T.M., Scardino, P. Salvage radical prostatectomy: outcome measured serum prostate specific antigen levels. J Urol 1995; 153: 104–110.
47. Shinohara, K., Connolly, J.A., Presti, Jr., J.C., Carroll, P.R. Cryosurgical treatment of localized prostate cancer (Stages T1 to T4): preliminary results. J Urol 1996; 156: 115–121.
48. Shuman, B.A., Cohen, J.K., Miller, Jr., R.J. Rooker, C.M., Olson, P.R. Histological presence of viable prostatic glands on routine biopsy following cryosurgical ablation of the prostate. J Urol 1997; 157: 552–555.
49. Stein, A., Smith, R.B., deKernion, J.B. Salvage radical prostatectomy after failure of curative radiotherapy for adenocarcinoma of the prostate. Urology 1992; 40: 197–200.
50. Tatsutani, K., Rubinsky, B., Onik, G., Dahiya, R. Effect of thermal variables on frozen human primary prostatic adenocarcinoma cells. Urology, 1996; 48: 441–447.

51. Wake, R.W., Hollabaugh Jr., R.S., Bond, K.H. Cryosurgical ablation of the prostate for localized adenocarcinoma: a preliminary experience. 1996; 55: 1663–1666.
52. Weider, J., Schmidt, J.D., Casola, G., van Sonnenberg, E., Stainken, B.F., Parson, C.L. Transrectal ultrasound-guided transperineal cryoablation in the treatment of prostate carcinoma: preliminary results. J Urol 1995; 154: 435–441.
53. Whittaker, D.K. Ice crystals formed in tissue during cryosurgery, I. Light microscopy. Cryobiology 1974; 11: 192–201.
54. Whittaker, D.K. Ice crystals formed in tissue during cryosurgery, II. Electron microscopy. Cryobiology 1974; 11: 202–217.
55. Widmark, A., Fransson, P., Tavelin, B. Self-assessment questionnaire for evaluating urinary and intestinal late side effects after pelvic radiotherapy in patients with prostate cancer compared with a matched control population. Cancer 1994; 74(9): 2520–2532.
56. Wong, W.S., Chinn, D.O., Chinn, M., Chinn J., Tom W.L., Tom W.L. Cryosurgery as a treatment for prostate carcinoma, results and complications. Cancer 1997; 79: 963–974.
57. Yamada, S., Tsubouchi, S. Rapid cell death and cell population recovery in mouse skin epidermis after freezing. Cryobiology 1976; 13: 317–327.
58. Zincke, H. Radical prostatectomy and exenterative procedures for local failure after radiotherapy with curative intent: comparison of outcomes. J Urol 1992; 147: 894–899.

Suggested Reading: Ultrasound Physics

1. Chivers R.C., Parry, R.J. Ultrasonic velocity and attenuation in mammalian tissues. J Acoust Soc Am 1978; 63: 940–953.
2. Christensen, E.E., Curry, T.S., Dowdey, J.E. Ultrasound. In: An introduction to the physics of diagnostic radiology, 2nd edition. Lea & Febiger, Philadelphia, 1978; pp. 361–394.
3. Goss, S.A., Johnston, R.L., Dunn, F. Comprehensive compilation of empirical properties of mammalian tissues. J Acoust Soc Am 1978; 64: 423–457.
4. Kremkau, F.W., Allen. A. Diagnostic Ultrasound: Principles and Instruments. W B Saunders Co, Philadelphia. 1998
5. Merritt CRB: Physics of Ultrasound. In: Rumack, C.M., Wilson, S.R., Charboneau, J.W. eds. Diagnostic Ultrasound. Mosby, New York, 1998; pp..2–23.
6. Merritt, C.R.B. Doppler US: The basics. Radiographics, 1991; 11:109–119.

13. Breast Cryosurgery

13.1 Cryosurgery for Breast Cancer

Nikolai N. Korpan

13.1.1 Primary Breast Cancer: Initial Cryosurgical Development

Breast cancer is on the increase world-wide. Secondary manifestations such as metastasis and local recurrence by the spread of cancer cells during diagnostic or surgical interventions can signify the death sentence for the patient.

A new way of thinking about the problem must therefore determine the future of cancer research and treatment. New methods of diagnosis and treatment will increase the cure rate for this disease.

Mammotomy is a new method of clarifying suspicious foci in the breast.

Modern breast cryosurgery is at present just at the start of its medico-technical development as well as of its international regard and spread. Good results can, however, already be demonstrated. They have also shown that the successful use of this method is really only made possible by high-performance medico-technical devices.

The following shows how the development and production of a modern mammotomy-cryosurgical instrument for diagnosis, prevention and treatment of breast cancer could be developed.

The "Universal Cryosurgical Mammotome" (UCM) has been submitted as a national and world-wide patent in Austria and consists of two systems:

1) Mammotome – this is already in production
2) Stationary Cryosurgical System consisting of a unit plus instruments and cryoprobes.

This high-tech device was developed and put into use in record time on the basis of our own know-how as well as on the basis of international theoretical, experimental and clinical knowledge in the area of mammotomic cryosurgery.

The subcutaneous cryosurgical operation for treatment of breast cancer is at present being researched and put into surgical practice (Figs. 13.1.1–13.1.10). Early clinical experience shows a good cure rate with a high quality of life.

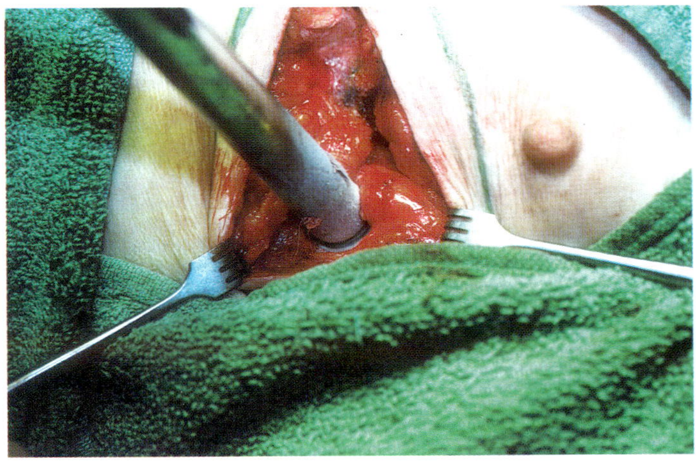

Fig. 13.1.1. Primary breast cancer on the left side in a 73-year-old woman. Infiltrating lobular carcinoma, mixed type (degree 1/2), clinical staging: pT2, pN0, pM0, tumor stage IIA. The technique is breast subcutaneous cryosurgery (BSC); shown is a disc probe and the rim of the cryozone, which forms the demarcation line between cryonecrosis and the healthy breast tissue. First cryosurgical session, using local anesthesia, with a disc cryoprobe with a diameter of 30 mm, which is placed on the tumor mass at a temperature of −180°C

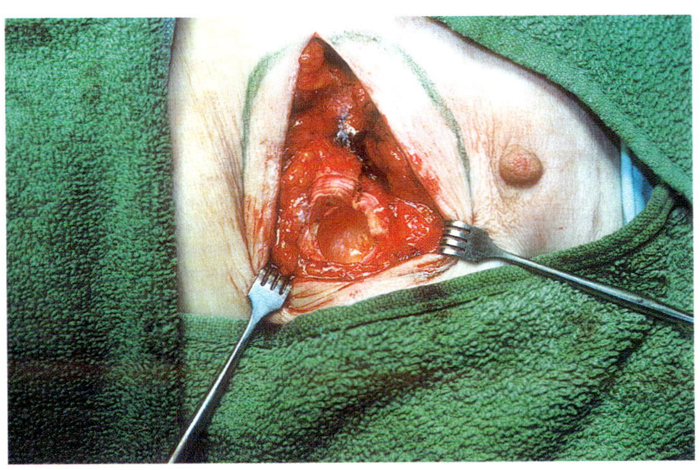

Fig. 13.1.2. BSC: The same patient. The formed post-cryosurgical zone is clearly circumscribed by a demarcation line

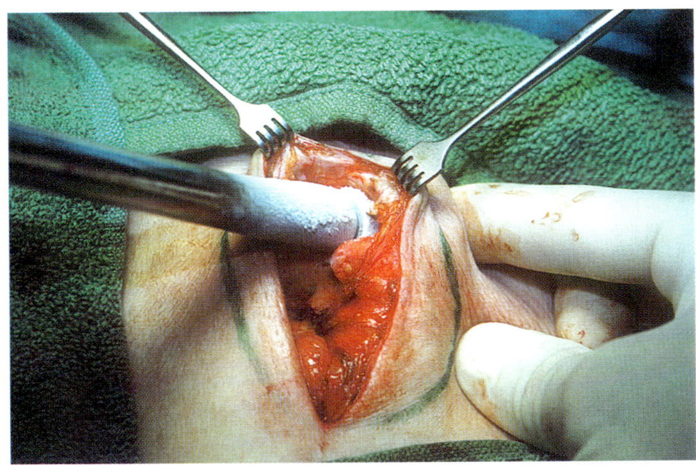

Fig. 13.1.3. BSC: The same patient. A second freeze-thaw cycle using the same disc cryoprobe (diameter of 30 mm at a temperature of −180°C)

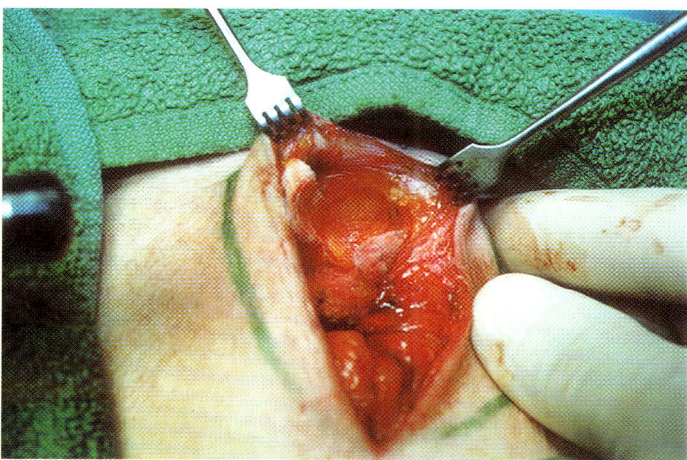

Fig. 13.1.4. BSC: The same patient. View of the post-cryosurgical zone after the second cryosurgical session immediately after the thaw of the cryoprobe

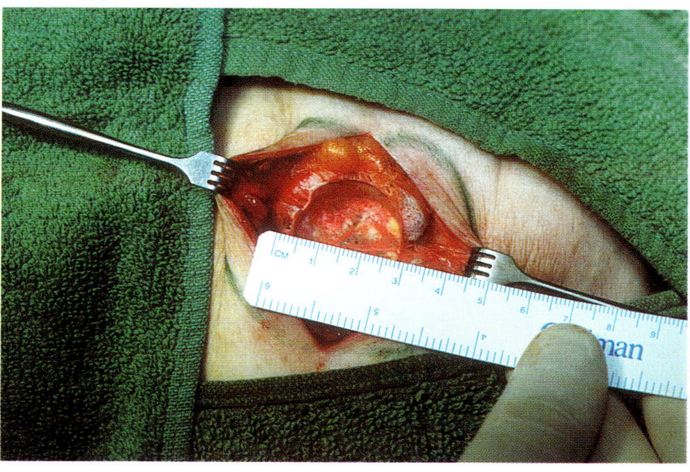

Fig. 13.1.5. BSC: The same patient. The post-cryosurgical zone measures 36 mm in diameter immediately after the thaw of the cryoprobe

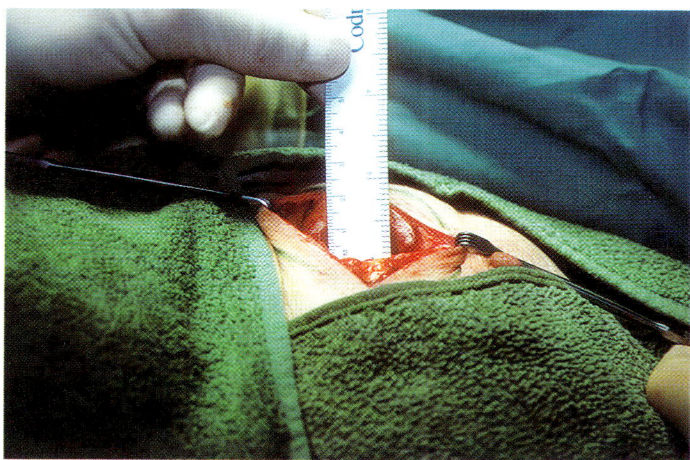

Fig. 13.1.6. BSC: The same patient. The post-cryosurgical zone measures 20 mm in depth immediately after the thaw of the cryoprobe. No postoperative bleeding

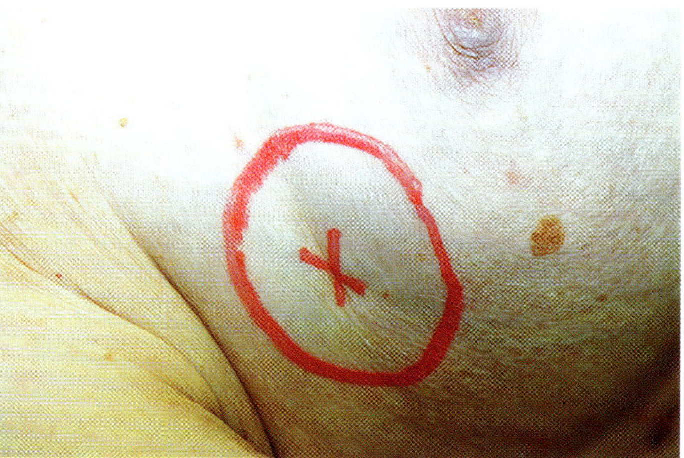

Fig. 13.1.7. Primary breast cancer on the right side in a 49-year-old woman. Breast subcutaneous cryosurgery (BSC): The breast lesion is preoperatively marked on the skin with the help of breast ultrasound

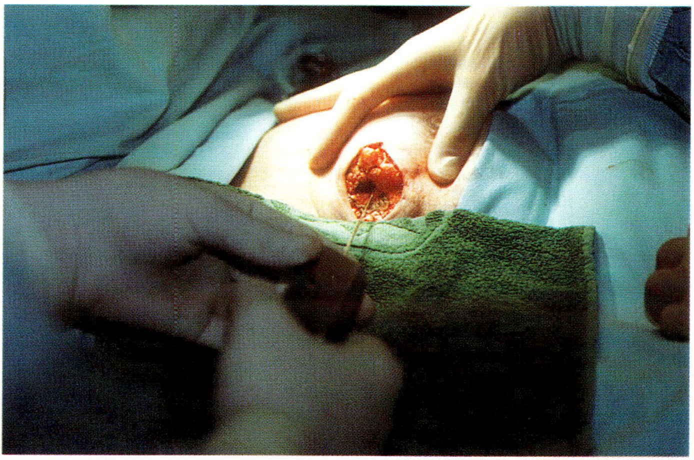

Fig. 13.1.8. BSC: Breast intraoperative biopsy (BIB) in the same patient under local anesthesia. This is a diagnostic tool used to evaluate and verify the breast tumor. The standard instrument for BIB - intraoperative tumor core-cutting needle biopsy - is the Tru-Cut (Bard-Magnum). Histological report: Invasive duct carcinoma, mixed type (degree 1), clinical staging: pT2, pN0, pM0, tumor stage IIA

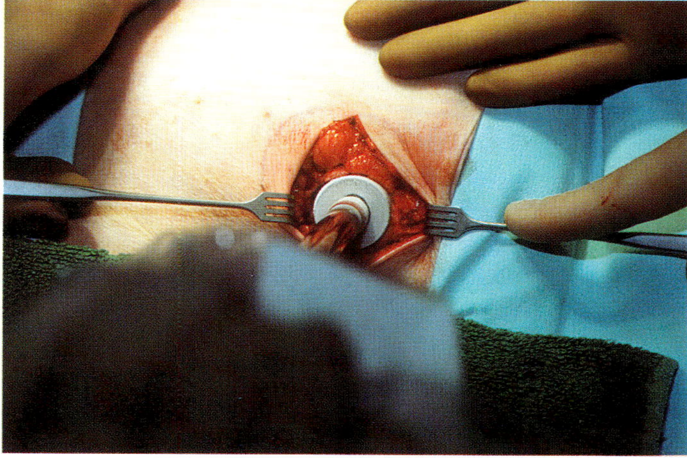

Fig. 13.1.9. BSC, which is continued under local anesthesia: The cryoprobe, 40 mm in diameter, is directed into the center of the lesion under direct vision at a temperature of −180°C for 7 minutes

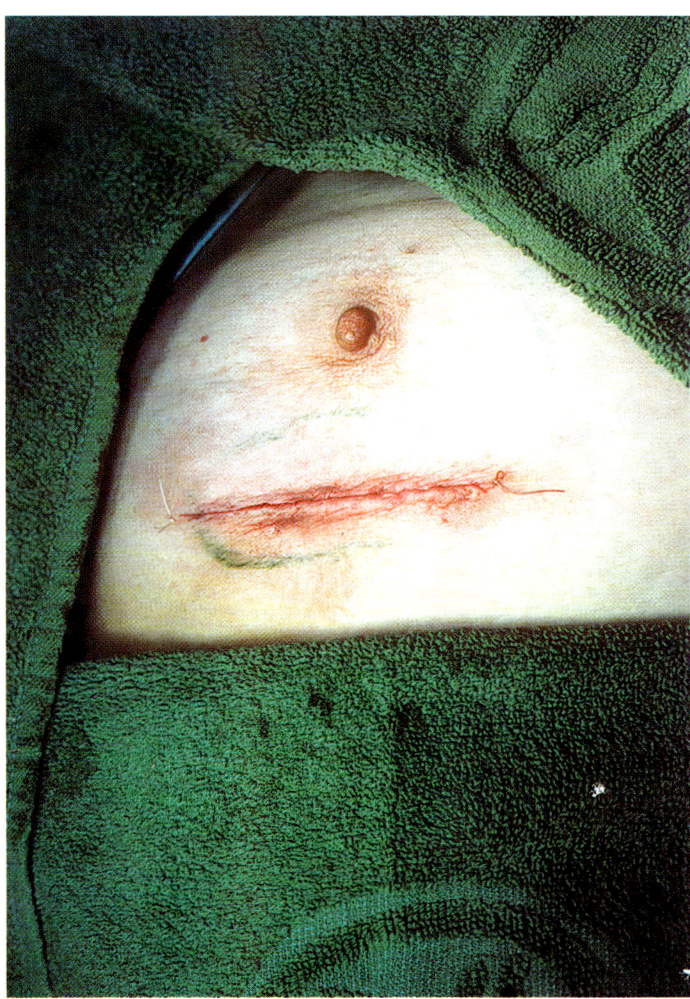

Fig. 13.1.10. BSC: Final local appearance, immediately after the cryosurgical treatment. View of the post-cryosurgical wound. No postoperative bleeding

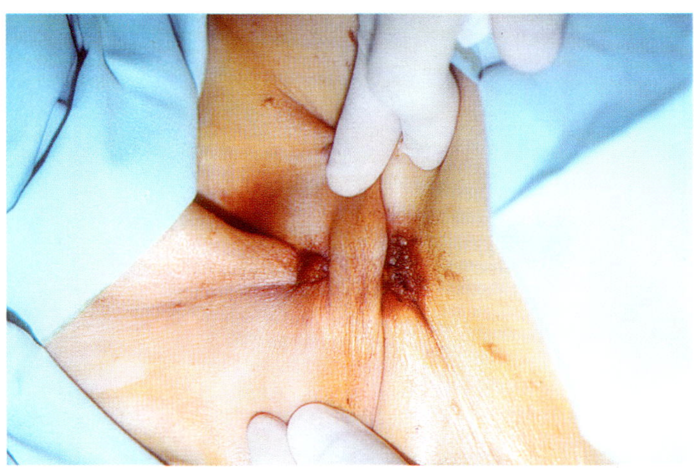

Fig. 13.1.11. Local-regional disease recurrence: Local-regional recurrence of breast cancer (cutaneous late recurrence of the infiltrating lobular carcinoma, mixed type (degree 1/2), clinical staging: pT3, pN1, pM0, tumor stage IIB) in a 78-year-old woman. Chest wall and skin overlying the involved chest wall after mastectomy. Preoperative view

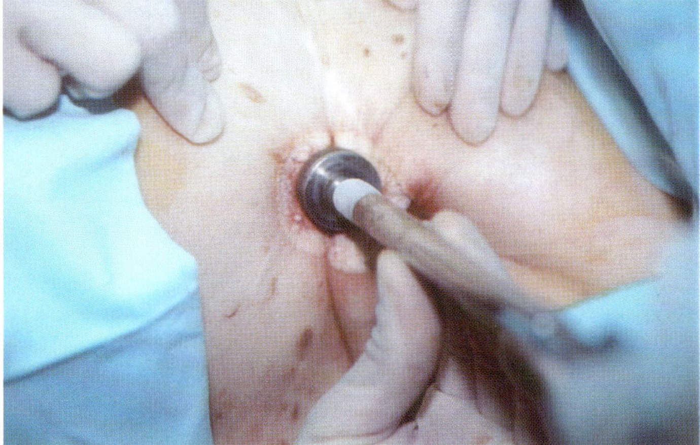

Fig. 13.1.12. Local-regional recurrence of breast cancer in the same patient. Breast cancer cryosurgery (BCC): Method of Application. The cryoprobe is applied on the recurrent breast lesion with involved skin at a temperature of −180°C for 7 min and a double freeze-thaw cycle is started without local or general anesthesia. Two treatment freeze-thaw cycles are usually needed

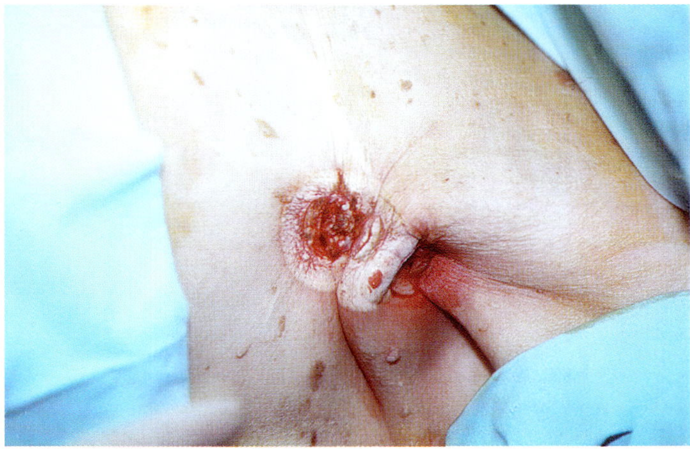

Fig. 13.1.13. The same patient. Base view of the post-cryosurgical zone immediately after the thawing of the cryoprobe. The rim of the cryozone forms a clear line of demarcation between the area that was cryosurgically destroyed, and which was followed by cryogenic necrosis, and the healthy skin. No postoperative bleeding

After preoperative breast marking (Fig. 13.1.7) the skin is incised and the tumorous lesion is exposed and removed. Biopsy is taken intraoperatively (Fig. 13.1.8) followed by two cycles of subcutaneous cryosurgery (Fig. 13.1.9). The operation is normally ended without a drain and the wound is closed by intracutaneous suture (Fig. 13.1.10).

13.1.2 Local Recurrence After Breast Cancer Surgery

One of the most effective surgical methods in patients with recurrences after surgery is surely the cryosurgical intervention.

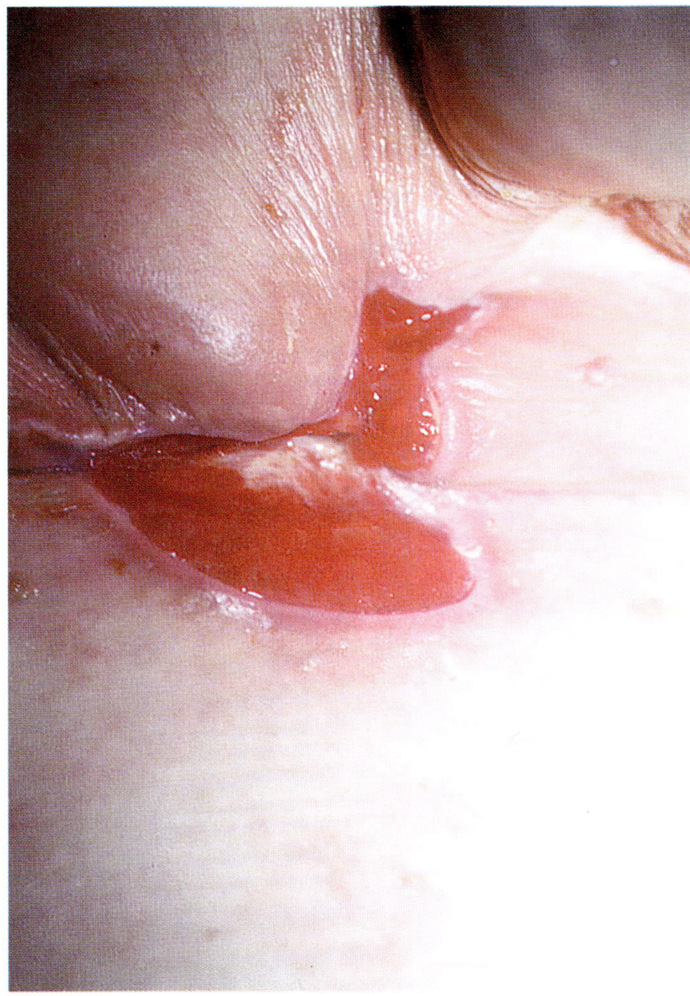

Fig. 13.1.14. BCC: Base view of the post-cryosurgical zone in the same patient: Wound healing. 8 weeks after cryosurgical treatment

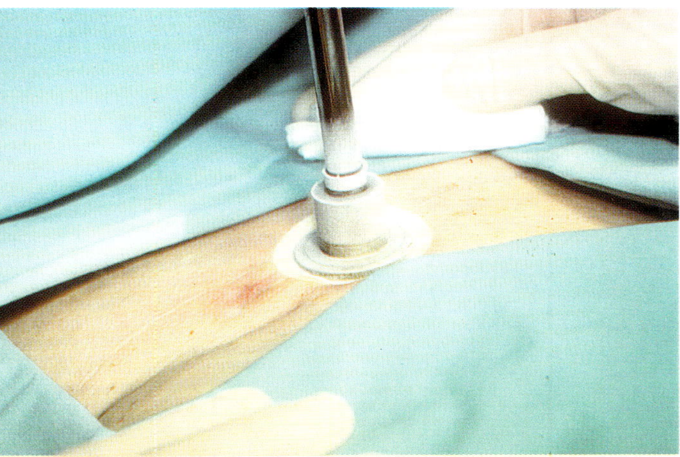

Fig. 13.1.16. Breast cancer: 69-year-old woman with multiple skin metastases after conventional breast cancer surgery, 9 months after right-sided mastectomy. Breast cancer cryosurgery (BCC): Method of Application: A double freeze-thaw cycle using a disc-shaped cryoprobe 50 mm in diameter which is placed on the skin metastases at a temperature of −180°C for 7 min without local or general anesthesia

The cryosurgical method is in these cases one of the most radical local treatment options, which we expect will in future be carried out in every hospital on a routine basis. At the same time, breast cryosurgery for the primary tumor serves as a preventive measure, in order to prevent metastasis in breast cancer patients. Cryosurgery is carried out under local anesthesia. Immediately before the cryosurgical intervention a biopsy is taken intraoperatively. The cryosurgical operation is usually carried out in two to three sessions, of 1–3 minutes' duration each (Figs. 13.1.11–13.1.15). The in-hospital stay is short – usually only two days. Further treatment and monitoring of the patient takes place on an out-patient basis.

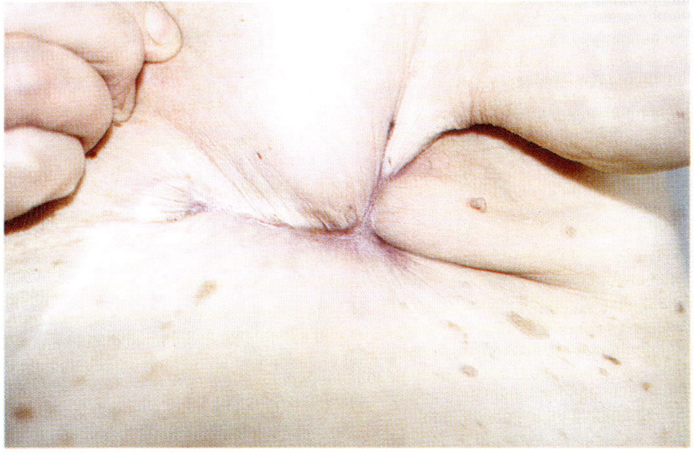

Fig. 13.1.15. BCC: Wound healing, 12 weeks after breast cryosurgery. Excellent cosmetic result. No recurrence or metastases following a 5-year observation period

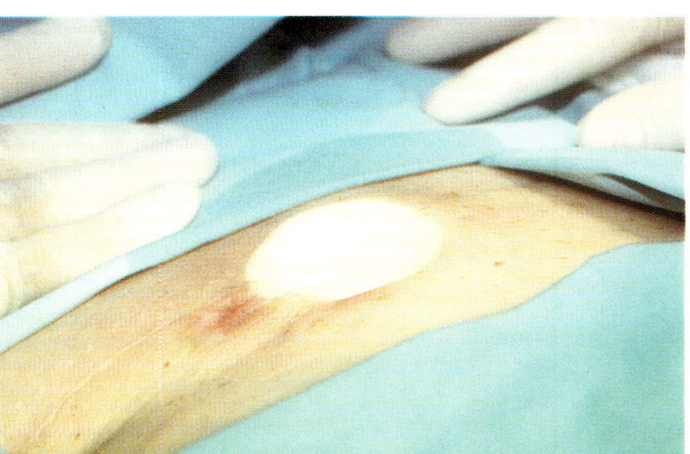

Fig. 13.1.17. BCC in the same patient. Typical view of the post-cryosurgical zone, which measures 68 mm in diameter. The formed post-cryosurgical zone is clearly circumscribed by a demarcation line. No postoperative bleeding

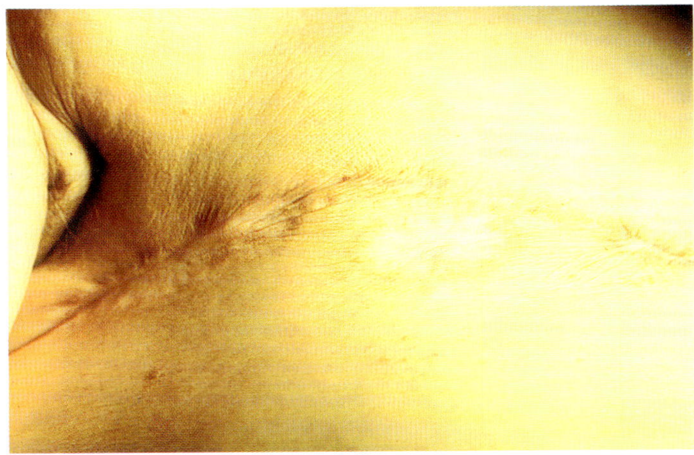

Fig. 13.1.18. The same patient. Excellent result: complete healing 10 weeks after cryosurgical treatment. The patient is disease-free 6 years after cryosurgery

13.1.3 Skin Metastases After Breast Cancer Surgery

Cryosurgical interventions are successful in patients with skin metastases (Figs. 13.1.16–13.1.18).

Skin metastases are removed in the same fashion, normally without local anesthesia. A special local cryoanesthesia is appropriate for the control of pain.

If numerous skin metastases appear, cryosurgical interventions can be carried out unproblematically and simultaneously in different foci. Normally these operations can be performed on an ambulatory basis. Post-surgical treatment and monitoring are carried out either in the out-patient department or in the private office.

13.2 Minimally Invasive Breast Cryosurgery

Yoed Rabin with a contribution by Thomas B. Julian and Peter Olson

13.2.1 Why Minimally Invasive Breast Cryosurgery?

The treatment of carcinoma of the breast has followed a fascinating evolution through the centuries. In the seventeenth century treatment consisted of a barbaric amputation and hot iron cauterization technique, without the aid of anesthesia. Both surgical technology and the understanding of the biology of breast cancer developed slowly until the twentieth century. Breast cancer treatment was one of anecdotalism applied to small numbers of patients without reproducible results.

During the twentieth century the treatment of breast cancer was dominated by the Halstedian principles of en bloc resection which mandated a radical mastectomy in order to control breast cancer. Halsted's belief that breast cancer spread systemically via contiguous involvement of muscle, fascia, and lymphatics was a strong one. Challenges to the Halstedian concept began to emerge and grow in the mid and late 1900's. These new concepts of local breast cancer control combined with a better understanding of the biological nature of the disease were incorporated into clinical trials. A landmark clinical trial from the NSABP B-06 provided data to support and propel breast conserving therapy forward (Fisher et al. 1995).

Currently, the utilization of breast conserving therapy has increased in the United States (Riley et al. 1999). As the information gained from a better understanding of the biological mechanism driving tumor cells is directed into new therapies which affect the cellular and subcellular level, breast conserving surgical procedures will take on a more significant role. Breast conserving therapy depends largely upon early detection, preoperative diagnosis and planning. Currently the best method for early detection is screening mammography (Tabar et al. 1985; Hendrick et al. 1997). Due to enhanced mammographic screening, it is estimated that by 2010 A.D. 50% of all new breast cancers discovered will be less than 10 mm in diameter (Cady et al. 1996), which represents 90,000 patients in the United States. Standard surgical treatments would require an open segmental resection, an operating room, anesthesia, and substantial cost.

The future, however, is bringing with it new tools which will undoubtedly increase the early detection of breast cancer and increase surgical intervention. On the horizon high resolution MRI is advancing rapidly in lesion detection, with sensitivities of nearly 100% (Harms et al. 1993; Orel et al. 1994). This technology may increase detection in the high risk population or of occult carcinomas. Digital mammography has the potential to improve detection and characterization of breast lesions.

Nuclear medicine scans utilizing scintimammography or PET are in both clinical and experimental use. Imaging may be achievable to a resolution of 1–2 mm. Each of these technologies has the ability to increase the detection of breast cancer and increase surgical removal of the disease at an earlier time.

The role of neoadjuvant chemotherapy is taking on an increasingly important role in breast cancer treatment. Results published from NSABP B-18 indicate a decrease in tumor size in 80% of patients with a modest conversion from mastectomy to lumpectomy (Fisher et al. 1998). Thus the use of preoperative chemotherapy can and has increased the role of breast conserving therapy. The effect of improving detection technology and preoperative therapies will ultimately increase segmental resections. The increase in surgical requirements will proportionally increase care costs.

Alternative methods of tumor removal or ablation for small malignancies are needed to complete the biological assault on breast cancer. A side benefit may be the lowering of treatment costs as well. Several technologies which have the ability to either remove tumor percutaneously or ablate tumor *in situ* percutaneously, are undergoing evaluation. Percutaneous tumor removal utilizing a vacuum-assisted stereotactic 11-gauge breast biopsy needle shows early promise (Liberman et al. 1999), but questions need to be answered concerning margin status.

Radiofrequency ablation has proved to be feasible in breast tissue and breast cancer (Bohm et al. 2000; Jeffrey et al. 1999). Interstitial laser coagulation in breast cancer is undergoing study with promising results (Harms 2000). Both techniques require intravenous or general anesthesia.

An additional alternative means is cryosurgery. Cryosurgery has been used successfully for more than three decades to treat benign and malignant neoplasms (Rand et al. 1968; Zacarian 1977; Ablin 1980; Orpwood 1981). To date, there is one reported case of primary breast cancer treatment with cryotherapy (Staren et al. 1997), which was followed up with ultrasound-guided biopsy and found negative for malignancy 12 weeks post-cryosurgery. Cryotherapy carries many benefits in addition to the attractive concept of minimally invasive surgery. Low temperatures generate anesthetic effect. Hemorrhage is reduced due to thrombosis of small blood vessels. Cryotherapy may cause stimulation of the body's immune system, which additionally augments local tumor destruction and may also induce a response in metastatic tumor sites (Rand et al. 1968; Ablin 1980; Ablin 1995; Suzuki 1995; Tonoka 1995).

Cryosurgery is still at a stage where art overshadows science. Most cryotherapy devices are bulky and somewhat complex to handle outside of a standard operating room. The ideal device would be small and compact. It should interface with the stereotactic biopsy table and ultrasound devices. Debate continues as to numbers and duration of freeze-thaw cycles needed to maximize the probability of cell destruction. Little information is known about the survival of the cell at the freeze front and the ability to regenerate. This leads to questions about the optimum tumor size and dimensions of the "ice ball". Investigations into these questions and technology developments are ongoing (Rabin et al. 1997; Gage and Baust 1998; Rabin et al. 1999a).

With multiple treatments such as neoadjuvant therapy, hormone therapy, and radiation, which have the ability to downsize primary cancers and treat small cancers, the use of lumpectomy can increase. Current diagnosis imaging trends are increasingly detecting small cancers ($\leq$1 cm). The minimization of surgical intervention to complement these trends is a natural progression of technology and understanding of the biological processes involved.

The use of minimally invasive percutaneous cryosurgery is a technology which might provide a substitute for an open surgical segmental resection (lumpectomy). This technique may decrease the disadvantages of lumpectomy while enhancing the cosmetic effect of breast conserving therapy and promote biologic and immunologic response. Further investigations will need to be undertaken in these areas.

13.2.2 Technological Background

James Arnott (1845) was probably the first to report on the destructive effect of freezing in the treatment of cancer. Since Arnott's first report, numerous cryodevices and techniques have been suggested. These have included pre-cooled metal blocks, dry ice applications, spray/pour freezing with compressed or liquefied gases (Kollner and Duczek 1974), refrigeration systems (Timmerhause 1989), thermoelectric methods and cryogenic heat pipes (Hamilton and Hu 1993), cryoneedles (Weshahy 1993), precooled needles (Gao et al. 1986), heat conducting needles (Stumpf and Andrea 1974), Joule-Thompson effect based cryoprobes (Rzasa and Wallach 1983; Bald 1984; Varney 1992; Goddard 1993; Homasson et al. 1994; Maytal 1997), boiling effect based cryoprobes (Cooper and Lee 1961; Lee 1967; Zimmer 1975; Fowle 1994; Rabin et al. 1996a; 1996b), and supercooled liquified gases (Rubinsky et al. 1994; Chang et al. 1994; Baust et al. 1996).

As a consequence of the high cooling power usually required for cryosurgery, and especially of internal organs, the boiling effect has been found to be the preferable cooling technique by most cryosurgeons since the 1930's, when technological developments enabled commercialization of liquefied gases. Some of the technical difficulties associated with Joule-Thomson cooling for cryosurgery have been solved in the past few years and devices based on this cooling technique are now competing with those based on boiling cooling (Kaplan et al. 1995; Hewitt et al. 1997; Rewcastle et al. 1999).

Some of the cryoprobes for invasive procedures combine a heating mechanism near the tip of the cryoprobe, in order to enhance the control of the cryoprobe temperature and, hence, to gain a better control over the ice ball formation (Van Gerven 1980; Merry and Smidebush 1990; Rabin 1996a). It has recently been suggested to combine temperature-controlled heaters (also termed Cryoheaters) within the cryotreated region, that are operated independently of the cryoprobes, in order to control the frozen region formation more precisely (Rabin et al. 1999b).

Cryosurgery can be monitored by ultrasound (Onik et al. 1985; Onik et al. 1988; Onik et al. 1991; Staren et al. 1997), CT (Isoda 1989; Quigley et al. 1992; Sandison et al. 1998), and MRI (Rubinsky et al. 1993; Gilbert et al. 1993; Hong et al. 1994), where ultrasound is most commonly used today. In addition, verification of temperatures and freezing front location can be achieved using point sensors such as impedance electrodes (Le Pivert et al. 1977; Novak and Craig 1984; Gage et al. 1985) and thermocouples (Rivoire et al. 1996; Abramovits et al. 1996). However, due to difficulties in sensor localization and uncertainty in measurements, point sensors are rarely a choice of practice in routine cryosurgery (Rabin 1998a).

Following is an up-to-date report on our research group efforts in development of a cryosurgical device for minimally invasive cryosurgery, experimental cryosurgery in sheep breast model, and long-term follow-up post cryosurgery.

13.2.3 A Compact Device for Breast Cryosurgery

For practical reasons of cost and simplicity, we chose liquid nitrogen boiling as the cooling technique for the development of a compact device and miniature cryoprobe for breast cryosurgery (Rabin et al. 1997). One of the key questions for thermal design is "What are the cooling capabilities required of such a system?" The ratio of the energy required to freeze a unit volume of tissue to the energy that can be absorbed by a unit volume of liquid nitrogen in boiling can be approximated by:

$$\eta = \frac{\int_{T_0}^{T_F} C_U dT + L_F + \int_{T_F}^{T_C} C_F dT}{L_{LN}} \tag{1}$$

where η is the energy ratio, T_0 is the initial temperature of the tissue (normal body temperature), T_F is the freezing temperature of the tissue, T_C is some minimal cryogenic temperature, T_{LN} is the liquid nitrogen boiling temperature, C_U is the volumetric specific heat of the unfrozen tissue, C_F is the volumetric specific heat of the frozen tissue, L_F is the latent heat of tissue freezing, and L_{LN} is the latent heat of liquid nitrogen boiling. Equation (1) is valid for cases of low blood flow rate, where the heat convection by blood is not significant. Nevertheless, Rabin and Shitzer (1998c) have shown theoretically that the frozen region size should not be affected significantly even in cases of high blood flow, as long as the cryotreatment is not being performed in the presence of a major blood vessel.

Applying the parameters listed in Table 13.2.1, Eq. (1) yields an energy ratio, η, in the range of 2 to 4. This means that, theoretically, freezing 1 ml of tissue requires only 2 to 4 ml of liquid nitrogen. It follows that, freezing a 1 cm spherical ice ball requires 1 ml to 2 ml of liquid nitrogen, freezing a 2 cm ice ball requires 8 ml to 16 ml of liquid nitrogen, and freezing a 5 cm ice ball requires 125 ml to 250 ml. Clearly, high thermal efficiency is a key parameter for the design of a compact cryodevice. Note that the parameter of thermal efficiency is typically overlooked in the design of cryodevices. Furthermore, liquid nitrogen-based cryodevices for internal organs are typically characterized by extremely high coolant consumption and, therefore, by low thermal efficiency.

A new device for minimally invasive cryosurgery, characterized by high thermal efficiency, has been presented by Rabin et al. (1997), and is describe in brief herein. The new minimally invasive cryoprobe comprises a U-shaped heat exchanger, a sharp pointed tip, and a thermal insulation jacket; one configuration of the cryoprobe is shown in Fig. 13.2.1.

The cooling process in the cryoprobe shown in Fig. 13.2.1 takes place as follows. Liquid nitrogen is forced from a small, hand held, container into the cryoprobe through feeding tube 9. The liquid nitrogen flows along the cryoneedle towards the

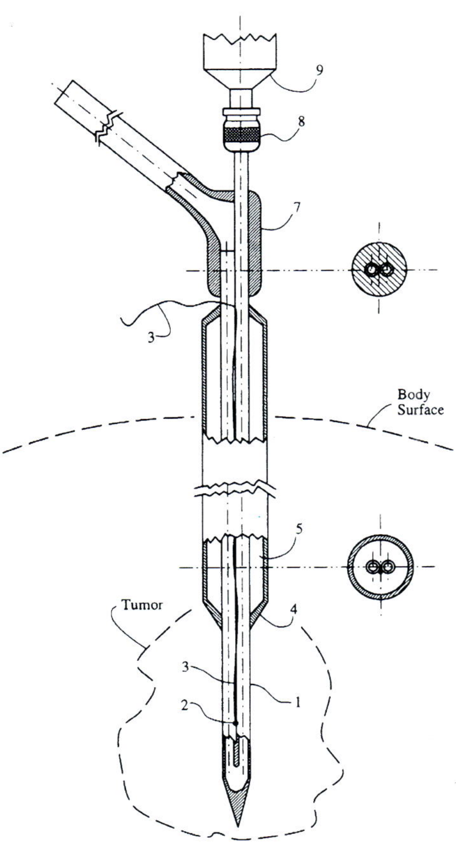

Fig. 13.2.1. Schematic illustration of a cross-section of a minimally invasive cryoprobe for breast cryosurgery (Rabin et al. 1997)

tip and then back, towards the outlet tube. Thermal insulation jacket 4 (achieved by vacuum in gap 5) prevents freezing of surrounding tissues. The only significant heat transfer occurs where the cryoneedle is in direct contact with the tissue, designated as the active surface, 1. Downstream heat convection driven by boiling effect takes place along the cryoprobe active surface, and causes freezing of the tissue. To achieve high thermal efficiency, the liquid nitrogen flow rate has to be controlled to ensure that no nitrogen droplets will escape to the surroundings through the venting tube 7.

Using an 18.5-gauge hypodermic needle, as construction material for the cryoneedle heat exchanger, and liquid nitrogen pressure of 30 psi, the typical variation of temperature at the cryoprobe active surface is: 37°C at the initiation of the procedure, −55°C after 15 sec, −82.5°C after 30 sec, −107.5°C after 45 sec, −116.5°C after 90 sec, and −140°C when approaching steady state. This cryoprobe and cooling protocol generates an average frozen region diameter of 22.3 mm within 5 min of operation in sheep breast tissue ($n = 21$). This cryosurgical device has a high thermal efficiency (43%). More detail with regard to the cryodevice setup and validation testing is presented by Rabin et al. (1997).

13.2.4 Cryoprobe Localization

Cryoprobe localization for internal applications can be performed using an imaging technique such as ultrasound or MRI, where the cryoprobe tip is simply maneuvered towards the center of the target area to be cryotreated. For example, the cryoprobe can be localized in a similar manner as in the well established process of needle localization technique, as a pre-process for conventional breast lumpectomy.

The flexibility of breast tissue increases the degree of complication in localization of a minimally invasive cryoprobe. In order to overcome this difficulty, one can use the highly accurate and well established technique of stereotactic localization for biopsy needles. In this procedure, the breast is imaged by two low-intensity X-ray images, at an angle of 15° from one another. The data is fed to a computer which generates a 3D image of the breast. Once the operator identifies a specific spot on these two images, the computerized device calculates the coordinates of the specific spot in space and the biopsy needle is automatically driven accordingly. Figure 13.2.2 shows 3 minimally invasive cryoprobes having thermal insulation jackets in a diameter of 3 mm and active surface length of 22 mm (upper, black), 32 mm

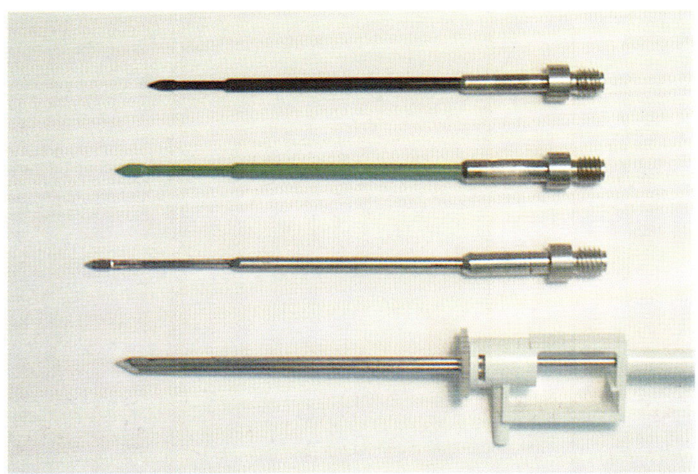

Fig. 13.2.2. Minimally invasive cryoprobes having a thermal insulation diameter of 3 mm, cryoneedle tube diameter of 1.5 mm, and active surface length of 22 mm (top, black), 32 mm (second from above, green), and 42 mm (third from above, stainless steel). Below, a biopsy needle from Biopsys Medical, Inc. (Mammotome Multi-Probe), having an oval cross-section of 3 × 4 mm

(second from above, green), and 42 mm (third from above, stainless steel). For comparison, Fig. 13.2.2 also shows a standard biopsy needle of Biopsys Medical, Inc. (below). One can see that the new cryoprobes can be easily designed to be compatible with the biopsy needle. It follows that stereotactic cryoprobe localization can be applied to breast cryosurgery.

13.2.5 Experimental Cryosurgery in a Sheep Breast Model

The animal model for this study is a recently pregnant sheep, 8 to 12 weeks post-lambing, and at least 4 weeks post-lactation. All animals in this study were about 5 years old, after 5 deliveries (once a year), having body weight in the range of 40 kg to 80 kg. Under these conditions the sheep breast is similar in size to the human breast. The importance of similarity arises from: (i) the need of large enough volume of untreated tissue surrounding the cryoinjured site, as the surrounding tissue is expected to take an important role in the recovery and regeneration process; and, (ii) the need of large size to make imaging practical.

All cryotreatments were performed on healthy breast tissue and not on a tumor model, the underlying assumption being that the recovery and regeneration processes following cryoinjury are not dependent on the pre-existence of a breast tumor. Based on the reported results of 100% tumor kill with cryosurgery of breast cancer in small animals (Staren et al. 1997), it is further assumed that cryodestruction of breast tumors is feasible. The authors are not aware of any tumor model for sheep breast, nor of any other tumor model of large animals which are similar in size and structure to the human breast. Therefore, the cryotreatment of healthy breast tissue is a choice of practice.

Cryoprocedures were performed in areas of dense breast tissue fibers and as far as possible from the dilated breast ducts. Identification of the different areas of the breast and monitoring of the ice ball formation were performed using a Doppler ultrasound (7 MHz linear array transducer). Figure 13.2.3 shows an ultrasound monitored cryoprocedure, where the ultrasound transducer is handheld from above, perpendicular to the cryoneedle center line, and above the middle of its active surface, with the animal lying on its back. The ultrasound images were videotaped for further analysis and measurements. In Fig. 13.2.3, the cryoprobe is inserted horizontally into the right breast. Figure 13.2.4 shows a closer view of the point of penetration into the breast, where a small cut (3 to 5 mm in length) in the skin was prepared prior to cryoprobe insertion and was closed with one suture at the end of the operation.

Figure 13.2.5 shows ultrasound images of the cryotreated site as the cryoprocedure progresses. Figure 13.2.5(a) shows the imaged cryoneedle prior to freezing, circled with a dashed line. Figure 13.2.5(a) also shows the shadow of the needle

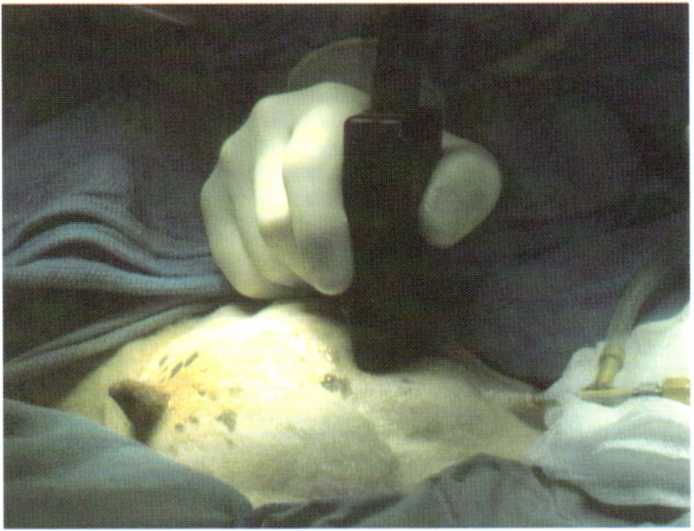

Fig. 13.2.3. Experimental cryosurgery in a sheep breast model. The animal is lying on its back. The ultrasound transducer is handheld from above. The cryoprobe is inserted horizontally and localized in an area of dense breast fibers

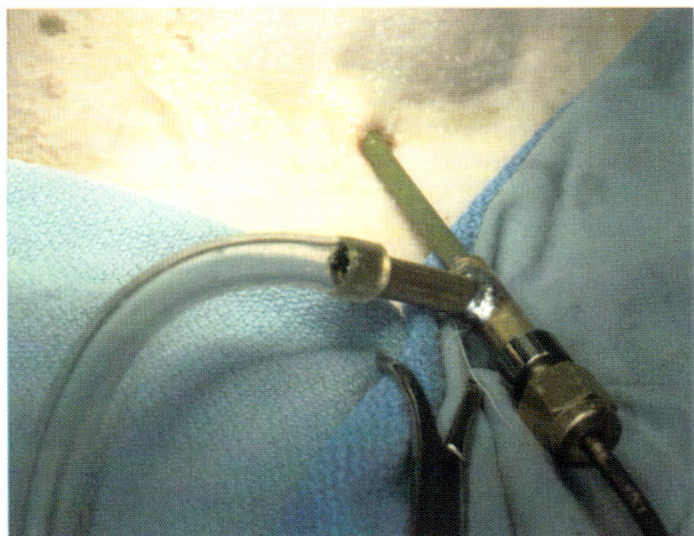

Fig. 13.2.4. A small skin cut of 3 to 5 mm is made to allow smooth cryoprobe penetration. The cryoprobe does not enhance the injury at the point of penetration. At the end of the cryoprocedure, one skin suture is applied to close the penetration point

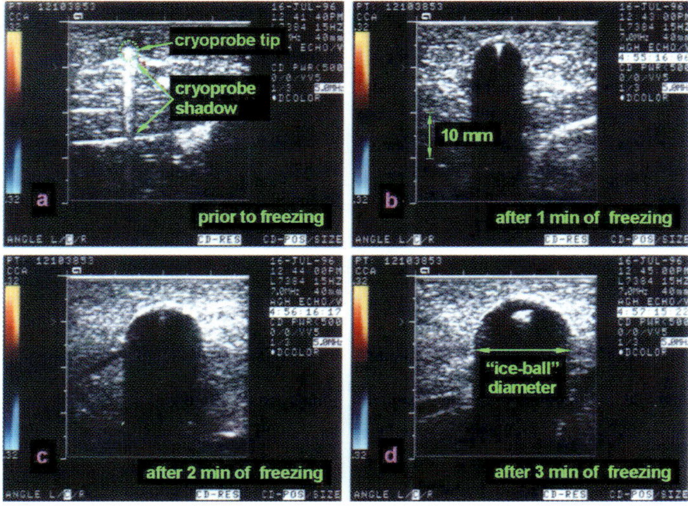

Fig. 13.2.5. Ultrasound imaged "ice ball" formation in a sheep breast model using 7 MHz linear array transducer. The frozen region appears as a dark area in the ultrasound image. The cryoprobe is placed perpendicular to the ultrasound transducer (to the monitor), the ultrasound transducer is applied from above and, therefore, the cryoprobe shadow is projected downwards, as illustrated in **a**. **b–d** show ultrasound images after 1, 2, and 3 min from the beginning of freezing. A measurement of the ice ball diameter is illustrated in **d**, which appears to be about 2 cm after 3 min of cryo-operation in this particular procedure

in ultrasound imaging. Shadowing is an inherent property of ultrasound imaging in the presence of solid objects. As the cryoprocedure progresses, a frozen region forms around the cryoprobe, appearing as a dark area, accompanied by a dark shadow projected downwards (the frozen tissue is solid). Figures 13.2.5(b), 13.2.5(c), and 13.2.5(d), show the ultrasound image after 1, 2, and 3 min from the beginning of cryo-operation. A length bar is illustrated in Fig. 13.2.5(b), while the frozen region diameter is illustrated in Fig. 13.2.5(d). It follows that, in this particular cryoprocedure, a frozen region diameter of about 10 mm, 16 mm, and 20 mm, was measured after 1 min, 2 min, and 3 min from the beginning of cryo-operation. This technique of frozen region diameter was repeated in 28 cases to generate a data base of the frozen region development in breast tissue under various conditions. The ultrasound imaged ice ball was compared with histology findings. For this comparison a staining technique was developed to assess the extent of cryoinjury, as discussed below.

13.2.6 Tissue Fixation and TTC Application as a Cryoinjury Indicator

The extent of cryoinjury was evaluated using the vital stain 2,3,5-triphenyltetrazolium chloride (TTC), an oxidation – reduction indicator that has been used effectively for histochemical analysis of infarct volume in ischemically injured tissues (Rabin et al. 1998b; 1999a). TTC, as a water soluble salt, is not a dye but is reduced by certain mitochondrial respiratory enzymes in normal tissue to a deep red, fat soluble, light sensitive compound (formazan) that turns normal tissue brick red and thereby delineates abnormal areas. TTC has been used extensively to stain tissues from humans and experimental animals and has been shown to reflect accurately the extent of irreversible ischemic damage.

Breast specimens were prepared for histological analysis by perfusion of the vital stain 2,3,5-triphenyltetrazolium chloride (TTC) followed by perfusion of formaldehyde *in situ* (Rabin et al. 1998b). In brief, all the major veins leading from the breasts were exposed and ligated (Fig. 13.2.6). The two major arteries leading to the breasts were exposed, cannulated, and connected to a controlled flow rate pump via a T connector. The breasts were perfused with 250 ml of TTC 2% in phosphate-buffered saline, at a rate of 18 ml/min, followed by 100 ml of 37.2% formaldehyde at a rate of 18 ml/min. The TTC and the animal's breasts

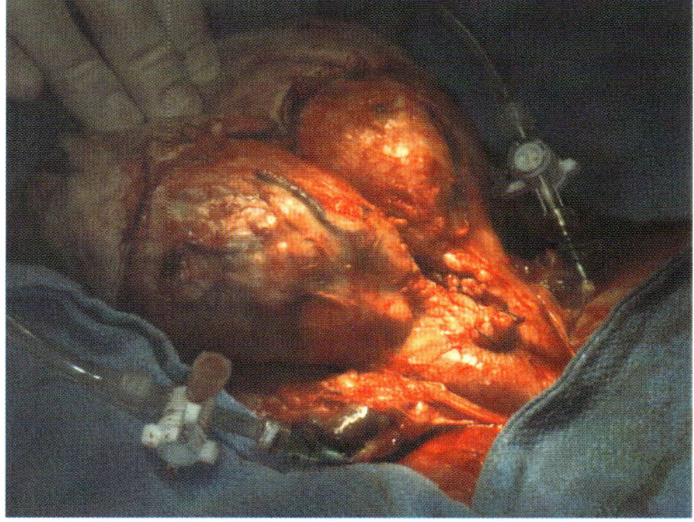

Fig. 13.2.6. Tissue fixation and staining with the vital stain 2,3,5-triphenyltetrazolium chloride (TTC): All the major veins leading from the breasts were exposed and ligated. The two major arteries leading to the breasts were exposed, cannulated and connected to a Harvard syringe pump via a T connector (the catheters are shown at both sides of the breasts). The breasts were perfused with 250 ml of 2,3,5-triphenyltetrazolium chloride (TTC) 2% in phosphate-buffered saline, at a rate of 18 ml/min, followed by 150 ml of 10% natural buffered formaldehyde at a rate of 18 ml/min. The animals were maintained at 37°C throughout the procedure for optimal histochemical enzyme reduction in the tissue. The breasts were immediately excised and immersed in the same formaldehyde solution for 24 h

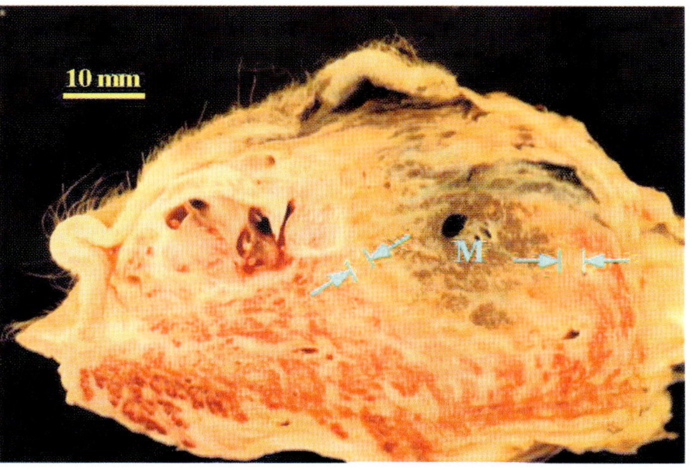

Fig. 13.2.7. Cross-section of a fixed breast specimen stained with TTC immediately after thawing. The main cryoinjured region is designated by *M*. The partly injured region, designated as the transition zone between the main cryoinjured region and the surrounding healthy tissues, is pointed out by blue arrows

were maintained at 37°C throughout the procedure for optimal histochemical enzyme reduction in the tissue using a temperature controlled thermal blanket. Skin temperature measurements were taken to verify temperature control, using 36 gauge hypodermic thermocouples. The breasts were excised immediately after and immersed in 10% neutral buffered formaldehyde solution for up to 24 h. The specimens were then bisected along the cryoneedle track, the color of the cut surface was observed and the cryoinjured (discolored) region was measured (Fig. 13.2.7).

Representative blocks of tissue from the cryotreated region were submitted for standard histological examination by light microscopy using hematoxylin & eosin stain (H&E), and Masson's trichrome stain. Representative histology cross-sections are presented.

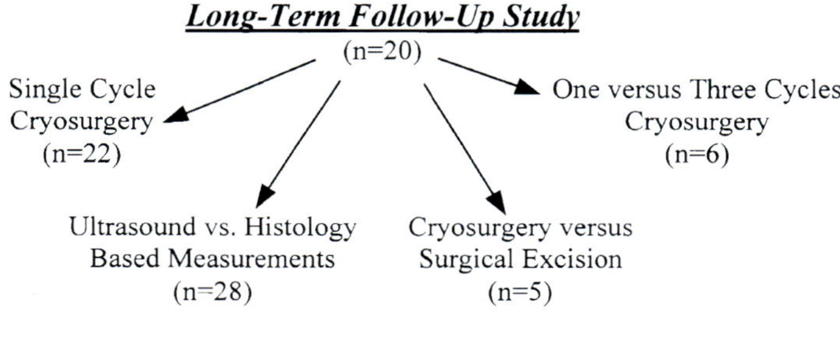

Fig. 13.2.8. Summary of animal work in the long-term follow-up study

13.2.7 Long-Term Follow-Up Post-Cryosurgery

The long-term follow-up study is described in detail by Rabin et al. (1999a). In brief, with reference to Fig. 13.2.8, a total of 20 animals were studied in six follow-up groups. Follow-up groups of immediate (n = 2), 1 week (n = 3), 1 month (n = 3), 2 months (n = 4), 3.5 months (n = 4), and 5 months (n = 4), were selected. The immediate follow-up experiments were performed to test the cryoprobes, to provide a baseline for the long-term follow-up, and to improve the application of the TTC perfusion and *in situ* fixation as described above.

A single cryoprocedure on one breast was compared with a three cycle cryoprocedure in the other breast in six animals of the 1- to 5-month follow-up groups. Five animals were used to compare the scar tissue developed as a result of a surgical excision with that developed after a single cycle cryoprocedure, for the same follow-up groups. The surgical excision procedure included incision in the skin to a length of 15 to 20 mm, followed by excision of tissue with an average diameter of 10 to 15 mm. One skin suture was applied to close the incision created for the cryoprobe, while about 4 sutures were applied to the surgical excision.

MRI and mammography were obtained about every 4 weeks in an effort to identify the sites of cryotreatment. The MRI was performed on animals from the 5-month follow-up group, under general anesthesia, with the animals lying on their backs, in a Siemens© MRI unit with 1.5 Tesla intensity. Mammography was performed on a larger number of animals from all follow-up groups, with 26 kV and between 56 and 63 MAS, in a Siemens© mammography unit. In some cases, the mammography was performed *in vivo* under general anesthesia, with the animals lying on their sides. In other cases, the mammography was performed on the breast specimens immediately after harvesting.

Figure 13.2.7 shows a cross-section of a fixed breast specimen stained with TTC from the immediate follow-up group. The main cryoinjured region is designated by the letter M. The partly injured region, designated as the transition zone between the main cryoinjured region and the surrounding healthy tissue, is pointed out by blue arrows. High power magnification of the main cryoinjured region is shown in the top right field of Fig. 13.2.11, and of the transition zone at the top left of Fig. 13.2.12. For comparison, the normal glands of the breast stained with H&E are shown at the top left of Fig. 13.2.11 (control).

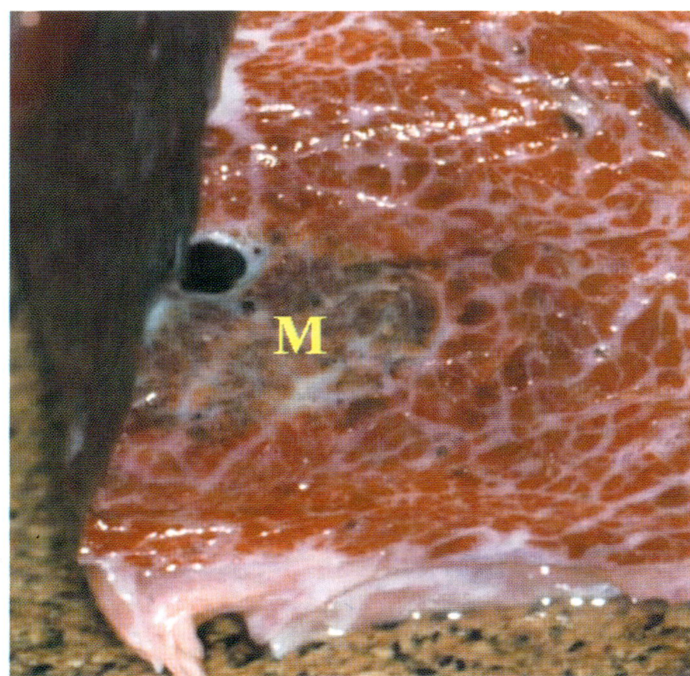

Fig. 13.2.9. Cross-section of a fixed breast specimen stained with TTC 7 days post-cryosurgery. The main cryoinjured region is designated by *M*

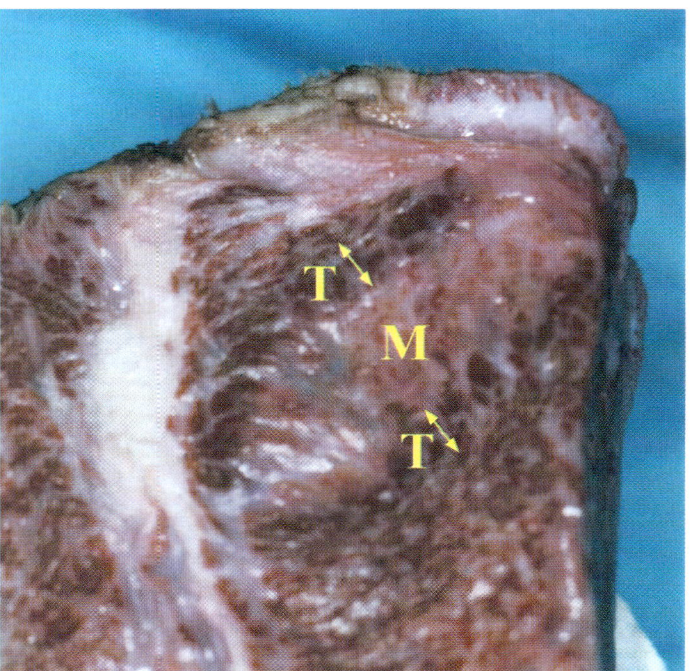

Fig. 13.2.10. Cross-section of a fixed breast specimen stained with TTC 1 month post cryosurgery. The main cryoinjured region is designated by *M*. The transition zone is designated by *T* and pointed out by the yellow arrows

Figure 13.2.9 shows a cross-section of a fixed breast specimen stained with TTC 7 days post-cryosurgery. The main cryoinjured region is designated by the letter M. Necrosis with complete loss of cellular detail is demonstrated at 1 week post-cryosurgery, bottom left field of Fig. 13.2.11.

Figure 13.2.10 shows a cross-section of a fixed breast specimen stained with TTC at 1 month post-cryosurgery. The main cryoinjured region is designated by the letter M. The transition zone is designated by the letter T and pointed out by the yellow arrows. The bottom right field of Fig. 13.2.12 shows regenerating duct in loose stroma, at 1 month post-cryosurgery (stained with Masson's trichrome stain). The Masson's trichrome stain is used to distinguish fibers within the scar. The trichrome dye stains collagen green, cytoplasm red, and nuclei black, in contrast to the standard H&E stain, which gives a pink color to both collagen fibers and cytoplasm of fibroblasts.

The cryoinjured site is very difficult to observe macroscopically at 5 months post-cryosurgery. However, microscopic findings show capillaries, fibroblasts, and bundles of collagen at 5 months post-cryosurgery (bottom right of Fig. 13.2.11), which indicate regeneration and recovery in progress.

13.2.8 Up-to-Date Summary

A minimally invasive cryosurgical device has been developed. The new cryosurgical device generates sufficient cooling power for breast cryosurgery with a relatively low coolant consumption, where 43% thermal efficiency has been demonstrated in gelatin. The new cryodevice can generate ice ball

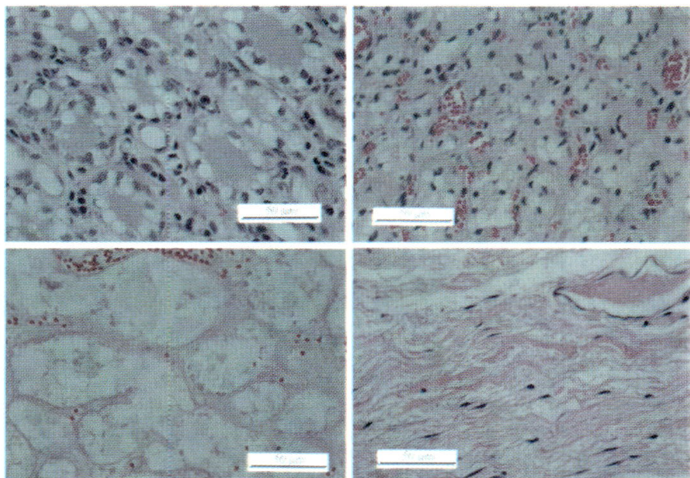

Fig. 13.2.11. Main cryoinjured region stained with H&E. Top left: Control tissue, normal glands of the breast. Top right: loss of cytoplasmic and nuclear detail immediately post-cryosurgery. Bottom left: necrosis with complete loss of cellular detail at 1 week post-cryosurgery. Bottom right: capillaries, fibroblasts, and bundle of collagen at 5 months post-cryosurgery (Fig. 13.2.11 is reproduced from Rabin et al. 1999a)

diameter of 20 mm within 3 to 5 min in breast tissue.

Experimental results indicate that the growth of the frozen region in sheep breast tissue is: (i) slower in larger breasts, (ii) slower in areas of large ducts and high fluid content, and (iii) faster in areas of fibrous breast tissue. When compared with liver cryosurgery, the frozen region growth in the sheep liver is 3 to 4.5 times faster than in the sheep breasts.

Ultrasound imaging of the ice ball formation leads to an underestimation of the cryoinjured region in the range of 2 to 5 mm. The cryoinjured region dimensions include a transition zone of partly damaged lobules having a typical thickness of 2 to 5 mm. A conservative application of the cryosurgical device developed for the current study in breast tissue suggests 5 mm safety margins in an ultrasound monitored cryoprocedure. It follows that a target tumor diameter of 10 mm requires an ice ball of 20 mm, which can be easily achieved within less than 5 minutes using the new cryosurgical device.

The cryoinjured region at 5 months post-cryosurgery is about one half the diameter of the imaged frozen region during the cryoprocedure. The reduction in cryoinjured region size over time is probably the result of contraction of the scar tissue within the area of injury as the scar develops, the post-injury healing process of the tissue, and the natural reduction of the sheep breast over time post-lambing. The cryotreatment site in a sheep breast model cannot be identified up to 5 months post-cryosurgery by means of ultrasound,

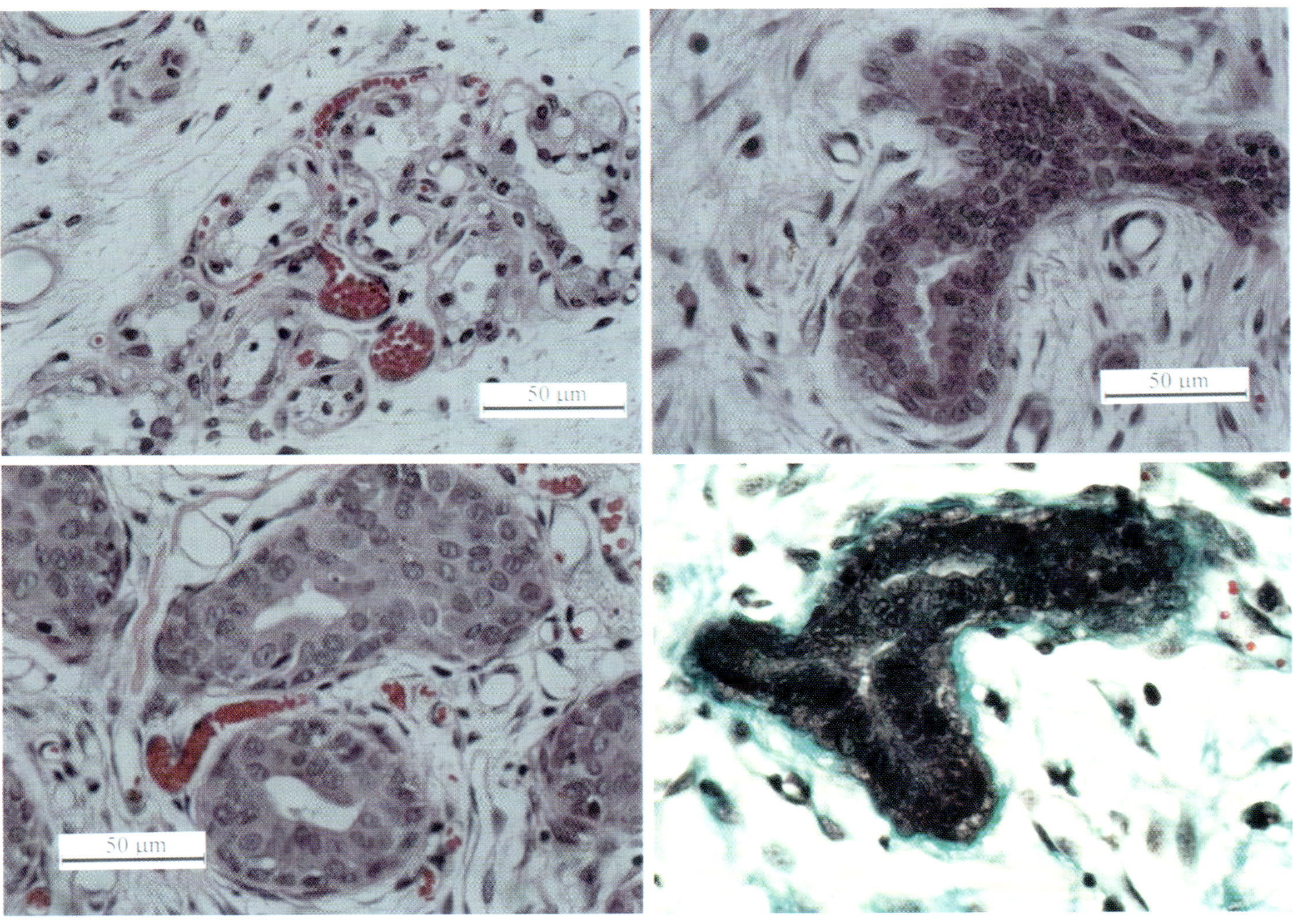

Fig. 13.2.12. Transition zone between the main cryoinjured region and the surrounding healthy tissues. Top left: glands with interstitial edema and vascular congestion with red blood cells immediately post-cryosurgery (H&E). Top right: regenerating duct in loose stroma at 1 month post-cryosurgery (H&E). Bottom left: regenerating duct, no secretory glands at 5 months post-cryosurgery (H&E). Bottom right: regenerating duct in loose stroma at 1 month post-cryosurgery (Masson's trichrome stain). The Masson's trichrome stain is used to distinguish fibers within the scar. The trichrome dye stains collagen green, cytoplasm red, and nuclei black, in contrast to the standard H&E stain, which gives a pink color to both collagen fibers and cytoplasm of fibroblasts. (Fig. 12.2.12 is reproduced from Rabin et al. 1999a)

mammography, or MRI. Using these standard imaging techniques, it is highly likely that the scar tissue will not be misinterpreted as a potential tumor in the long term.

The cryoprocedure produces an immediate injury which is characterized by cellular degeneration with vacuolization of the cytoplasm and loss of cellular and nuclear detail. This injury is associated with vascular congestion with red blood cells and edema. There is no gross or microscopic difference between lesions that have been subjected to one versus three freeze/thaw cycles. Either way, there is a main cryoinjured region that has uniform destruction of epithelium and healing scar formation, and a transition zone of damaged lobules without acining, which are surrounded by healthy tissue.

In terms of recovery and regeneration, surgical excision appears to have an advantage over cryosurgery, which is a more rapid healing process. The cryosurgical wound will catch up in establishing a fibrous scar in time, perhaps longer than one year. As a surgical procedure, however, cryosurgery has the advantages of substantial decrease in the risk of morbidity, simplicity of the procedure, minimal bleeding, anesthetic effect of low temperatures, low cost, minimal scarring, and possible stimulation of the body's immune system.

Acknowledgments

This study has been supported in part by Biopsys Medical, Inc. This study has also been supported in part by the Cancer Center of the Allegheny General Hospital. The authors would like to thank Mrs. Miriam Webber for her assistance in preparing this paper.

References

1. Ablin RJ (1980) Handbook of Cryosurgery. Dekker, New York.
2. Ablin RJ (1995) An appreciation and realization of the concept of cryoimmunology. In: Percutaneous Prostate Cryoablation, Quality Medical Publ, St Louis, MO, pp. 136–154.
3. Abramovits W, Pruiksma R, and Bose S (1996) Ultrasound-guided thermocouple placement for cryosurgery. Dermatol Surg 22(9): 771–773.
4. Arnott J (1845) On the present state of therapeutic injury. J Churchill, London, p. 35.
5. Bald WB (1984) A helium gas probe for use in cryosurgery. Cryobiology 21(5): 570–573.
6. Baust JG, Chang ZH, Finkelstein JJ (1996) Cryosurgical instrument with vent means and method using same. US Patent 5,520,682.
7. Bohm T, Hilger I, Muller W, et al. (2000) Saline-enhanced radio frequency ablation of breast tissue: an in vitro feasibility study. Invest Radiol 35(3): 149–157.
8. Cady B, Stone MD, Schuler SG, et al. (1996) The new era in breast cancer invasion, size and nodal involvement dramatically decreasing as a result of mammographic screening. Arch Surg 131: 301–305.
9. Chang Z, Finkelstein JJ, Ma H, Baust J (1994) Development of a high-performance multiprobe cryosurgical device. Biomed Instr & Tech 28: 383–390.
10. Cooper IS, Lee A (1961) Cryostatic congelation: a system for producing a limited controlled region of cooling or freezing of biological tissues. J Nerve Mental Dis 133: 259–263.
11. Fisher B, Anderson S, Redmond C, Wolmark N, Wickerham L, Cronin W (1995) Re-analysis and results after 12 years of follow-up in a randomized clinical trial comparing total mastectomy with lumpectomy with or without irradiation in the treatment of breast cancer. N Engl J Med 333: 1456–1461.
12. Fisher B, Bryant J, Wolmark N, et al. (1998) Effect of preoperative chemotherapy on the outcome of women with operable breast cancer. J Clin Onc 16: 2672–2685.
13. Fowle AA (1994) Entrained cryogenic droplet transfer method and cryosurgical instrument. US Patent 5,324,286.
14. Gage AA, Augustynowicz S, Montes M, Caruana JA, Whalen DA Jr (1985) Tissue impedance and temperature measurements in relation to necrosis in experimental cryosurgery. Cryobiology 22: 282–288.
15. Gage AA, Baust J (1998) Mechanisms of tissue injury in cryosurgery. Cryobiology 37, 171–186.
16. Gao XK, Sun DK, Sha RJ, Ding YS, Yan QY, Zhu CD (1986) Precooled, spring-driven surgical cryoneedle: a new device for cryohaemorrhoidectomy In: Proceedings of the 11th International Cryogenic Engineering Conference, IECE 11, Berlin, West Germany. pp. 825–829.
17. Gilbert JC, Rubinsky B, Roos MS, Wong STS, Brennan KM (1993) MRI-monitored cryosurgery in the rabbit brain. Magnetic Resonance Imaging 11: 1155–1164.
18. Goddard RW (1993) Cryosurgical apparatus. US Patent 5,224,943
19. Hamilton A, and Hu J (1993) An electronic cryoprobe for cryosurgery using heat pipes and thermoelectric coolers: a preliminary report. J Med Eng & Tech 17(3): 104–109.
20. Harms SE, Flamig DP, Hesley KL, Meiches MD, Jensen RA, Evans WP, Savino DA, Wells RV (1993) MR imaging of the breast with rotating delivery of excitation off resonance: clinical experience with pathologic correlation. Radiology 187: 493–501.
21. Harms SE (2000) Personal communication.
22. Hendrick RE, Smith RN, Ruteledge JH 3rd, Smort CR (1997) Benefit of screening mammography in women aged 40–49: a new meta-analysis of randomized controlled trials. J Natl Cancer Inst Monograph 22: 87–92.
23. Hewitt PM, Zhao J, Akhter J, Morris DL (1997) A comparative laboratory study of liquid nitrogen and argon gas cryosurgery systems. Cryobiology 35(4): 303–308.
24. Homasson JP, Thiery JP, Angebault M, Ovtracht L, Maiwand O (1994) The operation and efficacy of cryosurgical, nitrous oxide-driven cryoprobe. Cryobiology 31: 290–304.
25. Hong JS, Wong S, Rubinsky B (1994) MR imaging assisted temperature calculations during cryosurgery. Magnetic Resonance Imaging 12(7): 1021–1031.
26. Isoda H (1989) Sequential MRI and CT monitoring in cryosurgery – an experimental study in rats (Japanese). Nippon Igaku Hoshasen Gakkai Zasshi. Nippon Acta Radiol 49: 1499–1508.
27. Jeffrey SS, Birdwell RL, Ikeda DM, Daniel BL, Nowels KW, Dirbas FM, Griffey SM (1999) Radiofrequency ablation of breast cancer: first report of an emerging technology. Arch Surg 134(10): 1064–1068.
28. Kaplan SA, Greenberg R, Baust JG (1995) A comparative assessment of cryosurgical devices: application to prostatic disease. Urology 45(4): 692–699.
29. Kollner P, Duczek E (1974) Apparatus for cryosurgery. US Patent No. 3,794,039.
30. Le Pivert PJ, Binder P, Ougier T (1977) Measurement of intratissue bioelectrical low frequency impedance: a new method to predict peroperative by the destructive effect of cryosurgery. Cryobiology 14(2): 245–250.
31. Lee ASJ (1967) Freezing probe for the treatment of tissue, especially in neurosurgery. US Patent 3,298,371.
32. Liberman L, Zakowski MF, Avery S et al. (1999) Complete percutaneous excision of infiltrating carcinoma at stereotactic breast biopsy: how can tumor size be assessed? Am J Roentgenol 173: 1315–1322.

33. Maytal B-Z (1997) Multiprobe surgical cryogenic apparatus. US Patent 5,603,221.
34. Merry N, Smidebush M (1990) Apparatus for cryosurgery. US Patent 4,946,460.
35. Miller RH, Mazur P (1976) Survival of frozen-thawed human red cells as a function of cooling and warming velocities. Cryobiology 13: 404–414.
36. Novak SJ, Craig DL (1984) A low-cost impedance based cryosurgical temperature measurement unit. Australian Physical & Engineering Sciences in Medicine 7(3): 112–115.
37. Onik G, Gilbert J, Hoddick W, Filly R, Callen P, Rubinsky B, Farrel L (1985) Sonographic monitoring of hepatic cryosurgery in an experimental animal model. Am J Roentgenol 144(5): 1043–1047.
38. Onik G, Cobb C, Cohen J, Zabkar J, Porterfield B (1988) US characteristics of frozen prostate. Radiology 168(3): 629–631.
39. Onik G, Rubinsky B, Zemel R, Weaver L, Diamond D, Cobb C, Poterfield B (1991) Ultrasound-guided hepatic cryosurgery in the treatment of metastatic colon carcinoma - preliminary results. Cancer 67: 901–907.
40. Orel SG, Schnall MD, LiVolsi VA, Troupin RH (1994) Suspicious breast lesions: MR imaging with radiologic-pathologic correlation. Radiology 190: 485–493.
41. Orpwood RD (1981) Biophysical and engineering aspects of cryosurgery. Phys Med Biol 26(4): 555–575.
42. Quigley MR, Loesch DV, Shih T, Marquardt M, Lupetin A, Maroon JC (1992) Intracranial cryosurgery in a canine model: a pilot study. Surg Neurol 38: 101–105.
43. Rabin Y, Shitzer A (1996a) A new cryosurgical device for controlled freezing, part I: setup and validation test. Cryobiology 33: 82–92.
44. Rabin Y, Coleman R, Mordohovich D, Ber R, Shitzer A (1996b) A new cryosurgical device for controlled freezing, part II: in vivo experiments on rabbits' skeletal muscle hindlimb. Cryobiology 33: 93–105.
45. Rabin Y, Julian TB, Wolmark N (1997) A Compact Cryosurgical Apparatus for Minimal-Invasive Cryosurgery. Biomed Instr & Tech 31: 251–258.
46. Rabin Y (1998a) Uncertainty in temperature measurements during cryosurgery. Cryo-Letters 19(4): 213–224.
47. Rabin Y, Julian TB, Olson P, Taylor MJ, Wolmark N (1998b) Evaluation of post cryosurgery injury in a sheep breast model using the vital stain 2,3,5-triphenyltetrazolium chloride. Cryo-Letters 19(4): 255–262.
48. Rabin Y, Shitzer A (1998c) Numerical Solution of the Multidimensional Freezing Problem During Cryosurgery. ASME J Biomech Eng 120(1): 32–37.
49. Rabin Y, Julian TB, Olson P, Taylor MJ, Wolmark N (1999a) Long-term follow-up post-cryosurgery in a sheep breast model. Cryobiology 39: 29–46.
50. Rabin Y, Julian TB, Wolmark N (1999b) Method and apparatus for heating during cryosurgery. US Patent No. 5,899,897.
51. Rand RW, Rinret A, Von Leden H (1968) Cryosurgery. Thomas, Springfield, IL.
52. Rewcastle JC, Sandison GA, Saliken JC, Donnelly BJ, McKinnon JG (1999) Considerations during clinical operation of two commercially available cryomachines. J Surg Oncol 71(2): 106–111.
53. Riley GF, Potosky AL, Klaberode CN, Warren JL, Ballard-Borbooh R (1999) Stage at diagnosis and treatment patterns among older women with breast cancer: An HMO and fee for service comparison. JAMA 281: 720–726.
54. Rivoire ML, Voiglio EJ, Kaemmerlen P, Molina G, Treilleux I, Finzy J, Delay E, Gory F (1996) Hepatic cryosurgery precision: evaluation of ultrasonography, thermometry, and impedancemetry in a pig model. J Surg Oncol 61: 242–248.
55. Rubinsky B, Gilbert JC, Onik GM, Roos MS, Wong STS, Brennan KM (1993) Monitoring cryosurgery in the brain and the prostate with proton NMR. Cryobiology 30: 191–199.
56. Rubinsky B, Onik G, Finkelstein JJ, Neu D, Jones S (1994) Cryosurgical system for destroying tissue by freezing. US Patent 5,334,181.
57. Rzasa RP, Wallach RM (1983) Cryosurgical instrument. US Patent No. 4,377,168.
58. Sandison GA, Loye MP, Rewcastle JC, Hahn LJ, Saliken JC, McKinnon JC, Donnelly BJ (1998) X-ray CT monitoring of ice ball growth and thermal distribution during cryosurgery. Phys Med Biol 43: 3309–3324.
59. Staren ED, Sabel MS, Gianakakis LM, Wiener GA, Hart VH, Gorski M, Dowlatshahi K, Corning BF, Haklin MF, Koukoulis G (1997) Cryosurgery of breast cancer. Arch Surg 132: 28–33.
60. Stumpf JG, Andrea JF (1974) Cryosurgical device. US Patent 3,830,239.
61. Suzuki Y (1995) Cryosurgical treatment of advanced breast cancer and cryoimmunological responses. Skin Cancer 19: 19–26.
62. Tabar L, Fagerberg CJ, Gad A, et al. (1985) Reduction in mortality from breast cancer after mass screening with mammography: randomized trial from the Breast Cancer Screening Working Group of the Swedish National Board of Health and Welfare. Lancet 1:829:32
63. Timmerhause KD (1989) Trends to miniature cryogenic refrigeration systems and components. Int J Refrig 12: 246–254.
64. Tonoka S (1995) Cyrosurgical treatment of advanced breast cancer. Skin Cancer 10: 9–18.
65. Van Gerven H (1980) Cauterizing probes for cryosurgery. US Patent 4,202,336.
66. Varney KJ (1992) Cryosurgical probe. US Patent 5,078,713.
67. Weshahy AH (1993) Interlesional Cryosurgery: a new technique using cryoneedles. J Dermatol Surg Oncol 19: 123–126.
68. Zacarian SA (1997) Cryosurgical advances in dermatology and tumors of head and neck. Thomas. Springfield, IL.
69. Zimmer H (1975) Cryoprobe and flexible connector therefore. US Patent 3,910,277.

13.3 Cryosurgery for Advanced Breast Cancer

Shigeo Tanaka

13.3.0 Introduction

Cryosurgery has been developed since the 1960s (1, 4) to destroy benign and malignant tissues and is well established to treat a variety of neoplasms with minimal surgical risk. Thus it has been applied to control advanced cancer, in particular, to stop hemorrhage and malodorous discharge, reduction in tumor bulk with alleviation of intractable pain. Cryosurgery provides dual prominent features: destruction *in situ* of a tumor which otherwise is difficult to treat, and to elicit a potential tumor-specific immunologic reaction (9, 11, 14), (cryoimmunologic reaction) that in turn may control tumor remnants or distant metastases, if they exist.

However, application of cryosurgery for the treatment of advanced breast cancer does not seem to attract much attention (4) and has been performed by just a few active cryosurgeons (5,6,10–13).

As regards follow-up studies of three- and five-year survivals of primary cancer patients, who received cryosurgery as the primary method of treatment, only a few are known, e.g., for oral cancer (2), but none on breast cancer. Comparing the survival of advanced cancer patients by means of controlled clinical trials with other modalities of treatment on comparable cases is impossible at the moment, however.

In the author's series, of a total of 451 patients with malignancy, 52 had breast cancer: 10 primary advanced and 42 recurrent, who underwent cryosurgery in the period from July 1968 to January 2000. All the patients were referred to us as incurable cancer: advanced and unresectable, resistant to radiotherapy, chemotherapy, and endocrine therapy, or debilitated with associated systemic diseases. Although the number of the primary breast cancer is small in our series, three- and five-year survival was 40.0% (Table 13.3.1). This figure is not disappointing, given the patients' severe condition. Nevertheless, the advantages of cryosurgery have been well documented, and even cure could be attained. For inflammatory carcinoma (carcinoma erysipelatodes), which spreads rapidly, cryosurgery with the liquid nitrogen (LN_2) spraying technique is the only measure to stop the disease and salvage the patient.

Disadvantages inherent in cryosurgery include the time needed for the frozen tumor to slough off, extreme discharge during the course, and foul smell when the frozen tumor necrotizes. Another problem is anaplastic conversion of the tumor after cryosurgery. Though it is rarely seen and usually caused by insufficient freezing, even vigorous and drastic freezing that is thought to be sufficient still brings about anaplastic changes. Careful observation of the patient and countermeasures for this must be provided. To our present knowledge, anaplastic cancer and sarcoma are contraindicated for cryosurgery.

In view of the problems and prospects of cryosurgery, adjunctive use of the two innovative modalities, cryochemotherapy (7) and cryo-immunointensification therapy (8,11), are stressed in this chapter.

13.3.1 Indications

Any inoperable stages III and IV cancer, not indicated for conventional surgery, and recurrent breast cancer with multiple and wide-spread lesions, resistant to radio/chemo/endocrine therapy, and in particular, inflammatory carcinoma as mentioned above, are indicated for cryosurgery. Goals will vary from palliation of the disease to intention to cure. These will depend on the status of the tumor and general condition of the patient. Palliation includes arresting continuous hemorrhage from an ulcerating tumor, reducing malodorous discharge, reduction in the tumor bulk, and alleviating intractable pain. It deserves special mention that (1) this maneuver is safe even for patients debilitated with the disease, and (2) in an urgent problem, to stop very rapidly spreading disease, e.g., inflammatory cancer. In our experience, the only exception is anaplastic cancer. Cryosurgery for this may cause unexpected progression of the disease, thus is contraindicated as for anaplastic malignancies in other areas.

13.3.2 Cryosurgical Instrumentation

(1) For incurable cancer, LN_2 driven devices for heavy duty use with precision control units are mandatory to treat massive advanced cancer.
(2) Cryoprobes of closed-end type, 13 mm in outer diameter for large tumors, to a standard probe 8 mm in outer diameter are required.
(3) Probe-tip adaptors of various size and shape to be equipped with a cryoprobe, to obtain good contact with the tumor are selected.
(4) Cryosurgical device for spraying LN_2 (available as a portable unit). This is essential for the treatment of a widespread but not so deeply invasive lesion, such as inflammatory cancer,

Table 13.3.1. Survival in primary cancer patients–Tanaka Clinic and Shinsei Hospital (July 1968–January 2000)

Site of the lesion	No. of patients	Survival (year)		
		1	3	5
Head and neck (incl. thyroid cancer)	42	28 (66.7%)	25 (59.6%)	25 (59.6%)
Lung	1	1	0	0
Skin	46	42 (91.3%)	36 (78.3%)	27 (58.7%)
Anorectal	38	15 (39.5%)	4 (10.5%)	3 (7.9%)
Breast	10	8 (80.0%)	4 (40.0%)	4 (40.0%)
Female genital organs (vulva, uterine cervix)	4	3	2	1
Male genital organs (Prostate)	4	3	1	0
Teratocarcinoma	1	1	0	0
Total	146	101 (69.2%)	72 (49.3%)	60 (41.1%)

and is useful for the simultaneous combined methods of freezing, with contact and penetration, to expedite the freezing procedure.

(5) Thermocouple needles for tissue temperature monitoring are a prerequisite to achieve sufficient cryodestruction of the tumor and to protect adjoining normal tissue.

13.3.3 Procedure

(1) *Temperature Monitoring:* Before starting to freeze, thermocouple needles for tissue temperature monitoring are placed at multiple sites, at least at the three critical points: intratumor, basis of the tumor (invasive front), and juxtatumor normal skin (Figs. 13.3.1a,b) to achieve precise cryodestruction of the tumor and to protect adjacent normal tissue. Tissue temperature down to −50°C to −60°C or lower at the critical points is required to definitely destroy the tumor (3).

(2) *Freezing Temperature, Duration of Time, and Repetitive Freezing:* In the sequential freezing, the probe-tip temperature is set at −100°C to −180°C, and duration of the time is 3 minutes to 10 minutes. The ice front should be at least 1 cm beyond the margin of the tumor, and generally, two or three freeze-thaw cycles are necessary.

(3) *Freezing Technique:* (a) *Contact method*: The most frequently used and safe, with a variety of probe-tip adaptors to fit the size and shape of the tumor. If good contact cannot be obtained because of the rough surface of the tumor, Vaseline may be applied to cover and flatten the surface to obtain certain contact between the probe-tip adaptor and the tumor. Freezing sites are fractionated and overlapped when the tumor is large and wide.

(b) *Penetration method*: Used for a massive tumor. When the tumor surface is hard to penetrate, small cross incisions by an electric knife are made at several sites to introduce a cryoprobe. The penetration method is the best of all of the cryosurgical techniques for massive tumors, but dangerous bleeding from the penetrated wound can occur after thawing in tumors rich in blood vessels. To remedy this, the wound is packed with oxycellulose cotton and/or coagulative agents, and an elastic bandage around the chest, providing pressure on the bleeding tumor, is sometimes necessary as shown later. (c) *Contact method plus spraying method*: Frequently used safely for bulky and for wide-spread tumors, to expedite freezing. A heavy-duty apparatus and LN_2-spraying machine are utilized simultaneously (Fig. 13.3.2). A Vaseline embankment is prepared to prevent run-off of LN_2, which otherwise soaks into the surgical drapes, and thus protect normal skin from unnecessary cold injury when spraying liquid nitrogen (Fig. 13.3.3). (d) *Penetration method plus spraying method*: For massive tumors, it is the most powerful method, yielding the best depth of freezing. (e) *Spraying as the sole method*: For small tumors, e.g., skin metastases or recurrence, with a spray cone (closed spray) (Figs. 13.3.4a,b), or direct open spray onto the superficial lesion it is suitable to treat wide spread tumors in a short period of time. However, it must be remembered that the

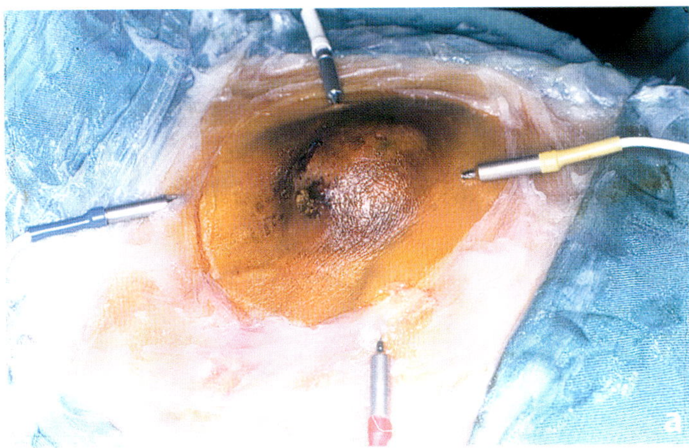

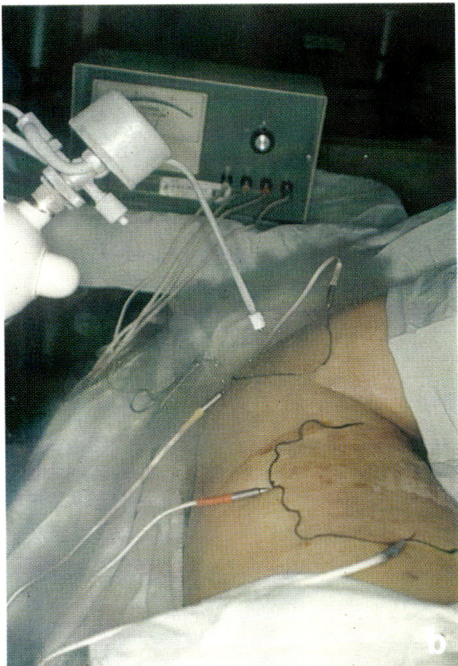

Fig. 13.3.1. a. Before cryosurgery, tissue temperature monitoring thermocouple needles are set in position. A recurrent breast cancer, right-sided, female, 55 y. **b.** Cryosurgery by LN_2-spraying method with subcutaneous temperature monitoring at multiple sites. Bilateral recurrent breast cancer, carcinoma erysipelatodes (inflammatory cancer), female, 49 y. [Reproduced with permission of *Skin Cancer*, Ref. (12)]

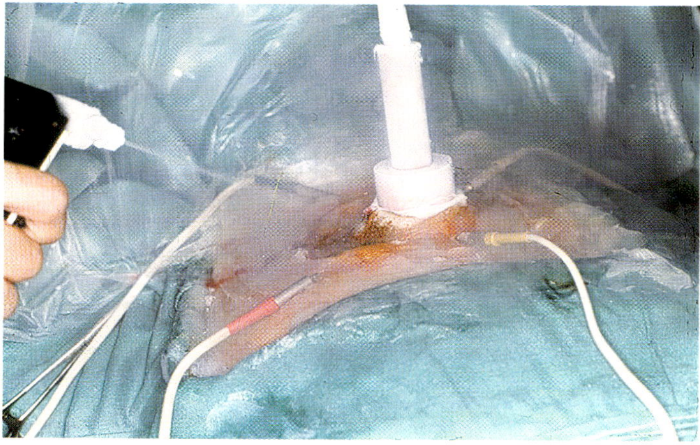

Fig. 13.3.2. Freezing by combined contact and LN_2-spraying method. The same patient as shown in Fig. 13.3.1a. Contact method with 40 mm ø cylindrical probe-tip adaptor, −160°C, 2 cycles, 5 + 10 min, and LN_2-spraying for 5 min

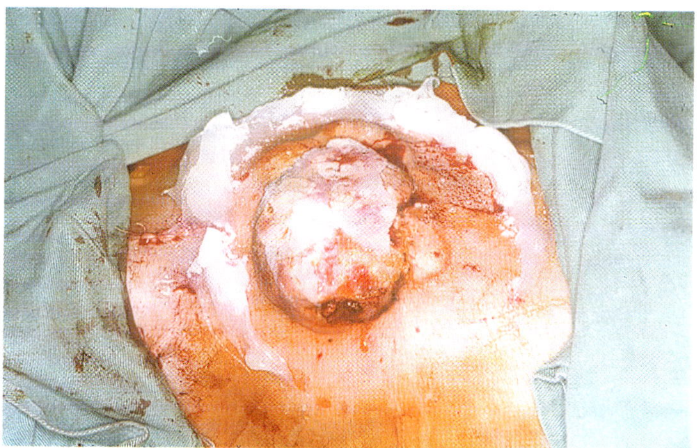

Fig. 13.3.3. A Vaseline embankment. Immediately after freezing by combined contact and spraying method of a solid tumor of a primary breast cancer, right-sided, female, 74 y. Vaseline is also frozen and appears white in the illustration

depth of freezing attained will be less than 1 cm, although there are some reports (5, 6) of successful aggressive freezing of bulky advanced cancer by the open spray alone.

(4) *Warming:* In most cases, the frozen tumor is thawed at room temperature: slow thawing. But sometimes it takes a longtime, therefore on occasion, warming by a microheater installed at the tip of the cryoprobe with the additional help of a hair dryer may be carried out. This maneuver is counter to the principle of "slow thawing", but in our experience, it does expedite the whole procedure, yet does not interfere with cryodestruction of the lesion.

(5) *Necrotomy and Mesh Skin Graft:* Two to three weeks after cryosurgery, necrotomy is done with scissors or an electric knife. At this point, bleeding is not seen or is minimal. Suspicious tumor remnants, if present, are frozen. A mesh skin graft (Fig. 13.3.5) follows to cover the skin defect, one month after the necrotomy. Time is required to observe and confirm no early recurrence of the tumor.

13.3.4 Postoperative Care

(1) *Pressure Bandage:* Postcryosurgical hemorrhage is often a problem. The wound is covered with a thick gauze dressing after topical application of an antibiotic ointment, and then with sterilized soft cotton sheet wadding, which is usually applied under cast fixation for bone fracture, wrapped in

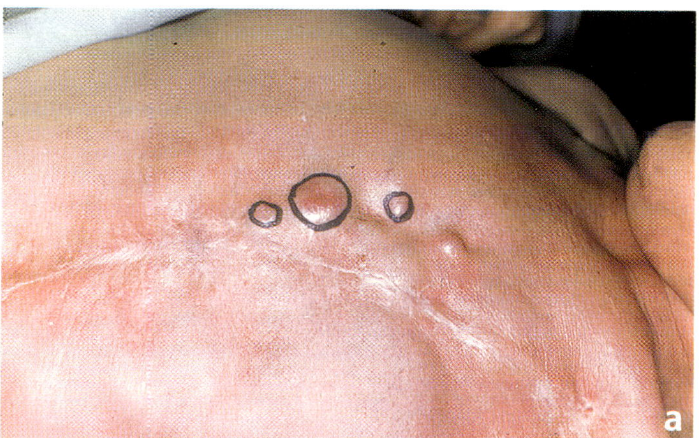

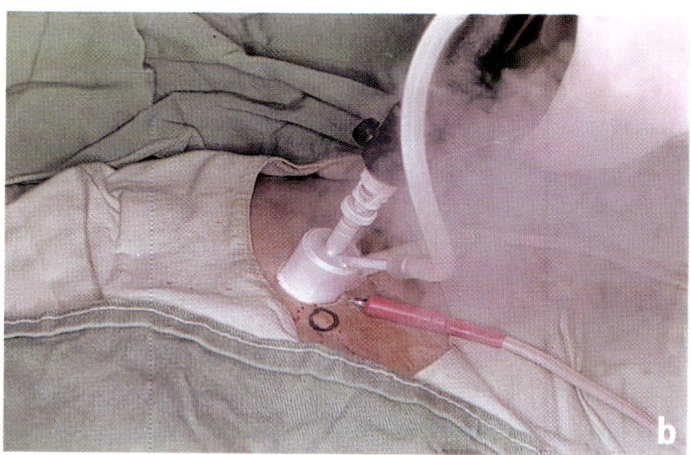

Fig. 13.3.4. **a** Spray-cone technique: Multiple local recurrence of the left-sided breast cancer, female, 75 y. Encircled spots indicate the lesions. **b** With temperature monitoring with thermocouples, LN_2 is sprayed directly into the spray-cone (closed spray), to the extent that the ice front just protrudes from the edge of the cup. [Reproduced with permission of Skin Cancer, Ref. (12)]

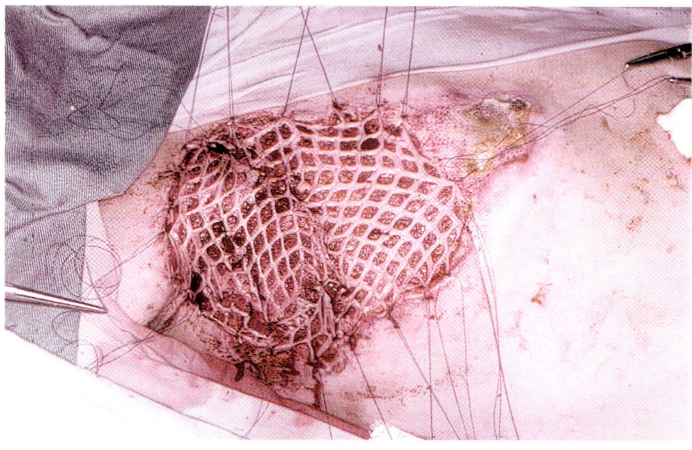

Fig. 13.3.5. A mesh skin graft covering the skin defect after removal of cryonecrotized tumor. A primary breast cancer, right-sided, female, 66 y. T4cN2MX, stage IIIB

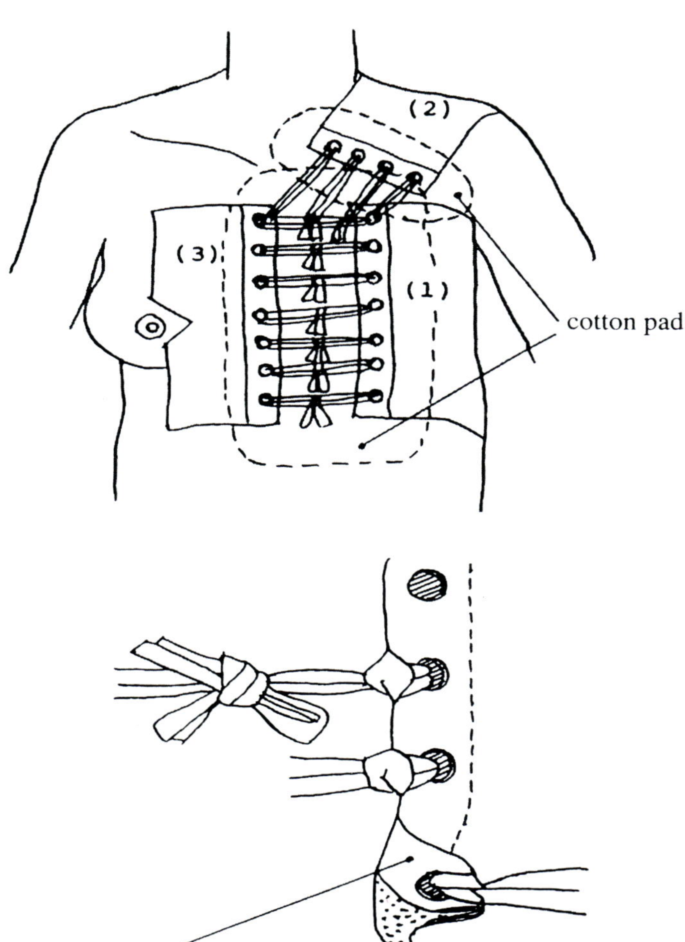

Fig. 13.3.6. A compression bandage after breast cryosurgery. (1)–(3): Wide adhesive plasters. Cotton tapes are tied over the cotton pads. Adhesive plasters are folded double at the edge, and holes are punched out. Cotton tapes are threaded and fixed. [Reproduced with permission of *Skin Cancer*, Ref. (13)]

gauze. Wide adhesive plasters with cotton tapes are prepared and applied. Pressure on the wound is given by tying the tapes to each other from three directions over the cotton pads, as depicted in Fig. 13.3.6, a compression bandage we have been using for advanced, unresectable breast cancer to prevent massive hemorrhage after cryosurgery.

(2) *Pleural Effusion:* After extensive cryosurgery of a breast cancer, the patient must be observed for pleural effusion and dyspnea one or two days after cryosurgical intervention.

(3) *Adjunctive Therapy:* Irradiation to the axillary region, parasternal region, or to the local skin; and standard chemotherapy, endocrine therapy, and immunotherapy are combined, if necessary.

13.3.5 Combination with Novel Modalities of Therapeutic Regimen

(1) *Cryochemotherapy:* A new mode of anticancer regimen, as described in the chapter "Cryochemotherapy". For example, mitomycin C is administered intravenously as a bolus or by drip infusion, either during cryosurgery or within one hour of the cryosurgery. The anticancer agent is trapped within or in the periphery of the tumor in high concentration, thereby the effect is multiplied in combination with the destructive effect of cryosurgery. Incidentally, adriamycin is not trapped in the tumor (7), indicating variable behavior of anticancer drugs. However, administration of the agents intratumorally or within the periphery of the tumor before the second cycle of the freezing is unproblematic and is recommended for the treatment of a solid tumor.

(2) *Cryoimmunointensification Therapy:* We have observed reduction in size of the unresected tumor or spontaneous regression of multiple metastatic lymph nodes (confirmed by biopsy) after cryosurgery (10, 11, 13). We have also observed that adjunctive use of proper biological response modifiers (BRM), (8) cryoimmunointensification therapy, resulted in growth arrest of the tumor in a patient with an advanced bilateral breast cancer, proved by immunohistochemical assessment: immunostaining of the encoded proteins of proto-oncogene, oncogene, and oncosuppressor genes (13).

13.3.6 Case Presentation

Case 1. An 83-year-old female with a primary advanced cancer of the left breast, showing a

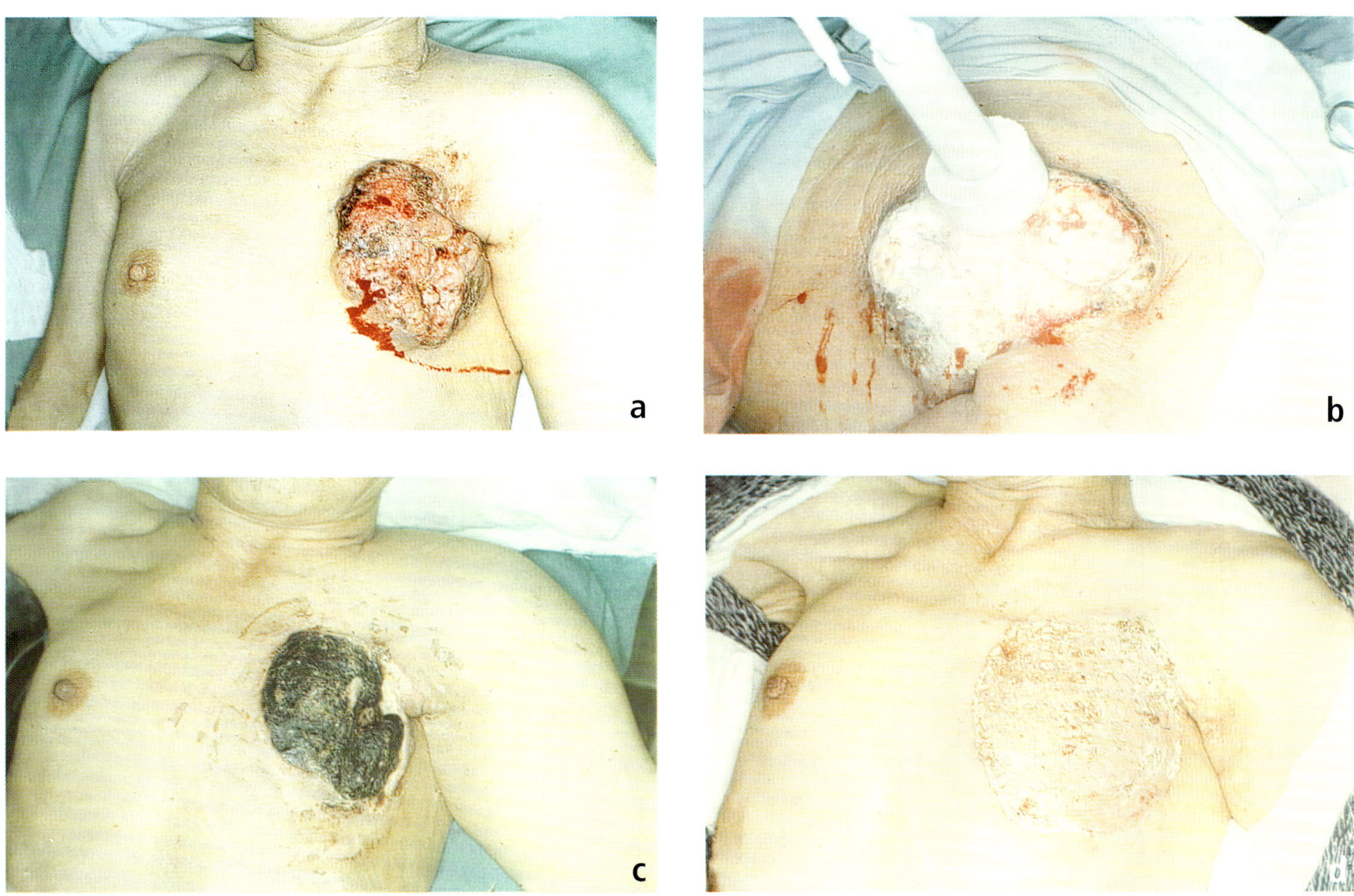

Fig. 13.3.7. a. Case 1. A primary advanced breast cancer, lt, female, 83 y. $T_{4c}N_2M_X$, stage IIIB, fixed to the chest wall, medullotubular carcinoma. **b**. Cryosurgery by contact method, with a 40 mm ø cylindrical probe-tip adaptor, for the fractionated 4 sites, −170°C, 3-cycle freezing, 5 min each, showing an ice ball covered the whole tumor. **c**. Three weeks later. The necrotized tumor is shrunk and crusting. **d**. After necrotomy, a mesh skin graft was performed and took well

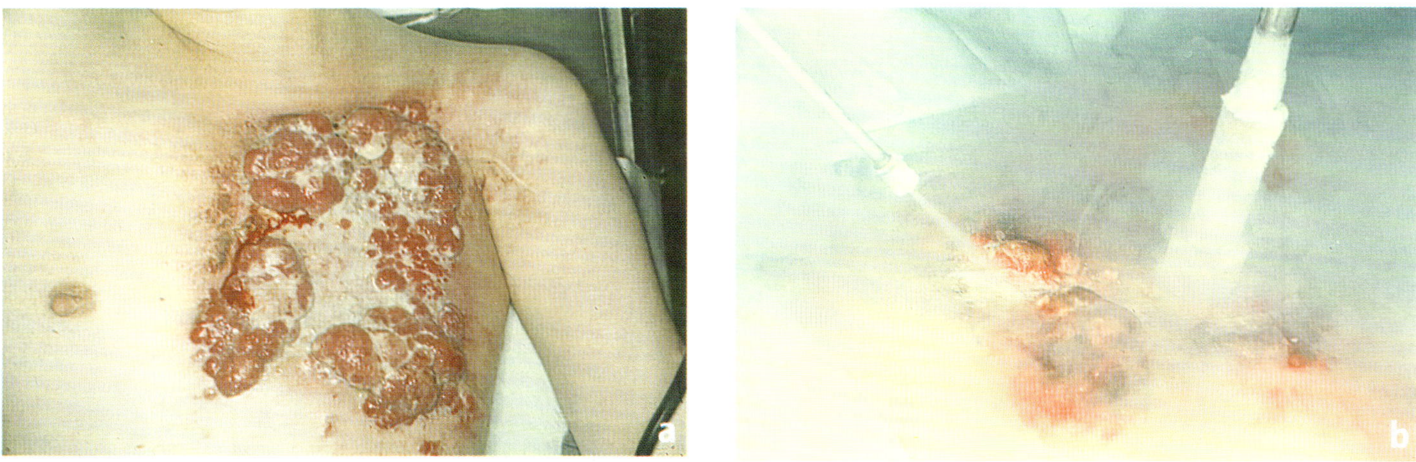

Fig. 13.3.8. a. Case 2. A locally recurrent and wide spread breast cancer, female, 53 y, ductal adenocarcinoma. **b**. Cryosurgery by combined contact and spraying method. Contact freezing with a 40 mm ø cylindrical probe-tip adaptor, for the fractionated 7 sites, −170°C, 2-cycle freezing, 5 min each, and LN_2 spraying for 7 min each of 3 cycles. **c**. Three weeks later, showing the tumor, completely necrotized

cauliflower-like solid tumor, fixed to the chest wall. T4cN2MX, stage IIIB (Figs. 13.3.7a–d). Biopsy revealed medullotubular carcinoma. Cryosurgery by the contact method was done with a heavy-duty device and the tumor was eradicated. After necrotomy, a mesh skin graft was performed and

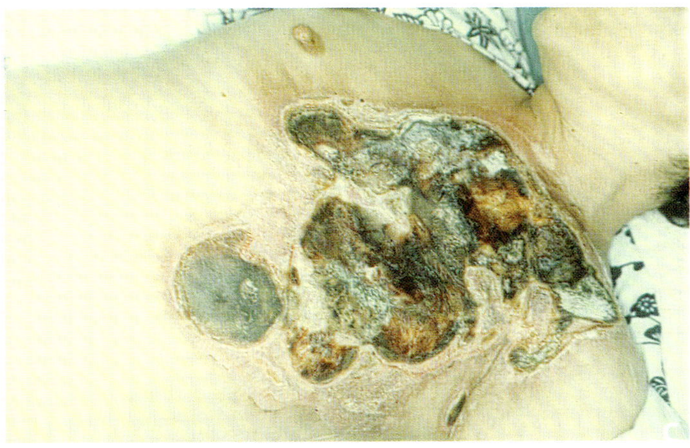

Fig. 13.3.8. (continued)

took well. No recurrence was observed after that, but the patient died of geromaasmus two years later.

Case 2. A 53-year-old female, with a locally recurrent, wide spread cancer of the left breast (Figs. 13.3.8a–c). Cryosurgery was performed by combined contact and spraying methods simultaneously: contact freezing for the fractionated 7 sites, and spraying liquid nitrogen. The tumor was destroyed completely and followed by a mesh skin graft. No recurrence was confirmed since then at least for 3 years, but the patient was lost to further follow-up.

References

1. Cooper IS (1963) Cryogenic surgery: A new method of destruction or extirpation of benign or malignant tissue. N Engl J Med 268: 743–749.
2. Gage AA (1976) Five-year survival following cryosurgery for oral cancer. Arch Surg 111: 990–994.
3. Gage AA, Caruana Jr JA, Montes M (1982) Critical temperature for skin necrosis in experimental cryosurgery. Cryobiology 19: 273–282.
4. Gage AA (1992) Cryosurgery in the treatment of cancer. Surg Gynecol Obstet 174: 73–92.
5. Gonçalves JCA (1986) Cryomastectomy for advanced cancer. Skin Cancer 4: 283–296.
6. Gonçalves JCA (1995) Cryosurgery of breast cancer. In: Lukas, L (ed): Cryosurgery–Mechanism and Applications. International Institute of Refrigeration, Paris, pp. 121–126.
7. Ikekawa S, Ishihara K, Tanaka S, Ikeda S (1985): Basic studies of cryochemotherapy in a murine tumor system. Cryobiology 22: 477–483.
8. Ohkuma T, Ikekawa T, Tanaka S (1982) Intensification of cryoimmunologic reaction by the hot water extract of *Flammulina velutipes* (Curt. ex Fr.) Sing in rabbits and mice. Cryothérapie suppl 10: 25–30 Lyon Méditerranée Médical.
9. Shulman S, Brandt EJ, Yantorno C (1968) Studies in cryoimmunology. II. Tissue and species specificity of the autoantibody response and comparison with isoimmunization. Immunology 14: 149–158.
10. Suzuki Y (1995) Cryosurgical treatment of advanced breast cancer and cryoimmunologic reaction. Skin Cancer 10: 19–26.
11. Tanaka S (1982) Immunological aspects of cryosurgery in general surgery. Cryobiology 19: 247–262.
12. Tanaka S (1995) Cryosurgical treatment of advanced breast cancer. Skin Cancer 10: 9–18.
13. Tanaka S, Ito M, Shinohara N (1998) Extensive cryosurgery and immunotherapy for advanced bilateral breast cancer. Immunohistochemical assessment and report of a case. Skin Cancer 13: 123–142.
14. Yantorno C, Soanes WA, Gonder MJ, Shulman S (1967) Studies in cryoimmunology. I. The production of antibodies to urogenital tissue in consequence of freezing treatment. Immunology 12: 395–410.

14. Cryosurgery for Bone Tumors

H. W. Bart Schreuder

14.0 Introduction

In 1968 Ralph C. Marcove introduced cryosurgery into orthopedic oncology for the treatment of primary and metastatic bone tumors by repetitive freezing. He was awarded the first prize in scientific research at the 162nd annual convention of the Medical Society of the State of New York (1). Since then more orthopedic surgeons dealing with skeletal tumors have adopted the technique, and the clinical results and experimental data of cryosurgery with specific reference to the skeletal system have been published regularly.

Cryosurgery utilizing liquid nitrogen is practised in orthopedic oncology for the treatment of primary benign and malignant bone tumors as well as for secondary metastases to bone. In benign and low-grade malignant stage IA skeletal tumors it is used as an adjuvant treatment to intralesional resection (curettage) to extend the surgical margin of resection. By this method the procedure can be considered to be marginal according to oncologic principles (2). The advantage of this kind of treatment, as compared to local resection, is that as much as possible of the supportive function of bone is preserved and that reconstructive surgery can be limited.

In high grade sarcomas, cryosurgery has been used as the primary treatment with variable results (3). Cryosurgery used in the treatment of bony metastases has to be considered as palliative and in this respect helpful in local control of the malignancy (4). Theoretically, adjuvant therapy may consist of systemic chemotherapy, radiotherapy and physical adjuvants like phenol, hypertonic saline merthiolate, polymethylmethacrylate (PMMA) cement applied locally, and cryosurgery.

Chemotherapy and irradiation therapy have an effect on mitotically-active cells. Their influence on benign bone tumors is limited and inappropriate because of the side-effects. Although benign bone tumors have been treated with radiation therapy, especially in sites of difficult surgical access, there is a growing concern about the risk of secondary sarcoma in the irradiated field.

Phenol is a non-selective cytotoxic agent and when applied directly to the surface of curetted bone tumors, it kills remaining residual tumor and normal cells. When phenol is used as an adjuvant after curettage of benign bone tumors, the reported recurrence rate is 12.5% to 20% (5,6). Recurrence is probably due to its superficial action and the impossibility of penetrating the periphery beyond the surgical margin.

The rationale for the use of PMMA cement as adjuvant treatment is based on its heating effect. Experiments have shown that a thermal lesion of at least −50°C is necessary for a cytotoxic effect. The maximum peripheral extent of a thermal lesion varies from 2.5 mm in cancellous to only 0.5 mm in cortical bone (7).

As compared to other adjuvant modalities cryosurgery has some major advantages. It is an active local adjuvant with no systemic side-effects, non-toxic to the patient and those working with it, extremely powerful, and above all the dosage can be controlled, so that the procedure can be customized to the specific type of bone tumor and location.

14.1 Cryosurgical Techniques for Bone Tumors

Progress in the attainment of low and very low temperatures is a reflection of technical inventions and advancements throughout history. When we look back, the apparatuses used in the early days of cryosurgery seem somewhat contrived. On the other hand modern cryosurgery instruments, which are perfectly equipped for successful treatment today, will probably be deemed inadequate tomorrow. In this, cryosurgery is comparable to every other advancement in medicine. Therefore continuing research to improve current techniques is necessary, in particular to respond to demands for safety and expanded indications.

14.2 Cryoprobe Design

The basic design of cryoprobes suitable for orthopedic oncological purposes can be divided into *open* and *closed* systems (8). Since today liquid nitrogen is most commonly used, this section will deal specifically with this particular cryogen.

In *open* systems liquid nitrogen is sprayed directly on tissue and has been shown to be an effective, if not the most effective, way of cooling. The liquid nitrogen cools the tissue by boiling, which occurs as heat is extracted from the tissue surface. When the liquid is forced out of the nozzle, the sudden drop of pressure causes partial vaporization, a phenomenon called "flashing". Liquid nitrogen drops in the spray will start boiling immediately when they come into contact with a higher surface temperature. The initial vaporized gas can form a vapor layer between the liquid nitrogen and the target tissue. This vapor layer or "film" acts as an insulator and prevents further cooling of the surface.

In general, *closed* systems employ two different principles for creating low temperatures at the end of a probe. The first principle applied in cooling a cryoprobe is to allow liquid nitrogen to boil at the end of the tip of the probe; by boiling it extracts latent heat from its surroundings, cooling it at the same time. As long as liquid nitrogen is passed through the tip fast enough to maintain boiling, the temperature at the tip of the probe will remain at the boiling point of liquid nitrogen: −196°C. The other principle used to cool the end of a cryoprobe in closed systems utilizes the Joule-Thomson effect. If a pressurized gas is allowed to expand to a much lower pressure, its temperature will drop. The magnitude of change in temperature depends on the change in pressure and the physical characteristics of the substance used. The most commonly used gas in this kind of probe is nitrous oxide.

The operational control of cryoprobes in general is carried out by simply stopping the flow of the cryogen. Stopping the cryosurgery is a decision made by the physician. The decision is mainly based on experience. In addition, monitoring devices are available, which will be described later.

14.3 Basic Technique

The basic technique of cryosurgery requires an effective use or exploitation of biological mechanisms leading to cell death under the influence of low temperature. It has been shown that the most effective way to achieve this is rapid freezing and slow thawing, done in repetitive cycles. To establish these suitable cryobiological circumstances an efficient technique is needed in situ to extract heat from the tissue.

The requirements for rapid freezing are:

- A cryogen suitable for the lesion, not only providing potential cooling power, but also in sufficient quantities.
- Furthermore it must be safe (nontoxic and nonflammable), easy to store and to transport, and preferably inexpensive. For orthopedic purposes only liquid nitrogen meets all these criteria, used either in closed probe systems or as a spray.
- The contact area between the lesion and the cryogenic device should be as large as possible, facilitating rapid transport of heat.
- The surface of a lesion in orthopedic oncology is always irregular and frequently large. These surface properties nearly always necessitate the use of a liquid nitrogen spray instead of a probe (Fig. 14.1). In orthopedic oncology closed cryoprobes are used in very small bones like those of the fingers (Fig. 14.2) and in "tricky" locations like the cervical spine (Fig. 14.3).

The principle for slow thawing requires only patience on the part of the surgeon. Ideally, frozen tissue should be allowed to completely thaw without assistance. While rapid freezing can be achieved in less than 30 seconds, spontaneous thawing in the orthopedic setting can take up to ten minutes or more. The thawing rate is most influenced by nearby heat sources such as blood vessels.

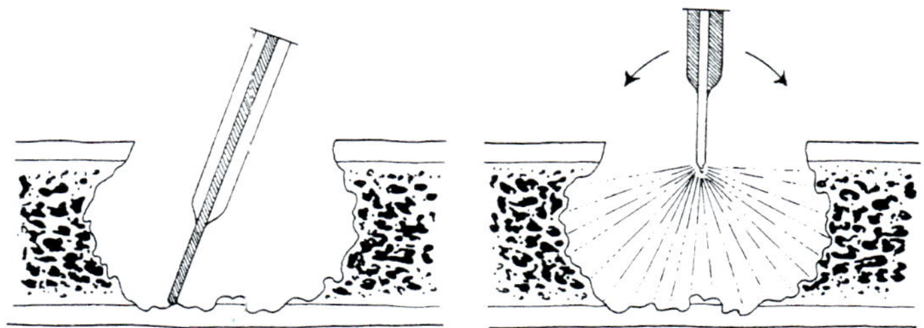

Fig. 14.1. A cryoprobe (left) is not able to freeze an irregular surface like spongiosa, a spray will wet the complete lesion (right)

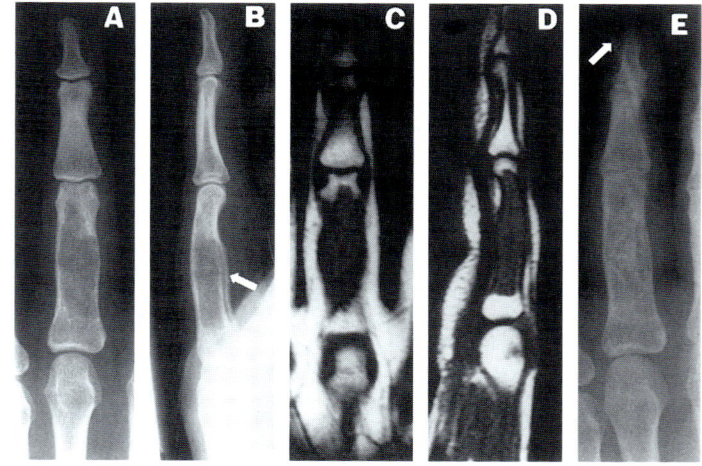

Fig. 14.2.1. Radiographs of painful enchondroma (**A**, **B**) located in first phalanx of digit 3 of a 30-year-old woman. Periosteal reaction (arrow). T1 weighted MRI: coronal (**C**) and sagittal (**D**). (**E**) Post-operative view after curettage, cryosurgery and autologous bone graft, wound drain in situ (arrow)

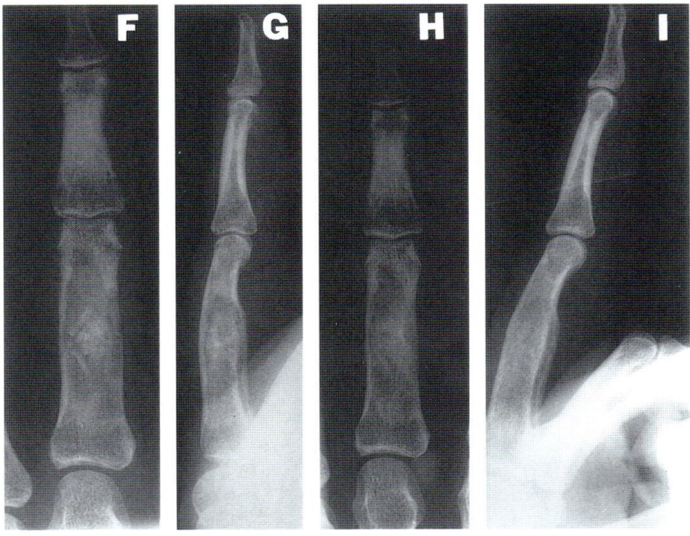

Fig.14.2.2. Seven weeks (**F** ,**G**) and 12 months (**H** ,**I**) postoperatively, progressive incorporation of bone graft, normal function

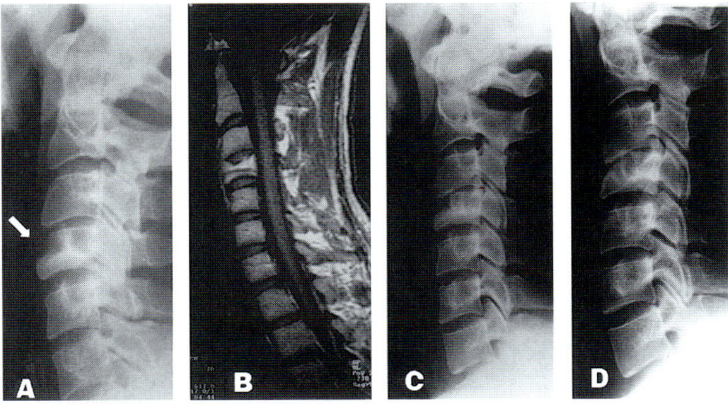

Fig. 14.3. Lateral radiograph of cervical spine of 23-year-old man. Eosinophylic granuloma of bone of body C4 (**A**). T1 weighted magnetic resonance image, partial collapse of body (**B**). Follow-up at 4 months after curettage, cryosurgery and autologous strut bone graft (**C**) and at 10 months (**D**)

It is necessary to repeat the freeze and thaw cycles several times, because living tissue is capable of resisting thermal injury and it is technically difficult to achieve optimal conditions for cell death in all areas of many lesions. To compensate, repetition of freeze/thaw cycles is a practical solution and provides safety especially at the periphery of the lesion. After the first cycle, thermal conductivity in the tissue is increased, and the specific heat capacity and vascularity are decreased. This preconditions the tissue, making the next cycles more effective by virtue of faster cooling and slower thawing rates. The benefit of repeat cycles is well established in the literature (9–12).

14.4 Surgical Technique

Standard orthopedic oncologic exposures are used. When the exact location of a lesion or the proximity of a growth plate is unclear, an image intensifier is used. To avoid inadvertent freezing of the skin, wide retraction is mandatory. The use of extremity tourniquets may be ill advised, because normal circulation decreases the risk of freezing nearby neurovascular bundles and skin. Normally it is not necessary to dissect the neurovascular bundle away from the lesion to be frozen.

A sufficient oval window is made in the cortex using a drill or saw. The tumor is resected as thoroughly as possible using a curette (Fig. 14.4B). Care is taken to avoid pushing tumor into the uninvolved medullary canal.

To monitor the cryosurgical process and local extent of the freeze, thermocouples are positioned in and around the lesion (see next section).

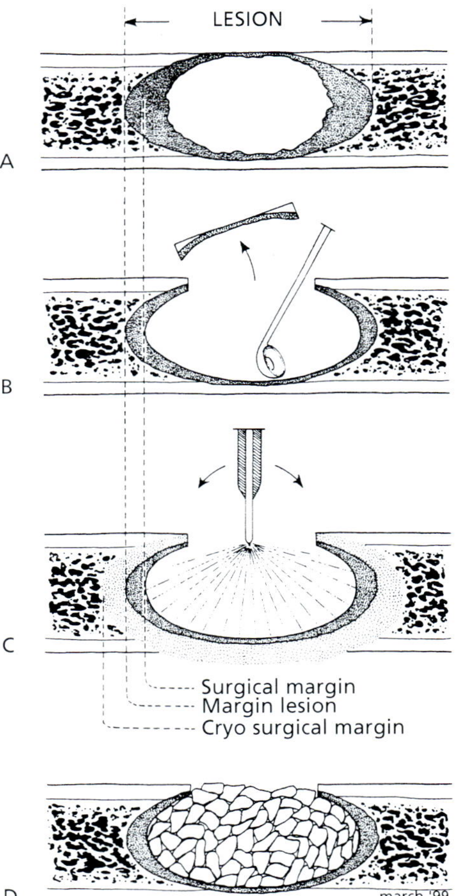

Fig. 14.4. The bone tumor (**A**) is exposed via a sufficient oval window made in the cortex (**B**). Intralesional resection or curettage is done with curettes resulting in a surgical margin. Three cycles of cryosurgery result in a cryosurgical margin (**C**).The defect remaining after curettage and cryosurgery is filled with autograft or allograft bone chips (**D**)

Cryosurgery is then performed (Fig. 14.4C). Three cycles of cryosurgery are performed using a machine producing a liquid nitrogen spray. This spray is directed into the lesion in every direction, until the whole cavity is wetted and becomes frosted. The nitrogen vapor clouding the view is waved away by hand. The duration of each freeze is based on the temperature readings and visual observation. Intralesional temperatures of at least −50°C are aimed for and are necessary to induce tissue necrosis (13,14). Warming up to 20°C takes place by spontaneous thawing.

The defect remaining after curettage and cryosurgery is filled with autograft or allograft bone chips. The cortical window is frozen as well and is replaced or used as a source of bone graft (Fig. 14.4D).

A careful soft tissue reconstruction is very important, restoring the periosteum, if possible, and covering the bone with muscle. A wound drain is always used and it should only be removed when drainage falls below 30 ml per 24 hours. Perioperative antibiotics are routinely used. If the strength of weightbearing bones, in particular the diaphysis of the femur, is compromised by the lesion and cryosurgery, prophylactic internal fixation is advised, using a plate and screws. An intramedullary enforcement is ill advised, because it has the risk of contaminating the entire intramedullary compartment with tumor cells. Partial weightbearing is usually necessary until three months after the operation.

14.5 Monitoring

A cryosurgical procedure with a satisfactory result can be achieved based only the physician's clinical judgement and experience. However, there are several reasons to use precise monitoring devices.

- To ensure that lethal temperatures are reached. The temperature of frozen tissue cannot be determined by its appearance, as frosted tissue looks the same at any freezing temperature.
- An accurate measurement of the depth of the freezing is important not only for obtaining adequate margins, especially if the lesion has a malignant nature, but also to avoid an unwarranted extension of the freezing and potential morbidity.
- Local temperature measurement enables a more precise determination of the ending of the thawing phase.
- Not only local monitoring is important, but systemic monitoring is also recommended, since cryosurgery has been associated with potentially lethal circulatory and pulmonary complications.
- Monitoring and preferably recording of the cryosurgical procedure enables the physician to evaluate the procedure itself, for instance the freezing rate, and better interpret follow-up results with respect to the procedure. Adjustments in technique can be developed and introduced. Scientific research on the data gathered will ultimately improve the quality of cryosurgery.

14.6 Local Monitoring

In orthopedic oncology procedures, tissues with different thermal characteristics are involved. These are cortical bone, intramedullary spongiosa, and soft tissues, mainly muscle. To supplement clinical judgement during cryosurgery, a range of monitoring devices and techniques has been developed, most of them to address monitoring needs for specific applications of cryosurgery. Measurement modalities are thermography (15), which involves very expensive equipment and provides only surface freezing evaluation, ultrasound which is not suitable for bony tissue (16, 17), and tissue impedance and resistance measurements (18–20), which raise concerns about accuracy. Computerized tomography and magnetic resonance imaging are capable of visualising frozen tissue, but their high cost and the logistics involved make them unsuitable for the orthopedic setting (21–24).

Thermocouples are by far the only suitable device for intraoperative (real-time) temperature monitoring during cryosurgery for bone tumors. Thermocouples are formed by a series of two dissimilar conductors in a closed circuit. When the junction of the two metals is subjected to a different temperature from the rest of the circuit, an electromotive force proportional to the difference in temperature is generated. This voltage can be measured. Thermocouples were first used to monitor cryosurgery of skin lesions. Their importance was recognized early in cryosurgical practice, particularly in establishing lethal temperatures. The accuracy of the thermocouple readings is important, as the effectiveness of treatment partially depends on it. Proper calibration and reliable hardware (good quality of thermocouple, wiring, electrical connections and display devices) are imperative. The thermocouples consist of a copper/copper-nickel alloy and are mounted in the tip of a 50-mm-long and 0.8-mm-diameter injection-like needle. Their accuracy is better than 0.1°C with a response time of 0.3 sec. Temperature data acquisition is done using a digital multimeter equipped with a thermocouple scanner card. Graphic real-time visualization of the course of the temperatures is accomplished by connecting the multimeter to a personal computer running appropriate software. Next to performing real-time display, this program stores all temperature data for later analysis (25). The locations of the thermocouples should be chosen from a strategic point of view as illustrated in Fig. 14.5.

Correct placement of the thermocouples and verification of their positions with radiographs is sometimes necessary, especially when structures have to be protected from a freeze injury, for instance joints and growthplates (Figs. 14.6 and 14.7).

Using the temperature measuring system with real-time graphic visualisation, it has been shown that in a cryosurgical system using a liquid nitrogen spray, intralesional temperatures of −150°C are achieved within seconds (freezing-rate >10°C/s^{-1}). Furthermore, the maintenance of a temperature of −50°C for 40 sec, and the tissue in the frozen state for 3 min, followed by spontaneous slow thawing and repetition of freeze/thaw cycles, are all of importance to maximize tissue destruction (26).

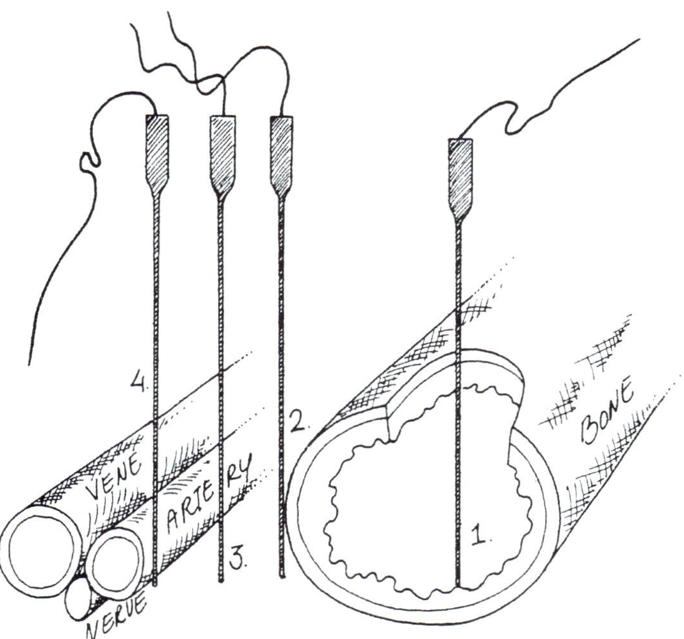

Fig. 14.5. Thermocouple 1 is situated intralesionally to ensure lethal temperatures to destroy tumor cells. Thermocouple 2 is located extracortically to monitor the extent of the freeze. Thermocouple 3 between the lesion and the vascular bundle and 4 close to the vascular bundle "guard" prevent damage to these structures

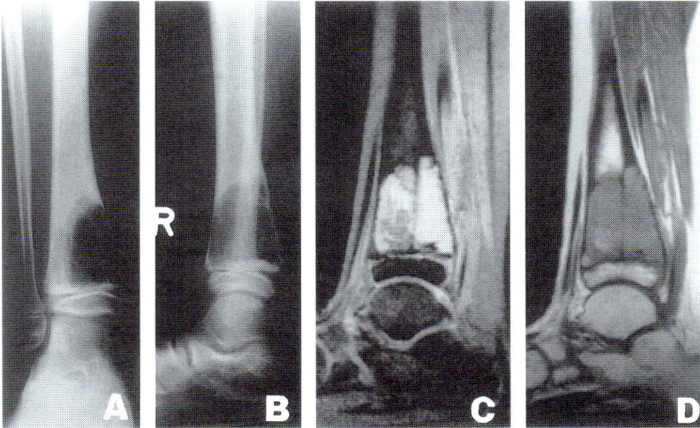

Fig. 14.6.1. Routine radiographs of an 11-year-old boy with aneurysmal bone cyst in the distal tibia, extending very close to the growth plate (**A**, **B**). Magnetic resonance imaging, T2 (**C**) and T1 (**D**), showing erosion of cortex and a fairly homogeneous intensity of the contents of the cyst consistent with fluid. The cyst seems not to have damaged the epiphysis

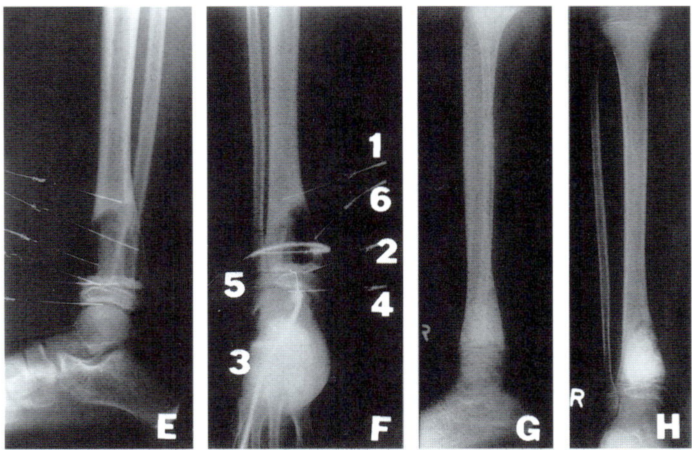

Fig. 14.6.2. Intraoperative radiographs showing localization of the temperature couples. Number 2 and 3 are situated in the growth plate, number 4 is intra-articular (**E**, **F**). The intralesional temperature couple number 7 was added later. After curettage and cryosurgery the cyst is filled with a homologous bone graft (**G**, **H**)

After spraying has been stopped and thawing is allowed, the extralesional thermocouples show a further lowering of temperature, representing the retraction of tissue heat, which is used for the thawing of the more central parts of the frozen lesion. The non-linear increase of the temperature in frozen tissue and its subzero plateau phase is explained by additional energy needed for the transition of ice into water, which halts the temperature increase temporarily. In Figs. 14.8 and 14.9 all these phenomena are shown next to almost identical patterns of the freeze/thaw cycles, indicating that cryosurgery utilizing a spray is a reproducible method.

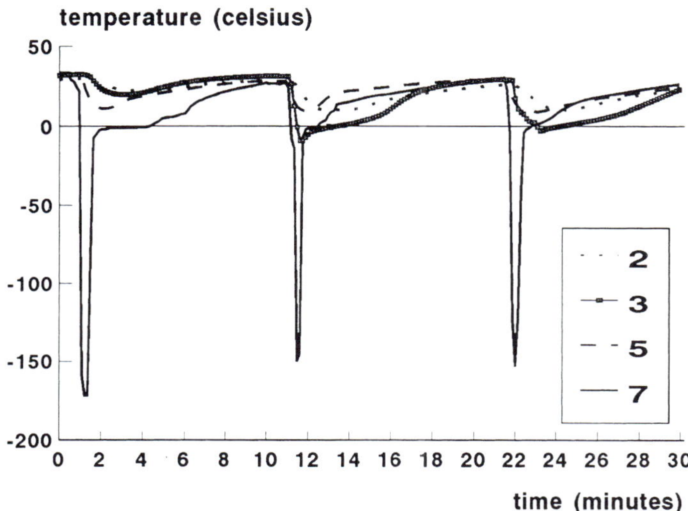

Fig. 14.7. Temperature recordings of patient in Fig. 14.6.1&2: numbers correspond with those in Fig. 14.6.2 E and F. The recording number 3, next to number 2 of the epiphysis, shows subzero levels during the second and third freeze cycle which may damage the epiphysis. The temperature measured by the thermocouples 1, 4 and 6 were at all times above 25°C. For reasons of clarity of the graph they are not shown

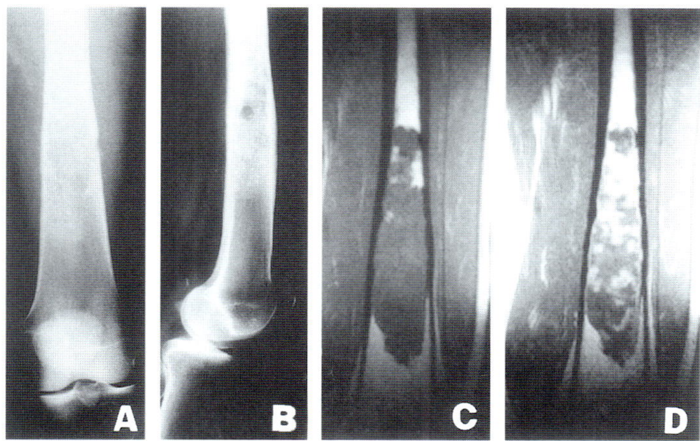

Fig. 14.8.1. Post-biopsy routine radiographs of a 29-year-old female with chondrosarcoma, grade 1, of diaphysis of the femur (**A**, **B**). Magnetic resonance imaging, T1 (**C**) and T2 (**D**) weighted showing erosion of cortex and an inhomogeneous signal intensity consistent with enchondroma or low-grade chondrosarcoma

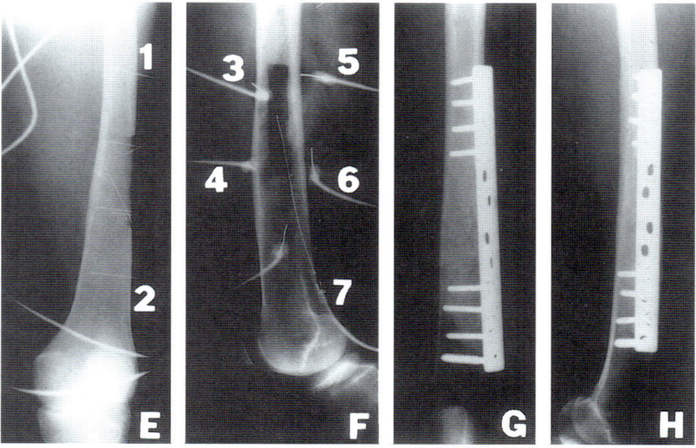

Fig. 14.8.2. Intra-operative radiographs of patient in Fig. 14.8.1 showing location of the temperature couples (E,F). Number 7 is situated in the curetted lesion. Numbers correspond to those in Fig. 14.9. After curettage and cryosurgery the cyst is filled with a homologous bone graft. To prevent postoperative fracture a prophylactic osteosynthesis was added (G,H)

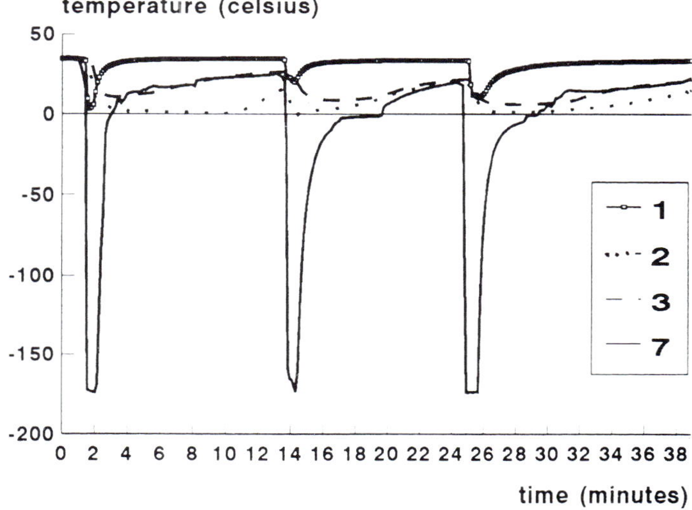

Fig. 14.9. Temperature recordings of patient in Fig. 14.8; numbers correspond to those in Fig. 14.8.2 E and F. The temperature measured by the thermocouples 4, 5 and 6 were at all times above 10°C. For reasons of clarity of the graph they are not shown

14.7 Systemic Monitoring

Whenever a gas is introduced into a body cavity there is always the hazard of intravascular introduction of gas bubbles, especially when pressure is allowed to develop. Gas emboli in the vascular circulation can cause serious hemodynamic complications (27–30). Therefore, in addition to routine systemic monitoring of the patient, end-tidal gas analysis is indicated using a mass spectrometer measuring inspired and end-tidal O_2, CO_2, N_2O, N_2 tensions and anesthetic vapor concentration. Using real-time recording of the gas analysis breath by breath makes detection of any exhaled N_2 possible, which is associated with venous nitrogen gas embolism. In this way one may be able to take appropriate action in time to prevent serious hemodynamic complications.

Monitoring the freeze/thaw cycles during a cryosurgical procedure with temperature recordings in and outside the lesion in orthopedic oncology is of importance and very helpful in facilitating an effective, reproducible cryosurgical procedure and in controlling the extent of the freeze avoiding local complications. Systemic monitoring is of paramount significance for the safety of the patient.

14.8 Clinical Results

In general the following orthopedic bone tumors are suitable for cryosurgery:

- simple bone cyst
- aneurysmal bone cyst
- giant cell tumor
- eosinophilic granuloma
- enchondroma and chondrosarcoma grade 1
- fibrous dysplasia
- miscellaneous.

In specific circumstances the technique can be of value for the treatment of malignant lesions of bone. These circumstances are:

- Marginal resection of the tumor is, due to its location, not possible or induces unacceptable morbidity, such as in vertebral (chordoma) and pelvic lesions.
- Marginal or wide resection is not indicated but beneficial for local control of the tumor, as with bone metastases.

Simple bone cyst: Simple bone cyst is a tumor of bone of unknown origin. It tends to occur in the metaphyses of long bones, particularly of the humerus and femur. Although histologically completely benign, it frequently weakens the integrity of bone resulting in pathological fracture, which is often the presenting feature. The treatment options for simple bone cysts include observation, injection and surgical curettage. Until Scaglietti et al. introduced the technique of steroid injections (31, 32), the most prevalent treatment method for simple bone cyst has been curettage followed by bone grafting, with recurrent rates that vary from 12 to 48% (33–42). Adjuvant therapy after curettage is indicated to destroy residual tumor cells and lower tumor recurrence.

A retrospective study in children with unicameral bone cysts treated with curettage, cryosurgery and bone grafting showed that 5 of 42 (12%) treated patients suffered a local recurrence with a mean clinical follow-up of 24.5 months (43). In another study of 13 patients 2 local recurrences were reported (44).

Aneurysmal bone cyst: Aneurysmal bone cyst is a rare benign tumor-like lesion of bone of unknown origin. There is controversy as to whether it is a distinctive radiological and pathological entity or a pathophysiological change superimposed on a preexisting lesion (45). Lack of understanding about its origin and growth makes treatment empirical. The most common treatment has been curettage with bone grafting which has a substantial rate of recurrence (33,46–49). Lower recurrence rates can be achieved by marginal or wide resection but are accompanied by loss of bone and the need for reconstruction (33,50,51).

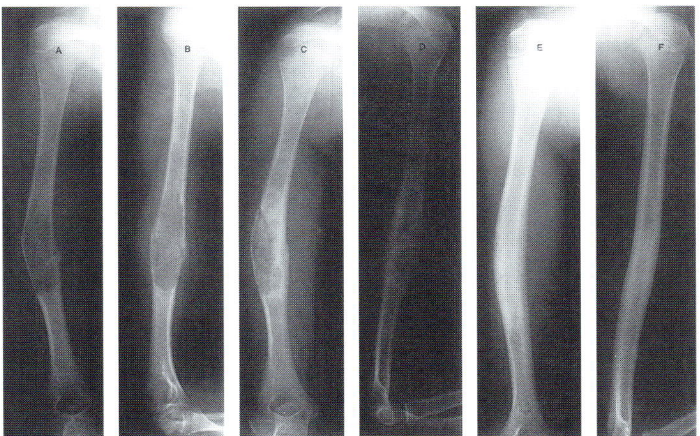

Fig. 14.10. Simple bone cyst of the humerus in an 11-year-old girl. Preoperative radiographs showing pathological fracture (**A**, **B**). Postoperative radiographs at two months after curettage, cryosurgery and bone grafting (**C**, **D**), and at 13 months demonstrating complete consolidation of the grafted site and humeral remodelling (**E**, **F**)

A review of the literature on the results of treatment modalities, including cryosurgery, is listed in Table 14.1.

The recurrence rates for irradiation with or without curettage are similar, 11.8% and 13.8%, respectively. Curettage with or without bone grafting is accompanied by a high recurrence rate of 30.8%. Cryosurgery as an adjuvant after curettage has a recurrence rate of 12.8%. In two series describing the use of cryosurgery as adjuvant treatment a local recurrence rate of 4% is reported in one. The other series reported a recurrence rate of 18%, which, after additional treatments with the same technique, decreased to 4% (48). It may be concluded that cryosurgery for aneurysmal bone cysts has comparable results to marginal resection in terms of control of the tumor (52). However, after marginal resection extensive reconstructive surgery is needed, with associated morbidity.

Giant cell tumor: Giant cell tumor is considered to be a benign lesion, however during its clinical course it shows very aggressive features with the potential for destruction of bone and joints and soft tissue intrusion. Furthermore, 3% of giant cell

Table 14.1. Different types of treatment (N) and recurrence (R) of aneurysmal bone cysts

Author	irradiation therapy		curettage + irradiation		curettage + or - bone graft		curettage + cryosurgery		marginal resection		wide resection		mean follow-up (months)	time to first recurrence (months)
	N	R	N	R	N	R	N	R	N	R	N	R		
Campanacci et al. (33)	8		15	3	91	19	–	–	47	0	–	–	84	2–72
Cole (50)	–	–	1	0	18	7	–	–	4	0	2	0	>24	75%< 24
Clough and Price (46)	1	0	2	0	15	8	–	–	3	0	–	–	79	5–48
Farcetti et al. (53)	–	–	3	0	11	2	–	–	–	–	6	0	116	3–4
Freiberg et al. (47)	–	–	–	–	7	5	–	–	–	–	–	–	>24	<14
Koskinen et al. (59)	–	–	1	0	14	2	–	–	–	–	5	0	54	–
Kreicbergs et al. (54)	–	–	–	–	21	8	–	–	–	–	–	–	>24	–
van Loon et al. (55)	1	0	–	–	8	3	–	–	–	–	1	0	102	7–15
Marcove et al. (48)	11	1	–	–	44	26	51	9	–	–	–	–	85	3–102
Nobler et al. (57)	6	1	1	0	18	6	–	–	4	2	4	0	–	–
Ruiter et al. (49)	2	0	–	–	82	28	–	–	17	4	4	0	80% > 24	–
Slowick et al. (56)	4	0	–	–	5	1	–	–	–	–	4	0	83	10
Szendröi et al. (51)	–	–	–	–	26	7	–	–	6	0	16	0	>24	14
Vergel De Dios et al. (58)	1	0	12	2	124	27	–	–	–	–	17	0	>24	90%<24
Schreuder et al. (52)	–	–	–	–	–	–	27	1	–	–	–	–	47	36
Total:	34	4	36	5	484	149	78	10	81	6	59	0		
Recurrence rates (%):	11.8		13.8		30.8		12.8		7.4		0			

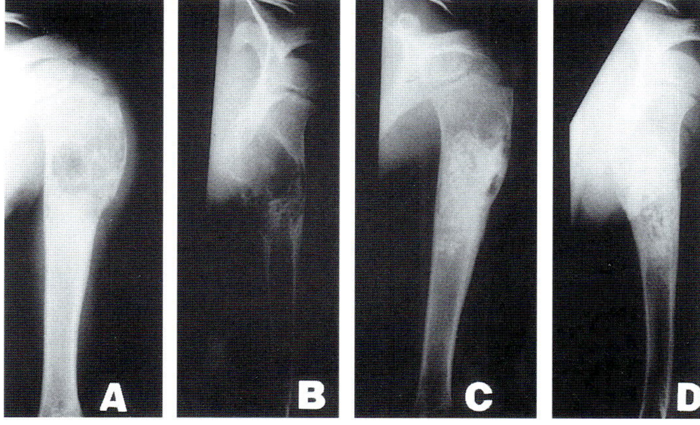

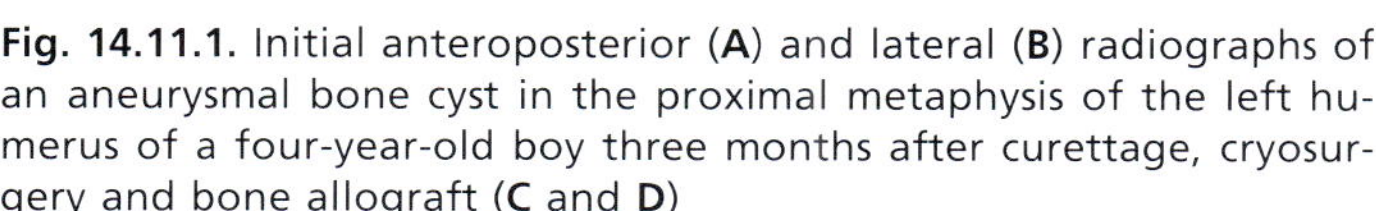

Fig. 14.11.1. Initial anteroposterior (**A**) and lateral (**B**) radiographs of an aneurysmal bone cyst in the proximal metaphysis of the left humerus of a four-year-old boy three months after curettage, cryosurgery and bone allograft (**C** and **D**)

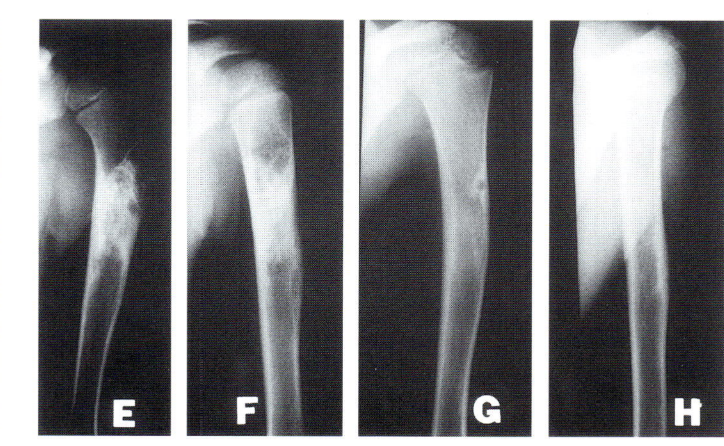

Fig. 14.11.2. Folow-up results of patient in Fig. 14.11.1 one year (**E** and **F**) and four years (**G** and **H**) later. The bone has completely remodelled and the appearance of the intramedullary space is almost normal

tumors are primarily malignant or will undergo malignant transformation and will metastasize either after radiation therapy or after several local recurrences. The anatomic locations in which giant cell tumors commonly occur are the femoral condyles, tibial plateau, proximal humerus and distal radius.

In view of the nature of this tumor, its treatment should be well thought through, sufficient, and in the hands of surgeons with experience dealing with this tumor. Expendable bones with giant cell tumor (proximal fibula, ribs) should be resected. Curettage (without an adjuvant treatment) will result in local recurrence rates of about 40% (60). Therefore, contained lesions are treated with curettage followed by local adjuvant treatment (cryosurgery, cytotoxic agents etc.) (Fig. 14. 12).

The treatment results published in the literature on curettage followed by cryosurgery of giant cell tumor are summarized in Table 14.2.

In the case of a joint destroyed by a giant cell tumor, commonly with an intra-articular pathological fracture, marginal resection and reconstruction are advised. However, preservation of the joint is possible in selected cases using curettage, cryosurgery, bone graft, cement and osteosyntheses (Fig. 14.13).

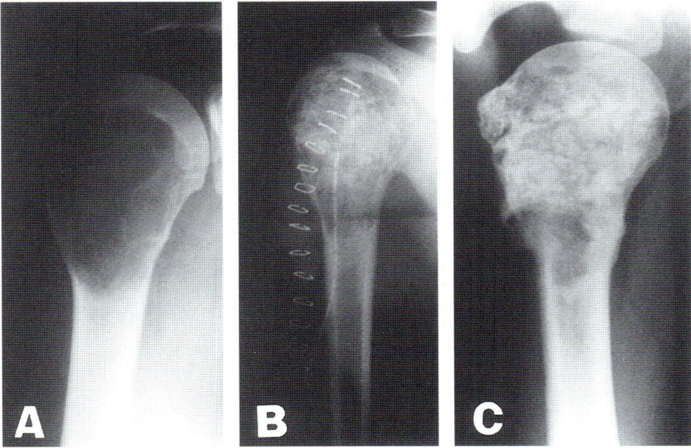

Fig. 14.12.1. Giant cell tumor in the proximal part of the humerus in a 24-year-old woman: only a thin layer of bone supporting the articular cartilage is preserved (**A**). Status after curettage, cryosurgery and homologous bone grafting (**B**) and at three months after the operation (**C**)

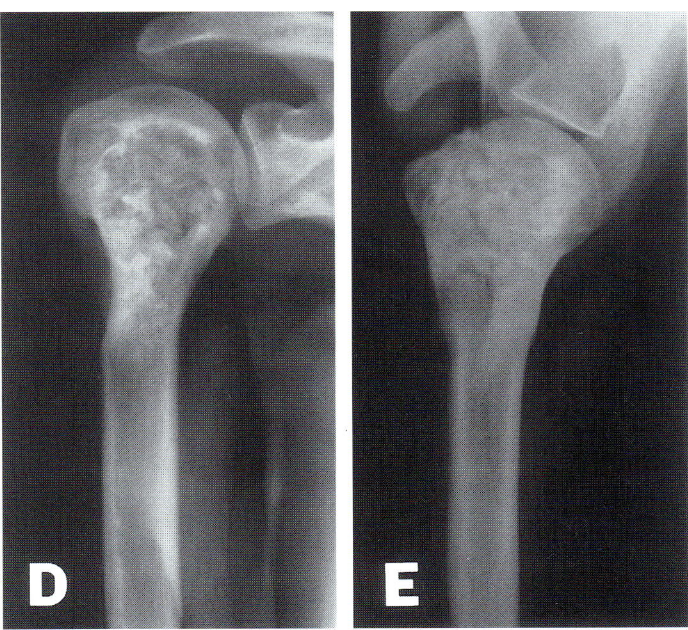

Fig. 14.12.2. One year postoperatively; no signs of arthrosis, excellent range of motion (**D**, **E**)

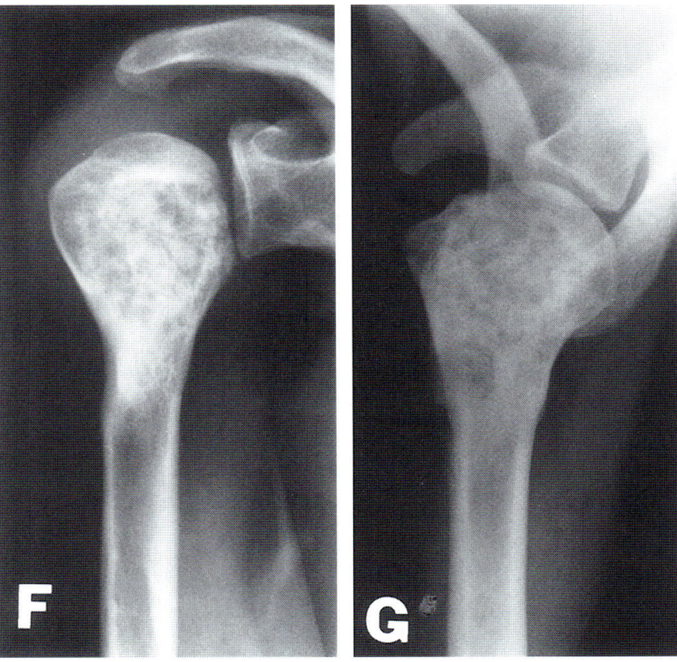

Fig. 14.12.3. 22 months after the operation. Arthrosis on the anteroposterior view (**F**), but not on the lateral view (**G**). The patient is currently asymptomatic, but should she develop severe osteoarthritis there is now sufficient bone stock, and the preservation of the rotator cuff musculature facilitates standard total shoulder arthroplasty

Eosinophilic granuloma of bone: Eosinophilic granuloma (EG) of bone is part of a spectrum of diseases known as Langerhans cell granulomatosis, all characterised by proliferation of specific histiocytes, designated as Langerhans type, in normal tissue. These histocyte proliferations, called eosinophilic granuloma, can occur unifocally or multifocally and be part of systemic illness known as Hand-Schüller-Christian disease and Letterer-Siwe disease (66, 67).

The etiology is unknown and therefore its treatment is empirical. Eosinophilic granuloma of bone was most commonly treated with chemotherapy, surgery and irradiation (68, 69). Currently intralesional instillation of steroids is the first choice of treatment, with good results (67,68, 70–72). However, some lesions fail to respond to steroid injection therapy or are unsuitable for injection therapy due to their size, location, loss of bony containment and/or soft tissue intrusion. Especially in case of cortical destruction with or without an impending pathological fracture and possible neurological damage in spinal cases (Fig. 14.3), a primary surgical treatment seems feasible. Schreuder et al. described six patients with eosinophilic granuloma of bone with these lesion characteristics and treated them with curettage, cryosurgery and bone grafting. No recurrences were reported (73).

Enchondroma and chondrosarcoma grade 1: Much controversy exists about the methods of evaluating, staging and final treatment of enchondroma, transient chondroid tumor and low-grade chondrosarcoma, because their accurate differentiation is hampered by their radiographic and histological similarity and clinical behavior. Therefore, the diagnostic distinction of enchondroma from transient chondroid tumor and chondrosarcoma grade 1 is one of the most difficult areas of bone tumor pathology, where particularly close co-operation

Table 14.2. Review of the literature on giant cell tumor treated with cryosurgery

Author	Year of publication	No.	Local recurrence	Comments
Marcove (61)	1973	25	9	
Marcove (62)	1978	27	3	
Jacops (63)	1985	12	2	
Malawer (64)	1991	14	1	
Aboulafia (65)	1994	6	1	
Malawer (60)	1999	86	2	primarily treated giant cell tumor with cryosurgery
Malawer (60)	1999	16	6	recurrent giant cell tumor treated with cryosurgery
Schreuder (44)	1999	13	4	two femoral local recurrences successfully treated with cryosurgery, two marginal resections of distal radius and ulna
Total:		199	28 (14%)	

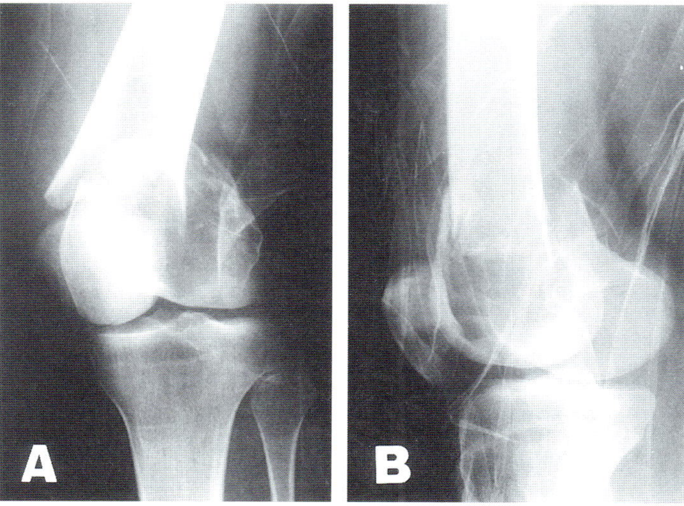

Fig. 14.13.1. Pathological intra-articular fracture due to giant cell tumor of the left distal femur in a young woman (**A**, **B**)

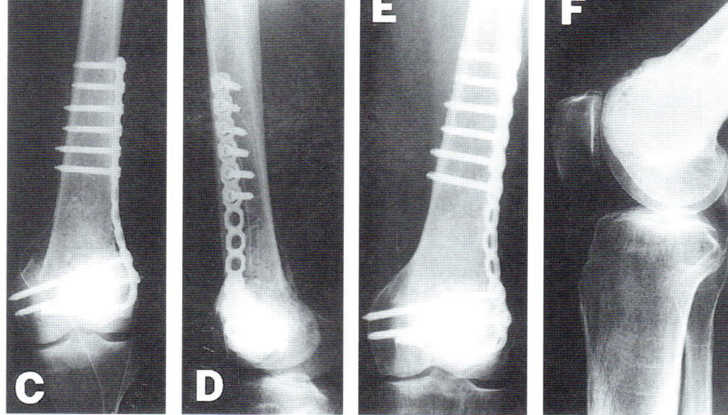

Fig. 14.13.2. Postoperative radiographs after reduction with some intentional shortening, cryosurgery, homologous bone graft in distal part of femur (in order to create bone stock), cementation of lateral femur condyle and titanium alloy osteosynthesis to achieve stability (**C**, **D**). Follow-up at 37 months after the operation, solid union and no recurrence, some (clinically asymptomatic) degenerative changes of the medial knee compartment (**E**, **F**)

between pathologist, radiologist and orthopedic surgeon is required. These diagnostic problems are the result of poorly defined criteria and subjective interpretation of clinical, radiological and histological features of enchondroma, transient chondroid tumor and chondrosarcoma grade 1 (74, 75). The continuous spectrum of biological behavior of these entities is unpredictable and best illustrated by the fact that histological appearances of a cartilage tumor in the pelvis, supporting the diagnosis of low-grade malignancy, can be safely ignored when the lesion is located in the tubular bones of hands and feet (Fig. 14.2) (76, 77). The correct diagnosis may further be hampered by sampling errors; histologic features of enchondroma, chondroid tumor and chondrosarcoma may coexist in the same lesion. It is established that a benign tumor such as enchondroma can undergo malignant transformation into secondary chondrosarcoma (75, 78, 79), especially in patients with multiple enchondromas as in Ollier disease and Maffuci syndrome (80).

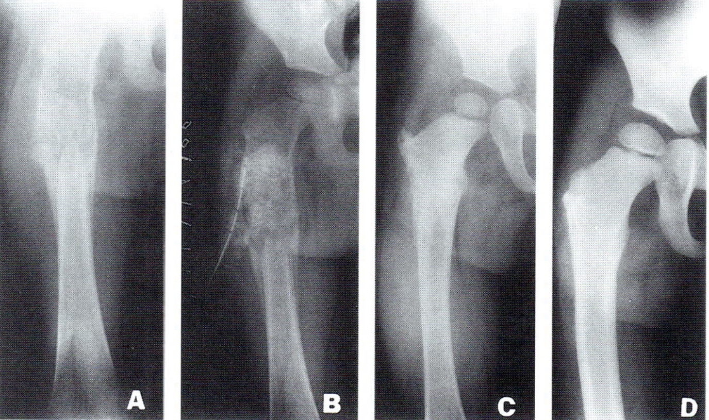

Fig. 14.14. Anteroposterior radiographs of right femur of a 6-year-old boy. Osteolytic lesion due to EG with impending pathological fracture (**A**). After curettage, cryosurgery and homologous bone graft (**B**). Follow-up at six (**C**) and 33 (**D**) months. A complete normalization of the proximal femur has occurred

Because of low risk of recurrence of enchondroma, transient chondroid tumor and low-grade chondrosarcoma in extremities, limited surgery with or without adjuvant therapy is advocated (81–83).

In view of the above, one of the advantages of cryosurgery is critical: since the dosage of this local adjuvant treatment can be well controlled, the extent of the cryosurgical margin can be adjusted to the worst case scenario of the chondroid lesion (Figs. 14.8, 14.16 and 14.17).

In a series of 21 patients with enchondroma and 15 with either transient chondroid tumor or chondrosarcoma grade 1, all located in the extremities, and with a follow-up of more than two

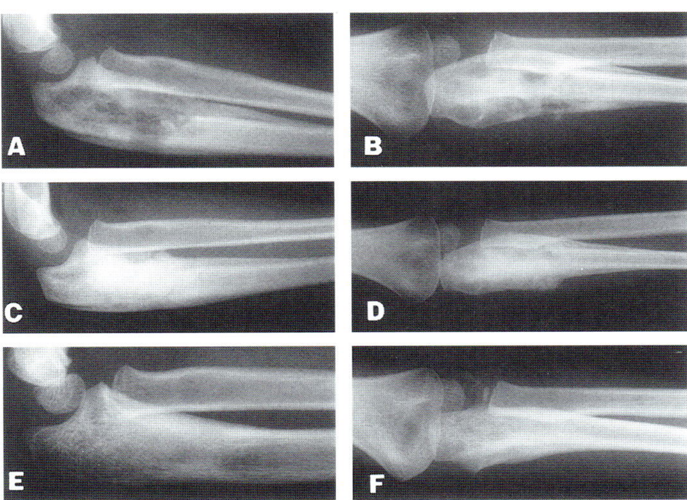

Fig. 14.15. Anteroposterior and lateral radiographs of left elbow of a 3.5-year-old boy. EG lesion close to joint (**A**, **B**). Follow-up at 7 months after curettage, cryosurgery and homologous bone graft (**C**, **D**) and at 15 months (**E**, **F**)

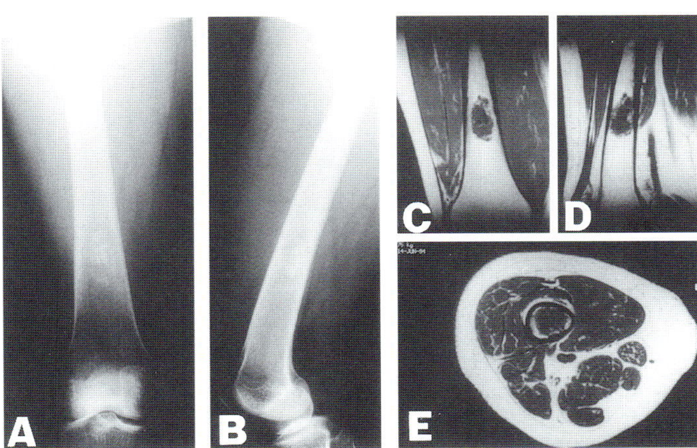

Fig. 14.16.1. Routine radiographs of a 34-year-old female with a symptomatic enchondroma in diaphysis of femur (**A**, **B**). T1 weighted MRI: coronal (**C**) and sagittal (**D**). On transversal (**E**) view some endosteal reaction is seen

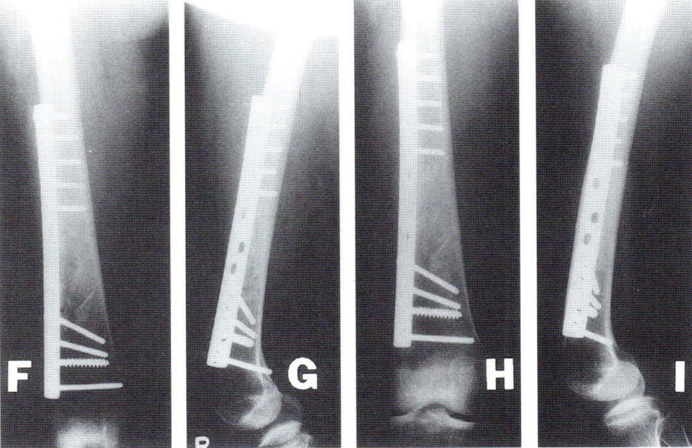

Fig. 14.16.2. Two (**F**, **G**) and 37 (**H**, **I**) months after curettage, cryosurgery and homologous bone graft. No evidence of recurrence

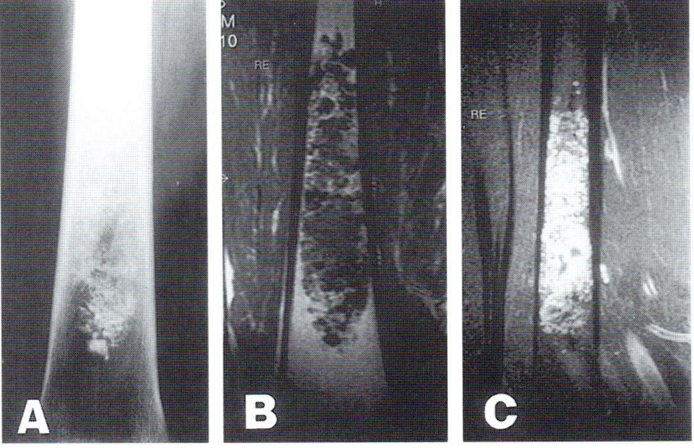

Fig. 14.17.1. 65-year-old man with a chondrosarcoma grade 1 of the right femur (**A**). Same lesion on T1 weighted MRI, coronal view (**B**) and T1 after administration of gadolinium, sagittal view (**C**)

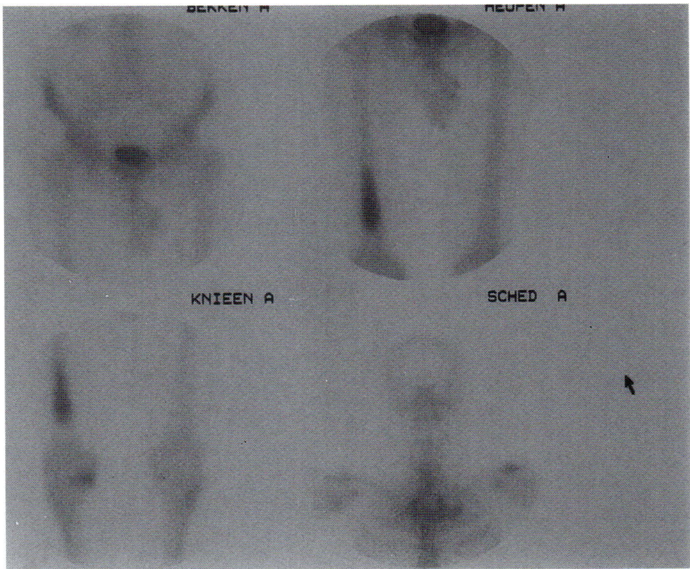

Fig. 14.17.2. Bone scan scintigraphy: the amount of activity in the femur is in concurrence with chondrosarcoma grade 1

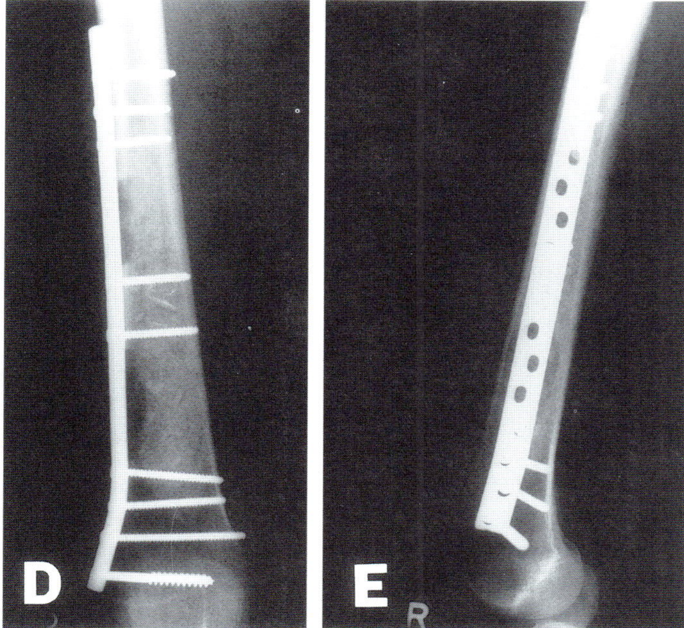

Fig. 14.17.3. Postoperative radiographs 4 months after curettage, cryosurgery, osteosynthesis and homologous bone grafting through two separated cortical windows (D, E)

years, there was one local recurrence of an enchondroma located in a finger (84).

Fibrous dysplasia: Fibrous dysplasia is a benign tumor-like lesion of immature fibrous connective tissue and poorly formed immature trabecular bone (85). Fibrous dysplasia can compromise the structural integrity of affected bones leading to recurrent fractures and skeletal deformities. The clinical picture of fibrous dysplasia is diverse. Its manifestation can be monostotic, polyostotic, or polyostotic in combination with skin pigmentation and dysfunction of the endocrine system (McCune-Albright syndrome).

Circumscribed lesions may remain asymptomatic for many years during adult age and need no further treatment. In most cases fibrous dysplasia presents with pain or a pathological fracture, usually noted between 5 and 20 years of age; the more extended the disease the earlier the onset of symptoms (85).

When operative treatment is indicated in circumscribed monostotic fibrous dysplasia, a single procedure of curettage, cryosurgery and bone grafting has shown satisfactory oncological results and functional outcome (86).

Extended lesions may result in bony deficiency or deformities necessitating additional internal fixation, massive allografts or corrective osteotomies. The beneficial effects of additional cryosurgery in extended lesions and particularly in McCune-Albright syndrome is unclear (86).

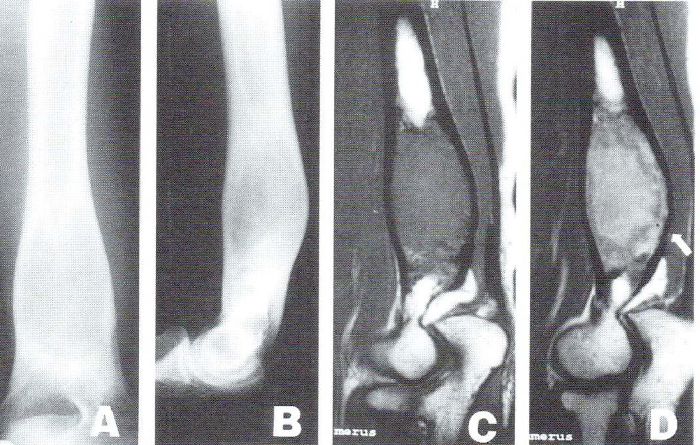

Fig. 14.18.1. Anteroposterior (A) and lateral (B) radiograph of the left distal humerus of a 20-year-old woman show an osteolytic expansile lesion with a ground-glass appearance. This image is characteristic for the circumscribed type of fibrous dysplasia. The MR images, T1 weighted, sagittal pre- (C) and post (D) gadolinium administration show the enhancement of the dysplasia and the endosteal irregularities (arrow)

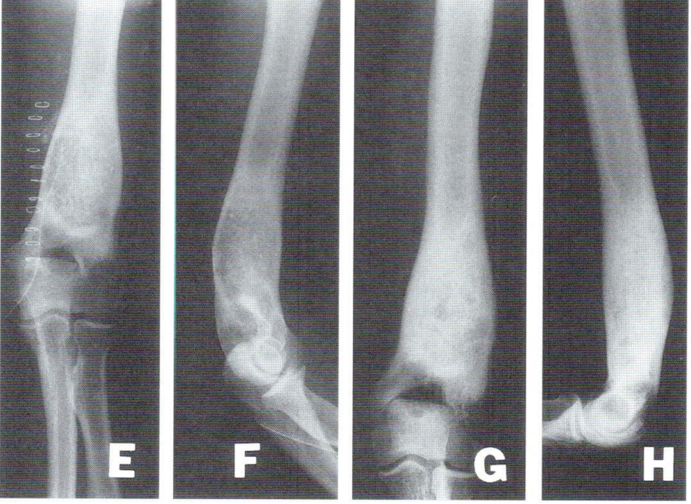

Fig. 14.18.2. After curettage, cryosurgery and bone grafting, the postoperative radiographs (E, F) show the graft that 17 months postoperatively (G, H) is being progressively incorporated into the bony structures

Miscellaneous: Chondroblastoma, chondromyxoid fibroma, intramedullary hemangioma and schwannoma are all very rare benign bone tumors suitable for curettage and local adjuvant therapy with cryosurgery. No data presenting series of patients with the results of cryosurgery with respect to these bone tumors are available in the literature.

14.9 Complications

Every surgical treatment, and especially a relatively new surgical treatment, will be accompanied by complications. Cryosurgery for bone tumors is no exception in this respect. In general, complications will diminish not only along the learning curve of physicians starting to implement the treatment, but also with improvement of the technique itself.

Wound infections: Intralesional resection (curettage) of an intramedullary tumor will leave behind a cavity with a lot of dead space. Cryosurgery results in an additional amount of tissue necrosis. Furthermore, most surgeons fill this defect with a "dead" homologous bone graft and sometimes an osteosynthesis is added as well. All these factors are strong mediators for developing a bacterial infection. The literature addressing infection related to cryosurgery is confusing because the criteria for the definition of wound infection are not clear. Delayed wound healing, persistent wound drainage with or without positive cultures, superficial and deep infection probably occur in about 4% of the skeletal tumors treated with cryosurgery (43, 44, 48, 60, 62, 64, 87).

As in all other operative procedures in which foreign bodies are implanted, postoperative wound infections are of major concern. Procedures in which cryosurgery is utilized are in that respect no exception. In general, infection rates decline along the learning curve and to avoid them after a cryosurgical procedure the following elements are of importance:

- The use of perioperative broad-spectrum antibiotics until 24 hours after the operation, comparable to regimens in use for prosthetic replacements.
- Adequate drainage of wound fluids. Clinical observation has taught that there seems to be some kind of reactive increased blood flow in the area of the cryosurgery. When this blood is allowed to form a hemathoma it may become infected.
- Adequate wound exposure with retraction of skin, and protection with gauze is necessary to avoid accidental freezing of the skin.
- Wound closure with sufficient soft tissue coverage.

Venous gas embolism: During cryosurgery liquid nitrogen is either sprayed or poured into the bony cavity and since its boiling point is −196°C, nitrogen gas bubbles are rapidly produced at room temperature. In general, whenever a gas is introduced into a body cavity there is the hazard of intravascular introduction of gas bubbles especially when pressure is allowed to develop. Gas emboli in the vascular circulation can cause serious hemodynamic complications (27, 28).

Dwyer et al. reported a presumed incident of venous gas embolism during a cryosurgical procedure in which a dramatically increased end-tidal nitrogen tension was noted, but without any hemodynamic complications (88).

In the literature, one fatal case due to venous gas embolism during cryosurgery has been described. The occurrence was explained by the blocking of the exit of gaseous nitrogen from the bone by intentional digital occlusion of the opening in the bone cortex (89).

De Vries conducted experiments in rats and rabbits to evaluate the problem of bone marrow embolism during cryosurgery. It was concluded that the intravasation of bone marrow was caused

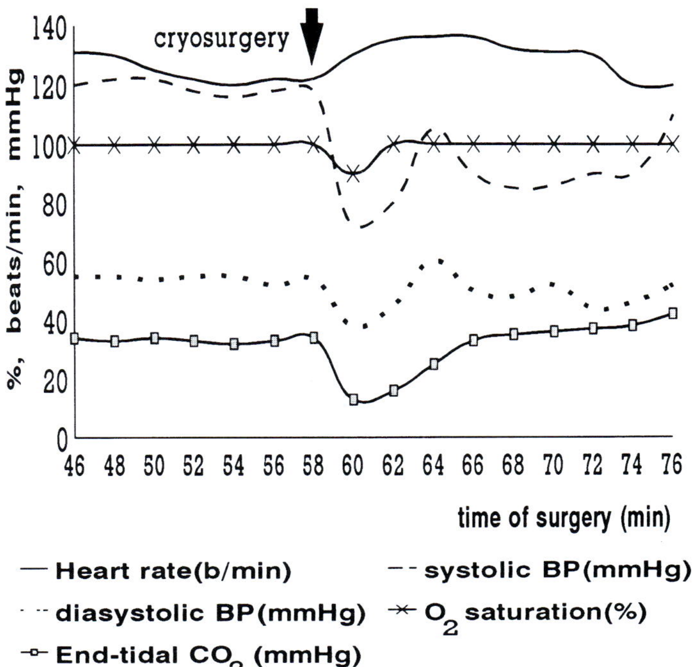

Fig. 14.19. Anesthetic records during a cryosurgical procedure. Three cycles of spraying liquid nitrogen for approximately 20 seconds and a thawing period of approximately 3 min were performed. During the last cycle, just when the nitrogen spraying was stopped, a decrease of O_2 saturation to 90% was noted. The blood pressure dropped to 70/40, and the heart rate increased. The end-tidal CO_2 tension decreased to 15 mm Hg. Close inspection of patient and equipment revealed no probable cause of this event other than a venous gas embolism. Nitrous oxide and halothane were stopped and 100% O_2 was administered. Within a few minutes vital signs returned to normal and the condition of the patient stabilized

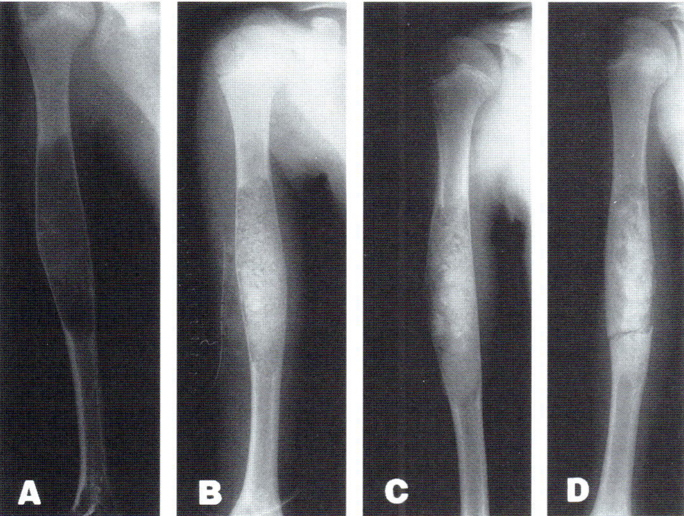

Fig. 14.20.1. Anteroposterior radiographs of simple bone cyst in the diaphysis of the right humerus of an 11-year-old girl (**A**). Curettage, cryosurgery and homologous bone graft (**B**). Six weeks postoperatively (**C**) and nondisplaced fracture six months after the operation (**D**), suspicion of local recurrence in proximal part of lesion

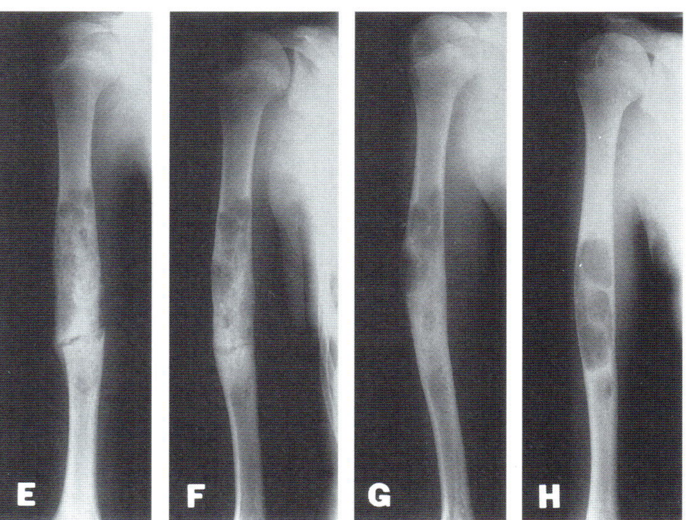

Fig. 14.20.2. Some callus formation at seven months (**E**), union at nine months after the operation (**F**). Local recurrence at 12 months (**G**) and 39 months (**H**) treated conservatively because at this point the lesion is asymptomatic, although the patient is not engaged in any sports

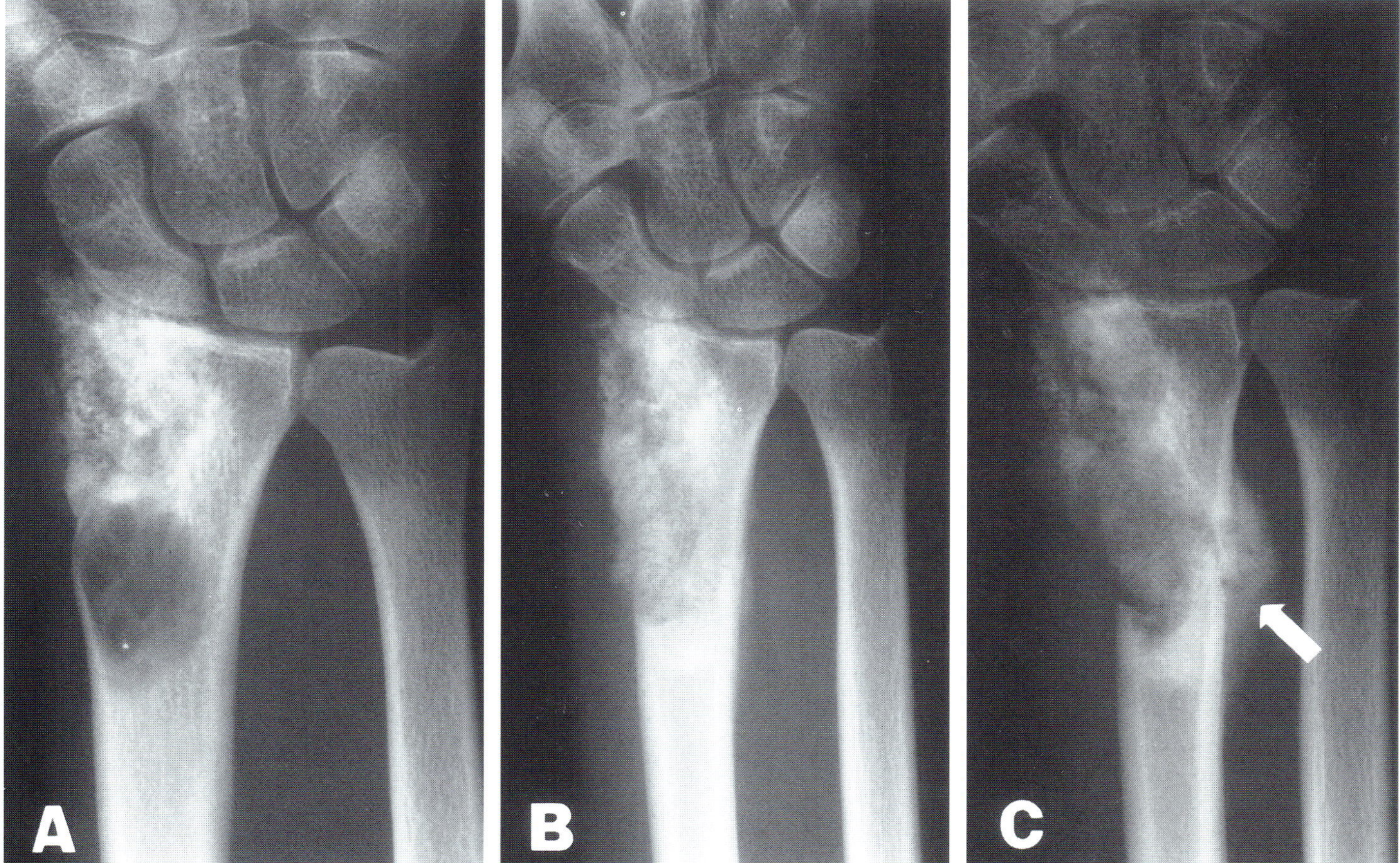

Fig. 14.21.1. Anteroposterior radiographs of right wrist of a 23-year-old woman. Recurrent giant cell tumor 5 months after curettage, cryosurgery and homologous bone grafting (**A**). One month after reoperation: curettage, cryosurgery and homologous bone grafting, a fissure may be visible (**B**). Evident fracture (arrow) and extensive callus formation 5 months after operation, some radial deformity (**C**)

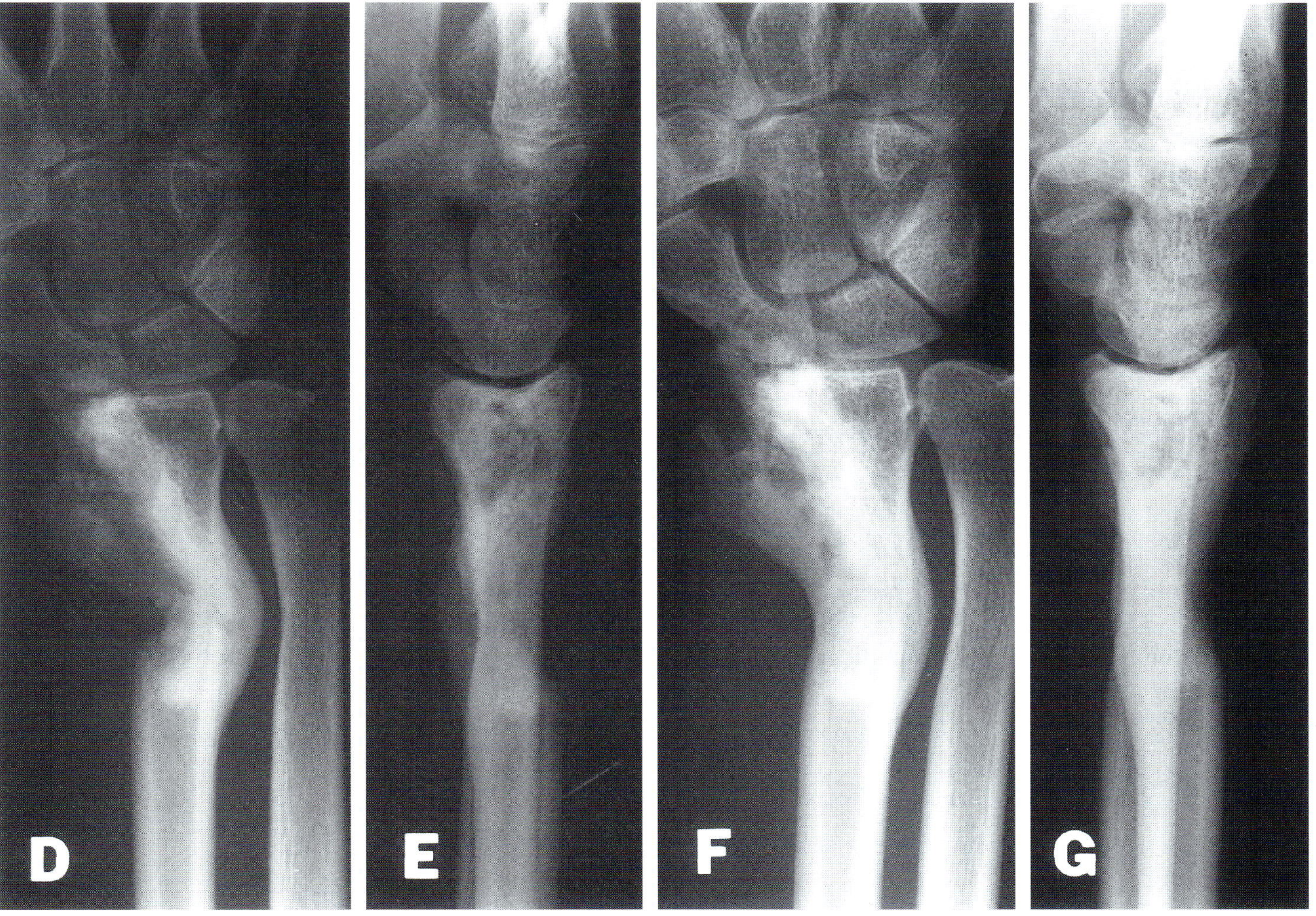

Fig. 14.21.2. Anteroposterior (AP) and lateral views, respectively, 7 (**D**, **E**) and 14 months (**F**, **G**) after operation; solid fracture healing, AP views suggest radio-carpal arthrosis, but on lateral views these degenerative changes are not extensive. Only minor impairment of range of movement. This patient suffered also from giant cell tumor around the right knee 10 years prior to her wrist lesion and is also suffering from a giant cell tumor located in the right acetabulum

by increased intramedullary pressure, and embolization of bone marrow was encountered but not on a large scale. Most of the bone marrow intravasations remained local in the extraosseous veins (90).

Schreuder et al. reported on two patients who showed signs of impairment of pulmonary circulation during cryosurgical procedures, as indicated by a sudden significant drop in end-tidal CO_2 and corresponding changes in blood pressure and heart rate. They suggested that these features represent venous gas embolism because of their rapid development at the same time as the instillation of the liquid nitrogen and the fact that the symptoms disappeared rather quickly after the cryosurgery was ended (Fig. 14.19) (30). Solid particle embolism by marrow or fat is less likely, because this kind of embolism is provoked by mechanical elevation of the intramedullary pressure as in intramedullary nailing and introduction of a prosthesis (91, 92).

In a clinical experiment Schreuder et al. used a mass spectrometer to perform end-tidal gas analysis in all patients who were treated by cryosurgery. The mass spectrometer measured inhaled and end-tidal O_2, CO_2, N_2O, N_2 tensions and anesthetic vapor concentration breath by breath. In 15 cases analyzed, they did not detect any exhaled N_2 during cryosurgery. Also, the measured O_2, CO_2, N_2O tensions and anesthetic vapour concentration were completely normal (30).

The mechanism of N_2 embolism is unclear. When during cryosurgery the surface of the cavity is becoming extremely cold, the additional sprayed liquid nitrogen will not be able to vaporize. Instead, the bone marrow develops properties comparable to a sponge and sucks the liquid nitrogen into small marrow spaces. This liquid

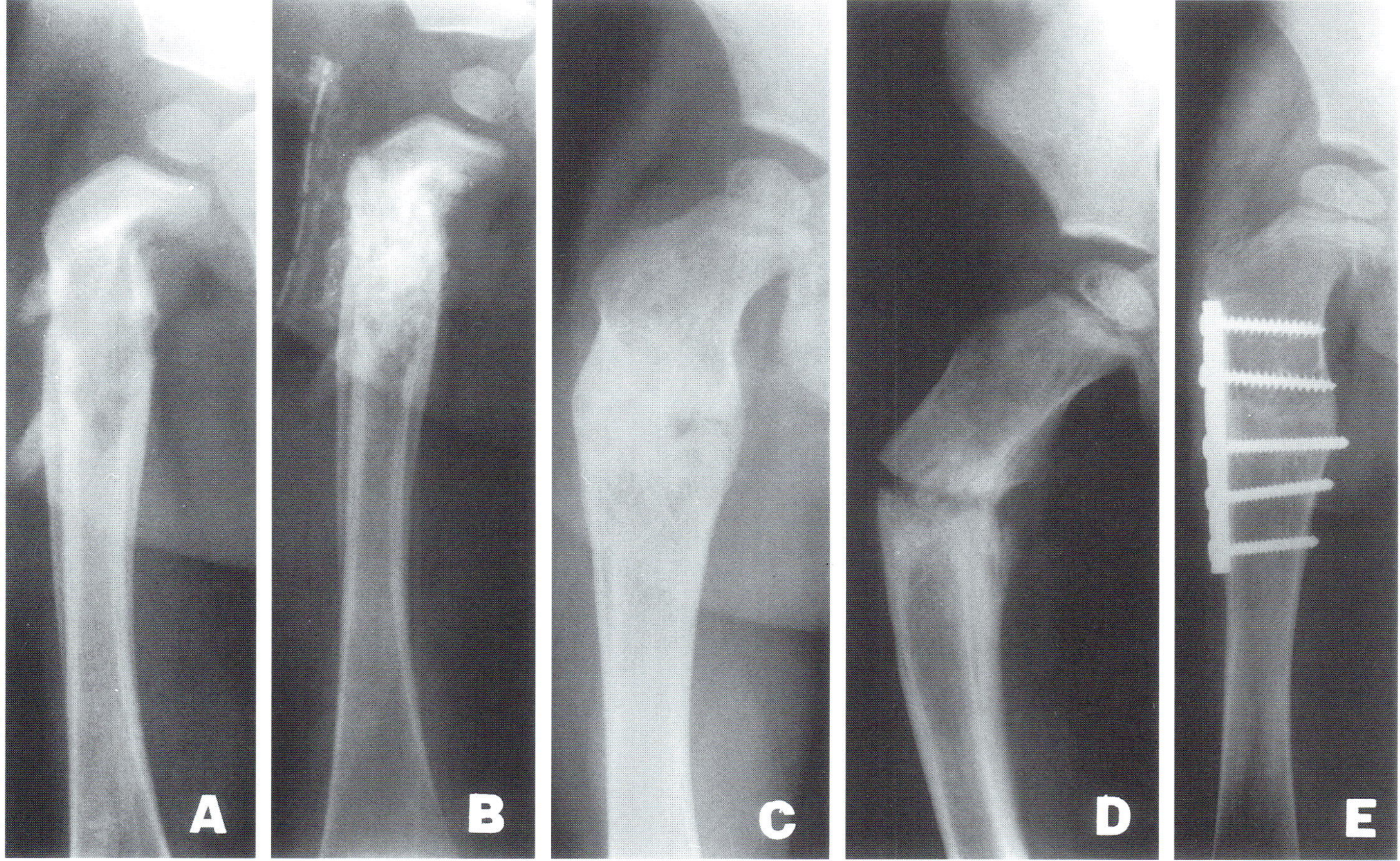

Fig. 14.22. Anteroposterior radiographs of the right femur of a 2-year-old girl. Osteolytic lesion due to eosinophilic granuloma of bone, preoperative (**A**). After curettage, cryosurgery and homologous bone graft (**B**). Follow-up at 5 months (**C**). Pathologic fracture 8 months after the operation, frozen sectioning during osteosynthesis did not show a local recurrence of eosinophilic granuloma (**D**). Solid consolidation 5 months after internal fixation with plate and screws (**E**)

nitrogen may get trapped in these marrow spaces. When thawing or a rise in the temperature is allowed, the trapped liquid nitrogen will boil and vaporize, building extremely high pressures. It may be possible that under these circumstances liquid nitrogen or gaseous nitrogen is pushed into the venous circulation. That N_2 dissolves in blood first is highly unlikely because of its very low Oswald solubility coefficient ($C = 0.015$ at 37°C). The risk is increased when the site of the tumor is located in a richly perfused area such as the metaphysis of the long bones where the major nutrient arterial and venous blood supply enters the medullar cavity. Unfortunately, the metaphysis is the location of preference for many bony tumors suitable for cryosurgical treatment.

When using cryosurgery, one should never block the entrance to the bony cavity.

Fractures: The tumor itself as well as the surgical exposure and resection jeopardize the structural integrity of the bone. Cryosurgery is said to further diminish bone strength by inducing necrosis of the local bone stock often leading to postoperative fractures. In the late sixties the pioneers of the cryosurgery used for bone tumors reported rather high fracture rates. In published series of 15 or more cases of bone tumors treated with cryosurgery, the postoperative fracture rate is 10% (43, 44, 48, 60–62, 64, 87, 93).

The effect of cryosurgery on the strength of bone was tested by Fisher et al. The mandibles of rats had a reduction in strength of approximately 30% eight weeks after cryosurgery. The gradual loss of strength in these bones paralleled observed radiographic osteolysis. At four months the mandibles had regained strength accompanied by clear radiographic evidence of sclerosis (94). Although not investigated in this experiment, the gradual loss and return of strength in cryosurgically treated bone also parallels histologic evidence of bone resorption, repair and remodelling (95, 96).

Postoperative fracture of the remodelling bone subjected to cryosurgery is not only very dis-

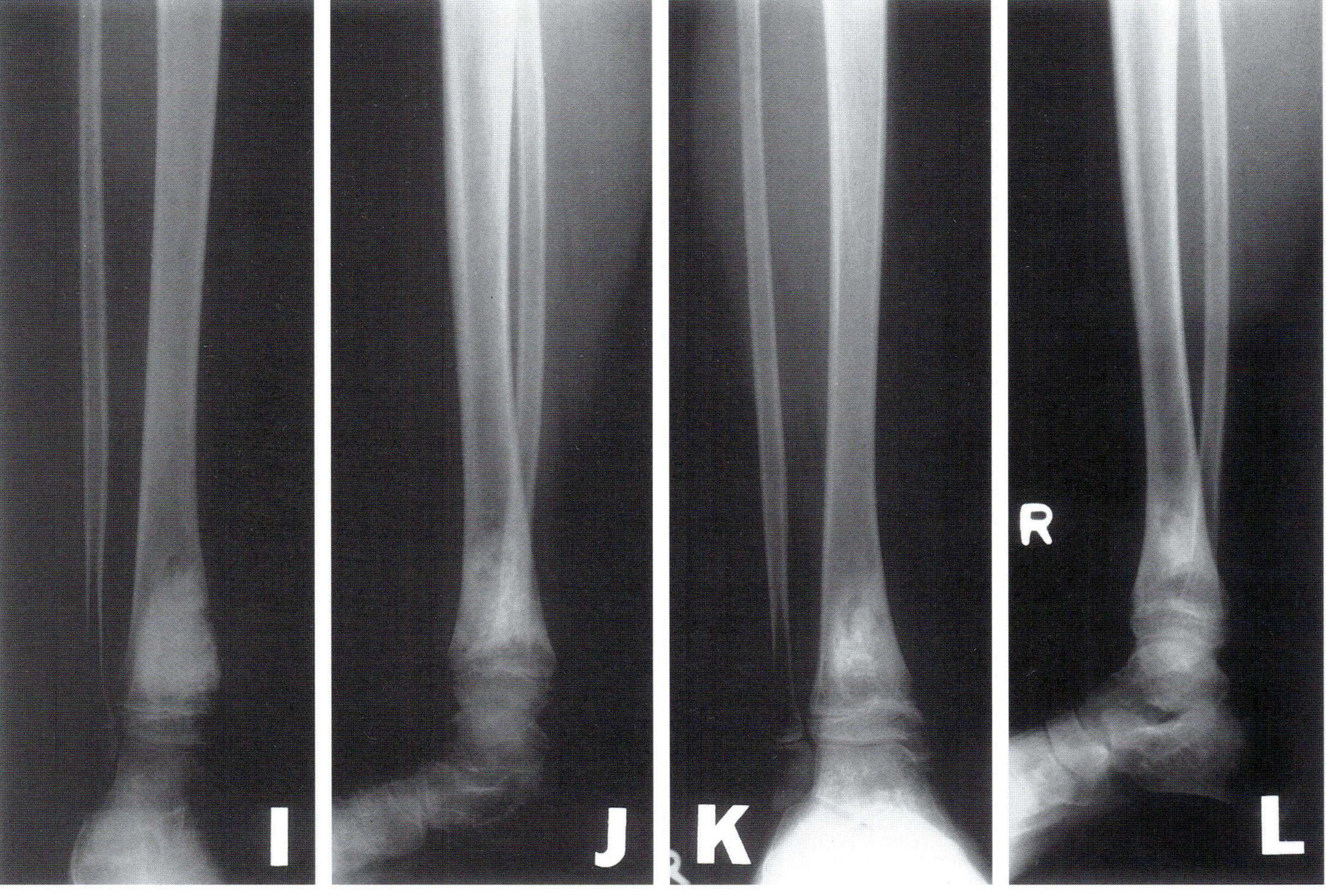

Fig. 14.23.1. Routine radiographs of the same patient as in Fig. 14.6 at 9 (**I**, **J**) and 16 (**K**, **L**) months postoperatively: suspicion of gradual closing of medial part of the distal epiphysis, but no evident varus bowing

tressing for the patient, but also compromises the orthopedic oncologic status; first there was intra-compartmental disease, because of the fracture it has now potentially changed to an extra-compartmental disease.

It seems that fractures are most likely to occur four to eight weeks after the cryosurgical treatment, but they can occur even 8 months after cryosurgery (Figs. 14.20–14.22). Diaphyseal lesions are most prone to fracture (Fig. 14.20). Therefore, prophylactic internal fixation is advised, but is mandatory when the femur is involved (Fig. 14.17). An intramedullary enforcement is ill advised, because it carries the risk of contaminating the entire intramedullary compartment with tumor cells. Titanium alloys are preferred because these implants create little interference on MRI, making tumor follow-up less difficult. Partial weightbearing is usually necessary until three months after the operation.

Experience and improvements in technique have reduced the fracture rate to an acceptable level. Since prophylactic osteosynthesis is used, sometimes in combination with cement and or auto/allo bone graft, fractures are no longer seen (60).

Damage to epiphysis: Benign bone tumors, especially simple bone cysts and aneurysmal bone cysts tend to occur in patients of immature skeletal age. Furthermore these tumors commonly develop in the metaphysis, often adjacent or very close to the epiphysis. Damage to the epiphysis either by the tumor itself or by the use of cryosurgery is very well possible and may result in arrest or disturbance of normal growth.

Malawer and Dunham reviewed 25 pediatric patients with aggressive benign tumors all treated by cryosurgery. They saw 2 patients with damage to the epiphysis necessitating epiphyseodesis of the contralateral side (64). During surgery no attempt was made to prevent the epiphysis from freezing, control of tumor was their first priority.

Schreuder and Conrad reported on 42 treated simple bone cysts of which 11 were located in the proximal metaphysis adjacent or close to the epiphysis. During surgery care was taken not to damage the adjacent physis by curettage and if the physis was exposed to the cyst, it was separated from freezing by several layers of surgical gel foam. No growth disturbances were seen, but two local recurrences were encountered (43).

Figure 14.23 demonstrates the long term follow-up of the patient in Fig. 14.6. Damage to an epiphysis is noted, even as the result of not very low temperatures.

Whether an epiphysis is damaged by the bone tumor or the treatment will not always become clear and in many cases may be the result of both. To minimize the risk of damage, protection of an exposed epiphysis by gel foam seems feasible, but on the other hand it lowers the effectiveness of the cryosurgery, which may result in a local recurrence of the bone tumor, which potentially will definitively damage the epiphysis.

Degenerative osteoarthritis: Some bone tumors occur almost always extremely close to the major joints, like giant cell tumor and chondroblastoma. Damage to the articular surface either by the tumor itself (intra-articular fracture) or treatment (cryosurgery) may be anticipated. Malawer et al. demonstrated in an experiment using dogs, that cryosurgery can produce bone necrosis 7 to 12 millimetres away from the surface of the cavity being treated, in contrast to the minimal zone of necrosis produced by the heat of polymerization of polymethyl-methacrylate. They found that cryosurgery had no effect on articular cartilage (97).

Aboulafia et al. described a technique for treatment of large subchondral tumors around the knee which extended to within two millimeters of the articular surface. Curettage, cryosurgery and composite reconstruction with bone graft, bone cement and osteosynthesis were used as an alternative to primary joint-sacrificing resection. Of nine tumors (six giant cell tumors, one chondroblastoma, one chondrosarcoma and one fibrosarcoma) there was one recurrence, retreated in the same fashion. All 9 patients had an excellent functional outcome. Only two patients had mild degenerative cartilage changes (65).

Among 120 cases all treated with cryosurgery and a follow-up of more than one year, Schreuder et al. saw 3 cases of secondary osteoarthritis, all giant cell tumors of which two were situated in the distal radius (Fig. 14.21) and one in the proximal humerus (Fig. 14.12.3) (44). Malawer et al. reported two of 48 patients with giant cell tumor around the knee joint developing radiographic and clinical evidence of degenerative changes (60).

It seems that articular cartilage can resist low temperatures to some degree. In practice local control of the tumor (especially in case of intra-articular pathological fracture) has priority, dealing with osteoarthritis seems in those circumstances to be of concern later (98).

Damage to nerves: Nerve palsy is a complication of cryosurgery which was recognized very early in the introduction of cryosurgery for bone tumors. Marcove saw in 128 patients, all treated for various types of bone tumors, nine (mostly transient) nerve palsies (48, 62, 87, 99). Schreuder et al. saw in 165 cryosurgical procedures seven nerve palsies; one peroneal nerve failed to regain its function. Not the cryosurgery but rather surgical traction was very likely the cause of this persistent palsy. Three patients with sacral lesions (two giant cell tumors and one chordoma) suffered perma-

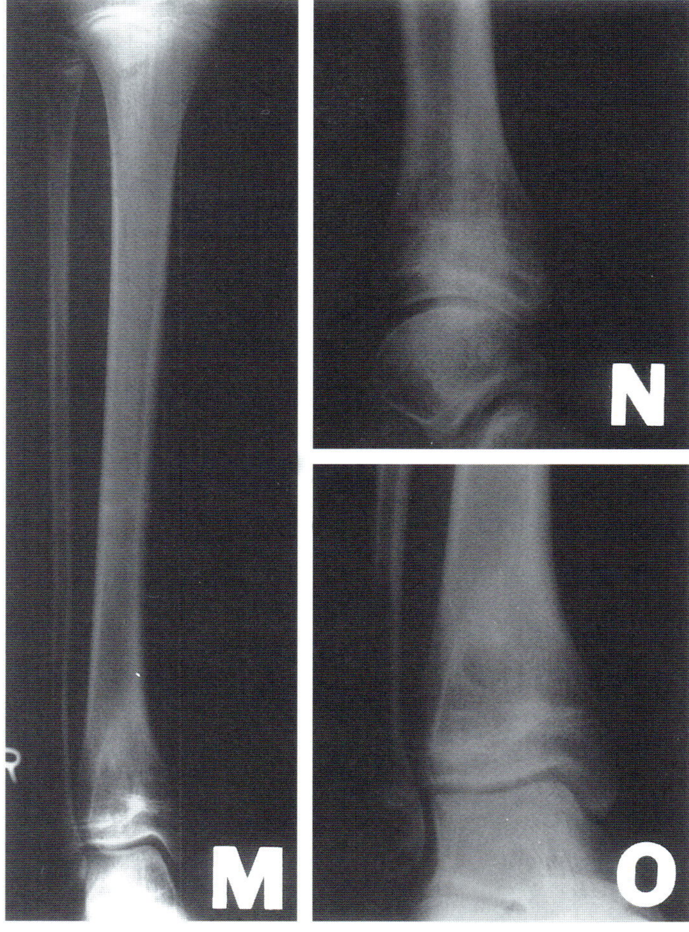

Fig. 14.23.2. Routine radiographs at 40 months postoperatively: closure of the medial part of epiphysis resulting in a varus deformity of 15° (**M, N, O**)

nent, only partially recovered loss of function of sacral roots. Two palsies of the radial nerve and one of the peroneal nerve were shown to be completely reversible.

The radial nerve seems especially at risk due to its proximity to the humeral bone (44).

If nerves are frozen their function is only temporarily impaired. Most neuropraxias resulting from freezing will resolve in 6 weeks to 6 months. Very likely, regenerating nerve fibers can grow down the nerve sheaths since they are left intact. Furthermore, the vital nerve cell nucleus is located at some remove in the dorsal root ganglion.

References

1. Marcove RC, Miller TR, Cahan WC. Treatment of primary and metastatic bone tumors by repetitive freezing. Bull N Y Acad Med 1968; 44: 532–544.
2. Enneking WF. A staging system of staging Musculoskeletal Neoplasms. Clin Orthop 1986; 204: 9–24.
3. Marcove RC, Zahr KA, Huvos AG, Ogihara W. Cryosurgery in osteogenic sarcoma: a report of three cases. Compr Ther 1984; 10: 52–60.
4. Marcove RC, Miller TR. Treatment of primary and metastatic bone tumors by cryosurgery. JAMA 1969; 207: 1890–1894.
5. Schiller CH, Ritschl P, Windhager R, Kropej D, Kotz R. Frequency of recurrence in phenolized and nonphenolized bone cavities following intralesional excisions of nonmalignant bone tumors. Z Orthop 1989; 127: 398–401.
6. Capanna R, Sudanese A, Baldini N, Campanacci M. Phenol as an adjuvant in the control of local recurrence of benign neoplasms of bone treated by curettage. Ital J Orthop Traumatol 1985; 11: 381–388.
7. Rock MG. Treatment of bone cysts and giant cell tumors. Curr Opin Orthopaed 1990; 1: 423–434.
8. Bradley PF. Cryosurgery of the maxillofacial region, Vol 1. Boca Raton, Florida, CRC Press, 1986 chapter 5.
9. Gill W, Frazer J, Carter D. Repeated freeze-thaw cycles in cryosurgery. Nature 1968; 219: 410–413.
10. Gage A. Experimental cryogenic injury of the palate: observations pertinent to cryosurgical destruction of tumors. Cryobiology 1978; 15: 415–425.
11. Neel HB, Ketcham AS, Hammond WG. Requisites for successful cryogenic surgery of cancer. Arch Surg 1971; 102: 45.
12. Berth-Jones J, Bourke J, Eglitis H, Harper C, Kirk P, Pavord S, Rajapakse R, Weston P, Wiggins T, Hutchinson PE. Value of a second freeze-thaw cycle in cryotherapy of common warts. Br J Dermatol 1994; 131: 883–886.
13. Gage AA. What temperature is lethal for cells? J Dermatol Surg Oncol 1979; 5: 459–460.
14. Gage AA, Guest K, Montes M, Caruana JA, Whalen Jr DA. Effect of varying freezing and thawing rates in experimental cryosurgery. Cryobiology 1985; 22: 175–182.
15. Bradley PF. Thermography. In: Bradley P (ed): Cryosurgery of the maxillofacial region, Vol 1. Boca Raton, Florida, CRC Press, 1986: 130–132.
16. Ravikumar T, Kane R, Cady B et al. Hepatic cryosurgery with intraoperative ultrasound monitoring for metastatic colon carcinoma. Arch Surg 1987; 122: 403–409.
17. Laugier P, Berger G. Assessment of echography as a monitoring technique for cryosurgery. Ultrason Imaging 1993; 15: 14–24.
18. Le Pivert P. The measurement of low frequency electrical impedance as a guide to effective cryosurgery. J Dermatol Surg Oncol 1977; 3: 395–397.
19. Gage AA, Augustynowicz S, Montes M. Tissue impedance and temperature measurements in relation to necrosis in experimental cryosurgery. Cryobiology 1985; 22: 282–288.
20. Gage A. Correlation of electrical impedance and temperature in tissue during freezing. Cryobiology 1979; 16: 56–62.
21. Moser R, Abbott I, Stephens C. Computerized tomographic imaging of cryosurgical iceball formation in brain. Cryobiology 1987; 24: 368–379.
22. Pease GR, Rubinsky B, Wong STS. An integrated probe for magnetic resonance imaging monitored skin cryosurgery. J Biomech Eng 1995; 117: 59–63.
23. Hong JS, Wong S, Pease G, Rubinsky B. MR imaging assisted temperature calculations during cryosurgery. Magn Reson Imaging 1994; 12: 1021–1031.
24. Matsumoto R, Selig AM, Colucci VM, Jolsz FA. MR monitoring during cryotherapy in the liver: predictability of histologic outcome. J Magn Reson Imaging 1993; 3: 770–776.
25. Schreuder HW, van Egmond J, van Beem HB, Veth RP. Monitoring during cryosurgery for bone tumors. J Surg Oncol 1997; 65: 40–45.
26. Bischof J, Christov K, Rubinsky B. A morphological study of cooling rate response in normal and neoplastic human liver tissue: cryosurgical implications. Cryobiology 1993; 30: 482–492.
27. Lowdon JD, Tidmore TL Jr. Fatal air embolism after gastrointestinal endoscopy. Anesthesiology 1988; 69: 622–623.
28. Jacoby J, Jones JR, Ziegler J. Pneumoencephalography and air embolism; Simulated anaesthetic death. Anesthesiology 1959; 20: 336.
29. Saha AK. Air embolism during anaesthesia for arthrography in a child. Anaesthesia 1976; 31: 1231–1233.
30. Schreuder HW, van Beem HB, Veth RP. Venous gas embolism during cryosurgery for bone tumors. J Surg Oncol 1995; 60: 196–200.
31. Scaglietti O, Marchetti PGM, Bartolozzi P. Final results obtained in the treatment of bone cysts with methylprednisolone acetate (Depo-Medrol) and a discussion of results achieved in other bone lesions. Clin Orthop 1982; 165: 33–42.
32. Scaglietti O, Marchetti PGM, Bartolozzi P. The effects of methylprednisolone acetate in the treatment of bone cysts. J Bone Joint Surg 1979; 61: 200–204.
33. Campanacci M, Capanna R, Picci P. Unicameral and aneurysmal bone cysts. Clin Orthop 1986; 204: 25–36.
34. Bovill DF, Skinner HB. Unicameral bone cysts. A comparison of treatment options. Orthop Rev 1989; 18: 420–427.
35. Pentimalli G, Tudisco C, Scola E, Farcetti P, Ippolito E. Unicameral bone cysts–comparison between surgical and steroid injection treatment. Arch Orthop Trauma Surg 1987; 106: 251–256.
36. Inoue O, Ibaraki K, Shimabukuro H, Shingaki Y. Packing with high-porosity hydroxyapatite cubes alone for the treatment of simple bone cysts. Clin Orthop 1993; 293: 287–292.
37. Oppenheim WL, Galleno H. Operative treatment versus steroid injection in the management of unicameral bone cysts. J Pediatr Orthop 1984; 4: 1–7.
38. Spence KF Jr, Bright RW, Fitzgerald SP, Sell KW. Solitary unicameral bone cyst: treatment with freeze-dried crushed cortical-bone allograft. A review of one hundred and forty-four cases. J Bone Joint Surg Am 1976; 58: 636–641.
39. Spence KF, Sell KW, Brown RH. Solitary bone cyst: treatment with freeze-dried cancellous bone allograft. A study of one hundred seventy-seven cases. J Bone Joint Surg 1969; 51: 87–96.
40. Neer CS II, Marcove RC, Terz and Carbonara PN. Treatment of unicameral bone cyst. A follow-up study of one hundred seventy-five cases. J Bone Joint Surg 1966; 48: 731–745.
41. Mylle J, Burssens A, Fabry G. Simple bone cysts. A review of 59 cases with special reference to their treatment. Arch Orthop Trauma Surg 1992; 111: 297–300.
42. Morton KS. Unicameral bone cyst. Can J Surg 1982; 25: 330–332.
43. Schreuder HW, Conrad EU, Bruckner JD, Howlett AT, Sorensen LS. Treatment of simple bone cysts in children with curettage and cryosurgery. J Pediatr Orthop 1997; 17: 814–820.
44. Schreuder HW, Keijser LC, Veth RP. Favourable results of cryosurgery in 120 patients with benign or low-grade malignant bone tumors. Ned Tijdschr Geneeskd 1999; 143(45): 2275–2281.
45. Kransdorf MJ, Sweet DE. Aneurysmal bone cyst: concept, controversy, clinical presentation, and imaging. Am J Roentgenol 1995; 164: 573–580.

46. Clough JR, Price CHG. Aneurysmal bone cysts: Pathogenesis and long term results of treatment. Clin Orthop 1973; 97: 52–63.
47. Freiberg AA, Loder RT, Heidelberger KP, Hensinger RN. Aneurysmal bone cysts in young children. J Pediatr Orthop 1994; 14: 86–91.
48. Marcove RC, Sheth DS, Takemoto S, Healey JH. The treatment of aneurysmal bone cyst. Clin Orthop 1995; 311: 157–163.
49. Ruiter DJ, van Rijssel ThG, van der Velde EA. Aneurysmal bone cysts. A clinicopathological study of 105 cases. Cancer 1977; 39: 2231–2239.
50. Cole WG. Treatment of aneurysmal bone cysts in childhood. J Pediatr Orthop 1986; 6: 326–329.
51. Szendröi M, Cser I, Konya A, Renyi-Vamos A. Aneurysmal bone cyst. A review of 52 primary and 16 secondary cases. Arch Orthop Trauma Surg 1992; 111: 318–322.
52. Schreuder HWB, Veth RPH, Pruszczynski M, Lemmens JAM, Schraffordt Koops H, Molenaar WM. Aneurysmal bone cysts treated by curettage, cryotherapy and bone grafting. J Bone Joint Surg (Br) 1997; 79: 20–25.
53. Farsetti P, Tudisco C, Rosa M, Pentimalli G, Ippolito E. Aneurysmal bone cyst. Long-term follow-up of 20 cases. Arch Orthop Trauma Surg 1990; 109: 221–223.
54. Kreicbergs A, Lonnqvist PA, Nilsson B. Curettage of benign lesions of bone. Factors related to recurrence. Int Orthop 1985; 8: 287–294.
55. van Loon CJ, Veth RP, Pruszczynski M, van Horn JR, Lemmens JA. Aneurysmal bone cyst. Long-term results and functional evaluation of 16 primary cases in 13 patients. Acta Orthop Belgica 1995; 61: 199–204.
56. Slowick FA Jr, Campbell CJ, Kettelkamp DB. Aneurysmal bone cyst. An analysis of thirteen cases. J Bone Joint Surg Am 1968; 50: 1142–1151.
57. Nobler MP, Higinbotham NL, Phillips RF. The cure of aneurysmal bone cyst. Irradiation superior to surgery in an analysis of 33 cases. Radiology 1968; 90: 1185–1192.
58. Vergel De Dios AM, Bond JR, Shives TC, McLeod RA, Unni KK. Aneurysmal bone cyst. A clinicopathologic study of 238 cases. Cancer 1992; 69: 2921–2931.
59. Koskinen EV, Visuri TI, Holmstrom T, Roukkula MA. Aneurysmal bone cyst: evaluation of resection and of curettage in 20 cases. Clin Orthop 1976; 118: 136–146.
60. Malawer MM, Bickels J, Meller I, Buch RG, Henshaw RM, Kollender Y. Cryosurgery in the treatment of giant cell tumor. Clin Orthop 1999; 2: 176–188.
61. Marcove RC, Lyden JP, Huvos AG, Bullough PG. Giant cell tumors treated by cryosurgery. A report of twenty-five cases. J Bone Joint Surg (Am) 1973; 55: 1633–1644.
62. Marcove RC, Weis LD, Vaghaiwalla MR, Pearson R. Cryosurgery in the treatment of giant cell tumors of bone. A report of 52 consecutive cases. Clin Orthop 1978; 134: 275–289.
63. Jacobs PA, Clemency Jr RE. The closed cryosurgical treatment of giant cell tumor. Clin Orthop 1985; 192: 149–158.
64. Malawer MM, Dunham W. Cryosurgery and acrylic cementation as surgical adjuncts in the treatment of aggressive (benign) bone tumors. Analysis of 25 patients below the age of 21. Clin Orthop 1991; 262: 42–57.
65. Aboulafia AJ, Rosenbaum DH, Sicard-Rosenbaum L, Jelinek JS, Malawer MM. Treatment of large subchondral tumors of the knee with cryosurgery and composite reconstruction. Clin Orthop 1994; 307: 189–199.
66. Makley JT, Carter JR. Eosinophilic granuloma of bone. Clin Orthop 1986; 204: 37–44.
67. Capanna R, Springfield DS, Ruggieri P, Biagini R, Picci P, Bacci G, Giunti A, Lorenzi EG, Campanacci M. Direct cortisone injection in eosinophilic granuloma of bone: a preliminary report on 11 patients. J Pediatr Orthop 1985; 5: 339–342.
68. Greis PE, Hankin FM. Eosinophilic granuloma. The management of solitary lesions of bone. Clin Orthop 1990; 257: 204–211.
69. Sartoris DJ, Parker BR. Histiocytosis X: rate and pattern of resolution of osseous lesions. Radiology 1984; 152: 679–684.
70. Cohen M, Zornoza J, Cangir A, Murray JA, Wallace S. Direct injection of methylprednisolone sodium succinate in the treatment of solitary eosinophilic granuloma of bone: a report of 9 cases. Radiology 1980; 136: 289–293.
71. Nauert C, Zornoza J, Ayala A, Harle TS. Eosinophilic granuloma of bone: diagnosis and management. Skeletal Radiol 1983; 10: 227–235.
72. Egeler RM, Thompson Jr, RC Voute PA, Nesbit ME Jr. Intralesional infiltration of corticosteroids in localized Langerhans' cell histiocytosis. J Pediatr Orthop 1992; 12: 811–814.
73. Schreuder HW, Pruszczynski M, Lemmens JA, Veth RP. Eosinophilic granuloma of bone: results of treatment with curettage, cryosurgery and bone grafting. J Pediatr Orthop B 1998; 7: 253–256.
74. Meachim G. Histological grading of chondrosarcomata. J Bone Joint Surg (Br) 1979; 61: 4–5.
75. Mirra JM, Gold R, Downs J, Eckardt JJ. A new histologic approach to the differentiation of enchondroma and chondrosarcoma of the bones. A clinicopathologic analysis of 51 cases. Clin Orthop 1985; 201: 214–237.
76. Giudici MA, Moser Jr, RP Kransdorf MJ. Cartilaginous bone tumors. Radiol Clin North Am 1993; 31: 237–259.
77. Bresser E, Roessner A, Brugg E, Erlemann R, Timm C, Grundman E. Bone tumors of the hand. A review of 300 cases documented in the Westphalian Bone Tumor Register. Arch Orthop Trauma Surg 1987; 106: 241–247.
78. Marcove RC. Chondrosarcoma: diagnosis and treatment. Orthop Clin North America 1977; 8: 811–820.
79. Healey JH, Lane JM. Chondrosarcoma. Clin Orthop 1986; 204: 119–129.
80. Schwartz HS. Zimmerman HB, Simon MA, Wroble RR, Millar EA, Bonfiglio M. The malignant potential of enchondromatosis. J Bone Joint Surg (Am) 1987; 69: 269–274.
81. Bauer HCF, Brosjö O, Kreicbergs A, Lindholm J. Low risk of recurrence of enchondroma and low-grade chondrosarcoma in extremities. 80 patients followed for 2–25 years. Acta Orthop Scand 1995; 66: 283–288.
82. Quint U, Pingsmann A. Surgical treatment of enchondroma in long tubular bones. Preservation of function versus extensive excision in the humerus. Arch Orthop Trauma Surg 1995; 114: 352–356.
83. Eriksson AI, Schiller A, Mankin HJ. The management of chondrosarcoma of bone. Clin Orthop 1980; 153: 44–66.
84. Schreuder HW, Pruszczynski M, Veth RP, Lemmmens JA. Treatment of benign and low-grade malignant intramedullary chondroid tumors with curettage and cryosurgery. Eur J Surg Oncol 1998; 24: 120–126.
85. Enneking WF. Fibrous dysplasia (84 cases). In: Enneking WF: Musculoskeletal tumor surgery. New York: Churchill Livingstone 1983: 855–867.
86. Keijser LCM, van Tienen TG, Schreuder HW, Lemmens JA, Pruszczynski M, Veth RP. Fibrous dysplasia of bone; management and outcome of 20 cases. Submitted.
87. Marcove RC, Stovell PB, Huvos AG, Bullough PG. The use of cryosurgery in the treatment of low and medium grade chondrosarcoma. A preliminary report. Clin Orthop 1977; 122: 147–156.
88. Dwyer DM, Thorne AC, Healey JH, Bedford RF. Liquid nitrogen instillation can cause venous gas embolism. Anesthesiology 1990; 73: 179–181.
89. Marcove RC. A 17-year review of cryosurgery in the treatment of bone tumors. Clin Orthop 1982; 163: 231–234.
90. de Vries J. Bonemarrow embolism and cryosurgery. Thesis, Groningen, 1983.
91. Pell AC, Christie J, Keating JF, Sutherland GR. The detection of fat embolism by transoesophageal echocardiography during reamed intramedullary nailing: a study of 24 patients with femoral and tibial fractures. J Bone Joint Surg (Br) 1993; 75-B: 921–925.
92. Christie J, Burnett R, Potts HR, Pell AC. Echocardiography of transatrial embolism during cemented and uncemented hemiarthroplasty of the hip. J Bone Joint Surg (Br) 1994; 76-B: 409–412.
93. Russe W, Kerschbaumer F, Bauer R. Kryochirurgie in der Orthopädie. Orthopäde 1984; 13: 142–150.
94. Fisher AD, Williams DF, Bradley PF. The effect of cryosurgery on the strength of bone. Br J Oral Surg 1978; 15: 215–222.
95. Gage AA, Emmings FG. Bone freezing in cryotherapy. J Barnabus Med Center 1967; 4: 314–319.

96. Schargus G, Winckler J, Schröder F, Schäfer B. Cryosurgical devitalization of bone and its regeneration. An experimental study with animals. J Maxillofac Surg 1975; 3: 128–131.
97. Malawer MM, Marks MR, McChesney D, Piasio M, Gunther SF, Schmookler BM. The effect of cryosurgery and polymethylmethacrylate in dogs with experimental bone defects comparable to tumor defects. Clin Orthop 1988; 226: 299–310.
98. Alkalay D, Kollender Y, Mozes M, Meller I. Giant cell tumors with intraarticular fracture. Two-stage local excision, cryosurgery and cementation in 5 patients with distal femoral tumor followed for 2–4 years. Acta Orthop Scand 1996; 67(3): 291–294.
99. Marcove RC, Sheth DS, Brien EW, Huvos AG, Healey JH. Conservative surgery for giant cell tumor of the sacrum. Cancer 1994; 74: 1253–1260.

15. Cryosurgery in the Treatment of Keloids and Hypertrophic Scars

Christos C. Zouboulis

15.0 Introduction

Cryosurgery – the well aimed and controlled destruction of diseased tissue by application of cold – is an effective and efficient method for treating various skin diseases (Graham 1993; Kuflik 1994; Zacarian 1994; Zouboulis 1998, 1999). The technique has several advantages and, especially in the treatment of keloids and hypertrophic scars, it provides good therapeutic and cosmetic results with few contraindications and a low incidence of complications (Zouboulis et al. 1993a; Rusciani et al. 1993; Ernst and Hundeiker 1995). The therapeutic effects of freezing on tissues have also been successfully used in the treatment of superficial atrophic acne scars (Table 15.1; Graham 1985; Röhrs 1997).

15.1 Cryobiological Background

The biological changes that occur in cryosurgery have been studied *in vitro* and *in vivo* and are caused by reduction of tissue temperature and consequent freezing (Farrant and Walter 1977; Orpwood 1981; Mazur 1984; Dawber 1988; Zouboulis 1999). Tissue injury is induced by direct physical effects of cell freezing and by the vascular stasis that develops in the tissue after thawing. The cryoreaction is, therefore, characterized by the physical and the vascular phases. A postulated third phase of cryoreaction, the immunologic phase, is still under investigation. The factors influencing the effects of freezing on tissue and their optimal parameters for the treatment of keloids and hypertrophic scars are shown in Table 15.2.

Table 15.1. Factors influencing the effects of freezing on tissue

	Optimum parameters for the treatment of keloids and hypertrophic scars
Speed of tissue freezing	Moderate speed (up to 100°C/min)
Speed of thawing	Slow speed (10°C/min, spontaneous rewarming)
Intra-/extracellular osmotic phenomena	Heterogenous and homogenous nucleation
Probe tip temperature	−85°C to −190°C
Tissue temperature	−20°C to −25°C
Duration of freezing	30 seconds
Repetition of freeze-thaw cycles	No
Vascular reaction	Yes
Immunologic reaction	Probable

Table 15.2. Cryosurgery of keloids and hypertrophic scars: clinical results

Cryosurgery as monotherapy					
	Number of patients	Significant to complete remission	%	Recurrences	
		Keloids			
Mende (1987)	7	5	71	–	
Zouboulis et al. (1993)	55	28	51	–	
Rusciani et al. (1993)	40	34	85	–	
Ernst and Hundeiker (1994)	234	158	68	9	
Zouridaki et al. (1996)	20	16	80	–	
Total	356	241	68	9	2%
		Hypertrophic scars			
Zouboulis et al. (1993)	38	29	76	–	
Ernst and Hundeiker (1994)	51	43	84	2	
Total	89	72	81	2	2%
Cryosurgery combined with intralesional corticosteroids					
	Number of patients	Significant to complete remission	%	Recurrences	
		Keloids			
Hirshowitz et al. (1982)	58	41	71	9	
Ernst and Hundeiker (1994)	56	38	68	2	
Zouridaki et al. (1996)	20	19	95	–	
Banfalvi et al. (1996)	25	21	84	–	
Total	159	119	75	11	7%

Very rapid freezing (100–260°C/min) leads to intracellular ice formation giving rise to cellular death due to an irreversible destruction of the cells known as homogenous nucleation. In the treatment of benign skin tumors, such as keloids and hypertrophic scars, cryosurgery does not have to be lethal, therefore, moderate freezing speeds (up to 100°C/min) can also be applied. Moderate freezing speeds lead to differential freezing in the different parts of the tissue, resulting in extracellular ice formation, hypertonic and sensitization damage. These phenomena which can also induce an irreversible destruction of the cells are known as heterogenous nucleation. Extracellular ice formation alone is not sufficient to kill cells, since disruption of cell membranes barely occurs despite the volume changes in the extra- and intracellular compartments. However, the temperature changes occurring in tissue by moderate freezing speeds are rapid enough to induce additional intracellular ice formation. When extracellular ice is formed, changing osmotic gradients between cells and extracellular fluid are produced which lead to a passage of electrolytes out of the cells, resulting in a decrease in cell volume. When a certain concentration of essential intracellular molecules is reached, they also pass out of the cell causing irreversible cell damage (hypertonic damage). However, gross cell damage can be observed even if the necessary hypertonic conditions are not achieved. This leads to the assumption that this "sensitization" damage is the result of phospholipid disruption in cell membranes.

A slow thawing speed (10°C/min) induces volume changes in the extra- and intracellular compartments leading to an increase of the intracellular water content. Rapid electrolyte transfer has been incriminated as the cause of damage to cell proteins and enzyme systems. Reverse osmotic gradients during thawing may give rise to "sensitization" damage. In addition, intracellular recrystallization of ice is responsible for tissue destruction. The latter process is as important as the initial freezing in causing cell death. Adequate freezing has been performed when the thawing time is 1.5 times the freezing time or longer.

Freezing takes place in the tissue at −0.6°C but this not the lethal temperature. Different cell populations present a differing ability to tolerate cold, with fibroblasts being rather resistant to cold, dying at −30°C to −35°C (Gage et al. 1979, 1982; Shepherd 1979). Therefore, it is difficult to avoid killing other cells during cryosurgery of keloids and hypertrophic scars. Theoretically, formation of ice crystals in tissue and, therefore, tissue freezing, starts from temperatures lower than −21.8°C, which is the eutectic temperature of sodium chloride solutions (Orpwood 1981). Therefore, an optimal cryosurgery of benign skin lesions, such as keloids and hypertrophic scars, requires tissue temperatures of −20°C to −25°C (Kuflik 1994).

Cell death rates have been shown *in vitro* to increase not only with lower temperatures but also with longer freezing times (Farrant and Walter 1977). However, the effect of freezing on cell viability reaches a maximum at about 100 sec followed by a plateau in cell death rates over time.

The importance of more than one freeze-thaw cycle in causing increased rates of cell death has been demonstrated in several *in vitro* and animal studies (Farrant and Walter 1977; Breitbart and Schaeg 1990). However, repeated freezing-thawing cycles are not essential in the treatment of keloids and hypertrophic scars (Zouboulis et al. 1993).

Cryogenic injury leads to vascular stasis and inevitable tissue anoxemia resulting in ischemic necrosis (Zacarian 1985). Microscopic examination of injured tissue in animals has shown that edema, focal capillary damage, hemorrhages and isolated microthrombi begin to occur after 2 hours and that by 5–8 hours focal or segmental necrosis of blood vessels is present. Thrombosis of terminal arteries leading to gangrene appears between 1 and 7 days, but only when injury is severe. Even after mild cold injuries, the initial circulatory impairment is irreversible, thus implicating delayed progressive thrombosis as the main factor producing tissue loss (Kulka 1965; Sebastian and Scholz 1993). Thrombosis in 65% of the capillaries and 35–40% of the arterioles and venoles already occurs at tissue temperatures of 11°C to 3°C, while thrombosis of all vessels is detectable at −15°C to −20°C in tissue (Rinfret 1962; Zacarian et al. 1970). In an attempt to explain exudation which occurs after cryosurgery, ultrastructural studies of endothelial cells have shown that cell damage in the first hour after freezing and thawing includes rupture of cell membranes, thinning and later condensation of ground substance and swelling of rough endoplasmic reticulum and mitochondria (Rabb et al. 1974).

15.2 Cryosurgery in the Treatment of Keloids and Hypertrophic Scars

Keloids and hypertrophic scars are benign cutaneous lesions produced by uncontrolled synthesis and deposition of dermal collagen as a result of abnormal wound healing. They usually follow injury to the skin of predisposed individuals but can also occur spontaneously. The chest, the shoulders, the head-neck area and the upper back are the most susceptible regions of the body (Datubo-Brown 1990; Muir 1990). While keloids have a strong tendency to grow beyond the confines of the previous wound, hypertrophic scars remain within the borders of the original dermal trauma (Peacock et al. 1970; Ehrlich et al. 1994). In contrast to hypertrophic scars, keloids do not regress with time and do not provoke scar contractures. Keloids contain large, thick collagen fibers composed of numerous fibrils closely packed together. In contrast, hypertrophic scars exhibit modular structures in which fibroblastic cells, small vessels, and fine, randomly organized collagen fibers are present (Ehrlich et al. 1994).

The primary cell in keloids has been shown to be the myofibroblast with prominent rough endoplasmic reticulum and bundles of myofilaments with focal densities in the cytoplasm (James 1980; Matsuoka et al. 1988; Ehrlich et al. 1994; Lee and Vijayasingam 1995). Enhanced secretory activity was reflected in the prominence of the Golgi apparatus and the frequent presence of intracellular collagen within the tubular membranes (Lee and Vijayasingam 1995). Proliferating dermal fibroblasts in the periphery of the keloid tissue have been shown; their numbers were increased in comparison with hypertrophic scars and normal skin (Nakaoka et al. 1995; Appleton et al. 1996). In contrast, no proliferating cells were found in the central region of the keloid (Appleton et al. 1996). Northern blot analysis of total RNA obtained from keloids with high growth tendency *in vivo* and immunohistochemistry of keloids and hypertrophic scars showed a marked induction of the small proteoglycan biglycan and collagen-a1 (I) expression in comparison with normal skin (Scott et al. 1995; Hunzelmann et al. 1996). In another study, increased levels of a1 (I)- and a1 (III)-collagen mRNA were observed in fibroblasts from the edge and outside of hypertrophic scar tissue, while normal levels were noted in fibroblasts from the center of this tissue. In addition, decreased levels of collagenase mRNA were found in the hypertrophic scar fibroblasts, suggesting that decreased expression of collagenase in hypertrophic scar fibroblasts may be one possible cause for the excessive accumulation of collagen in the skin lesions of hypertrophic scars (Arakawa et al. 1996). On the other hand, increased collagen synthesis by normal collagen degradation has been found in keloid fibroblasts *in vitro* (Diegelmann et al. 1979). Tenascin, a large extracellular matrix glycoprotein, was shown to be strongly expressed in keloids, demarcating their borders in tissue (Wulff et al. 1995; Dalkowski et al. 1997). Significantly increased levels of tenascin expression were also found in keloidal fibroblasts in comparison to normal cells *in vitro*. As *in vivo*, normal and keloidal fibroblasts have been shown to exhibit similar basal rates of fibrin matrix gel contraction *in vitro*, while fibroblasts from hypertrophic scars exhibited a consistently higher basal rate of fibrin matrix gel contraction than other fibroblasts (Younai et al. 1996). Furthermore, only nodules of hypertrophic scars contained a-smooth muscle actin-expressing myofibroblasts when compared to keloid and normal skin tissue (Ehrlich et al. 1994). The presence in hypertrophic scar myofibroblasts of a-smooth muscle actin, the actin isoform typical of vascular smooth muscle cells, may represent an important element in the pathogenesis of increased contraction in hypertrophic scars.

Patients wish treatment mainly for cosmetic reasons; pruritus, pain and restriction of movement by lesions close to joints are often additional ones. A variety of therapeutic regimens has been used with unsatisfactory final results because these lesions, especially keloids, are notoriously recurrent (Peacock et al. 1970; Brown et al. 1986; Rudolph 1987; Kelly 1988; Datubo-Brown 1990; Berman and Bieley 1995). In several studies in recent years, cryosurgery was found to be effective and safe in keloids and hypertrophic scars. Due to its major advantage of rarely occurring recurrences, the technique, either as monotherapy or as combination therapy, has been established as the treatment of choice for keloids and hypertrophic scars.

Effects of freezing on connective tissue: An advantage of cryosurgery often cited is that of minimum scarring. The collagen fiber network of the dermis has been shown to remain largely undamaged by the standard cryosurgical procedures performed by clinicians (Shepherd 1979). Using the young domestic pig as the model and two 1-min freeze-thaw cycles, no alteration was found in the periodicity of fibrillar cross-banding nor fracturing or distortion of collagen fibrils. In a study on rats, wound contraction after freeze injury was minimal in contrast to burn damage in which contracture was the rule (Ehrlich and Hembry 1984).

Effects of freezing on keloidal fibroblasts: Fibroblasts are rather resistant to freezing (Shepherd 1979; Dalkowski 1997), and cryosurgery was shown to increase their proliferation *in vivo* (Dawber 1988) and *in vitro* (Wulff et al. 1996; Dalkowski 1997). Suspended fibroblast cultures established from keloids and normal skin samples incubated in sterile cryotubes were frozen in precooled ethanol (−75°C) and consequently seeded on culture dishes. The proliferation of keloidal fibroblasts significantly increased immediately after cryotherapy *in vitro* in 4 of 6 cultures tested. After subcultivation, persistence of significantly increased proliferation was determined in 3 of 4 cultures. On the other hand, the proliferation of normal fibroblasts decreased in 3 of 6 cultures immediately after cryotherapy but returned to higher rates after subcultivation. These data correspond to the increase in the number of dermal fibroblasts observed 3 weeks after cryosurgery of the young domestic pig skin (Dawber 1988). Furthermore, cryosurgery induced a significant reduction of collagen I synthesis in 2 of 4 cultures examined after being frozen in comparison to non-frozen cultures, while increased synthesis of collagen IV was found in 2 of 4 cultures (Wulff et al. 1996; Dalkowski 1997). No uniform changes of collagen III and fibronectin synthesis were detected. After subcultivation, increased collagen IV synthesis of keloidal fibroblasts persisted in 2 of 2 cultures, while the synthesis of collagen I was no more suppressed. Collagens I and III represented more than 90% of the total collagen amount produced by keloidal fibroblasts *in vitro*. Normal fibroblasts showed no uniform changes of collagen and fibronectin synthesis either immediately after cryotherapy or after subcultivation. It is likely that cryotherapy exerts a temporary inhibitory effect on the synthetic activity of keloidal fibroblasts, while it does not affect the activity of normal cells.

Structural changes in keloids and hypertrophic scars after cryosurgery: Significant skin thickening was found to occur 3 weeks after cryosurgery of pig skin which corresponded to an increase in the number of fibroblasts, followed by significant thinning at 6 months, probably due to the chronic ischemia induced by cryosurgery (Dawber 1988). In man, neovascularization, regular linear arrangement of collagen bundles, increased fibroblasts in a stroma running parallel to the skin surface, and mononuclear cells mostly arranged at the perivascular area were found in clinically responding lesions after cryosurgery (Zouboulis et al. 1993a). In a prospective, randomized study of 40 patients with keloids, which compared the clinical and histological effects of cryosurgery as a single regimen or combined with intralesional steroids, the major structural changes observed were increased vessel number and lumen dilatation in both groups and a reduction of the number and the length of rete ridges in the monotherapy group (Zouridaki et al. 1996). Immunohistologically, enhancement and diffusion of tenascin expression in the entire treated dermal region and depletion of IFNg expression, indicating immune regulation, were found (Zouboulis et al. 1996). These histological and immunohistological studies indicate that cryosurgery can induce changes in keloids which are compatible with a rejuvenation of the scars.

Clinical results: Cryosurgery was initially applied in the treatment of keloids and hypertrophic scars as a weak cryotherapy regimen prior to intralesional corticosteroids in order to induce tissue edema and to facilitate intralesional injections (Ceilley and Babin 1979). Cryosurgery as a therapeutic monotherapy regimen was first used by Shepherd and Dawber (1982): They treated 17 patients with keloids with a single cryosurgical session, achieving 80% improvement of the lesions; however, they observed a high recurrence rate of 33%. With the exception of case or technical reports (Meltzer 1983; Muti and Ponzio 1983; Cirne de Castro et al. 1986), further monotherapy studies were probably delayed by the rather disappointing recurrence rate, until Mende (1987) and Zouboulis and Orfanos (1990) showed that repeated cryosurgical sessions can exert a beneficial effect on keloids and hypertrophic scars and additionally prevent relapses.

Cryosurgery was shown to exhibit significantly better results than intralesional triamcinolone (5 mg/lesion) in a randomized study with 11 patients with multiple acne keloids, especially in early, vascular lesions (Layton et al. 1994). It is nowadays regarded as an established treatment for keloids and hypertrophic scars (Drake et al. 1994), possibly being the treatment of choice (Zouboulis 1998). The following techniques are established or currently under evaluation.

Cryosurgery as monotherapy: In 241 of 356 patients (68%) with keloids and 72 of 89 (81%) patients with hypertrophic scars a greater than 50% improvement or complete regression has been observed (5 studies; Mende 1987; Zouboulis et al. 1993a; Rusciani et al. 1993; Ernst and Hundeiker, 1995; Zouridaki et al. 1996) (Table 15.3). Acne keloids also showed a 73% improvement or complete regression in 16 patients treated (Röhrs 1997). To achieve these results 1 to more than 20 sessions of an average of 30 seconds each applied once monthly using the contact method of treatment have been required. Progression or recurrence were rare (2%). The number of sessions, the dia-

Table 15.3. Variables affecting the outcome of cryosurgery in keloids and hypertrophic scars

Factors that influence the outcome of cryosurgery in keloids and hypertrophic scars	
Diagnosis	Hypertrophic scars respond significantly better than keloids
Number of sessions	Better responses were seen in subjects treated with 3 or more sessions than in subjects treated once or twice
Age of the lesion	Lesions younger than 2 years responded better than older ones
Factors that do not influence the outcome of cryosurgery in keloids and hypertrophic scars	
Age of the patient	
Sex of the patient	
Size of the lesion	
Location of the lesion	
Pretreatment	

gnosis and the duration of lesions significantly correlated with the result of the treatment. The age and the sex of the patient, the size and the location of lesions and pretreatment with another method did not influence the outcome of cryosurgical treatments (Zouboulis et al. 1993a). The cryosurgical treatment was generally well tolerated and only minor complications occurred. About one third of the patients treated complained of mild local pain which was easily managed, when necessary. 12–100% of the subjects experienced lesional hypopigmentation and 1–8% skin atrophy. The complications were dependent on the duration of freezing and the number of freeze-thaw cycles applied (Mende 1987; Zouboulis et al. 1993a; Rusciani et al. 1993).

Cryosurgery combined with intralesional corticosteroids: Initially performed in 1982 by Hirshowitz et al. (1982) with the impressive result of 71% complete remission in 58 patients with keloids, the combination of cryosurgery prior to or following intralesional corticosteroids exhibited significant regression of keloids in 78 of 101 patients (77%) treated in 3 further studies (Ernst and Hundeiker, 1995; Banfalvi et al. 1996; Zouridaki et al. 1996) (Table 15.3). Cryosurgery performed prior to corticosteroid treatment induces tissue edema and facilitates intralesional injections. However, in a randomized trial with 40 patients with keloids the combined therapy was not superior (in 90%, >50% reduction of lesion volume) to monotherapy (in 83%, >50% reduction of lesion volume) (Zouridaki et al. 1996).

Surgical debulking prior to cryosurgery with or without intralesional corticosteroids: Lesions refractory to cryosurgery or cryosurgery combined with intralesional corticosteroids can be surgically removed, and postsurgical cryoprevention with or without intralesional corticosteroids can be applied in order to avoid recurrences. This regimen is unavoidable in large keloids although recurrences are not rare, despite the promising initial result (Glazer et al. 1985; Lubritz 1985; Sebastian and Scholz 1990; Zouboulis et al. 1993b). Intramarginal excision is advisable because it is followed by a lower recurrence rate when compared to extramarginal excision (Engrav et al. 1988). Removal of the lesion by surgery and by carbon dioxide laser yield similar recurrence rates (Stern and Lucente 1989); however, the carbon dioxide laser provides a high degree of hemostasis and avoidance of sutures.

Intralesional cryosurgery: A method of intralesional cryosurgery for keloids and hypertrophic scars developed by modification of the technique by Weshahy (1993) is under evaluation in our department.

Cryopeeling: The freezing peel (cryopeeling) is a full face, superficial cryosurgical treatment for atrophic acne scarring that is especially useful in patients with mild to moderate circinate scars. Results are similar to those obtained with chemical peeling but not as good as those obtained with dermabrasion. Repeated sessions, sometimes over 2 to 3 years, are required for obtaining optimum results (Röhrs 1997).

15.3 Cryosurgical Equipment and Treatment Techniques

The simplest cryosurgical modality, still in current use, is the cotton-tipped applicator method which applies small or large swabs soaked in liquid nitrogen. This modality lacks the capacity of active freezing and therefore can only induce a slow freezing speed which limits its application in the treatment of keloids and hypertrophic scars. In addition, large swabs create large frozen surfaces, generally overriding the limits of the area intended for treatment in small lesions, while small swabs have a limited liquid nitrogen reservoir capacity. A modification of the classic cotton-tipped applicator is the "hard tail" dip-stick which has been devised in an attempt to avoid these disadvantages (Simon 1986). The "hard tail" dip-stick is made out of a standard large cotton-tipped applicator. At its end, a tiny amount of cotton is pinched between the index finger and thumb and strongly twisted in order to obtain the so-called "hard tail". The distal part of the tail is cut down so that the total tail does not exceed 5 mm. This dip-stick is soaked in liquid nitrogen. Since a large swab is used, a large amount of liquid nitrogen is absorbed by the cotton reservoir. Only the tail of the swab is brought into contact with the lesion. Liquid nitrogen is slowly released at the pointed end of the swab, producing an accurate freezing effect. The method does not induce temperatures low enough for sufficient cryosurgery of dermal benign lesions, such as keloids and hypertrophic scars. However, it can be used as an alternative technique when other cryosurgical devices are not available or with very small scar lesions (smaller than 5 mm).

Nowadays many well-functioning cryosurgical units with different design, function and performance characteristics are commercially available (Torre 1985; Ferris and Ho 1992). Sufficient cold for cryosugery can be produced by direct or indirect application of a solid or liquid cryogen stored at low temperatures, by lowering the pressure of a gas (Joule-Thompson effect), electromechanically, or simply by refrigeration. The devices are mainly characterized by the applied cryogen and the manner of cryogen application to the skin (Zouboulis 1999).

The methodology of cryosurgery is nowadays sophisticated and the techniques standardized. There are at present three different techniques used for the treatment of keloids and hypertrophic scars.

The contact technique: The contact method uses metallic probes which function on the principle of temperature exchange. A gas cryogen circulates through these probes. As the tip removes heat from the tissue, the tissue gradually cools. The size, material, composition and temperature of the probe tip determine its tissue cooling capacity. Other factors, such as tissue moistness, extent of tissue contact, the duration of freeze and pressure exerted on the probe, affect heat diffusion. When the cryosurgical unit is activated and the probe is placed in firm contact with the tissue, an area of frozen tissue or ice ball may be observed extending radially from the cryoprobe tip. The interface between the ice ball and unfrozen tissue represents the 0°C isotherm, which is the line connecting the points at a temperature of 0°C at the given time. The longer the duration of the freeze, the farther the iceball radiates from the cryoprobe tip margin (Farrant and Walter 1977). The distance between the tip margin and the 0°C isotherm represents the lateral spead of freeze. The depth of the 0°C isotherm from the tip indicates the depth of freeze. Although variable, the lateral spread of freeze approximates the depth of freeze by a ratio of 1:1.3 (Torre 1979). The volume of tissue located between the −22°C isotherm and the probe tip is called the lethal zone. Cells within this zone undergo cryonecrosis (Orpwood 1981). Those cells situated in the warmer region between the −22°C isotherm and the 0°C isotherm generally survive the freeze. This important zone represents the recovery zone. Although the depth of freeze is time related, as the duration of freeze extends towards 100 sec the lethal zone flats. The contact method is the method of choice in the treatment of keloids and hypertrophic scars, since it provides controllable as well as reproducible results. The results can additionally be modulated by cryoprobe pressure and can induce vessel contraction.

The spray technique: The spray technique uses an open freezing system with freeze-secure vents. It emits a fine spray of a cryogen directly at the target area. It is particularly useful for irregular lesions and lesions with a curved surface. For large lesions to be treated in one session, a paint-brush or spiral pattern of spray can be used (Lubritz 1978). The spray is emitted from a distance of 1 to 2 cm from the target site and at 90-degree angle to it. The depth of the freeze may be judged by the lateral spread of freezing on the surface; it is about half the radius of the surface area (Elton 1985). An intermittent spraying of liquid nitrogen is desirable since it results in a more uniform temperature in the ice ball and greater depth, while it limits lateral spread. The depth of freeze can only reach 10 mm (Elton 1985) and, therefore, it is not the appropriate technique for voluminous keloids and hypertrophic scars. There are two variants of the spraying procedure, the described open-spray technique and the confined-spray technique. The latter directs the spray into cones (Torre 1985), individually prepared plastic moulages, or other materials which are open at both ends with one end placed on the skin. The confined-spray technique restricts the spray to the lesion and avoids wide freezing of the healthy peripheral tissue; however, it makes clinical evaluation of the depth of freeze impossible.

Intralesional cryosurgery: The inability of skin surface cryosurgery to freeze beyond 20 mm in depth (Gage 1982) led Weshahy (1993) to develop a method for applying cryosurgery in depth. One or more needles are introduced into the skin from one point, run through the deeper tissues of the lesion and appear on the surface at the opposite border. A sprayed cryogen is then passed through the needle by inserting the spray tip of the cryosurgical device into the head piece of the needle. The cryogen is passed through the lumen, exiting to the atmosphere at the other end of the needle. An ice cylinder is formed around the embedded part of the needle within the deeper tissues. The distance of extension of freezing can be clinically estimated by the degree of extension of the whitish ice balls formed around the points of contact between the skin surface and the visible portions of the needle. The needles can be angled, curved and hook-shaped. Compression of the lesions is accomplished by pulling up the visible parts of the needle. We are currently evaluating intralesional cryosurgery in the treatment of keloids and hypertrophic scars. We have developed a device consisting of a small liquid nitrogen Dewar flask engaging a single-use, 20-gauge needle instead of a tip, to spray liquid nitrogen through, connected by a flexible, long metallic cryoprobe stem. The cryoprobe stem is luer-locked to the needle. The shape of the cryoprobe stem is variable so that the Dewar flask can stay upright during freezing. The shape of the needle can also be changed in order to form a hook. The main advantages of intralesional cryosurgery compared with the contact and spray techniques could be the minimal surface destruction, which can be further reduced by using peripherally insulated needles.

15.4 Practical Procedures

In the following, the practical procedures for the cryosurgical treatment of keloids and hypertrophic scars are described step-by-step. Although the techniques seem rather simple, the physician using cryosurgery has to be a certified dermatologist in order to correctly diagnose the disease and have knowledge of the skin and subcutaneous tissues. In addition, the physician should have had training in cryosurgery. Prior to treatment the following general measures have to be taken:

I. The patient has to be informed about the procedure, the reported results of the technique, and the personal experience of the cryosurgeon, as well as the complications which may occur. In sensitive patients lidocaine-prilocaine 1:1 creme (Juhlin et al. 1980) has to be prescribed and be occlusively applied by the patient on the lesion(s) to be treated one hour prior to cryosurgery. Instead of long explanations about the technique which may confuse the patient, simplified written information on cryosurgery can be prepared and distributed to the patients before their treatment.
II. The cryoprobe tips have to be desinfected after every treatment either by soaking them in ethanol solution or by dry sterilization.
III. Gloves have to be worn during the procedures.
IV. The lesion to be treated has to be disinfected using sterile gauze soaked in ethanol solution.

Contact technique: A cryoprobe tip is chosen that fits the size of the lesion in order to avoid freezing the healthy peripheral tissue. The size of probe tips should be the same as or, even better, a little smaller than the size of the lesion, taking into consideration that an ice ball is formed during freezing which spreads laterally from the lesion.

When using a liquid nitrogen hand unit with silicone exhaust tubing, the tubing has to be frozen at a position away from the patient and the physician, otherwise the tubing will flail and finally freeze to a position that may disturb the treatment.

The time of freezing for each lesion or a part of it has to be controlled. For keloids and hypertrophic scars a single freeze-thaw session of 20 to 60 seconds is used, depending on the volume of the lesion.

Large scars can be treated with specially formed cryoprobes, such as a flat linear probe for a linear scar (Meltzer 1983), or with classical small probes in order to induce significant pressure and vasocontraction on fragments of the lesion.

As mentioned above, the optimal use of the technique allows exact freezing of the lesion without any freezing of the peripheral healthy tissue.

If there is no intervention after cryosurgery, the physical course of the cryoreaction is:

i. Peripheral erythema, occurring immediately to 30 minutes after cryosurgery.
ii. Edema of the lesion, occurring between a few minutes and some hours after treatment.
iii. Bulla formation, usually presenting between one and three days after treatment.
iv. Exudation, lasting between a few to 14 days after cryosurgery.
v. Mummification, in which a serum crust builds from the second to the fourth posttreatment week.
vi. Healing, with a flat slightly atrophic scar.

In order to minimize erythema and edema after cryosurgery a mild, non-atrophogenic steroid cream (e.g., hydrocortisone aceponate, hydrocortisone buteprate, hydrocortisone-17-butyrate, methylprednisolone aceponate, prednicarbate) is applied on the lesion immediately after treatment, especially in areas that are prone to react with strong edema (e.g., facial areas).

The patient is requested to visit the physician again when the bulla is formed so that the physician or his assistant can aspirate the serum content with a sterile fine needle (e.g., 26-gauge). The bulla roof is left on the lesion as a natural protection film. The bulla is disinfected using sterile gauze soaked in ethanol solution before aspiration.

A disinfectant-drying solution (e.g., Castellani colorless solution, merbromine 2%, polyvidone-iodine 10%) or a lotion (e.g., chlorhexidine 1% in lotio alba aquosa) is prescribed, to be used by the patient once daily on the lesion.

A new appointment is given the patient for evaluating the results and performing the next session of treatment 4 weeks later. The treatment is repeated once monthly, if required. A total of 3 or more sessions significantly increase the response rates and minimize recurrences.

The clinical results to be obtained by the technique are shown in Figs. 15.1 to 15.11.

Spray technique: The spray technique is not advisable for the treatment of keloids and hypertrophic scars. However, the physician who prefers to apply this technique based on his experience, has to use the confined-spray technique following a procedure similar to the one described for the contact technique. The following additional measures have to be taken:

I. The spray is emitted from a distance of 1 to 2 cm from the target site and at a 90-degree angle to it.
II. A single freeze-thaw session of 20 to 60 seconds is used, depending on the volume of the lesion.
III. If the open-spray technique is used, two freeze-thaw sessions of 20 to 30 seconds are required in order to limit the ice ball radius and to obtain results similar to those obtained by the contact method.

Point-spraying yields better results in keloids and hypertrophic scars than a paint-brush or spiral pattern of spray.

Cryosurgery combined with intralesional corticosteroids

Lesions, mostly keloids, that are refractory or respond minimally after at least 6 sessions to cryosurgery performed as monotherapy, may improve by a combination of cryosurgery and intralesional steroids. Intralesional betamethasone or triamcinolone injections (up to 2 mg/cm^2 lesional surface) are applied by a luer-locked 26-gauge needle 30 to 60 minutes after cryosurgical treatment, performed as described above. This delay is required in order to allow the lesions to enter the edematous phase of cryoreaction, which

i. makes intralesional injections easier and
ii. leads the fluid to the area of minor resistance which is in this case the lesion due to the edema.

If, in contrast, intralesional injections were given prior to cryosurgery or as monotherapy, the lesion would resist accepting the fluid volume, leading to a concentration of the fluid at the healthy periphery of the lesion and finally to the well-known perilesional atrophy after intralesional corticosteroid injections in keloids. In addition, the corticosteroid concentration of up to 2 mg/cm^2 lesional surface has also been defined in order to avoid perilesional atrophy. On the other hand, corticosteroid injections in keloids are painful, and, therefore, there is better acceptance if the injections are performed in edematous tissue. In patients who continue to feel pain during the corticosteroid injection despite this improved

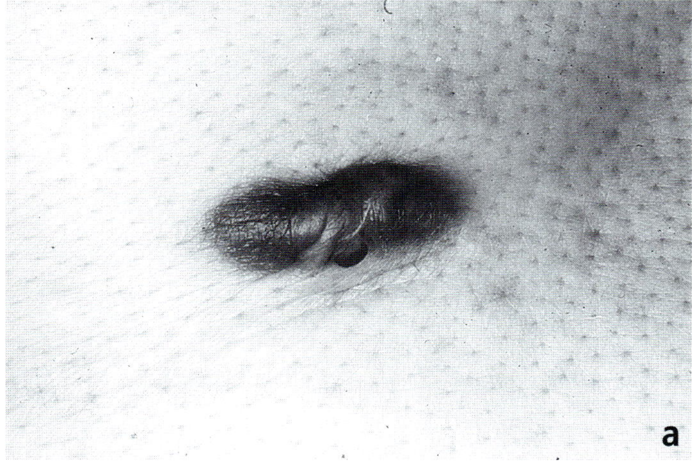

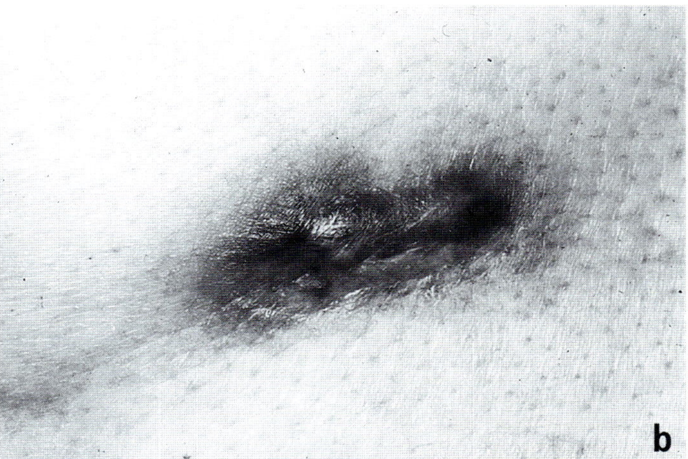

Fig. 15.1. Keloid on the chest of a patient before (**a**) and 2 months after (**b**) a single session of cryosurgery with nitrous oxide, 30 seconds, contact technique. A reduction of the lesional volume of more than 50% can be observed (from Zouboulis and Orfanos 2000)

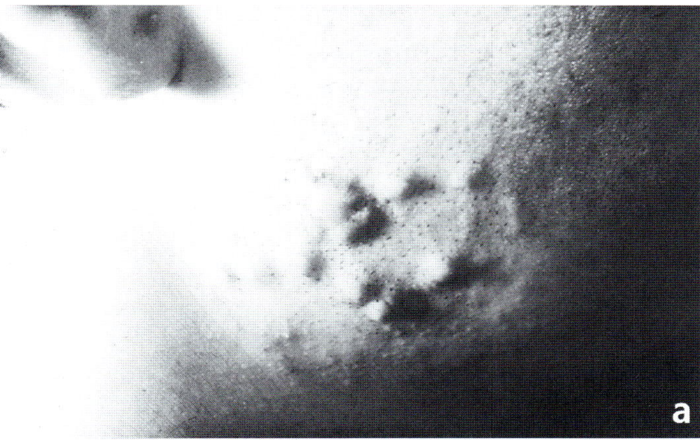

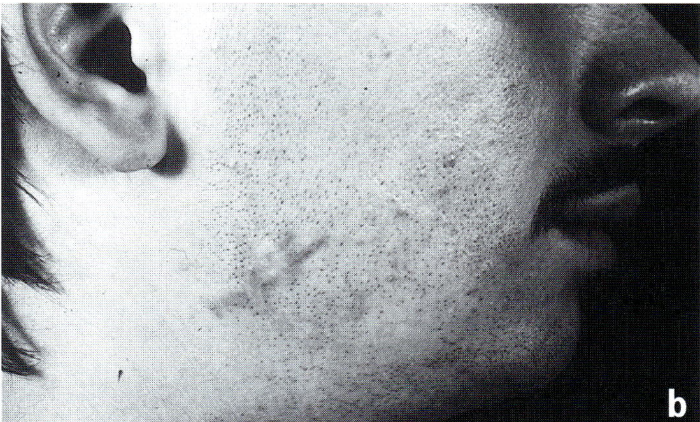

Fig. 15.2. Two-year-old post acne keloids on the right cheek of a patient before (**a**) and 8 months after (**b**) the last of seven sessions with liquid nitrogen, 30 seconds/lesion, contact technique (from Zouboulis et al. 1993a)

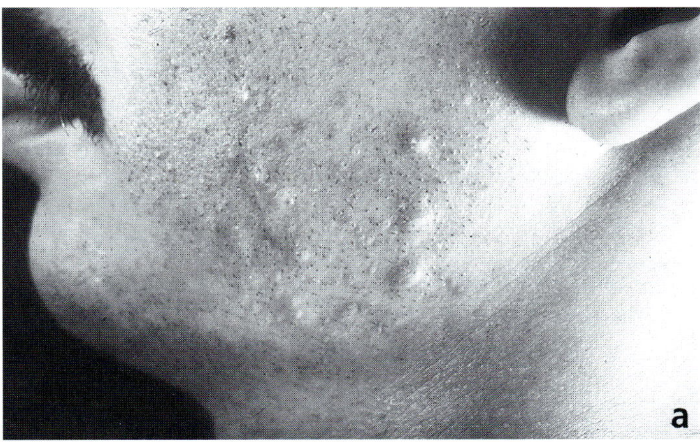

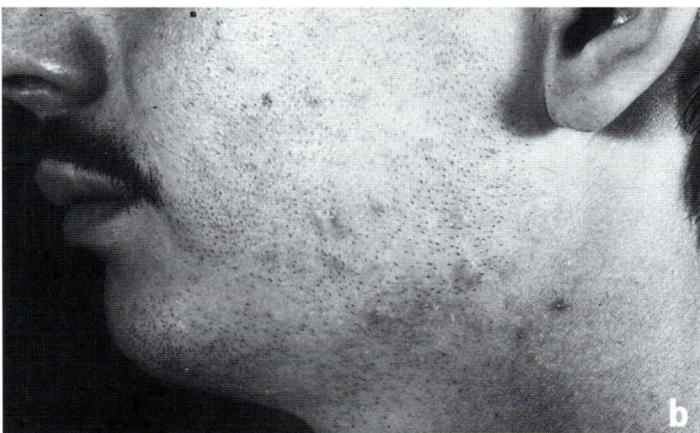

Fig 15.3. The left cheek of the same patient before (**a**) and 8 months after (**b**) the last of seven sessions with liquid nitrogen, 30 seconds/lesion, contact technique (from Zouboulis and Orfanos 2000)

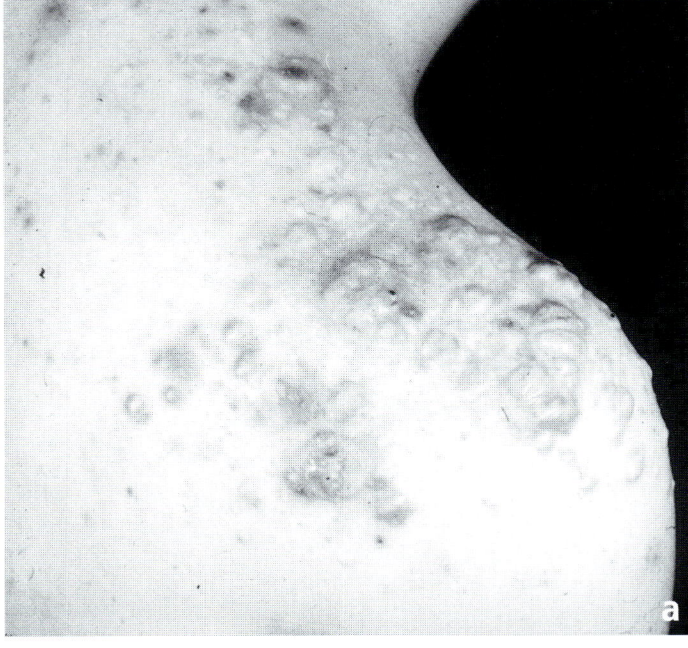

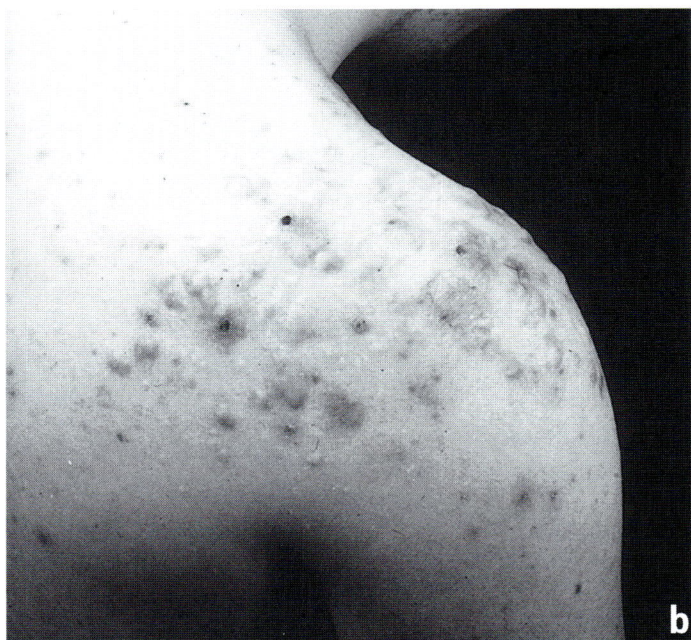

Fig. 15.4. Large acne keloids on the right shoulder of an 18-year-old male patient before (**a**) (from Zouboulis and Orfanos 2000) and 2 months after (**b**) 12 sessions with nitrous oxide, 40–60 seconds/lesion, contact technique (from Zouboulis and Orfanos 1990)

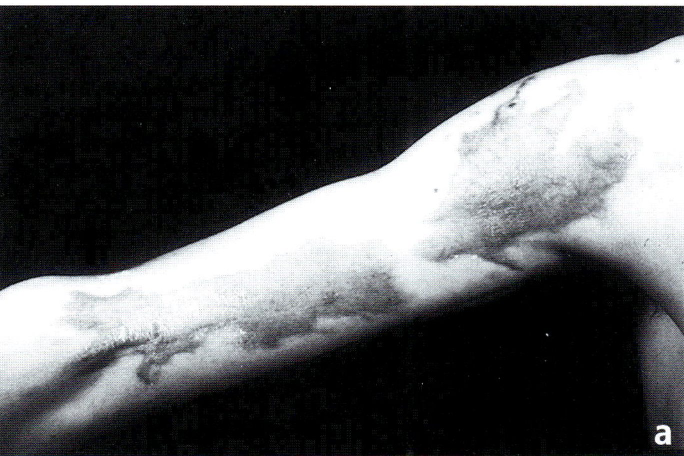

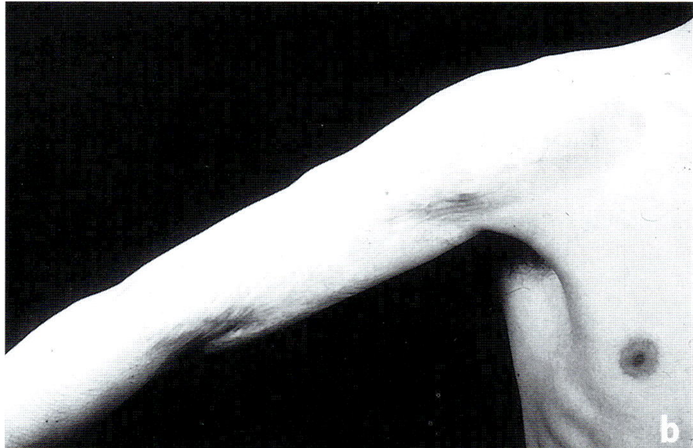

Fig. 15.5. Huge keloids after chemical burn with sulphuric acid and contraction of the right elbow joint in a 21-year-old male patient before (**a**) and one year after 9 sessions initially with liquid nitrogen (4 sessions) and finally with nitrous oxide (5 sessions), 30 seconds/lesion, contact technique (**b**). Elbow mobility is again complete (from Zouboulis 1998)

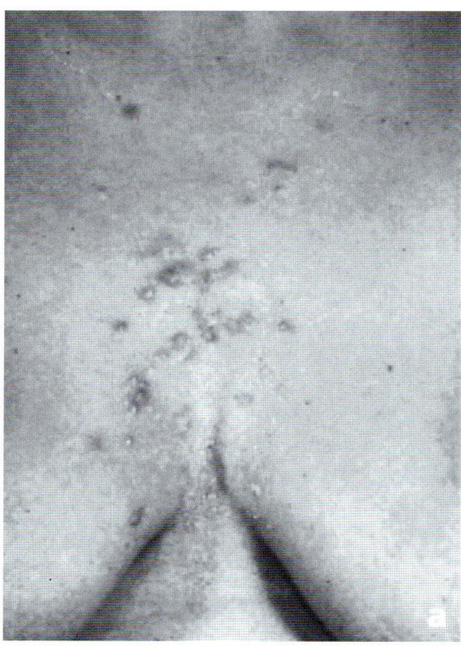

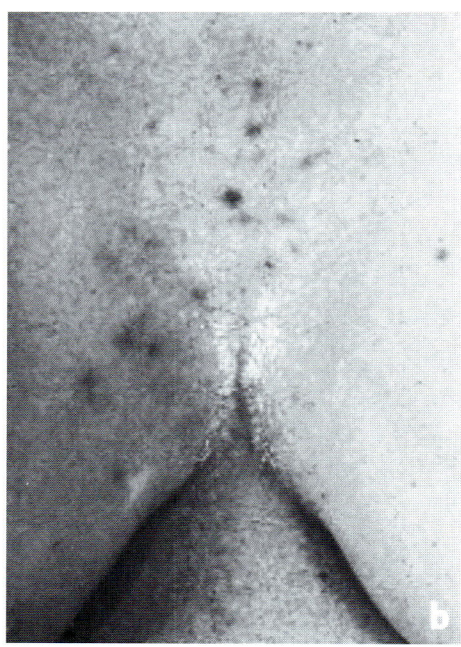

Fig. 15.6. Acne scars on the chest of a 22-year-old female patient before (**a**) and one month after (**b**) the last of 9 sessions with nitrous oxide, 30 seconds/lesion, contact technique (from Zouboulis and Orfanos 2000)

procedure, a mixture of corticosteroid-lidocaine 1% 1:1 can be injected. Results of the technique are shown in Fig. 15.12.

Surgical debulking prior to cryosurgery: Cryosurgery of large-volume keloids is a difficult task. These lesions are better removed surgically, with post-surgical cryoprevention, with or without intralesional corticosteroids, applied in order to decrease the recurrence rate. However, recurrences are unavoidable. Before surgery is performed, the following points have to be considered:

i) Intramarginal excision is advisable because it is followed by a lower recurrence rate than is extramarginal excision (Fig. 15.13).
ii) Removal of the lesion by the carbon dioxide laser provides a high degree of hemostasis and obviates sutures.

The carbon dioxide laser setting is 11 Watts, 2 mm beam diameter, continuous discharge, energy 350 Watt/cm^2.

Cryoprevention (20 to 30 seconds at −86°C or −196°C) has to be performed on the resultant fresh

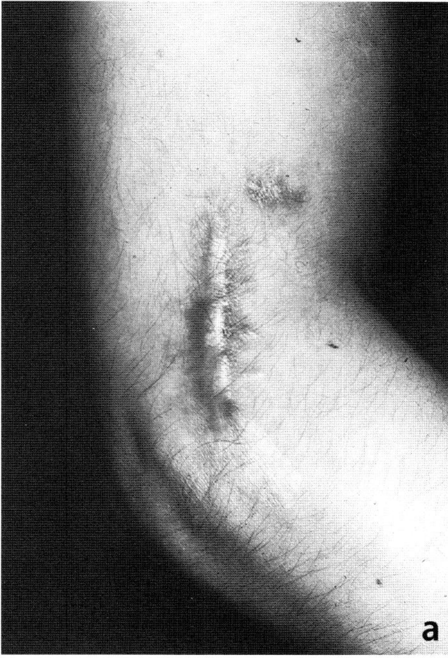
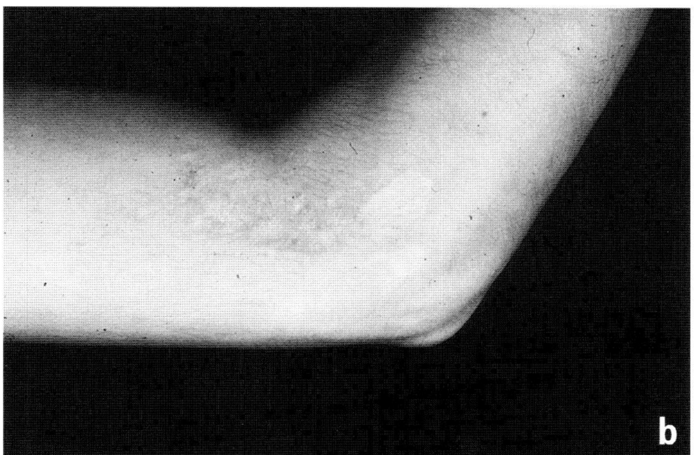

Fig. 15.7. Two-year-old hypertrophic scar before (**a**) and 2 months after (**b**) the last of 4 sessions with liquid nitrogen, 30 seconds/lesion, contact technique (from Zouboulis et al. 1993a)

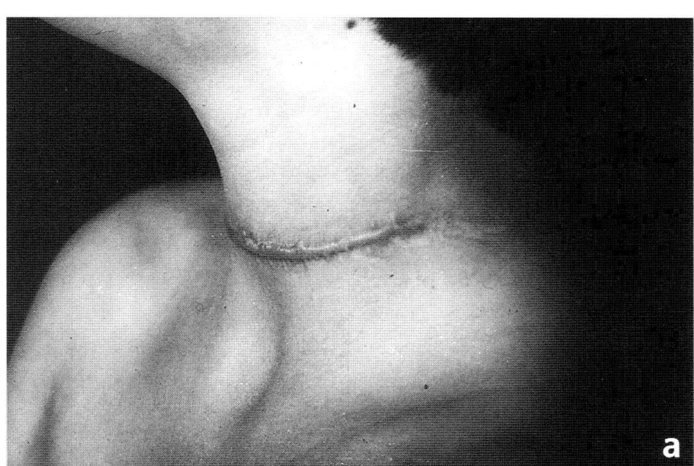
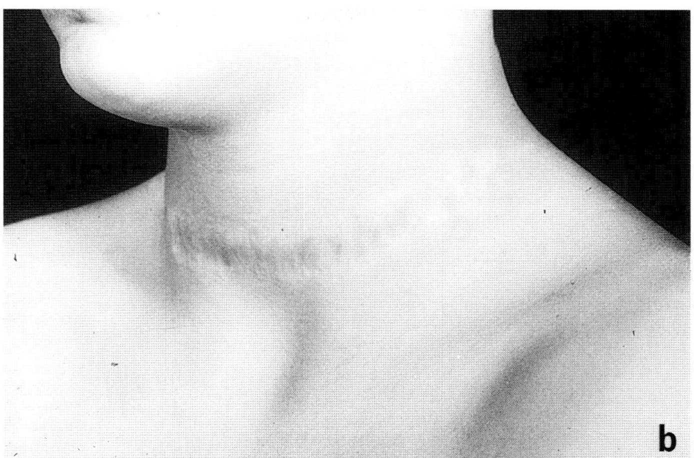

Fig. 15.8. Six-month-old 22 cm long hypertrophic scar before (**a**) and 6 months after (**b**) the last of 5 sessions with liquid nitrogen, 30 seconds, contact technique (from Zouboulis et al. 1993b)

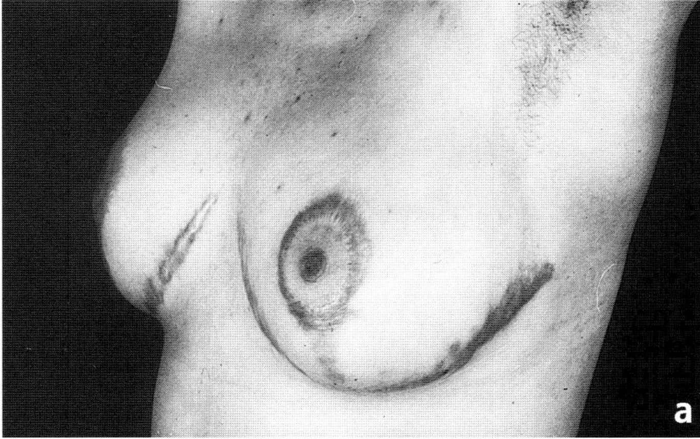
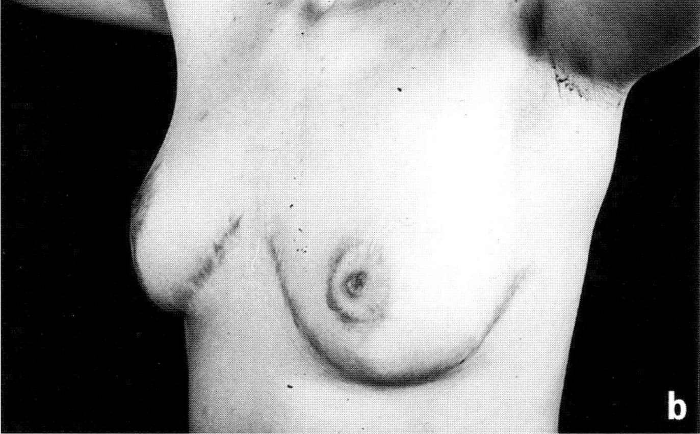

Fig. 15.9. Two-year-old hypertrophic scars before (**a**) and 10 months after the last of 6 sessions (**b**), initially with liquid nitrogen (2 sessions) and finally with nitrous oxide (4 sessions), 30 seconds/lesion, contact technique (from Zouboulis and Orfanos 2000)

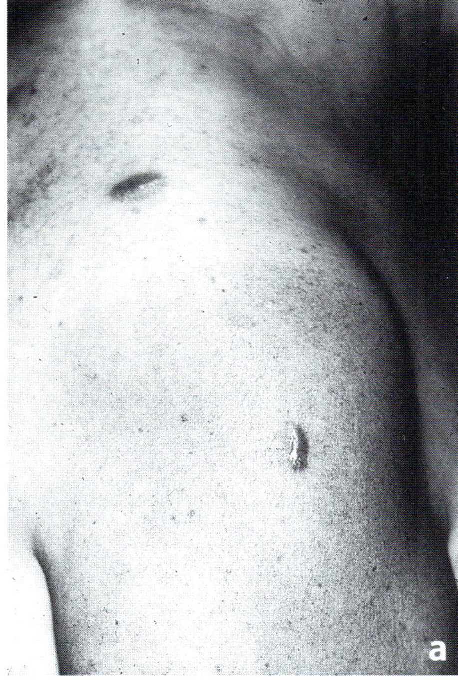
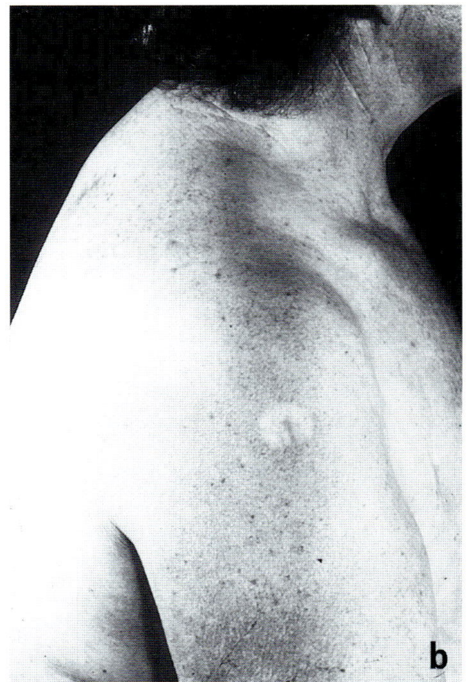

Fig. 15.10. Five-month-old hypertrophic scars before (**a**) (from Zouboulis and Orfanos 1990) and one year after 3 sessions with nitrous oxide, 30 seconds/lesion, contact technique (**b**) (from Zouboulis and Orfanos 2000). In the lesion on the arm long-term hypopigmentation is observed due to cryosurgery; interestingly the second lesion on the shoulder is not hypopigmented

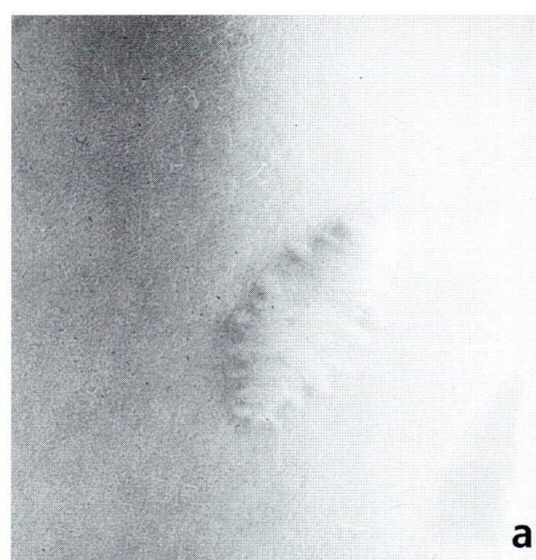
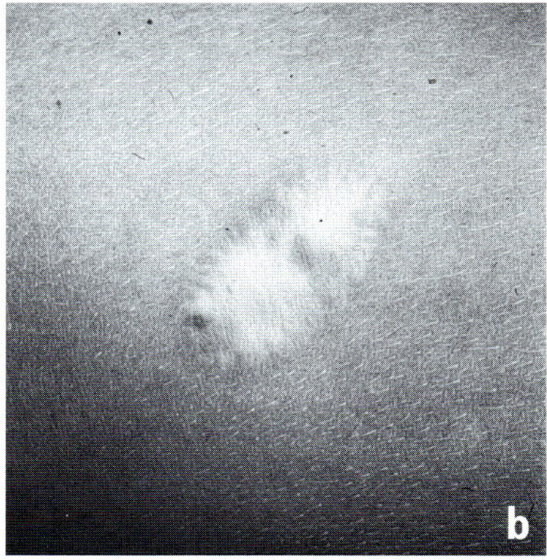

Fig. 15.11. Hypertrophic scar on the upper arm of a 22-year-old female patient before (**a**) and 3 months after (**b**) the last of 7 sessions with liquid nitrogen, 30 seconds, contact technique. An excellent clinical result but also lesional hypopigmentation and slight peripheral hyperpigmentation can be seen (from Zouboulis and Orfanos 2000)

scar after healing, repeated every 4 weeks for at least 6 months. If intralesional corticosteroids are additionally applied, the first injection has to be given intraoperatively, followed by injections once monthly combined with cryosurgery according to the procedure described above. Results can be seen in Figs. 15.14 and 15.15.

Intralesional cryosurgery: The lesion is disinfected and perilesional anesthesia is performed by lidocaine 1% solution. The lesion is grasped between the fingers and a single-use 20-gauge needle is introduced into the skin at one border of the lesion and exits at the surface at a point on the other border of the lesion. The needle has to be directed in a way which rules out that the cryogen spray will come into contact with healthy patient skin during treatment. The needle is connected to the cryoprobe stem and this is connected to the liquid nitrogen Dewar flask. Compression of the lesion is

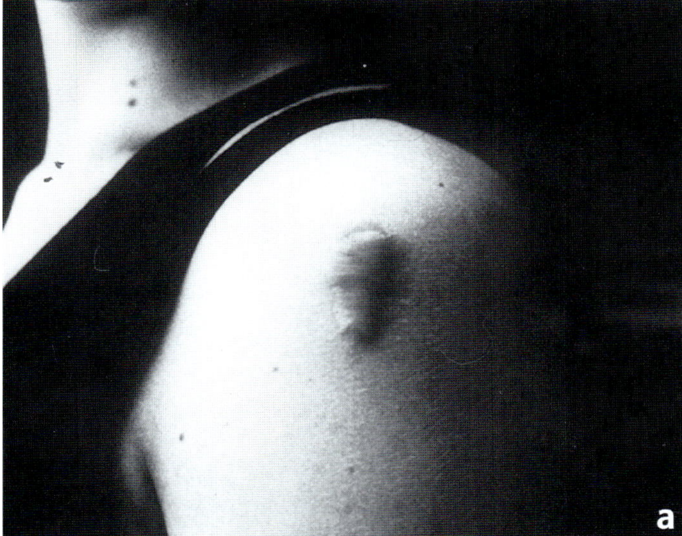
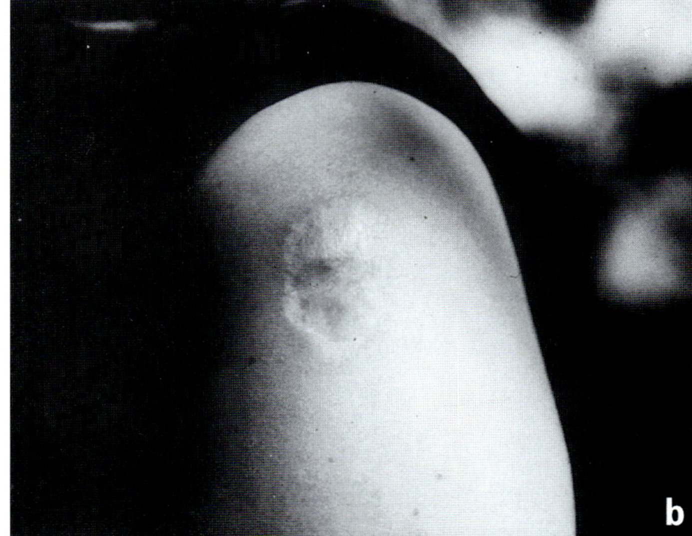

Fig. 15.12. Hypertrophic scar (**a**) treated with 3 sessions of combined cryosurgery (liquid nitrogen, 30 seconds, contact technique) and intralesional corticosteroid injections (betamethasone, 2 mg/cm^2 lesional surface). Good clinical result, but also characteristic skin atrophy extending beyond the borders of the initial scar is seen as a side-effect of the applied corticosteroid (**b**) (Courtesy of E. Zouridaki; from Zouboulis and Orfanos 2000)

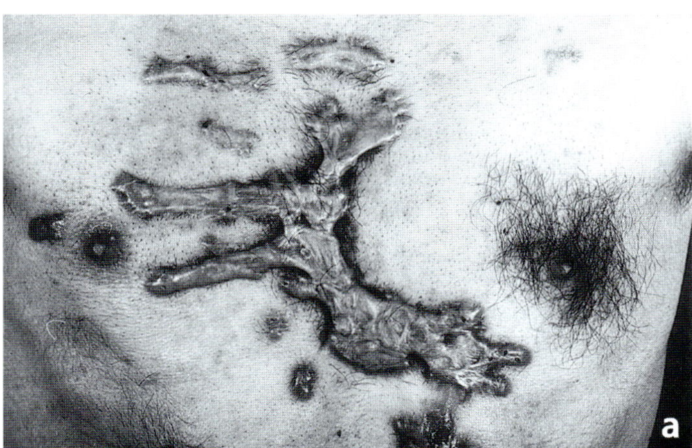
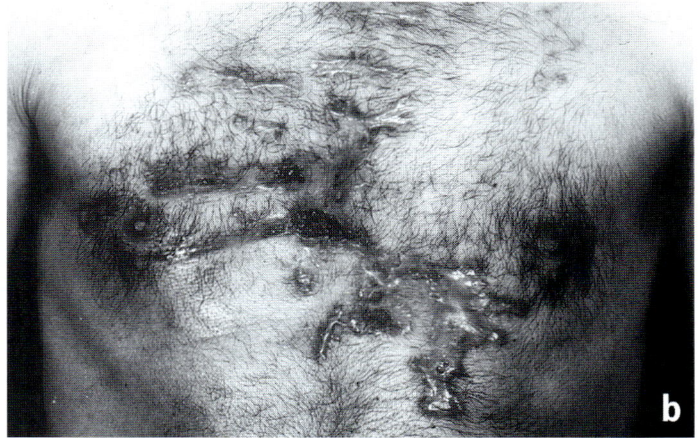

Fig. 15.13. Intramarginal removal of huge keloids (**a**) with the carbon dioxide laser and intraoperative application of intralesional corticosteroid injections into the scars followed by 3 sessions of cryoprevention (liquid nitrogen, 30 seconds/lesion, contact technique) (**b**) (from Zouboulis and Orfanos 2000)

accomplished by pulling the visible parts of the needle up with the help of the connected cryosurgical device.

The cryogun is activated and liquid nitrogen is passed through the needle lumen, exiting to the atmosphere from the other end of the needle. At the beginning of freezing, two ice balls are formed at the sites of contact between the visible portions of the needle and the skin (Fig. 15.16). These circles increase in diameter by continuation of freezing. In addition, an ice cylinder is formed around the embedded part of the needle in the deeper tissue. This is visible through the skin and gradually spreads towards the surface. The procedure ends when the whole lesion is frozen, independently of the duration of the freeze. The needle is left to thaw and is then pulled out of the lesion.

Since some bleeding may occur after thawing a sterile firm dressing has to be applied. Postsurgical care is similar to that described above. The treatment has to be repeated every 3 weeks. The optimal number of sessions to obtained best results is still under investigation.

Cryopeeling: Patient exclusion criteria are: dark white-skinned patients, patients who do not refrain from sunbathing during the month before treatment, during the treatment period and two

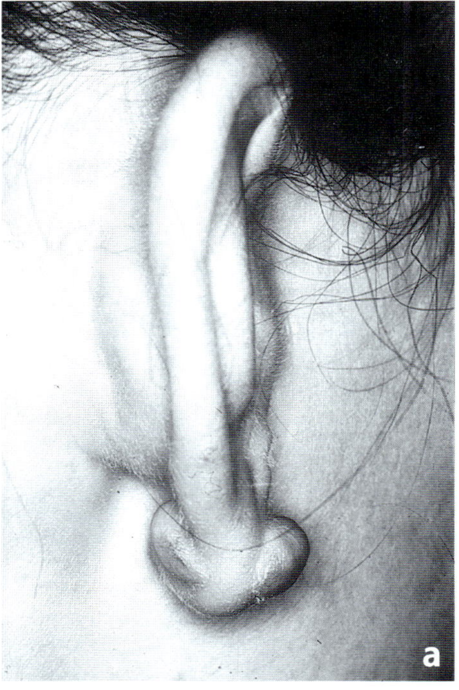

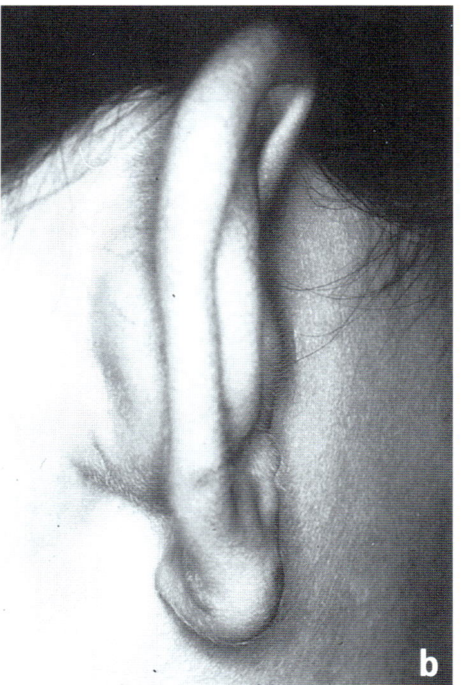

Fig. 15.14. Earlobe keloid before (**a**) and 2 months after (**b**) intramarginal excision with the carbon dioxide laser followed by 4 sessions of cryoprevention initially with liquid nitrogen (one session) and finally with nitrous oxide (3 sessions), 30 seconds/lesion, contact technique (from Zouboulis et al. 1993b)

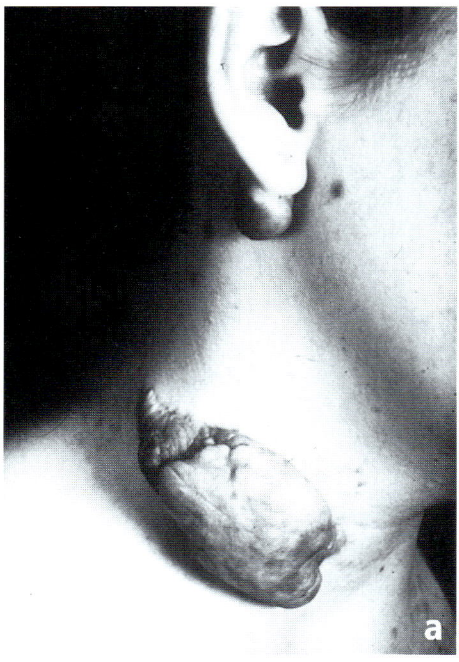

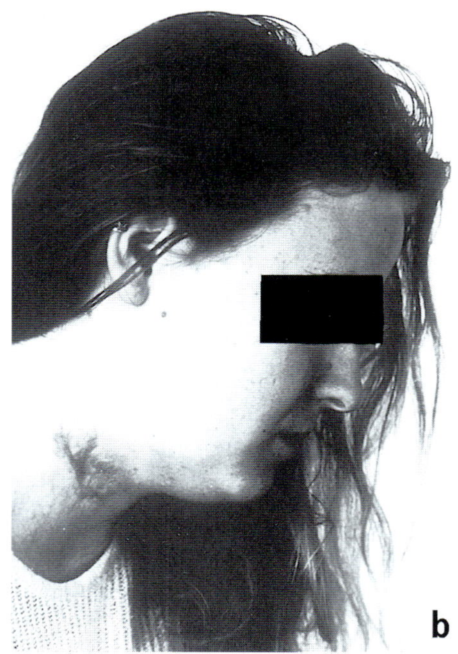

Fig. 15.15. Huge keloids on the neck and the earlobe (arrow) before (**a**) and after (**b**) intramarginal excision with the carbon dioxide laser with general anesthesia and intraoperative intralesional corticosteroid injections followed by 12 sessions of cryoprevention (liquid nitrogen, 30 seconds/lesion, contact technique) and intralesional corticosteroids (triamcinolone, 2 mg/cm^2 lesional surface) (from Zouboulis and Orfanos 2000)

months after treatment, patients taking drugs that induce hyperpigmentation, and patients who want to experience immediate results.

During treatment the patient lies in a reclining armchair and the physician sits at the patient's head. No sedation or premedication is required. The patient's eyes can be covered by a pair of goggles. The facial skin is cleaned with gauze soaked in ethanol solution. The ethanol is left to evaporate before the treatment is started. A nitrous oxide cryosurgical device (contact method) with a round cryoprobe tip 2 cm in diameter is used for cryopeeling. Cryopeeling proceeds horizontally from the middle of the forehead in either direction and continues according to the plan shown in Fig. 15.17. The cryoprobe tip is slowly moved over the skin in order to leave a fine ice film on it. The skin is stretched and held tight to ensure even application of the ice film. Individual deeper scars are treated for a longer period of time to increase depth of cryosurgery. The entire facial skin surface has to be treated in order to limit borderline post-inflammatory hyperpigmentation, which is one of the unpleasant side effects.

The skin reacts with erythema and light edema immediately after cryopeeling, which lasts up to 24 hours. A mild, non-atrophogenic steroid cream (e.g., hydrocortisone aceponate, hydrocortisone buteprate, hydrocortisone-17-butyrate, methylprednisolone aceponate, prednicarbate) can be applied on the lesion immediately after treatment in order to reduce the erythematous reaction. After 2 to 3 days a fine scaling of the superficial epidermis is observed.

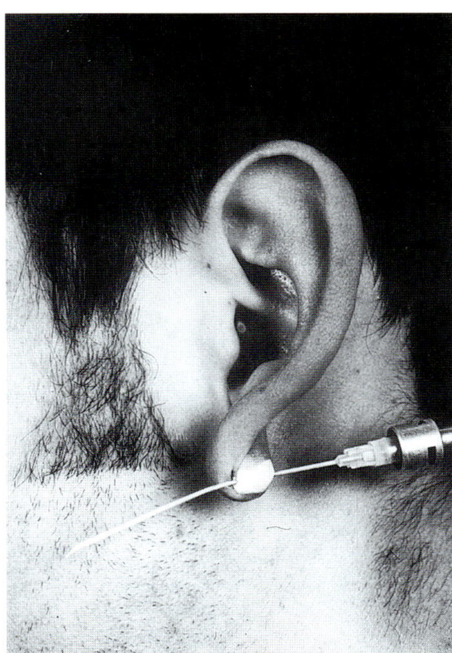

Fig. 15.16. Intralesional cryosurgery. A single-use 20-gauge needle is introduced into the skin at one border of the lesion to exit at the surface at a point on the diametrically opposite border of the lesion. The needle is connected to the cryoprobe, the cryogun is activated and liquid nitrogen is passed through the needle lumen, exiting to the atmosphere from the other end of the needle. Two ice balls are formed at the sites of contact between the visible portions of the needle and the skin. In addition, an ice cylinder is formed around the embedded part of the needle in the deeper tissue, which is visible through the skin and gradually spreads towards the surface (from Zouboulis and Orfanos 2000)

Treatment is repeated once monthly during the winter (October to April in the northern hemisphere, six sessions per year) and can last 2 to 3 years. A sunscreen has to be worn during the interval between treatments.

The results of the treatment are shown in Fig. 15.18. A more aggressive cryopeeling procedure has been described by Graham (1985) and Chiarello (1992) using liquid nitrogen spray in the paint-brush technique for 5 to 30 seconds on 8 cm^2 facial skin fragments. This technique leads to long-lasting erythema. In our opinion cryopeeling should be a mild technique, since dermabrasion with or without punch excision and punch elevation is more adequate and better controlled in the treatment of deeper atrophic scars.

15.5 Complications and Contraindications

Of the various temporary or permanent complications described after cryosurgery (Graham 1985; Drake et al. 1994; Kuflik 1994; Zouboulis 1998), the major side effects occurring in the treatment of keloids and hypertrophic scars are local pain during and/or shortly after treatment and lesional hypopigmentation and/or peripheral hyperpigmentation (Figs. 15.11–15.12). Large local edema, wound infection, local hypoesthesia, local necrosis and formation of milia have been reported in individual patients (Zouboulis et al. 1993). Delayed wound healing is an additional side effect mostly

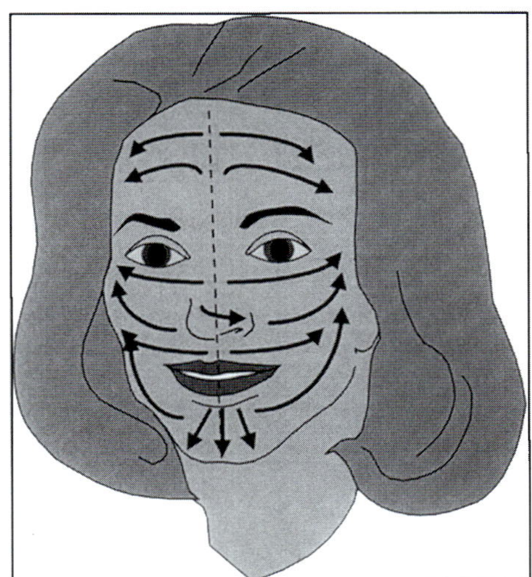

Fig. 15.17. Cryopeeling starts from the forehead and ends at the chin. The cryoprobe tip is slowly moved from the middle of the face towards the periphery in both directions in order to leave a fine ice film on the skin. The skin is stretched and held tight to ensure even application of the ice film. The treatment is applied to the entire facial area (from Zouboulis and Orfanos 2000)

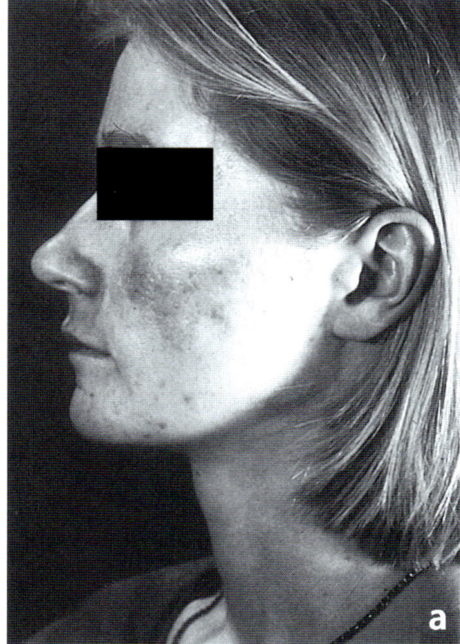

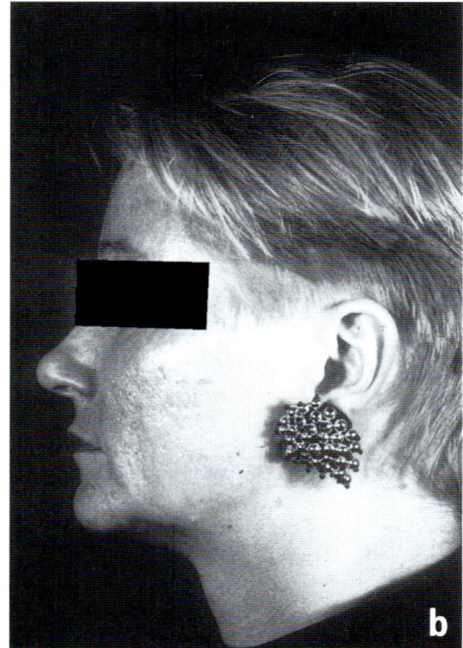

Fig. 15.18. Atrophic acne scars before (**a**) and 6 months after cryopeeling (12 sessions in 2 years) (**b**) (from Zouboulis and Orfanos 2000)

occurring after combined cryosurgery and intralesional corticosteroids (Zouridaki et al. 1996). There are a few absolute contraindications including cold-inducible urticaria, cryoglobulinemia, cryofibrinogenemia and Raynaud's disease (Zouboulis 1998). Reported relative contraindications are collagen diseases, lesions at the extremities of elderly patients and black skin due to long-term depigmentation following melanocyte death.

References

1. Appleton I, Brown NJ, Willoughby DA. Apoptosis, necrosis, and proliferation: possible implications in the etiology of keloids. Am J Pathol 1996; 149: 1441–1447.
2. Arakawa M, Hatamochi A, Mori Y, Mori K, Ueki H, Moriguchi T. Reduced collagenase gene expression in fibroblasts from hypertrophic scar tissue. Br J Dermatol 1996; 134: 863–868.
3. Banfalvi T, Boer A, Remenar E, Oberna F. Treatment of keloids (review of the literature, therapeutic suggestions). Orv Hetil 1996; 137: 1861–1864.
4. Berman B, Bieley HC. Keloids. J Am Acad Dermatol 1995; 33: 117–123.
5. Breitbart EW, Schaeg G. Electron microscopic investigation of the cryolesion. In: Breitbart EW, Dachow-Siwiec E (eds) Clinics in dermatology: advances in cryosurgery. New York: Elsevier, 1990: 30–38.
6. Brown LA Jr, Pierce HE. Keloids: scar revision. J Dermatol Surg Oncol 1986; 12: 51–56.
7. Ceilley RI, Babin RW. The combined use of cryosurgery and intralesional injections of suspensions of fluorinated adrenocorticosteroids for reducing keloids and hypertrophic scars. J Dermatol Surg Oncol 1979; 5: 54–56.
8. Chiarello SE. Full-face cryo- (liquid nitrogen) peel. J Dermatol Surg Oncol 1992; 18: 329–332.
9. Cirne de Castro JL, Pereira dos Santos A, Morais Cardoso LP, Ribeiro R. Cryosurgical treatment of a large keloid. J Dermatol Surg Oncol 1986; 12: 740–742.
10. Dalkowski A. Immunhistochemische Untersuchungen an Keloiden und keloidalen Fibroblasten und der Einfluß der Kryotherapie auf Proliferation, synthetische Aktivität und Immunphänotyp humaner keloidaler und normaler Fibroblasten *in vitro*. Dissertation, The Free University of Berlin, Berlin, Germany, 1997.
11. Datubo-Brown DD. Keloids: a review of the literature. Br J Plast Surg 1990; 43: 70–77.
12. Dawber R. Cold kills! Clin Exp Dermatol 1988; 13: 137–150.
13. Diegelmann RF, Cohen IK, McCoy BJ. Growth kinetics and collagen synthesis of normal skin, normal scar and keloid fibroblasts *in vitro*. J Cell Physiol 1979; 98: 341–346.
14. Drake LA, Ceilley RI, Cornelison RL, Dobes WL, Dorner W, Goltz RW, Lewis CW, Salasche SJ, Chanco Turner ML, Lowery BJ, Graham GF, Detlefs RL, Garrett AB, Kuflik EG, Lubritz RR. Guidelines of care for cryosurgery. J Am Acad Dermatol 1994; 31: 648–653.
15. Ehrlich HP, Hembry RM. A comparative study of fibroblasts in healing, freeze and burn injuries in rats. Am J Pathol 1984; 117: 218–224.
16. Ehrlich HP, Desmouliere A, Diegelmann RF, Cohen IK, Compton CC, Garner WL, Kapanci Y, Gabbiani G. Morphological and immunochemical differences between keloid and hypertrophic scar. Am J Pathol 1994; 145: 105–113
17. Elton RF. Epilogue. In: Zacarian SA (ed) Cryosurgery for skin cancer and cutaneous disorders. St Louis: CV Mosby, 1985: 313–322.
18. Engrav LH, Gottlieb JR, Millard SP, Walkinshaw MD, Heimbach DM, Marvin JA. A comparison of intramarginal and extramarginal excision of hypertrophic burn scars. Plast Reconstr Surg 1988; 81: 40–45.
19. Ernst K, Hundeiker M. Ergebnisse der Kryochirurgie bei 394 Patienten mit hypertrophen Narben und Keloiden. Hautarzt 1995; 46: 462–466.
20. Farrant J, Walter CA. The cryobiological basis of cryosurgery. J Dermatol Surg Oncol 1977; 3: 403–407.
21. Ferris DG, Ho JJ. Cryosurgical equipment: a critical review. J Fam Practice 1992; 35: 185–193.
22. Gage A, Meenaghan M, Natiella J, Greene G. Sensitivity of pigmented mucosa and skin to freezing injury. Cryobiology 1979; 16: 348–361.
23. Gage AA. Deep cryosurgery. In: Epstein E, Epstein E (eds) Skin Surgery. Springfield: Charles C Thomas, 1982: 857–877.
24. Gage AA, Caruana JA Jr, Montes M. Critical temperature for skin necrosis in experimental cryosurgery. Cryobiology 1982; 19: 273–282.

25. Glazer SF, Sher AM. Adjunctive cryosurgery in the surgical approach to keloids. In: Zacarian SA (ed) Cryosurgery for skin cancer and cutaneous disorders. St Louis: CV Mosby, 1985: 91–95.
26. Graham G. Cryosurgery for acne. In: Zacarian SA (ed) Cryosurgery for skin cancer and cutaneous disorders. St Louis: CV Mosby, 1985: 59–76.
27. Graham GF. Cryosurgery. Clin Plast Surg 1993; 20: 131–147.
28. Hirshowitz B, Lerner D, Moscona AR. Treatment of keloid scars by combined cryosurgery and intralesional corticosteroids. Aesth Plast Surg 1982; 6: 153–158.
29. Hunzelmann N, Anders S, Sollberg S, Schonherr E, Krieg T. Coordinate induction of collagen type I and biglycan expression in keloids. Br J Dermatol 1996; 135: 394–399.
30. James WD, Besaucenaey CD, Odom RB. The ultrastructure of a keloid. J Am Acad Dermatol 1980; 3: 50–57.
31. Juhlin L, Evers H, Broberg F. A lidocaine-prilocaine cream for superficial skin surgery and painful lesions. Acta Derm Venereol (Stockh) 1980; 60: 544–546.
32. Kelly AP. Keloids. Dermatol Clin 1988; 6: 413–424.
33. Kuflik EG. Cryosurgery updated. J Am Acad Dermatol 1994; 31: 925–944.
34. Kulka JP. Cold injury of the skin. The pathogenic rate of microcirculatory impairment. Arch Environ Health 1965; 11: 484–497.
35. Layton AM, Yip J, Cunliffe WJ. A comparison of intralesional triamcinolone and cryosurgery in the treatment of acne keloids. Br J Dermatol 1994; 130: 498–501.
36. Lee YS, Vijayasingam S. Mast cells and myofibroblasts in keloid: a light microscopic, immunohistochemical and ultrastructural study. Ann Acad Med Singapore 1995; 24: 902–905.
37. Lubritz RR. Cryosurgical spray patterns. J Dermatol Surg Oncol 1978; 4: 138–139. Lubritz RR. Cryosurgical approach to benign and precancerous tumors of the skin. In: Zacarian SA (ed) Cryosurgery for skin cancer and cutaneous disorders. St Louis: CV Mosby, 1985: 41–58.
38. Matsuoka LY, Uitto J, Wortsman J, Abergel P, Dietrich J. Ultrastructural characteristics of keloid fibroblasts. Am J Dermatopathol 1988; 10: 505–508.
39. Mazur P. Freezing of living cells: mechanisms and implications. Am J Physiol 1984; 247: 125–142.
40. Meltzer L. A cryoprobe for the therapy of linear keloid. J Dermatol Surg Oncol 1983; 9: 111–112.
41. Mende B. Keloidbehandlung mittels Kryotherapie. Z Hautkr 1987; 62: 1348–1355.
42. Muir IFK. On the nature of keloid and hypertrophic scars. Br J Plast Surg 1990; 43: 61–69.
43. Muti E, Ponzio E. Cryotherapy in the treatment of keloids. Ann Plast Surg 1983; 11: 227–232.
44. Nakaoka H, Miyauchi S, Miki Y. Proliferating activity of dermal fibroblasts in keloids and hypertrophic scars. Acta Derm Venereol (Stockh) 1995; 75: 102–104.
45. Orpwood RD. Biophysical and engineering aspects of cryosurgery. Phys Med Biol 1981; 26: 555–575.
46. Peacock EE Jr, Madden JM, Trier WC. Some studies on the treatment of keloids and hypertrophic scars. Southern Med J 1970; 63: 755–760.
47. Rabb JM, Renaud ML, Bradt PA, Witt CW. Effect of freezing and thawing on microcirculation and capillary endothelium of the hamster cheek pouch. Cryobiology 1974; 11: 508–518.
48. Rinfret AP. Cryobiology. In: Vance RW (ed) Cryogenic technology. New York: John Wiley & Sons, 1962.
49. Röhrs H. Dokumentation therapeutischer und kosmetischer Ergebnisse bei der kryochirurgischen Behandlung von Hauterkrankungen. Dissertation, The Free University of Berlin, Berlin, Germany, 1997.
50. Röhrs H, Orfanos CE, Zouboulis ChC. Cryosurgical treatment of acne keloids. J Invest Dermatol 1997; 108: 396.
51. Rudolph R. Wide spread scars, hypertrophic scars, and keloids. Clin Plast Surg 1987; 14: 253–260.
52. Rusciani L, Rossi G, Bono R. Use of cryotherapy in the treatment of keloids. J Dermatol Surg Oncol 1993; 19: 529–534.
53. Scott PG, Dodd CM, Tredget EE, Ghahary A, Rahemtulla F. Immunohistochemical localization of the proteoglycans decorin, biglycan and versican and transforming growth factor-beta in human post-burn hypertrophic and mature scars. Histopathology 1995; 26: 423–431.
54. Sebastian G, Scholz A. Unsere Erfahrungen mit konservativen Therapiemethoden bei hypertrophen Narben und Keloiden. Dt Derm 1990; 38: 872–877.
55. Sebastian G, Scholz A. Histopathology of the cryolesion. Dermatol Monatsschr 1993; 179: 237–241.
56. Shepherd JP. The effects of low temperature on dermal connective tissue components. Dissertation, University of Oxford, Oxford, United Kingdom 1979.
57. Shepherd JP, Dawber RPR. The response of keloid scars to cryosurgery. Plast Reconstr Surg 1982; 70: 677–681.
58. Simon CA. A simple and accurate cryosurgical tool for the treatment of benign skin lesions: The "hard tail" dip-stick. J Dermatol Surg Oncol 1986; 12: 680–682.
59. Stern JC, Lucente FE. Carbon dioxide laser excision of earlobe keloids. A prospective study and critical analysis of existing data. Arch Otolaryngol Head Neck Surg 1989; 115: 1107–1111.
60. Torre D. Understanding the relationship between lateral spread of freeze and depth of freeze. J Dermatol Surg Oncol 1979; 5: 1–3.
61. Torre D. Instrumentation and monitoring devices in cryosurgery. In: Zacarian SA (ed) Cryosurgery for skin cancer and cutaneous disorders. St Louis: CV Mosby, 1985: 31–40.
62. Weshahy AH. Intralesional cryosurgery. A new technique using cryoneedles. J Dermatol Surg Oncol 1993; 19: 123–126.
63. Wulff A, Zouboulis ChC, Blume-Peytavi U, Schuppan D, Orfanos CE. Tenascin: Ein Marker für die Charakterisierung von Keloiden *in vivo* und von keloidalen Fibroblasten *in vitro*. In: Gollnick H, Blume U, Zouboulis ChC, eds. Abstracts of the 38th Meeting of the German Dermatological Society. Herford: Busse, 1995: 385.
64. Wulff A, Zouboulis ChC, Blume-Peytavi U, Sommer Ch, Schuppan D, Orfanos CE. Cryotherapy modifies proliferation and collagen synthesis of keloidal fibroblasts. Arch Dermatol Res 1996; 288: 303.
65. Younai S, Venters G, Vu S, Nichter L, Nimni ME, Tuan TL. Role of growth factors in scar contraction: an *in vitro* analysis. Ann Plast Surg 1996; 36: 495–501.
66. Zacarian SA, Stone D, Clater M. Effect of cryogenic temperature on the microcirculation of the golden Syrian hamster cheek pouch. Cryobiology 1970; 7: 22–29.
67. Zacarian SA. Cryogenics: the cryolesion and the pathogenesis of cryonecrosis. In: Zacarian SA (ed) Cryosurgery of skin cancer and cutaneous disorders. St Louis: CV Mosby, 1985: 1–30.
68. Zacarian SA. Cryosurgery in the management of cutaneous disorders and malignant tumors of the skin. Compr Ther 1994; 20: 379–401.
69. Zouboulis ChC, Orfanos CE. Kryochirurgische Behandlung von hypertrophen Narben und Keloiden. Hautarzt 1990; 41: 683–688.
70. Zouboulis ChC, Blume U, Büttner P, Orfanos CE. Outcomes of cryosurgery in keloids and hypertrophic scars. A prospective consecutive trial of case series. Arch Dermatol 1993a; 129: 1146–1151.
71. Zouboulis ChC, Blume U, Orfanos CE. Keloids and hypertrophic scars: cryosurgical treatment and postsurgical cryoprevention. Dermatol Monatsschr 1993b; 179: 278–284.
72. Zouboulis ChC, Zouridaki E, Wulff A. The treatment of keloids, hypertrophic and atrophic scars. J Eur Acad Dermatol Venereol 1996; 7(Suppl. 2): 22.
73. Zouboulis ChC. Cryosurgery in dermatology. Eur J Dermatol 1998;8: 466–474.
74. Zouboulis ChC. Principles of cutaneous cryosurgery: An update. Dermatology 1999;198: 111–117.
75. Zouboulis ChC, Orfanos CE. Cryosurgical treatment. In: Hatahap M (ed) Surgical techniques for cutaneous scar revision. New York: Marcel Dekker, 2000: 171–234.
76. Zouridaki E, Trautmann Ch, Alvertis H, Katsambas A, Orfanos CE, Zouboulis ChC. Cryosurgery alone and cryosurgery combined with intralesional steroids are equally effective on keloids but induce different histological changes: results of a prospective randomised study. J Eur Acad Dermatol Venereol 1996; 7 (Suppl. 2): 87.

16. Plastic Cryosurgery: Cryosurgery and its Cosmetic Effect

Biological Mechanism of Liquid Nitrogen Cryotherapy for Nevus Ota and its Clinical Advantages

Yoshiaki Hosaka

16.0 Introduction

Nevus Ota is a congenital or acquired facial dermal melanosis that is rather rare in Caucasians but is observed frequently in Mongolian races (Kukita et al. 1981, Yamauchi et al. 1981). The pigmentation is usually unilateral and most pronounced on the eyelids and in the zygomatic and maxillary regions. It is composed of light brownish-blue to deep purplish-blue macules caused by an abnormal occurrence of melanocytes within the connective tissue. In Japan, this disorder is estimated to affect approximately 0.4 percent of the dermatology outpatient population (Yoshida 1952) and 2.6 percent of plastic surgery outpatients (Suzuki 1991). The ratio of male to female patients is reported to be approximately 1:3 (Kukita et al. 1981, Suzuki 1991).

As nevus Ota is not only stigmatic and disfiguring but also can be sociopsychologically devastating, various treatment modalities have been contemplated and developed. Among them, until recently, carbon dioxide snow cryotherapy had been used most frequently to treat this disorder. However, the results were not always satisfactory and often left scarring after treatment. In Japan, liquid nitrogen has become preferred to carbon dioxide snow in cryotherapy because of its ease of handling and its lower temperature during surgery.

Over the past 20 years, we have developed a treatment modality using CRYO-MINI, a liquid

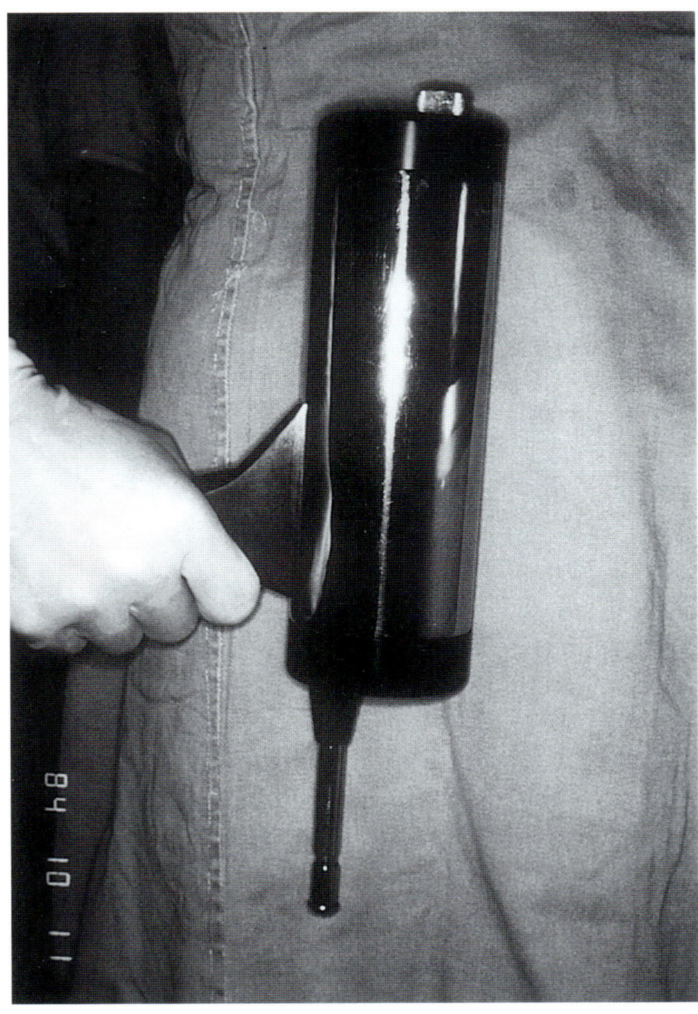

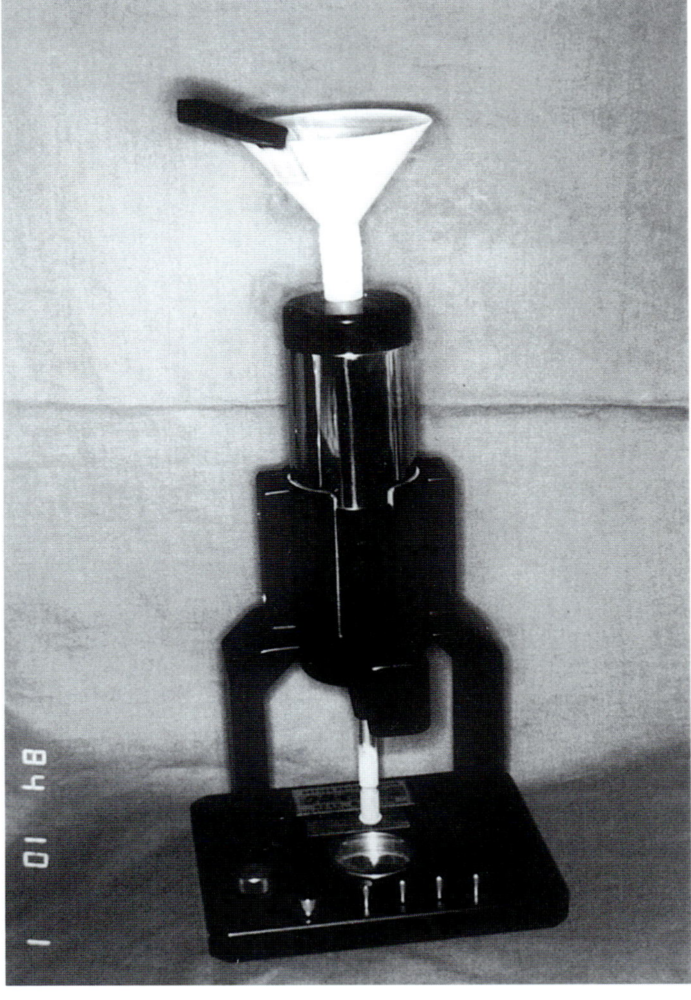

Fig. 16.1. Outside view of the CRYO-MINI cryogenic instrument. Liquid nitrogen is used as the cryogen

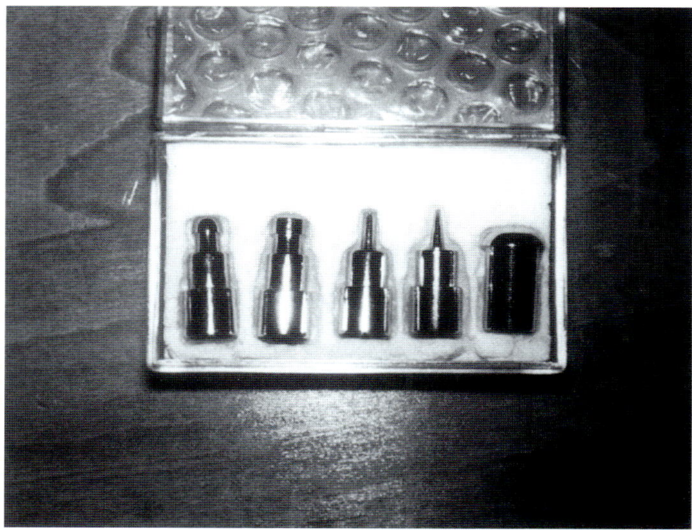

Fig. 16.2. Removable copper disk tips available for CRYO-MINI: Disk diameter ranges from 1 mm to 1 cm

Table 16.1. Treatment response of facial pigmented lesions to liquid nitrogen cryotherapy using CRYO-MINI

Type of lesion	No. of patients	Results
Nevus Ota	164	Excellent-good
Nevus Ota-like melanosis	15	Good[1]
Nevus spilus	34	Good-fair[2]
Blue nevus	12	Good
Senile lentigines	237	Excellent-good
Nevus pigmentosus	138	Good-fair

[1]Postoperative pigmentation is more likely to occur than in nevus Ota.
[2]Recurrence of the lesion is frequently observed, and postoperative pigmentation often follows.

Table 16.2. Treatment response of nevus Ota to liquid nitrogen cryotherapy using CRYO-MINI

Severity of nevus Ota	No. of patients	Average no. of treatments	Results		
			excellent	good	fair
Intensive	45	4.2	34	7	4*
Moderate	58	2.4	50	6	2
Mild	29	1.3	23	6	0
Palpebral only	32	1.5	20	7	5*

Partial scarring was left after surgery in some of the patients.

nitrogen cryogenic instrument with a removable disk-shaped metal tip (Figs. 16.1 and 16.2), and treated a total of 600 Japanese patients with facial pigmentation disorders at Showa University Hospital, Hatanodai, Tokyo (Tables 16.1 and 16.2). We have found this method to be simple and extremely effective in the treatment of nevus Ota (Hosaka et al. 1982, 1987, 1995) and senile lentigines, as well as for delayed nevus spilus and blue nevus (Hosaka and Onizuka 1991). In this chapter we discuss the suggested biological mechanism of cryosurgery for nevus Ota and present our techniques and the results achieved in the treatment of eight representative patients who had deeply situated or superficially situated types of nevus Ota.

16.1 Pathology and Clinical Diagnosis

The pathology of nevus Ota is an increase of melanin granules (melanosomes) caused by active epidermal and dermal melanocytes (nevus cells). Based on the distribution and extent of pigmentation in the affected skin, dermatologists have generally classified patients with nevus Ota into four types: mild, type I; moderate, type II; intensive, type III; and bilateral, type IV (Kukita et al. 1981). To diagnose correctly the pathological state of nevus Ota for treatment, biopsy is indispensable. However, to some extent, it is possible to speculate about the type of this disorder and the depth of dermal melanocytes by observing the color distribution of the pigmentation carefully. In a superficially situated type of nevus Ota, a brownish color is usually predominant because of increased melanogenesis in the epidermis and the upper layer of the dermis. In contrast, in a deeply situated type, a purplish-blue tinge is prominent because of increased melanogenesis in the lower layer of the dermis.

According to a study by Hidano et al. (1967), there are two peaks in the onset of nevus Ota: one in early childhood and the other in the teens. This finding indicates that there is a possibility that the activity of dermal melanocytes is restimulated in adolescence, making the therapy for young patients with this disorder difficult and complicated. For this reason, we advise preadolescent patients to undergo cryosurgery after age 20. In severe cases, however, we begin treatment in early childhood because of the sociopsychological effects of a disfiguring discoloration of the face.

16.2 Assumed Biological Mechanism of Liquid Nitrogen Cryotherapy and its Clinical Advantages

The purpose of employing cryotherapy for treatment of nevus Ota is both to suppress the melanin synthesis in epidermal melanocytes and to destroy dermal melanocytes selectively while minimizing the formation of scar tissue. In the past, dermabrasion and cryosurgery were interpreted as being used only to obscure the disfiguring pigmentation. However, Yamazaki and Tezuka (1984, 1985) studied the biological mechanism of cryosurgery using carbon dioxide snow and showed that it decreases the number of dermal melanocytes as a result of cryonecrosis. Their suggested mechanism involves degeneration of dermal melanocytes as a result of direct freezing. The cell membrane breaks and melanosomes are dispersed in the dermis. Dermal melanocytes and melanophages affected slightly by direct freezing are attacked by secondarily activated lysosomal enzymes and are vacuolated. Some of the dispersed melanosomes are dispersed to the exfoliating crusts when tissue damage is relatively severe, but most of them are taken up in the histiocytes by phagocytosis and are carried to regional lymph nodes and excreted. Some of the melanosomes remain phagocytized in the histiocytes located around capillary blood vessels. Eventually, the number of dermal melanocytes and the amount of dermal melanin granules decreases. The biological mechanism of liquid nitrogen cryotherapy for nevus Ota is assumed to be the same as that of carbon dioxide snow cryotherapy (Fig. 16.3).

Although there is no critical difference in the biological mechanisms between the cryotherapies with carbon dioxide snow and liquid nitrogen, liquid nitrogen can generate far lower temperatures on the skin surface: −180°C for liquid nitrogen versus −50 to −60°C for carbon dioxide snow (Table 16.3). This difference, however, was found

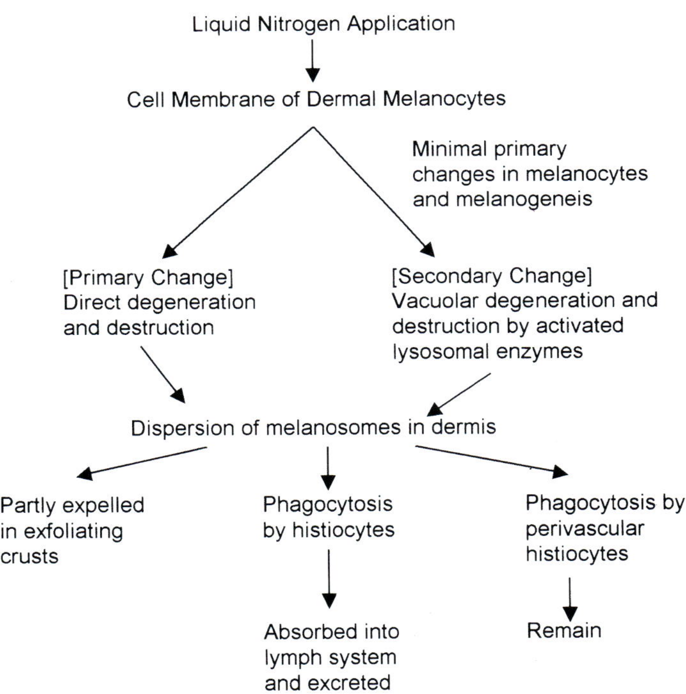

Fig. 16.3. Assumed biological mechanism of liquid nitrogen cryotherapy for nevus Ota

Table 16.3. Cryogens and the temperatures generated on the surface of the treated skin

Cryogen	Attainable temperature	Temperature generated on the surface of the treated skin
Dry ice (carbon dioxide only)	−78°C	−50 ~ −60°C
Liquid nitrogen	−195°C	−180°C

to represent a profound improvement in the treatment of facial pigment lesions, compared with that of carbon dioxide snow cryosurgery. In carbon dioxide snow cryosurgery, there is a tendency for wider and deeper tissue cryonecrosis to be produced in surrounding normal skin because of the relatively longer freeze time. Conversely, in liquid nitrogen cryosurgery, the surface of the treated skin is frozen in a much shorter time, thus making it possible to minimize the damage to surrounding normal skin and to produce less scarring after surgery. Because liquid nitrogen can have a more destructive effect on deeper sites of the skin in a much shorter time, the number of repetitions of the treatment can be reduced to one-third to one-quarter those needed for carbon dioxide snow cryotherapy. Also, a topographical study using replicas revealed that the texture of the skin surface treated by liquid nitrogen cryotherapy is much improved and closer to that of normal skin (Hosaka et al. 1987).

16.3 Methods of Liquid Nitrogen Cryosurgery with CRYO-MINI

Instrument: A portable gun-type cryogenic apparatus called CRYO-MINI (Nagai Manufacturing Company, Ltd., Tokyo, Japan) was used in the therapy. This instrument is 6.7 cm in diameter, 30 cm in length, and 980 gm in weight; it is composed of a stainless steel cylindrical container that can store 180 ml of liquid nitrogen and has a removable disk-shaped copper tip that can be cooled by liquid nitrogen circulating in the storage unit. There are tips available in flattened, rounded, and fine-pointed shapes for different treatment purposes. The temperature of the tip drops to −180°C about 1 minute after liquid nitrogen is poured into the cylinder, and it stays unchanged until the stored liquid nitrogen is completely vaporized. The maximum time available for cryosurgery when the container is filled with liquid nitrogen is 20 minutes. The tip can lower the temperature of the lesion in a matter of seconds when placed

Table 16.4. Application time of the liquid nitrogen cryoprobe of CRYO-MINI for treatment of Japanese patients with nevus Ota

Involved sites/ severity of nevus Ota	Eyelid	Cheek	Forehead/nose
Adult			
Mild case	3–5 sec	6–8 sec	8–9 sec
Intensive case	4–7 sec coagulation	7–9 sec abrasion	9–10 sec abrasion
Child			
Mild case	2–3 sec	3–4 sec	4–5 sec
Intensive case	3–4 sec	4–5 sec	4–5 sec

in contact with it. This apparatus is light and easy to handle, thus allowing a much greater degree of control of the destructive cryolesion than do other, cruder methods using a cotton-tipped applicator dipped in liquid nitrogen or a liquid nitrogen spray apparatus.

Application Time and Procedure: Application time of the cryogenic probe to the lesion is determined by taking into consideration the age and sex of the patient, depth of dermal melanocytes, and thickness of the skin to be treated. Table 16.4 shows the optimal application times we generally employ for treatment of Japanese patients with different nevus Ota conditions. These were obtained by increasing the application time incrementally by 1 second. For relatively thick skin, such as that on an adult's forehead and cheeks, 7 to 10 seconds are appropriate; for thinner skin, such as eyelids, 5 to 7 seconds are recommended. Because the temperature generated by liquid nitrogen is extremely low, it is likely to cause freeze damage to surrounding healthy skin as well as to the lesion if the exposure

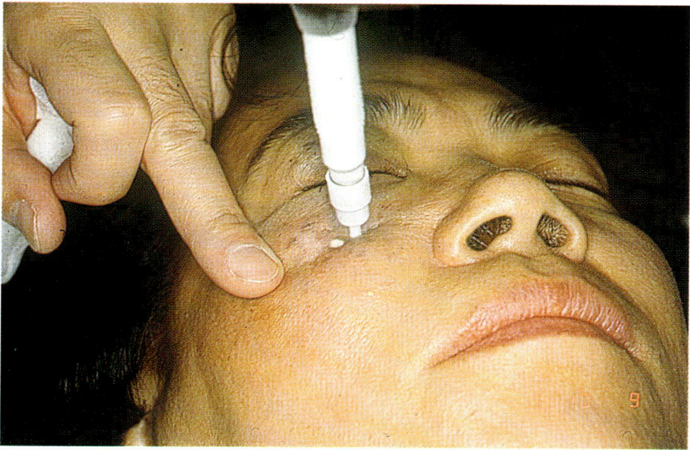

Fig. 16.4. Cryosurgery using CRYO-MINI. A view of the tip area is shown. The cryoprobe is applied to involved skin with only the pressure necessary to hold the instrument. The contacted skin is frozen

is excessive. Therefore it is important to make the application time as short as possible, to hold the instrument lightly, and to place as little pressure as possible on the lesion (Fig. 16.4). Because children have thinner skin than adults, the application time for a child is shortened to about two-thirds of the time for an adult. Usually, one application is administered to each lesion site during a session. In severe and extensive cases, however, patients may receive two applications to the same site during a session. In such cases, the second application time is shorter than the first. The cryoprobe tip is disk shaped, thus an arrangement should be made for the verges to overlap to ensure a continuous appearance after surgery.

Anesthesia: Since liquid nitrogen is both anesthetic and hemostatic once tissue is frozen, anesthesia with xylocaine is optional, and the use of local anesthetics is recommended only for apprehensive patients and novice cryosurgeons who have not yet developed skill at cryosurgery (Biro and Brand 1983). We usually administer local anesthetics, which seem less offensive to the patients and are effective for reduction of postoperative pain. For this purpose, epinephrine-containing anesthetics are potent and long lasting. In extensive cases with deep pigmentation that requires dermabrasion, we administer general anesthesia.

Treatment: Because the low temperature generated by liquid nitrogen is immediately conducted to and affects dermal melanocytes, one application of liquid nitrogen is sufficient to produce good results in most cases of superficially situated nevus Ota. For treatment of the deeply situated type, however, repeated applications of liquid nitrogen in combination with dermabrasion are usually required. As a rule, dermabrasion is employed lightly immediately after cryosurgery at the first session and is repeated in later sessions, if necessary. The main objective in employing dermabrasion for treatment of severe cases of nevus Ota is to accelerate excretion of destroyed melanin granules by facilitating the excretion of the exudates. Therefore, light dermabrasion is performed after cryosurgery, to the extent required to shave off just the epidermis. Although it is virtually impossible to completely destroy dermal melanocytes from outside the skin by liquid nitrogen cryotherapy, even in combination with dermabrasion, none of the patients we have treated has experienced recidivation during a 5-year follow-up period.

For treatment of extensive lesions, we usually conduct trial tests in advance on one side of the

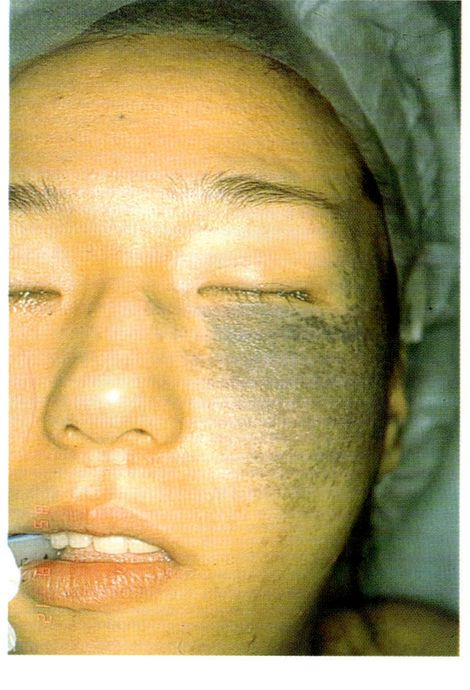

a

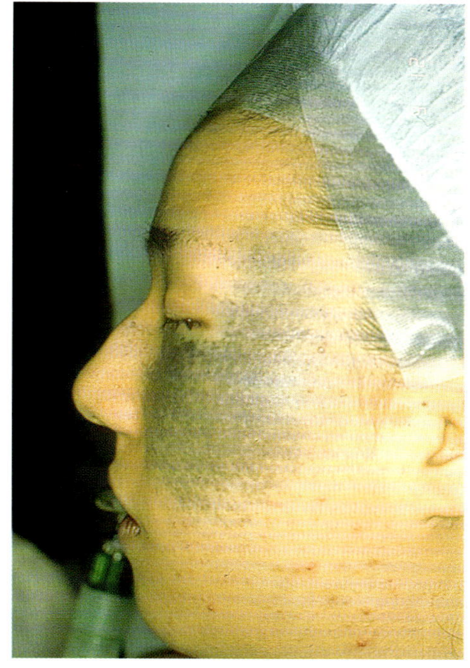

b

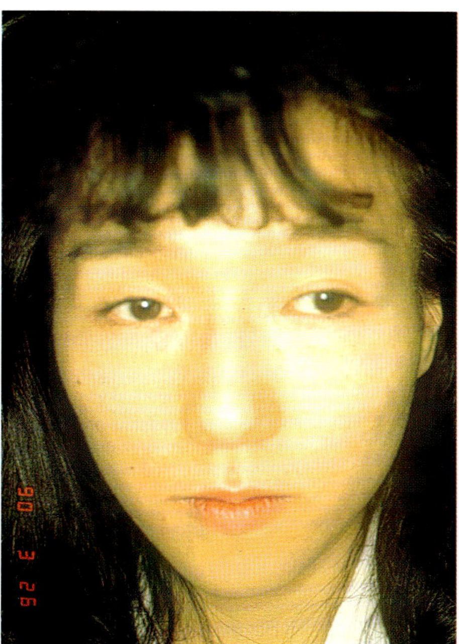

c

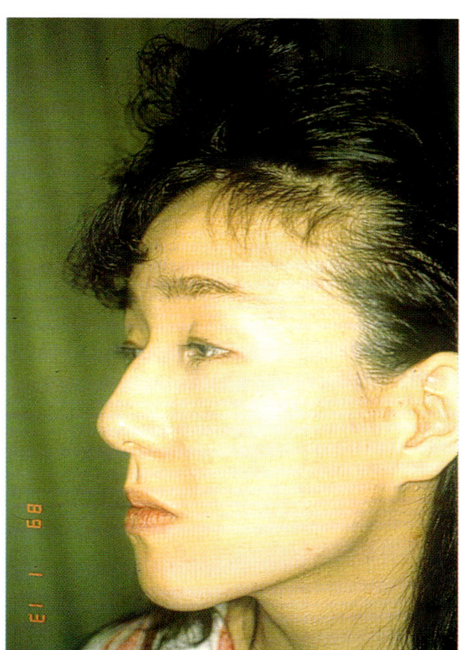

d

Fig. 16.5. Patient 1. A 21-year-old woman with nevus Ota. **a**, **b** Frontal and lateral views, preoperative. Intensive pigmentation spread over the zygomatic region. **c**, **d** Frontal and lateral views, 2 years after the fourth therapy

head, usually covered by hair, and then proceed to treatment of the whole lesion. Patients with deep pigmentation in the palpebral area are the most difficult to treat. Because the palpebral skin is thin and excessive treatment leads easily to necrosis of the skin (with a tendency toward scarring), it is risky to abrade this area. To avoid the potential hazard of injury to the eyelids, excessive treatment should be avoided and only the area of pigmentation should be treated. The cryoprobe is applied to the orbital rim rather than to the eyelids directly, and the application time is shorter than for lesions on the cheeks. Because dermal melanocytes often reach as far as the muscle layer, it is very hard to destroy all the cells by cryosurgery alone. Therefore, we have developed a new technique to

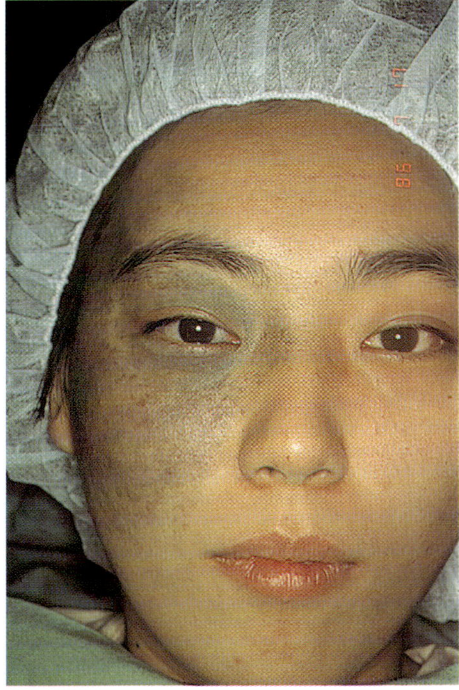

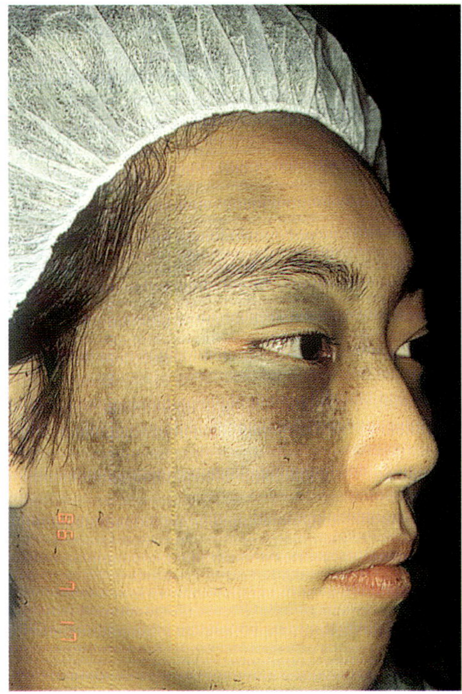

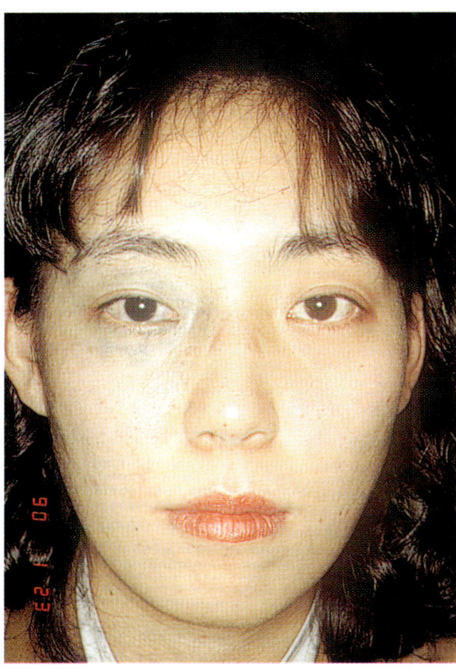

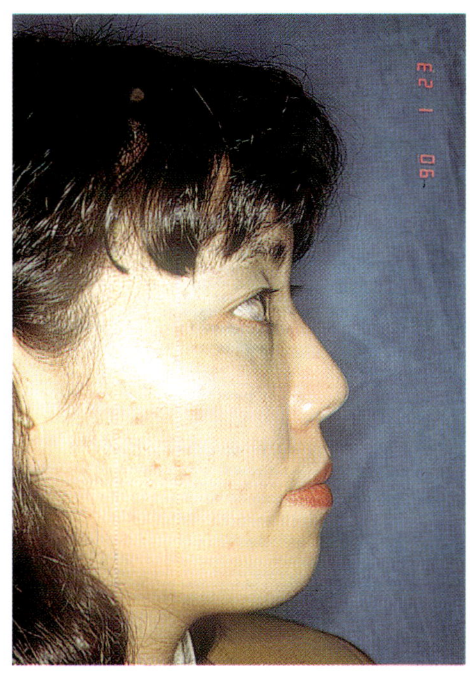

Fig. 16.6. Patient 2. A 21-year-old woman with nevus Ota. The pigmentation spreads over eyelid, forehead, and cheek regions. **a**, **b** Frontal and lateral views, preoperative. **c**, **d** Frontal and lateral views, 2 years and 5 months after the fifth therapy.

desiccate the lesion by electrocoagulation using a specially designed hair-removing needle (Hosaka et al. 1982). This needle is coated with silicone except at the tip, thus enabling the tip to be heated. This is a very useful tool, and it is convenient for burning dotted lesions remaining on the cheeks.

Aftercare: When cryosurgery is over, the treated area is kept cold with gauze soaked in physiological saline, in combination with an ointment containing steroids and antibiotics, and covered by Torex (silicone-coated gauze; Fuji Systems Corporation, Tokyo, Japan), or Sofratulle (sterilized

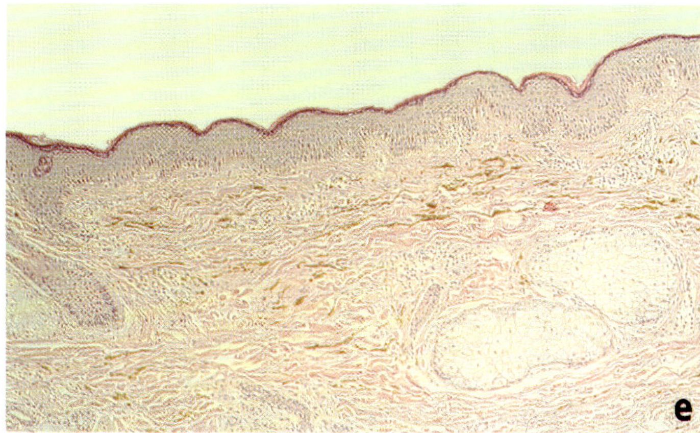

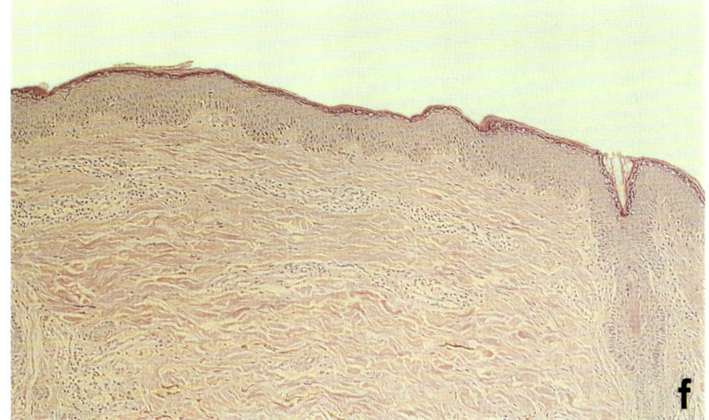

Fig. 16.6.e. Histopathology of the periocular region, preoperative. (H&E stain ×100) **f** Histopathology of the periocular region, after the fourth treatment. (H&E stain ×100)

bactericidal dressing; Roussel Laboratories Corporation, England). Then the entire treated area is covered with regular gauze. On the following day, small blisters are formed but are left untouched, and only the outermost gauze is changed. When dermabrasion is performed, only the outermost gauze is changed. The bulla dries in 7 to 10 days. The crusts that form fall off spontaneously. About 2 weeks after surgery, the patients are allowed to wash their faces. For at least 3 months, they are advised not to expose the treated area to solar radiation, covering it with gauze, and protecting it with sunscreen preparations and/or covering it with cosmetics. Exposure to sunlight causes brownish pigmentation in the treated area. If this occurs, patients are advised to avoid further exposure to solar radiation, to take vitamin C tablets, and to wait for the pigmentation to fade gradually.

16.4 Results of the Treatment

Most of the patients with nevus Ota we have treated at Showa University Hospital over the past 20 years were females. Their age distribution was 0–9 years (2 percent), 10–19 (8 percent), 20–29 (80 percent), 30 years and older (10 percent). The majority of the patients were in their 20s. Figures 16.5–16.12 show clinical pictures before and after use of this therapy for eight representative Japanese patients. All the patients had nevus Ota from early childhood, but dark pigmentation appeared and developed in adolescence, except for patient 7.

Patient 1 is a 21-year-old woman with intensive pigmentation over the zygomatic region. She underwent cryosurgery four times from September 1985 through March 1987. At each session, she received two applications of the cryoprobe. Dermabrasion was performed at the first three sessions. At the fourth session, the remaining dotted lesions were burned by electrocoagulation using the specially designed needle. Figures 16.5a and 16.5b show frontal and lateral views of the patient before cryotherapy. Figures 16.5c and 16.5d show results 2 years after the fourth treatment.

Patient 2 is a 21-year-old woman. Intensive pigmented spots were distributed over the lower and upper eyelids, and the periocular, zygomatic, and temple regions. She received liquid nitrogen cryotherapy five times from July 1986 through November 1988. In the first three sessions, treatment consisted of two applications of the cryoprobe and dermabrasion. Figure 16.6 shows frontal and lateral views before the therapy (a, b) and 2 years and 5 months (c, d) after the fifth therapy. In this case, pigmentation over the periocular region was not completely removed, but the patient was satisfied with the result, and thus the therapy was discontinued. Histological examination of biopsy specimens obtained from the periocular regions both before and after the fourth therapy showed a markedly decreased number of dermal melanocytes in the connective tissue, although some melanocytes still remained in the lower layer of the dermis (Figs. 16.6e and 16.6f).

Patient 3 is a 20-year-old man. The distribution of pigmentation was almost the same as in patient 2 except for the upper eyelid area. He received liquid nitrogen cryotherapy four times. Dermabrasion was performed at the first two sessions. Figure 16.7 shows his preoperative views (a, b) and postoperative views (c, d).

Patient 4 is a 26-year-old female. She received liquid nitrogen cryotherapy twice. Dermabrasion

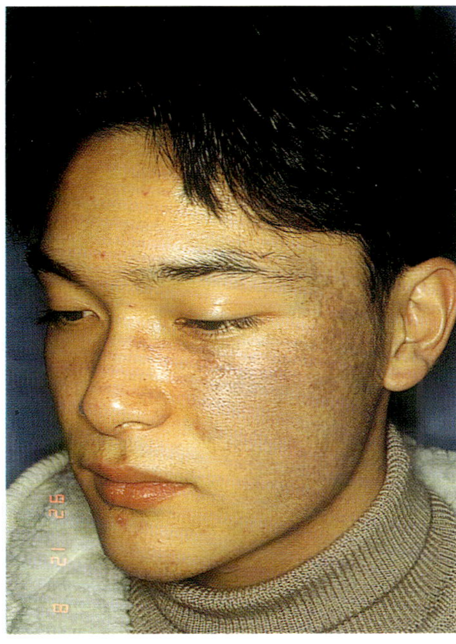
a

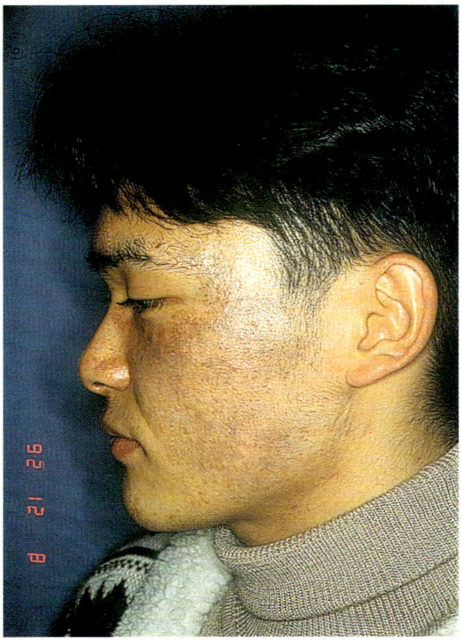
b

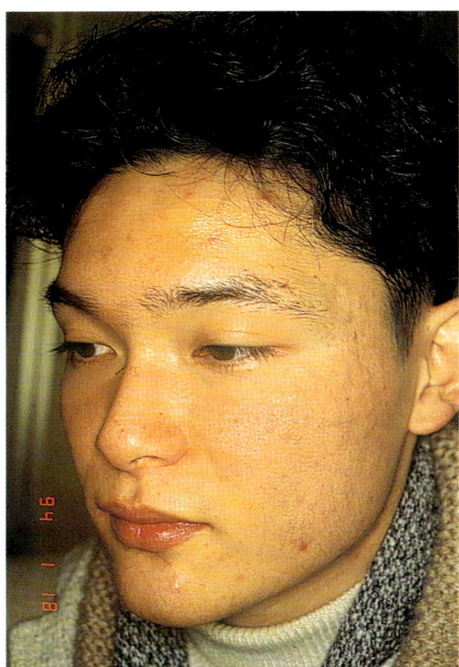
c

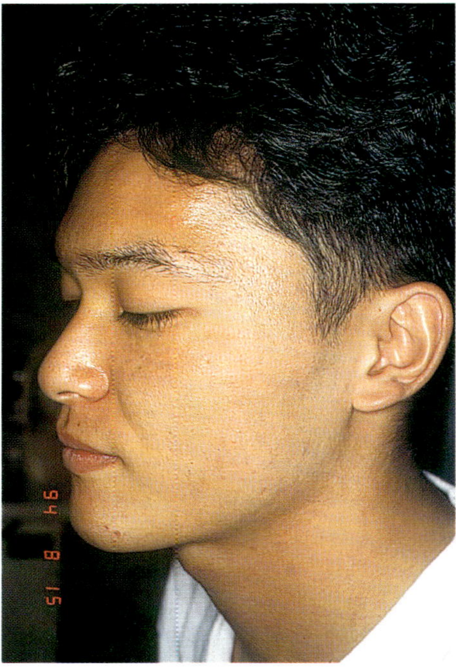
d

Fig. 16.7. Patient 3. A 20-year-old man with nevus Ota. The distribution of pigmentation was almost same as in patient 2 except for upper eyelid area. **a, b** Preoperative view. **c, d** After the fourth cryotherapy with two dermabrasions

was employed at both sessions. Figure 16.8 shows her frontal and lateral views before the therapy (a,b) and 5 months after the second therapy (c,d). Figures 16.8e and 16.8f are four years after the second therapy. Substantial reduction of pigmentation was observed in part.

Patient 5 is a 22-year-old female. She received liquid nitrogen cryotherapy three times. Dermabrasion was performed at the first two sessions such that only the outermost skin (epidermis) of the bullae formed on the following day was removed. Figure 16.9a is her preoperative view and 16.9b shows the postoperative view.

Patient 6 is an 18-year-old female. This is the case of the superficially situated nevus Ota. In this case, only one application of liquid nitrogen was

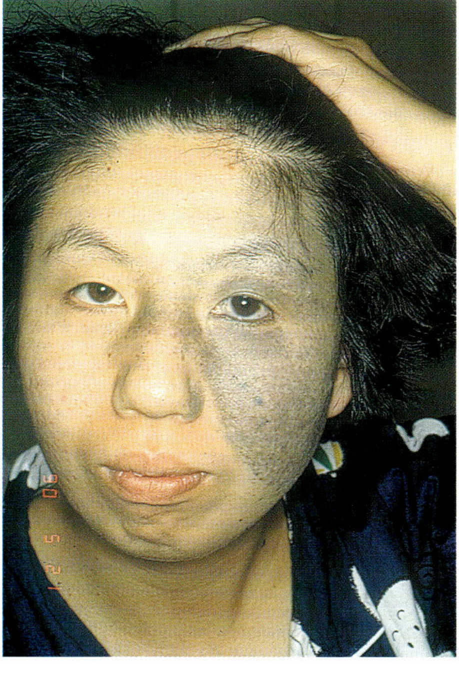
a

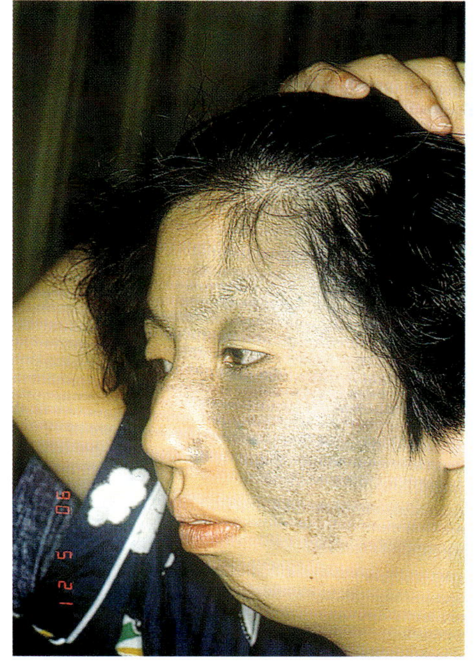
b

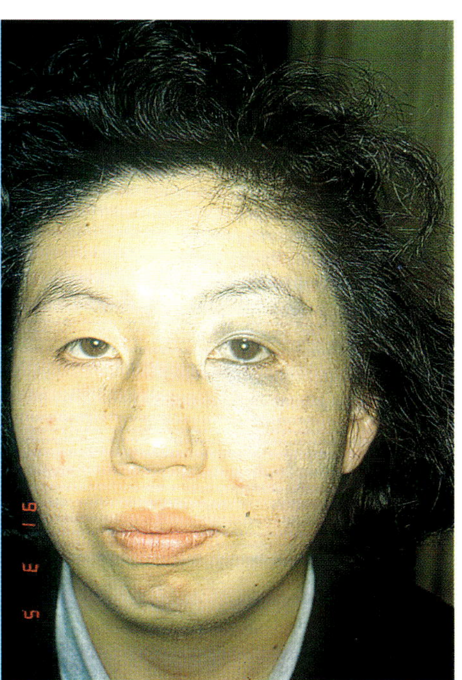
c

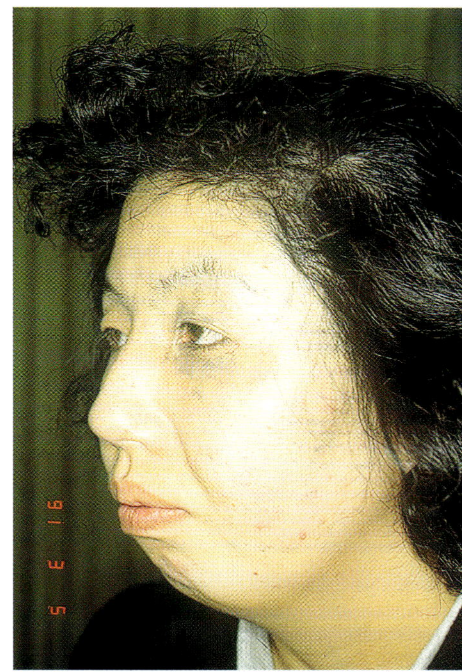
d

Fig. 16.8. Patient 4. A 26-year-old female with nevus Ota, **a, b** Frontal and lateral views, preoperative, **c, d** Five months after the second therapy with two dermabrasions, **e, f** Four years after the second cryotherapy

administered. Figure 16.10a is her preoperative view and Fig. 16.10b shows the postoperative view.

Patient 7 is a 6-year-old boy with nevus Ota. This is a special case: slate-bluish pigmentation was observed on half of his face, extending from the zygomatic region to the cheek and maxillary region. The patient received liquid nitrogen cryotherapy five times from June 1987 through December 1989. Dermabrasion was performed only at the first session. Figures 16.11a and 16.11b are frontal and lateral views before the therapy. Figure 16.11c is immediately after the dermabrasion, and 16.11d is one month after. Figure 16.11e shows the histopathology after skin biopsy, which was undertaken at the second therapy. Dermal

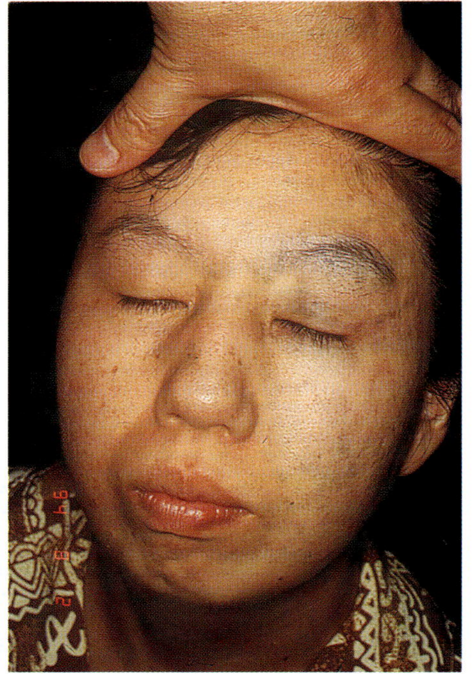
e

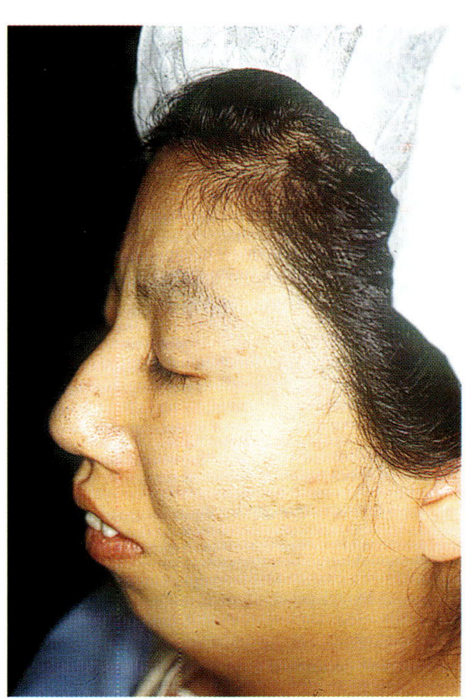
f

Fig. 16.8 (continued)

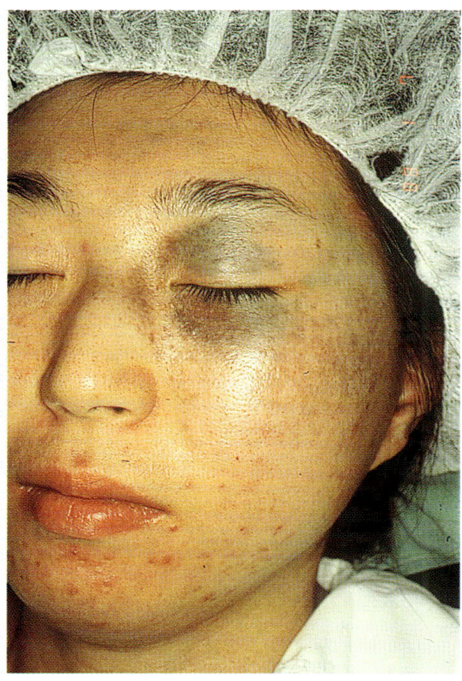
a

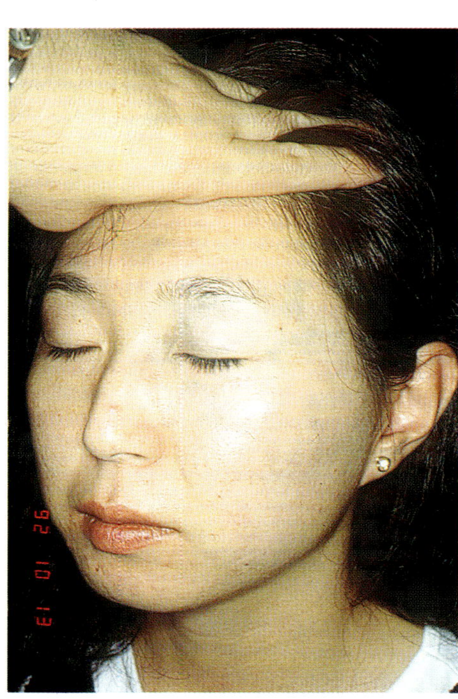
b

Fig. 16.9. Patient 5. A 22-year-old female with nevus Ota. **a** Preoperative. **b** After the third cryotherapy with two dermabrasions

melanocytes were still observed from dermis toward subcutaneous tissue. Figures 16.11g and 16.11f show the results 3 years after the fifth cryotherapy.

Patient 8 is a 19-year-old male. First, we attempted trial laser surgery but at the patient's request, two liquid nitrogen cryosurgeries were performed. Thereafter the skin lesions where pigmentation still remained were exposed to Q-switched ruby laser three times. Figure 16.12a is the preoperative view, 16.12b after the first cryotherapy, 16.12c after the second cryotherapy, and

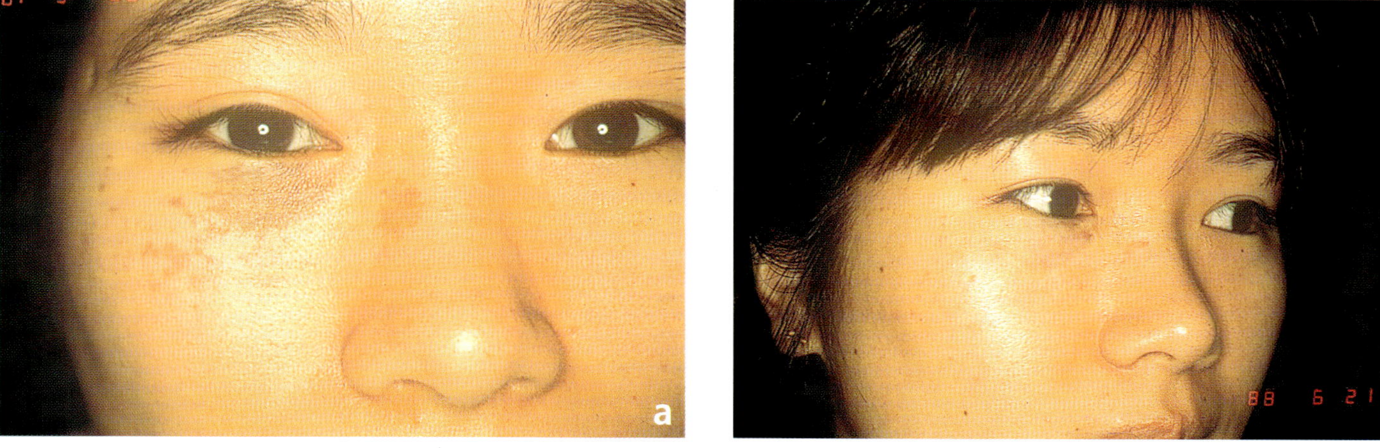

Fig. 16.10. Patient 6. An 18-year-old female with superficially situated nevus Ota. **a** Preoperative. **b** After the first cryotherapy

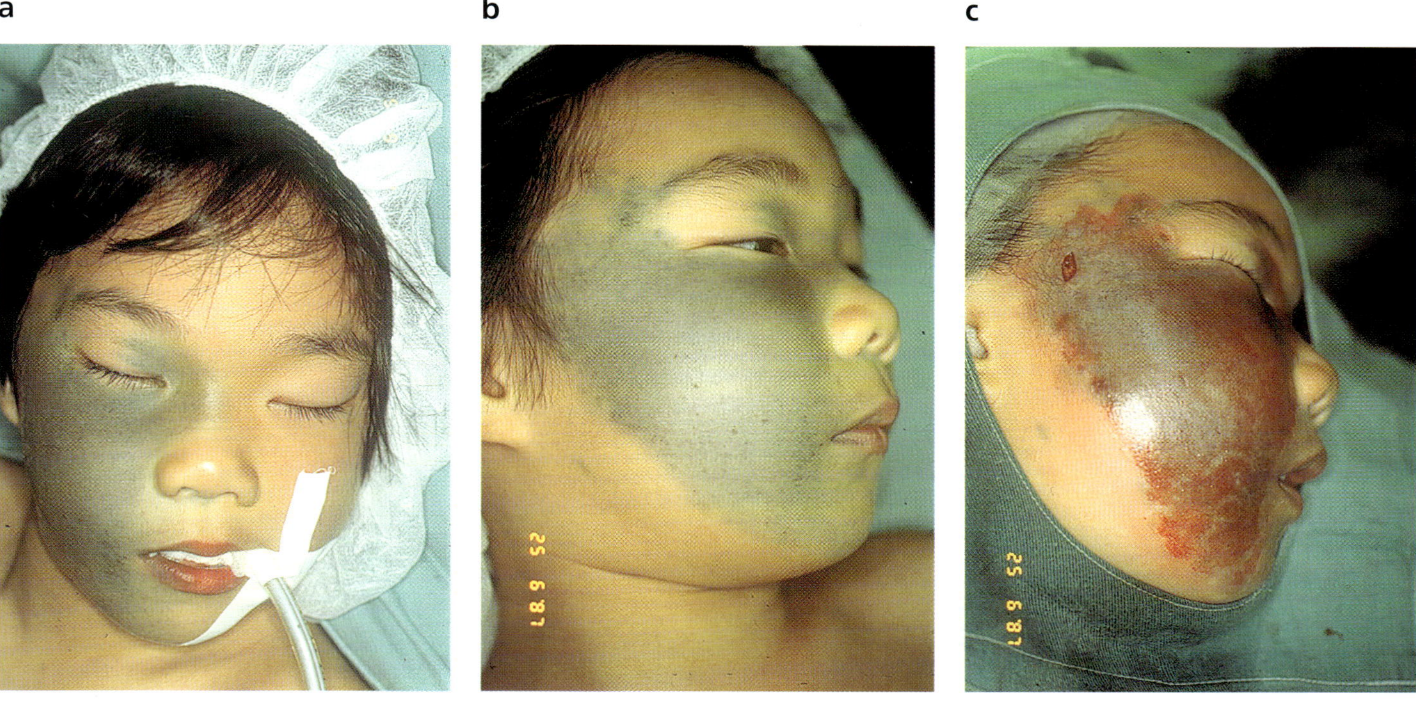

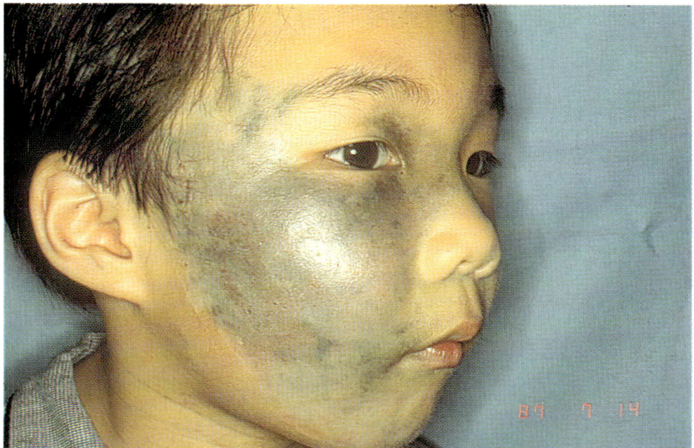

d

Fig. 16.11. Patient 7. A 6-year-old boy with nevus Ota. This is a special case in which slate-bluish pigmentation extended from the zygomatic region to the cheek and maxillary region. **a, b** Frontal and lateral views, preoperative. **c** Immediately after dermabrasion. **d** One month after the dermabrasion. **e** Skin biopsy site. Histopathology of the biopsied skin. (H&E stain, ×100). **f, g** Three years after the fifth cryotherapy

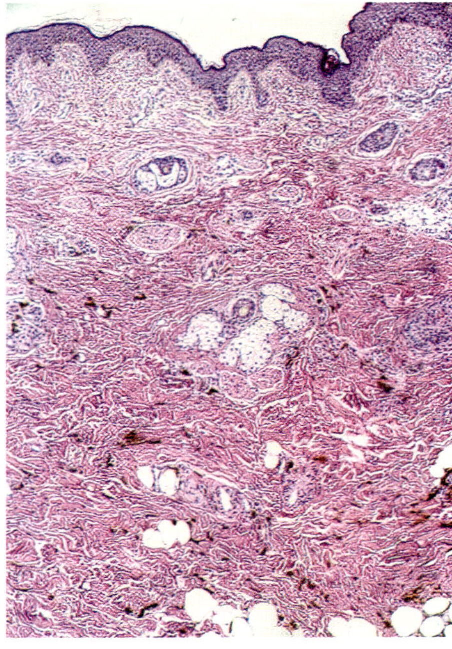
e

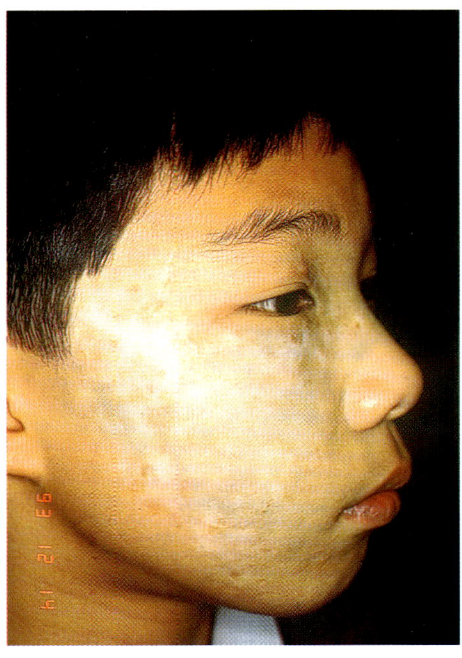
g

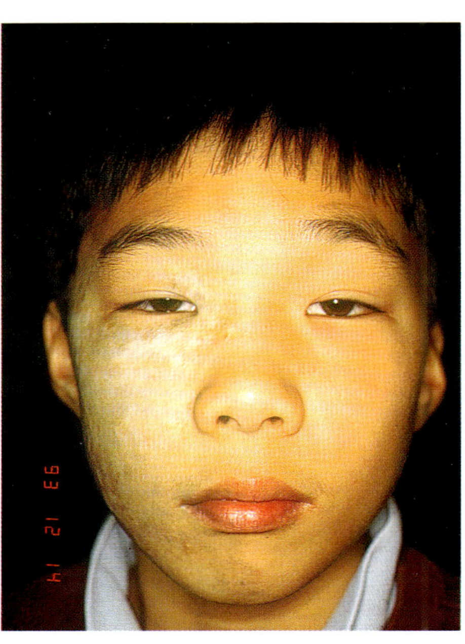
f

Fig. 16.11 (continued)

16.12d after three exposures to the Q-switched ruby laser.

16.5 Discussion

Results of cryosurgery are not apparent immediately. Melanin granules released from destroyed melanocytes are assumed to be excreted mainly through lymphatic vessels. This process is thought to take 3 to 4 months, thus it is our practice to set intervals of at least 4 to 5 months between cryosurgery treatments and to examine the results of previous cryosurgery before repeating it. Although some patients require one or more years as an interval, this delay does not seem to cause any particular treatment problems. In the case of female patients, it is sometimes observed that the treated skin appears to have lost melanin pigment after cryosurgery but looks slightly darkened, depending on physiological (hormonal) state. In such situations, continuation of the treatment leaves only scarring and is useless, thus further therapy is discontinued.

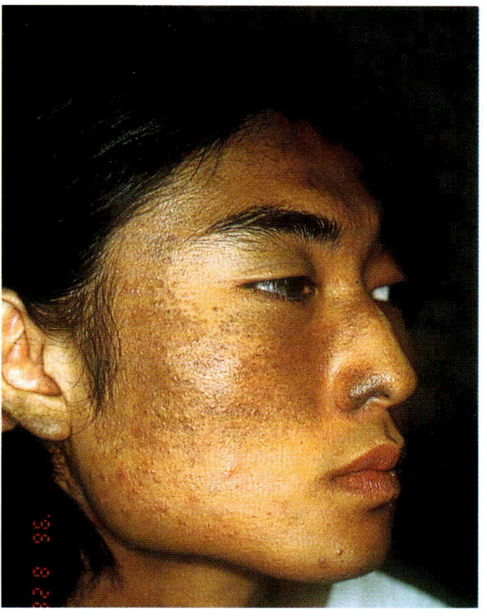
a

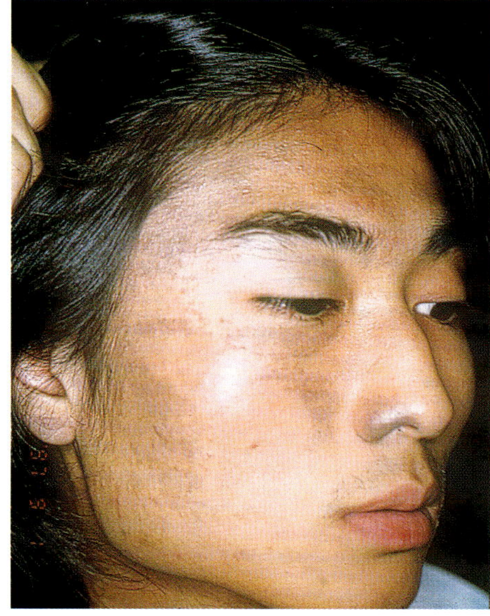
b

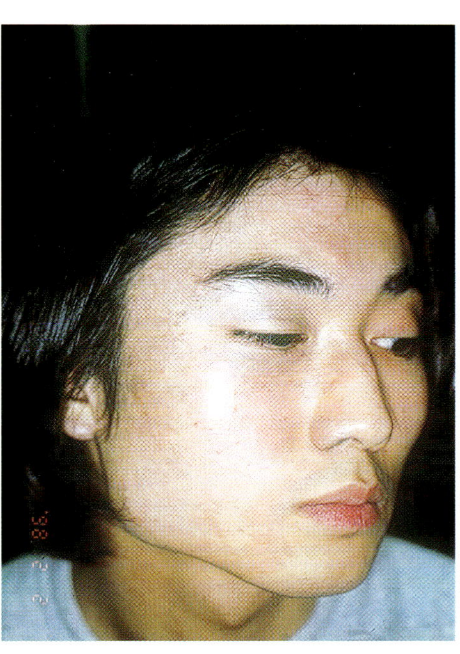
c

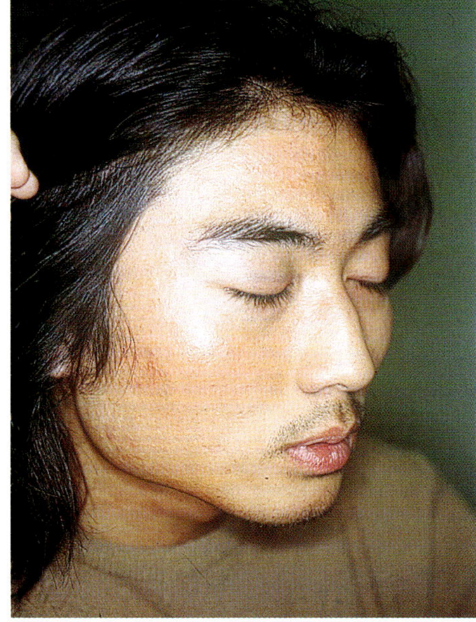
d

Fig. 16.12. Patient 8. A 19-year-old man with nevus Ota. **a** Preoperative. **b** After the first cryotherapy. **c** After the second cryotherapy. **d** After three exposures to Q-switched ruby laser

Recent studies have shown the successful use of the Q-switched ruby laser in the treatment of nevus Ota (Goldberg and Nychay 1992, Geronemus 1992, Pfeiffer 1993, Lowe et al. 1993, Hayashi et al. 1993). Its wavelength (694 nm) is highly selective for melanin and does not cause vascular injury, and reportedly, it penetrates deeply into the dermis to destroy the abnormal melanocytes of nevus Ota but only damages the normal melanocytes. Thus, the nevus does not recur and transient hypopigmentation is reversed (Goldberg and Nychay 1992).

In our clinical experience using this modality, it was suggested as the treatment of choice for the superficially situated to moderately diffused types of nevus Ota because it results in excellent clearance with less edema formation and less postoperative pain compared with liquid nitrogen cryotherapy. In contrast, the results thus far obtained for treatment of the deeply situated type were not always successful. Recurrence of the lesions was observed often in the treated area within a few months after the surgery; postoperative histological examination revealed that dermal melanocytes in the lower layer of the dermis were only partially destroyed, and many of them remained even after repeated exposures. At present it is still unclear whether recurrence of the original pigmentation will return over time as a consequence of the residual nevus cells in the deep dermis (Geronemus 1992). In addition, the pulsed dye lasers now in use are very expensive and require considerable space. In this sense, we believe that liquid nitrogen cryotherapy is not only simple and effective but advantageous and beneficial in the treatment of the extensive and deeply situated type of dermal pigmentary lesions.

References

1. Biro L, Brand AJ (1983) Cryosurgery combined with scissor excision. J Dermatol Surg Oncol 9: 185.
2. Geronemus RG (1992) Q-switched ruby laser therapy of nevus of Ota. Arch Dermatol 128: 1618.
3. Goldberg DJ, Nychay SG (1992) Q-switched ruby laser treatment of nevus of Ota. J Dermatol Surg Oncol 18: 817.
4. Hayashi Y, Yasuda Y, Tsukada S (1993) Q-switched ruby laser treatment of Ota's nevus. Jpn J Plast Reconstr Surg 13: 705.
5. Hidano A, Kajima H, Ikeda S, Mizutani H, Miyasato H, Niimura M (1967) Natural history of nevus Ota. Arch Dermatol 95: 187.
6. Hosaka Y, Udagawa K, Ichinose M, Tsurukiri K, Onizuka T, Dokoh S (1982) Treatment of nevus Ota by liquid nitrogen cryotherapy in combination with a specially designed hair removing needle. Jpn J Plast Reconstr Surg 2: 693.
7. Hosaka Y, Haraguchi K, Onizuka T, Sato Y, Yoshimoto S, Shinomiya S, Ohmura Y, Hori S, Ichinose M (1987) Liquid nitrogen cryotherapy for treatment of nevus Ota and the topographical changes of the postoperative skin surface. Jpn J Plast Reconstr Surg 7: 783.
8. Hosaka Y, Onizuka T (1991) Treatment of nevi by liquid nitrogen cryotherapy. Operation (Japan) 45: 916.
9. Hosaka Y, Onizuka T, Ichinose M, Yoshimoto S, Okubo F, Hori S, Keyama A (1995) Treatment of nevus Ota by liquid nitrogen cryotherapy. Plast Reconstr Surg 95: 703–711.
10. Kukita A, Hori Y, Ohhara K, Kawashima M, Takehara K (1981) Nevus of Ota. In: Fitzpartick TB, Kukita A et al. (eds.): Biology and Diseases of Dermal Pigmentation, University of Tokyo Press, Tokyo, pp. 67–76.
11. Lowe NJ, Wieder JM, Sawcer D, Burrows P, Chalet M (1993) Treatment with high energy fluences of the Q-switched ruby laser. J Am Acad Dermatol 29: 997
12. Pfeiffer N (1993) Q-switched ruby laser used to remove pigmented lesions. J Clin Laser Med Surg 11: 147
13. Suzuki T (1991) Studies of Ota's nevus – statistical and photomicroscopic observations. Jpn J Plast Reconstr Surg 11: 532.
14. Yamauchi A, Okawa M, Okawa Y, Ito M (1981) Electron microscopy of dermal melanocytes in nevus of Ota. In: Fitzpartick TB, Kukita A et al. (eds.): Biology and Diseases of Dermal Pigmentation, University of Tokyo Press, Tokyo, pp. 67–76.
15. Yamazaki H (1984) The mechanism of the action of the dry ice press therapy for the pigmented lesion of nevus Ota. 1. Histological investigation. Nishinihon J Dermatol 46: 1140.
16. Yamazaki H, Tezuka T (1985) The mechanism of the action of the dry ice press therapy for the pigmented lesion of nevus Ota. 2. Electron microscopic investigation. Nishinihon. J Dermatol 47: 33.
17. Yoshida K (1952) Studies on melanin. VII. Nevus Fusco-caeruleus ophthalmo- maxillaris Ota. Tohoku J Exp Med 55 (Suppl.): 34

17. Cryosurgery in Otorhynolaryngology

Marco Scala with contributions by G. Margarino, P. Mereu and M. Gipponi

17.0 Introduction

Cryosurgery can be a suitable treatment for many benign and precancerous lesions of the oral cavity, as well as in selected patients with squamous cell carcinoma. Although the use of cryosurgery in oral disease is still limited, its advantages can modify this attitude and, in the near future, it is likely to become a new standard of treatment due to:

- the easy access to the oral cavity by means of different types of probes;
- the possible use of an anesthetic cream by topic application;
- the treatment of high-risk-surgical patients and/or with clotting deficit;
- the treatment of wide lesions with higher possibility of functional rehabilitation;
- the relatively painless postoperative course, with only a mild edema, which requires a limited use of analgesics, and a soft diet that can be taken during the first postoperative days;
- the direct visual inspection of the area of cryonecrosis, and the possibility of repeating freeze cycles on the residual disease.

17.1 Equipment and Technique

Cryosurgery is a relatively simple technique but the proper instruments as well as respect for codified procedures are required. The freezing capability of nitrous protoxide (−89.5°C) is limited to a depth of about 5 mm, but liquid nitrogen (−196°C) can freeze to a substantially greater depth.

Thus, adequate treatment of oral cavity lesions requires two cryogenic instruments: one with nitrous protoxide, for superficial spreading benign lesions, and the other one with liquid nitrogen for malignant tumors due to the more pronounced vascular supply and the deep infiltration of surrounding tissues, which require a higher freezing power. Oral lesion freezing should consider the following parameters:

The probe: it should fit perfectly into the irregular surfaces of the oral cavity; the more proximal ending should be isolated in order to avoid any damage to the labial commissures or to the anterior part of the cheek.

Pressure on the tissue: in order to obtain a deep cryonecrosis, pressure with the probe on the tissue is required to reduce the amount of blood within the lesion.

Modality of freeze delivery: in benign lesions, a single cycle of freezing is required, while malignant lesions need repeated freeze cycles.

Technique of freezing applied: the choice of the technique depends on the site, kind and extent of the lesion: the *contact* technique shouid be used for superficial spreading lesions; the *spray* technique in wide, very superficial lesions with irregular margins, and the *insertion* technique in malignant lesions or those with a high fibrous component. The probe surface, in the contact technique, should perfectly fit the shape of the lesion, and the "ice ball" should be assessed under direct vision and by palpation. Care should be taken to avoid freezing of the *Stenone's* and *Warthon's* ducts which would cause postoperative salivary retention. As regards the spray technique, it is well tolerated in the anterior part of the oral cavity while in the posterior area the "run-off" of the gas cannot be well controlled, and this may damage surrounding normal tissues. In our experience, the use of thermocouples to control freezing is not necessary for the treatment of oral cavity lesions.

17.2 Precancerous Lesions

Precancerous lesions include local abnormalities associated with a systemic disease as well as solitary lesions produced by pathogenic factors for the oral mucosa. Clinically, they can appear as whitish plaques (*leukoplakia*), reddish mucosal abnormalities (*erythroplasia*) due to the inflammatory reaction, or whitish plaques with a reticular aspect, possibly associated with erythema and ulcerated areas. *Leukoplakia* can be distinguished in three forms:

- homogeneous leukoplakia: a flat, whitish lesion or with raised and sharp margins;
- speckled leukoplakia: a white lesion with reddish areas, rather soft, with undistinguished borders, which can be associated with inflammatory reaction; verrucous leukoplakia is included in this subset;

- erosive leukoplakia: whitish and reddish lesions with areas deprived of the epithelial surface, soft and with irregular, undefined margins.

These morphologic differences correspond to peculiar histologic patterns, ranging from *cheratosis* to *dysplasia, Lichen Ruber Planus,* up to *carcinoma in situ*. All these lesions do not show those biological and histological features specific to malignant tumors but are at potential risk of malignant transformation (1). This risk is 10–15% for *leukoplakia*, up to 30–91% for *erythroplasia*, which is defined, by some authors, as an obliged precancerous lesion. The term dysplasia of grade I, II and III, as for female genital lesions, has recently been changed into *Oral Intraepithelial Neoplasia* (OIN) of low or high grade, depending on morphologic aspects, which can evolve into carcinoma *in situ*.

A biopsy should always precede the cryosurgical treatment because the histology of the lesion can modify the therapeutic planning. The biopsy should include the margins of the lesion with a rim of normal tissue to evaluate the infiltration of surrounding tissues. Vital dyes can be effective for marking the most suitable site for biopsy; in fact, vital dyes are retained within the DNA of high-rate proliferating tissues, and may detect areas of malignant transformation within benign-looking lesions. Every suspicious, raised or ulcerated lesion should undergo biopsy, as well as those that are marked by the dye. In our experience, cryosurgery is the treatment of choice of precancerous lesions of the oral cavity due to easy treatment, the short time required, the possibility of sparing normal tissue, and the reduced rate of postoperative complications (i.e., bleeding, wound infections, etc.). As compared to other modalities, such as electrocoagulation or laser ablation, the time of healing is longer but the wound is better because it is more elastic, with satisfactory functional and esthetic results. The patient's compliance is optimal and the postoperative discomfort is minimal. An exception is represented by *Lichen Ruber Planus* because of its different pathogenesis, which is related to immunological disorders, which make it more amenable to systemic medical treatment. We perform topical anesthesia by means of an anesthetic cream for superficial lesions (EMLA). It is applied 10 min before cryosurgery, and the operation is performed on an outpatient basis. The treatment requires firm contact of the cryoprobe with the surface of the lesion; the freezing should include a small rim of normal tissue; if the lesion is limited to the epithelium, the depth of freezing should not exceed 1 mm. Freezing time should consider the histology, the site, and the degree of cryosensitivity (Table 17.1). The postoperative course does not require antibiotic therapy but only a mild analgesic during the first 1–2 days. The patient should consume a cold, soft diet for the first 3 days. Within 10 days, granulation tissue will cover the wound, and within 3 weeks the complete *restitutio ad integrum* will be accomplished.

Table 17.1. Modalities of cryosurgical treatment for precancerous lesions of the oral cavity

Histology	Gas	Technique	Time of application	No. of cycles
OIN low grade	N_2O	Cryoprobe	15–30 minutes	1
OIN high grade	N_2O	Cryoprobe	45–60 minutes	1

At the Division of Surgical Oncology of the National Institute for Cancer Research (IST) in Genoa (Italy), 76 patients with precancerous lesions of the oral cavity underwent cryosurgery; 75 completely healed while one patient (1.3%) developed a verrucous carcinoma on the site of a previously treated lesion. On the whole, 8 recurrences developed in patients with *Lichen Ruber Planus;* moreover, 18 new lesions developed in different sites as compared to the index lesion. Thus, cryosurgery can achieve satisfactory local control of precancerous lesions, although it has no impact on the pathogenesis of the disease and, consequently, does not reduce the risk of relapse at a different site nor the onset of malignant lesions. For this reason, a chemoprevention regimen with 13-cis retinoic acid (0.5 mg/kg/d for three months) has been proposed because the treatment planning cannot be limited to the local problem but should consider the pathogenesis of the disease, with the aim of stimulating cellular differentiation and inhibiting neoplastic transformation. Hong (1986) and Stick (1988) have well defined the role of chemoprevention in precancerous lesions of the oral cavity, suggesting the benefit of carotenoid and retinoid compounds in this subset of patients (2–3).

17.3 Benign Tumors

Benign neoplasms of the oral cavity are particularly amenable to cryosurgery due to its easiness and low complication rate. The diagnostic work-up should include a preliminary biopsy; the freezing should be extended to include a small rim of normal tissue; sometimes, repeat freeze cycles are required due to the well represented fibrous component or vascular supply. The most used technique is contact probe application or the insertion

Table 17.2. Management of precancerous lesions of the oral cavity

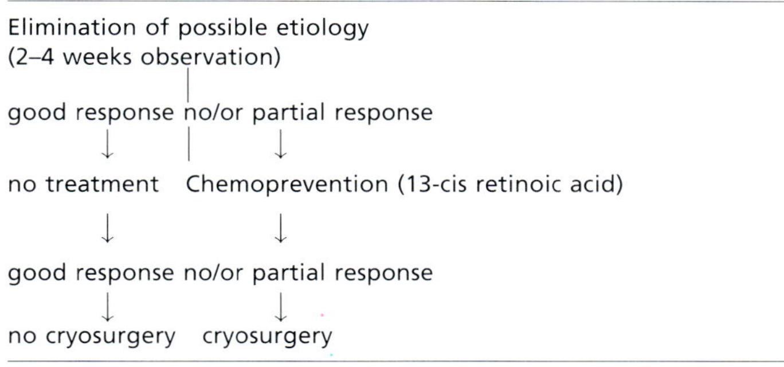

technique. The cryoprobe should be selected in order to include the whole lesion; then, it should be applied firmly to the surface with the aim of reducing the amount of blood within the lesion and decreasing its thickness. The freezing time should be 2–3 minutes; wider lesions may require repeat freeze cycles or a second treatment after 14–20 days.

17.4 Oral Cancer

Squamous cell carcinoma is the most frequent malignancy of the oral cavity; it shows progressive local growth with a tendency towards deep infiltration of the surrounding tissues, with a high risk of regional nodal metastasis. It can appear as an ulcerated or vegetating lesion over the oral mucosal layer. Hematogenic distant spread is rather infrequent, although there are differences related to the site and stage of the disease; such differences can also modify the therapeutic planning, and surgery may be preceded (neoadjuvant) or followed by chemo-radiation therapy (4).

Cryosurgery may represent an alternative modality of treatment; as palliation in high-surgical-risk patients or after failure of conventional surgery, radiation therapy or chemotherapy. In selected patients, cryosurgery may even represent the treatment of choice. In an advanced stage of the disease, pain, bleeding, necrotic and fouling secretions, and difficulty in taking in an oral diet are very invaliding factors; in such cases, cryosurgery may interrupt sensitive neural fibers, thus reducing the pain as well as the need for analgesics; the tumor burden is reduced as well as local invaliding symptoms, thus allowing for a transient but almost normal lifestyle.

Recurrences following conventional surgery and/or chemotherapy are rather frequent, and the patients are usually non-responders to second-line drugs, while radiation therapy would often exceed the limiting dose. These are the most suitable patients amenable to cryosurgery. The selection of patients for primary cryosurgery should be restricted to patients without lymph node metastasis, and with the following co-morbidity factors:

- patients with inoperable malignant tumors at other sites (i.e., second cancer in the lung, larynx, or with a short-term poor prognosis);
- high-surgical-risk patients due to cardiac or pulmonary insufficiency, or with serious clotting deficits;
- AIDS patients with a high morbidity rate.

In any case, the cryosurgical treatment should be aggressive, in order to produce an "ice ball" including at least 5 mm of apparently normal tissue surrounding the primary tumor site; the insertion technique should be used whenever deep infiltration occurs. In order to freeze the whole lesion, different cryoprobes can be inserted at the same time, using (preferably) liquid nitrogen with repeated freeze cycles, with a long thawing period to improve cryonecrosis. Postoperative edema is rather serious, and a postoperative tracheostomy may be required in some patients with large tumors or with tumors in the posterior part of the oral cavity. In such cases careful observation of the respiratory functions should be performed during the postoperative course. A soft diet is required and some patients may also need a naso-gastric tube for feeding. Although rare, post-treatment bleeding may occur due to the high vascular supply of oral cancer; moreover, the slough of necrotic tissue may occur 10 to 20 days after cryosurgery, and the bleeding may be controlled by electrocoagulation of small vessels. Modalities and times of cryoprobe applications are shown in Table 17.3.

Airoldi et al. (1985) have confirmed the advantage of cryosurgery in patients with oral cancer (5).

Eighty-four non pre-treated patients with T_{1-4} N_0M_0 oral cancer underwent multimodality treat-

Table 17.3. Cryosurgery for oral cancer

Type of gas	No. of cycles	No. of applications	Application time	Type of cryoprobe
Liquid nitrogen	2–4	2–4, followed by a slow heating procedure	4′–7′	contact cryoprobe

ment including cryosurgery, chemotherapy and external beam radiation therapy. Cryosurgery was performed in T_{1-2} patients in 1 or 2 cycles, and in T_{3-4} patients in 3 to 4 cycles; chemotherapy included a CMF regimen (Cyclofosfamide, Methotrexate, 5-Fluorouracil). 15–20 days after cryosurgery and chemotherapy, patients underwent radiation therapy 850 Gy on the tumor site and regional lymph nodes in T_1 patients, with a boost on the tumor site of 10–15 Gy in T_{2-4} patients. A complete response was achieved in 76 out of 84 patients (90.5%) within 4 months of treatment. After a follow-up of more than 3 years, the survival rate was 59.6% for the series as a whole; 70.3% for T_{1-2} patients, and 50% for T_{3-4} patients. As reported, these results are encouraging, especially in T_{3-4} patients, coupled with a lesser degree of anatomic and functional impairment.

17.5 Other Malignant Neoplasms

17.5.1 Head and Neck Mucosal Melanoma

Cryosurgery can be effective in the treatment of mucosal melanoma of the head and neck. Mucosal melanoma of the upper digestive tract includes 2–27% of all melanomas. The site of origin may be normal mucosa or a pre-existing pigmented lesion; it is usually a black, soft, easily bleeding lesion with an irregular shape and width. Nasal cavity, paranasal sinus, hard palate, alveolar ridge, gingival fornix, tongue, and floor of the mouth are decreasingly the most frequent sites. The prognosis is poor, similar to ano-rectal melanoma but worse than cutaneous melanoma, with a 5-year survival rate of 4.5–40% (6). Cryosurgery is a good palliative procedure for inoperable or recurrent disease; the peculiar features of this neoplasm makes it particularly freeze-sensitive so that the application of the cold temperature very selectively destroys the neoplastic tissue as compared to other tumors. Moreover, cryosurgery seems to promote an immunostimulating effect due to the unmasking action of tumour-antigens by tissue necrosis, as suggested by the detection of specific antineoplastic antibodies (7). The disease-free survival, the complication rate, and the satisfactory esthetic and functional results occurring in our patients underscored the effectiveness of cryosurgery in this clinical setting (8).

17.5.2 Epidemic Kaposi's Sarcoma

Epidemic *Kaposi's Sarcoma* is associated with AIDS; more than one agent is involved in the pathogenesis of the disease, such as environmental, viral, or genetic factors. The lesions are more frequently multiple than unique; their appearance is nodular or papular, sometimes ulcerated.

Disease progression is variable, although in most cases it is usually very rapid; relevant prognostic factors are represented by CD4+ count, and opportunistic infections; mean survival is about 20 months (9). The therapeutic planning of Kaposi's Sarcoma requires a careful staging and evaluation of the disease progression. When the site of the disease is unique, a simple surgical excision may have merit, but systemic disease requires the use of interferon, chemotherapy and radiation therapy.

Cryosurgery has been proposed as a palliative measure in localized disease due to the possibility of performing the treatment under local anesthesia, the easiness of subsequent cryosurgical applications, and the limited postoperative pain or bleeding complications. We use the contact probe technique with mean application time of one minute for oral lesions (10).

References

1. Van der Waal I, Schepman KP, Vander Meij, Smeele LE (1997) Oral Leukoplakia: Clinicopathological Review. Oral Oncol 33: 291–301.
2. Stick HF, Rosin MP, Hornby AP (1988) Remission of oral leukoplakias and micronuclei in tobacco/betel chewers treated with beta-carotene plus vitamin A. Int J Cancer 42: 195–199.
3. Hong WK, Endicott J, Itri LM (1986) 13-cis retinoic acid in the treatment of oral leukoplakia. N Engl J Med 315: 1501–1505.
4. Leonard JR, Hass AC (1970) Management of cancer of the oral cavity: the trend toward combined radiotherapy and surgery. Am J Surg 120: 514–521.
5. Airoldi M, Fazio M, Gandolfo V, Ozzello F, Pedani F, Camoletto D, Negri L (1985) Combined cryosurgical, chemotherapeutic, and radiotherapeutic management of T1-4 N0 M0 oral cavity cancers. Cancer 56: 424–431.
6. Blatchford S (1986) Mucosal melanoma of the head and neck. Laryngoscope 96: 929–934.
7. Fazio M, Airoldi M, Negri L, Marchesa P, Gandolfo S (1900) Specific immunological stimulation induced by cryosurgery in patient with squamous cell carcinoma of the oral cavity. J Max Surg 12: 153–155.
8. Scala M, Gipponi M, Comandini D, Franzone P, Fabiani P, Del Bello A (1994) Cryosurgery alone or in combination with Radiotherapy and Hyperthermia in the treatment of head and neck mucosal and cutaneous melanoma. J Exp Clin Cancer Res 13: 243–246.
9. Groopman JE (1987) Biology and therapy of epidemic Kaposi's sarcoma. Cancer 59: 633–640.
10. Scala M, Canavese G, Catturich A, Schenone G, Gipponi M, Canessa A, Ropolo F, Moresco L (1992) Cryosurgery and Epidemic Kaposi's Sarcoma. Proceedings of the 8th Intern. Congress of Cryosurgery, Buenos Aires (Argentina).

18. Cryosurgery for Malignant Melanoma

Shigeo Tanaka

18.0 Introduction

Malignant melanoma is not seldom and its prognosis is notoriously bad. Treatment of the disease has proved difficult for many years, and even the results of treatment with new therapeutic agents have been disappointing. The fast neutron therapy has been recently introduced, but its indication is limited. Problems include: (1) initially, misdiagnosis of the lesion and careless biopsy lead to rapid general metastases, and (2) though controversies about diagnosis (6, 7) and regional lymph node dissection (2, 4) still exist, a wide excision and frequent sacrificing of the patient's limb are generally accepted as surgical treatment. For this reason, when the lesion is suspected of malignancy, *cryobiopsy*, immobilizing tumor cells by cryosolidification of the lesion and resection should be the first choice. That is, the suspicious lesion is frozen by the contact method until the ice boundary encompasses at least 10 mm beyond the tumor margin, then the lesion is excised while it is in the frozen state, followed by immediate histological examination. Experimental contact freezing of an acrylamide gel mold forms a shallow hemispherical ice ball (8), yet with sufficient depth to excise the lesion three-dimensionally. Thus rapid freezing prevents dissemination of the tumor cells, thereby avoids excessive surgical intervention, and the patient's limb may be saved. It is indispensable for the patient's quality of life after surgery.

In this chapter, (1) the importance of cryobiopsy at the first step of the diagnosis and treatment, and (2) effectiveness of cryosurgery to treat even an advanced malignant melanoma, and (3) cryosurgery for the tumor difficult to access, located at an anatomically critical area, are presented.

18.1 Study of Patients with Malignant Melanoma Treated by Cryosurgery

Of the patients with malignant melanoma who received cryosurgery in our institution, 10 cases were studied. This study was confined to only those cases revaluated by and matched to the UICC Classification determined in 1997. Location of the lesions included 5 skin, 2 fingers, 1 palate, and 2 nasopharynx. Three were resected immediately after cryosolidification of the lesions. Cryodestruction of the lesion was performed on 7 patients. Of these, 4 (stages I and III) are alive with no evidence of recurrence or developing metastases, the two longest for more than 20 years.

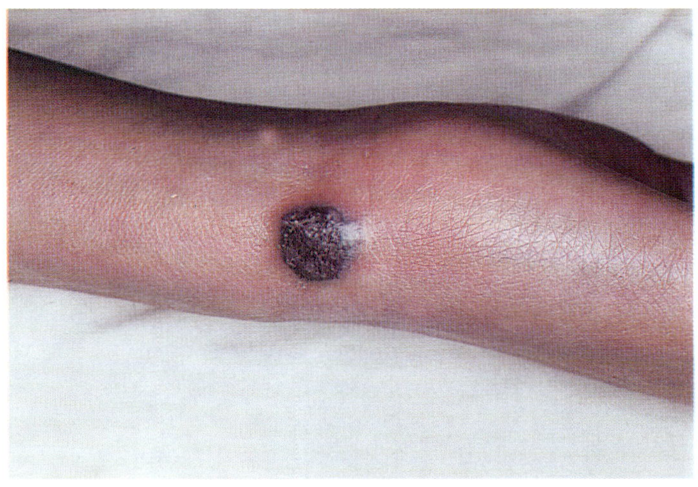

Fig. 18.1a. Case 1. Female, 42 y, with a melanoma 11 mm in diameter on the left forearm

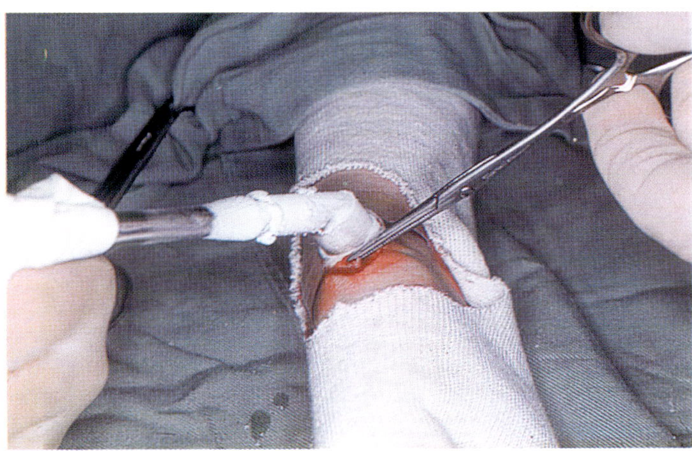

Fig. 18.1b. Extirpation of the tumor while freezing under cryosolidification, by contact method. Histological examination proved the tumor to be a stage I malignant melanoma. pT2pN0pM0

Case 1. A 42-year-old female, with an easily bleeding, melanoma, 11 mm in diameter, on the left forearm (Fig. 18.1a). As malignancy was suspected, an excisional biopsy was performed upon cryosolidification of the lesion (Fig. 18.1b). Histological examination proved the tumor to be a stage I

---

*Figs. 18.1–18.4 are reproduced with permission of *Skin Cancer* (10: 43–52, 1995)

malignant melanoma. Consequently, the patient underwent wide local resection. Later axillary dissection revealed no metastases, pT2pN0pM0. The patient is alive with no evidence of recurrence for more than 20 years.

Case 2. A 76-year-old female, with a stage III tumor, pT4pN2bpM0, occupying the palate (Fig. 18.2a). The patient complained of difficulty in swallowing. Cryosurgery was performed with intention of palliation, but in fact it resulted in total eradication of the tumor. After the main tumor had sloughed off, remaining pigmented spots on the palate and oropharynx disappeared spontaneously one year later. Since no effective chemotherapeutic agents were available at that time, and cryosurgery was the only treatment done, a cryo-mmunologic reaction against the tumor is strongly

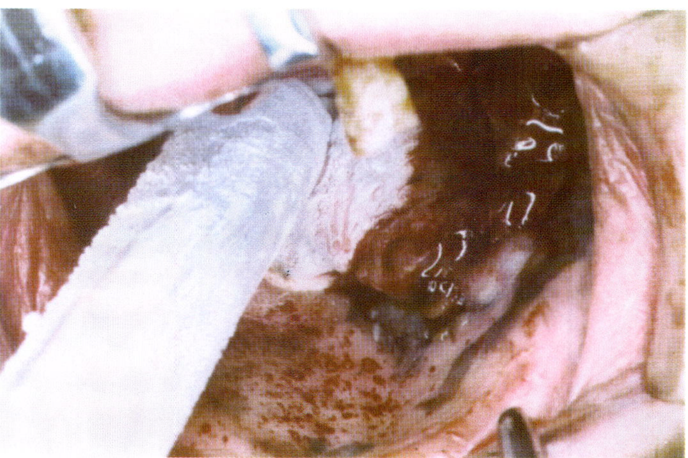

Fig. 18.2c. Freezing of the right half of the tumor, the melanotic portion. A cryoprobe for a large tumor, equipped with a doglegged special probe-tip adaptor devised for oral tumors, −160°C, 2 cycles, 5 + 3 min, LN_2

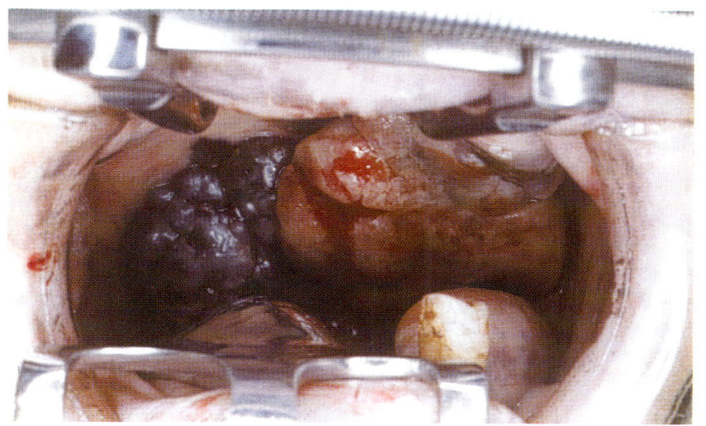

Fig. 18.2a. Case 2. Female, 76 y, with a stage III tumor occupying the palate. The right half is melanotic, and the left half amelanotic

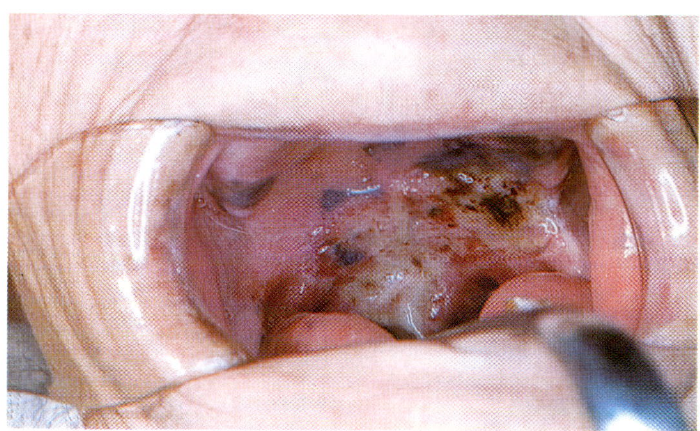

Fig. 18.2d. Three weeks later. The main tumor has already sloughed off, and many pigmented spots remain on the palate

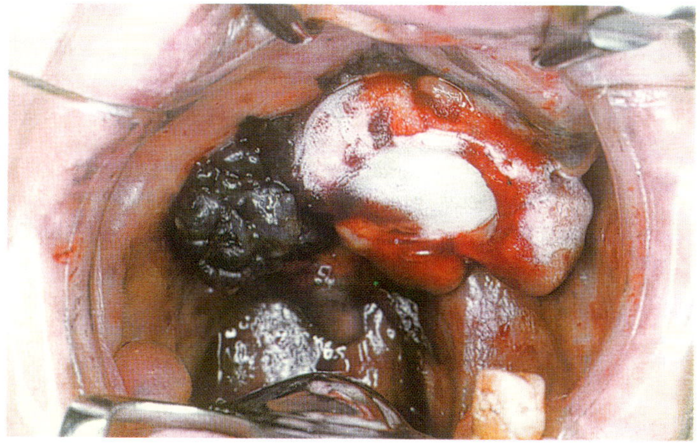

Fig. 18.2b. Immediately after freezing of the left half of the tumor, the amelanotic portion. Diffuse black pigmentation over the uvula and oropharynx is observed

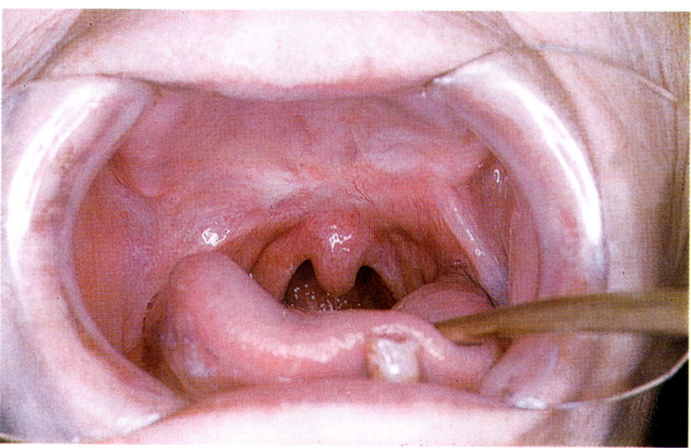

Fig. 18.2e. One year later. All pigmentation on the palate, uvula and oropharynx has disappeared spontaneously

suggested. Thirteen months after the first treatment, a tumor was noticed in the left neck, growing rapidly. The extirpated tumor looked like a blood-containing cyst. Histological examination proved the tumor to include a metastasis of malignant melanoma, thus a bilateral modified neck dissection was performed. About 20 lymph nodes were dissected, mostly black in color, yet no metastases were detected. Thereafter the patient achieved a two-year disease-free interval. Then suddenly, metastatic tumors appeared in the right neck, soon thereafter in both lungs. Immunotherapy, intratumoral injection of Nocardia cell-wall-skeleton (200–600 g, five times) and others failed to control the disease. The patient's survival period after the initial treatment was 3 years and 7 months. Although the immunologic survey was unsatisfactory in this case, an elevation of the N/L ratio, s_2-globulin and IgG, in contrast to a decrease in the IgM level, relevant to recurrence of the disease, were noted.

Case 3. A 71-year-old male, with a stage III tumor, pT4bpN0pM0, on the left sole (Fig. 18.3a). The patient noticed black pigmentation on his sole in January 1992. Diagnosed as malignant melanoma clinically at the first visited hospital, the patient underwent immunochemotherapy (DAV + INF-cl) once, and he was told that his leg should be amputated. The patient refused amputation surgery and was admitted to our hospital to receive cryosurgery in June 1992. The main tumor was 20 × 10 mm in size with 45 × 30 mm of tumor infiltration, and accompanied by multiple satellite lesions. Cryobiopsy was performed in order to assess the stage of the disease, immediately after

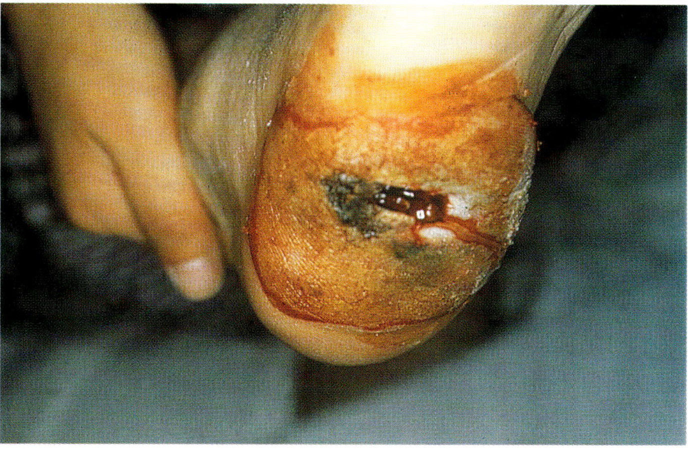

Fig. 18.3b. The lesion after cryobiopsy, before the second cycle of freezing. Cryosurgery was performed by combined contact and spraying method with LN_2, at −160°C for 5 to 7 min, four freeze-thaw cycles

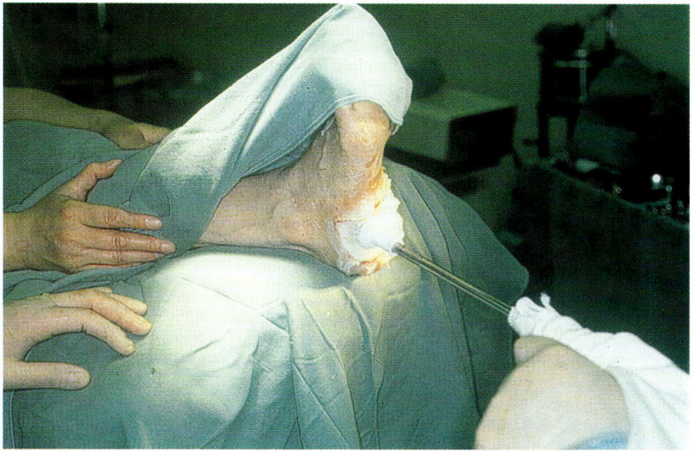

Fig. 18.3c. At the termination of the cryosurgery. The ice boundary is well beyond the margin of the tumor, about 2 cm

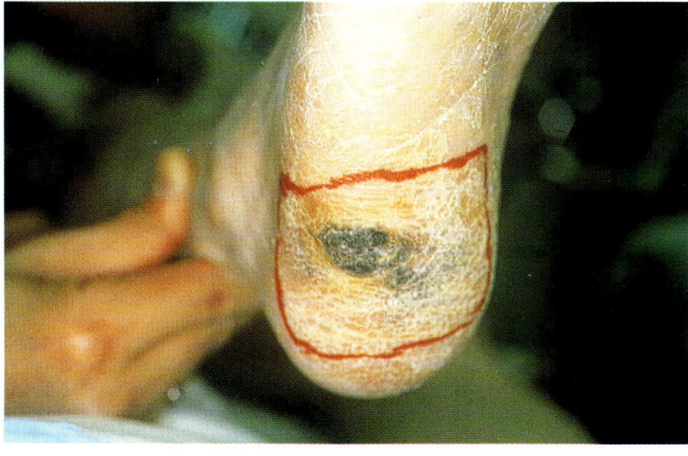

Fig. 18.3a. Case 3. Male, 71 y, with a stage III tumor on the left sole. Main tumor, 20 × 10 mm, with 45 × 30 mm of tumor infiltration and satellite lesions. The red marker indicates the provisional boundary of freezing

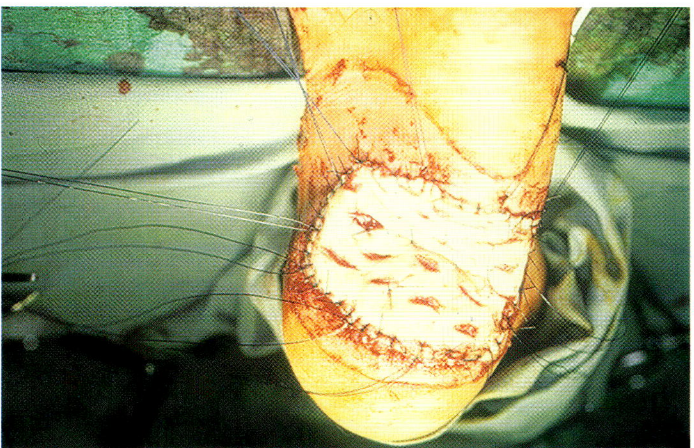

Fig. 18.3d. After necrotomy, a full-thickness free skin graft was performed

the first cryosurgery and before the second cycle of freezing, while the tumor was in the frozen state (Fig. 18.3b). Three weeks after cryosurgery, the necrotized lesion was removed, followed by a left groin dissection, which revealed no evidence of lymph node metastases. A full-thickness free skin graft was performed in July 1992 (Fig. 18.3d) successfully. The patient has been well and disease-free for 8 years to date, and *his leg was saved*.

Case 4. A 72-year-old male, with stage III tumor, pT4apN1pMX, in the nasopharynx, a difficult case to treat (Figs. 18.4a–d) because it was hard to access the lesion. Cryosurgery was performed through both the oral route (Fig. 18.4c) and nasal route simultaneously. This maneuver was surprisingly effective and resulted in total eradication of the tumor 2 weeks after the treatment. He received bilateral radical neck dissection a week later. Postsurgical recovery appeared smooth; however, the patient died of acute renal insufficiency 3 months after the initial treatment. Autopsy was refused, and the cause of the renal failure remained obscure.

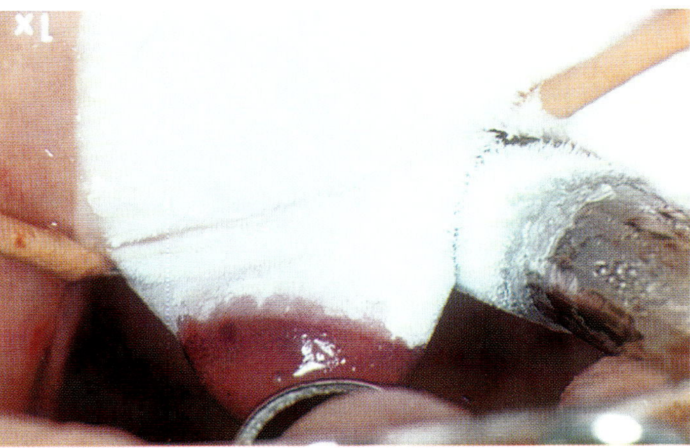

Fig. 18.4c. Freezing of the right epipharyngeal tumor through the oral route, by the contact method, with an 8 mm ø cryoprobe equipped with a doglegged cylindrical probe-tip adaptor, at −100°C for 5 min, plus at −140°C for 5 min with an L-shaped probe-tip adaptor

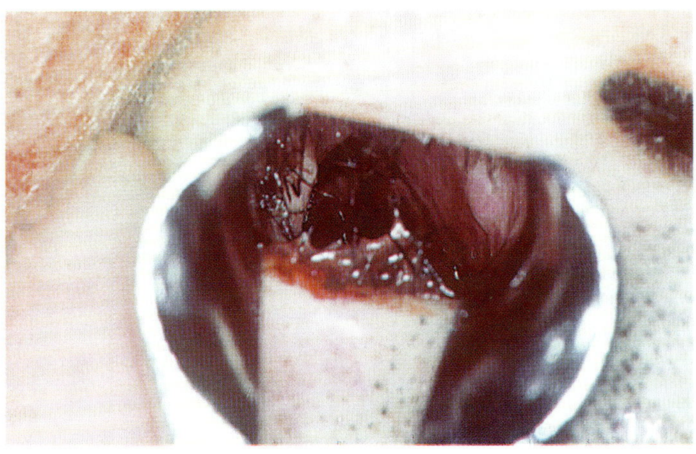

Fig. 18.4a. Case 4. Male, 72 y, with a stage III tumor in the right nasopharynx

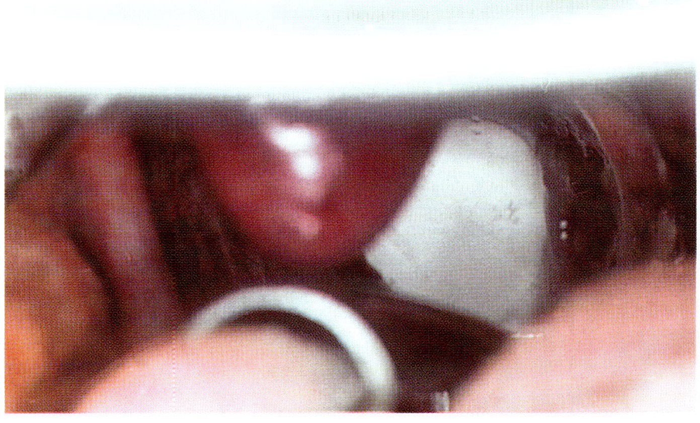

Fig. 18.4d. Immediately after freezing. The tumor frozen in white is seen by posterior rhinoscopy

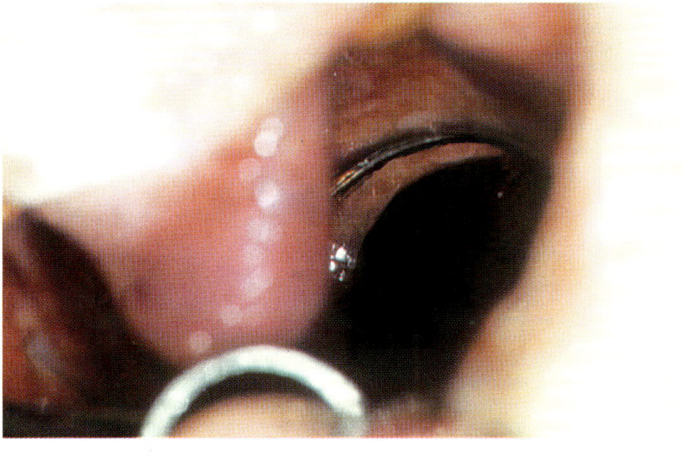

Fig. 18.4b. An epipharyngeal melanoma is observed by posterior rhinoscopy

18.2 Comments

The author has rarely treated malignant melanoma patients by cryosurgery, because most of them were referred to me from other institutions with considerable difficulties: associated with systemic diseases, or already carrying distant metastases, or difficulty in accessing the lesion. In this presentation on the small series of patients with malignant melanoma from 1971 to 1999, who received cryosurgery as the initial treatment method, cryodestruction was intended in 7 of the 10 patients: 1 stage I, 1 stage II, 4 stage III, and 1 stage, IV. Of these, 4 patients of stages I and III are alive and well (excluding 2 cases lost to our follow-up) with no signs of recurrence.

The difficulty was to eradicate tumors in the advanced stages. Even though primary tumors disappeared, recurrence or metastases soon occurred, and the follow-up revealed no 5-year survivors in the stage IV group. However, a number of reports emphasizing the superiority of cryosurgery for the treatment of malignant melanoma have been published. Barton (1) treated malignant melanoma of mucosal origin on the head and neck, known for its poor prognosis. Cryosurgery was judged quite effective, since 3 cryosurgically treated patients achieved 5-year survival among a total of 11 cases.

Prospects of cryosurgery include tumor-specific cryoimmunologic reaction elicited by freezing of the targeted tumor. Besides the destruction of resistant tumors, this is another beneficial effect to be expected, since malignant melanoma is known for its high immunogenicity (as is prostatic cancer). Case 2 was referred to the author from the otorhinolaryngology department and treated by cryosurgery for palliation. Unexpectedly, it yielded complete eradication of the main tumor and spontaneous disappearance of the numerous black spots and diffuse pigmentation over the uvula and oropharynx, suggesting a cryoimmunologic reaction against the tumor. Bilateral modified radical neck dissection proved no metastases in about 20 lymph nodes, mostly black in color. Retrospectively, it is thought reasonable that many of the lymph nodes in the neck should have contained metastases, but the tumor cells might have been destroyed by the cryoimmunologic reaction. Indeed, the neck tumor first extirpated contained metastases, but breakdown of the tumor and central necrosis might have led to intralesional bleeding, resulting in rapid enlargement of the tumor in appearance. Kärjä et al. (5) also achieved an excellent result with cryosurgery in a patient with a large malignant melanoma of the palate. Although the patient died of lung metastases 3 years later, no local recurrence was observed. Our case 2, stage III, with a large tumor of the palate, achieved a 2-year disease-free period, but finally died of multiple metastases 3 year and 7 months after the initial treatment. In view of this evidence, the cryoimmune state may be maintained a maximum of about 2 or 3 years. Accordingly, cryoimmunointensification therapy (9) and/or intermittent immunochemotherapy are essential, particularly in treating patients with the late stages, III and IV. These regimens during the disease-free interval might have helped to prevent recurrence in Case 2. Cryochemotherapy (3), a novel modality of anticancer strategy, may also be of help as the initial procedure.

In conclusion, our consensus for the treatment of malignant melanoma is as follows:

(1) Cryosolidification of the suspicious lesion is mandatory not only when performing biopsies, but also when doing conventional wide excision as the first treatment.

(2) Cryosurgery should be the first choice in treating stages I and II. Cryosurgery is particularly indicated for the head and neck and for mucosal lesions in anatomically critical sites.

(3) For stages III and IV, cryosurgery may be a choice for palliation. A beneficial effect owing to cryoimmunologic reaction may be expected.

References

1. Barton RT (1975) Mucosal melanoma of the head and neck. Laryngoscope 85: 93–99.
2. Conrad CFG (1972) Treatment of malignant melanoma. Wide excision alone vs lymphadenectomy. Arch Surg 104: 587–593.
3. Ikekawa S, Ishihara K, Tanaka S, Ikeda S (1985) Basic studies of cryochemotherapy in a murine tumor system. Cryobiology 22: 477–483.
4. Kapelanski DP, Block GE, Kaufman M (1979) Characteristics of the primary lesions of malignant melanoma as guide to prognosis and therapy. Am Surg 189: 225–235.
5. Kärjä J, Jokiner K, Palva A (1975) Experience with cryotherapy in otolaryngological practice. J Laryngol Otol 89: 519–526.
6. McGovern VJ (1976) Malignant melanoma: clinical and histological diagnosis. J Wiley, New York.
7. Rouge F, Aubert C (1979) A new approach to differential diagnosis of human malignant melanoma. Cancer 44: 199–209.
8. Tanaka S (1981) Cryosurgery for the treatment of malignant melanoma. Cryothérapie, No. 4, suppl. Lyon Méditeranée Med 17: 4–13.
9. Tanaka S (1982) Immunological aspects of cryosurgery in general surgery. Cryobiology 19: 247–262.

19. Neck Cryosurgery. Experimental and Clinical Experience for the Treatment of Thyroid Cancer

Shigeo Tanaka

19.0 Introduction

Papillary cancer of the thyroid gland is generally gentle in nature, growing very slowly or even remaining in a stationary state for a long period of time, and it is not rare to see long survival. However, in our experience, once the tumor starts its rapid growth, one can hardly control the disease by conventional means, particularly large, necrotizing and bleeding tumors with intractable pain and compression symptoms owing to the tumor.

Cryosurgery is feasible for reduction of tumor bulk without bleeding, while preserving major blood vessels and alleviating intractable pain, which would otherwise be difficult to treat by conventional means.

Cryosurgery of advanced or recurrent thyroid cancer, though, inevitably involves freezing injury to the adjacent vital organs of the neck: trachea, recurrent laryngeal nerve, and common carotid artery. Basic studies on the effect of cryosurgical intervention on the blood vessels have been well documented (3,5,6,14). However, in view of the lack of sufficient information on the vital organs of the neck other than major blood vessels, experimental studies on the trachea and recurrent laryngeal nerve of animals were carried out prior to clinical application of cryosurgery for the treatment of advanced thyroid cancer. In the following are presented the summarized results of the animal experiments done by Masui and the author et al. (1975, 1976) (7,8). With the evidence obtained in mind, we proceeded to clinical application.

19.1 Experimental Studies on Cryosurgical Intervention to the Trachea and Adjacent Vital Organs of the Neck

Trachea: Fourteen mongrel dogs, 12 adult (6 each male and female) and 2 puppies (female) were used. Freezing of the trachea was performed after its exposure by the 3-dimensional contact method at $-170°C$ for $5+5$ or $3+3$ minutes (2-cycle freezing) using a liquid nitrogen (LN_2) driven cryosurgical device. It froze the entire circumferential tracheal segments including 5 to 7 rings (Fig. 19.1). Histological observations were made immediately after freezing, and at the time intervals of 24 hours, 3 days, 1, 2, and 3 weeks, and 3 months (Figs. 19.2a–d). The results revealed damage to the mucous membrane of the trachea immediately after freezing, and its regeneration in a week. As for the cartilagenous portion, degeneration began one week after freezing, and was most prominent in the 3rd week, in contrast to the complete regeneration of the mucosa. Narrowing of the trachea was observed only in the puppies 3 months after cryosurgery (Fig. 19.3), although it never occurred in the adult dogs. It was suspected that the growth disturbance of the trachea was due to poor microcirculation at the frozen site. During

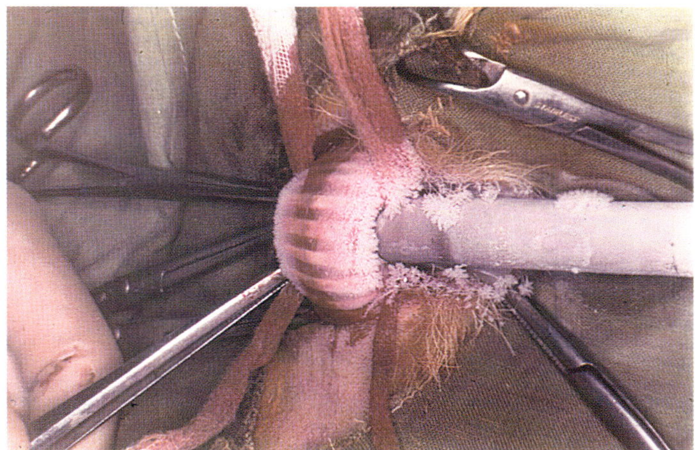

Fig. 19.1. Experimental freezing of a canine trachea. Contact method with a cryoprobe 8 mm in diameter, −170°C, 2 cycles, 5 + 3 minutes

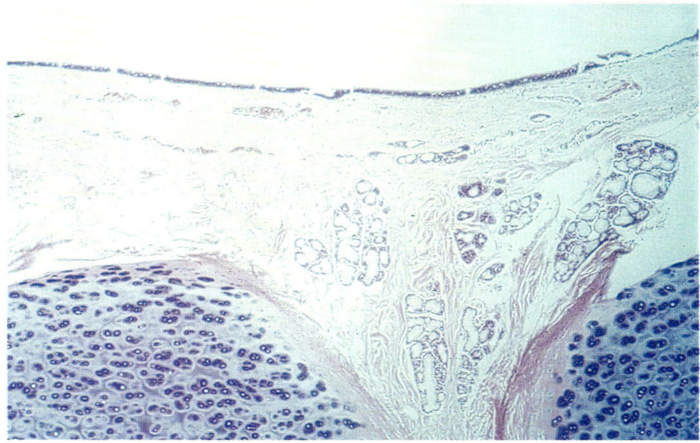

Fig. 19.2a. Histology of canine trachea, a photomicrograph of the normal tracheal wall. Hematoxylin & Eosin (H.E.)

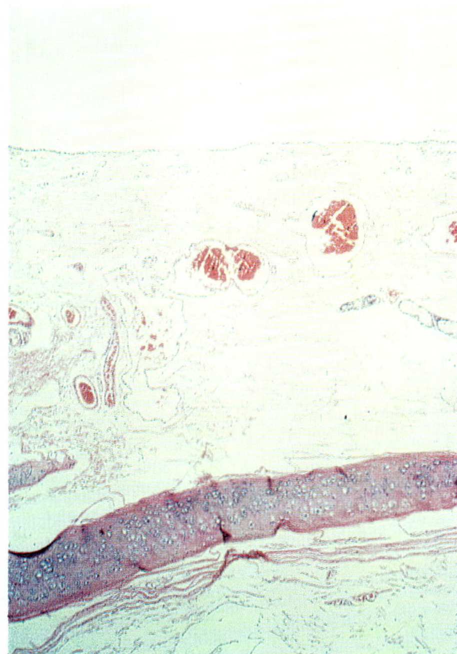

Fig. 19.2b. Immediately after cryosurgery. Mucosa is already lost

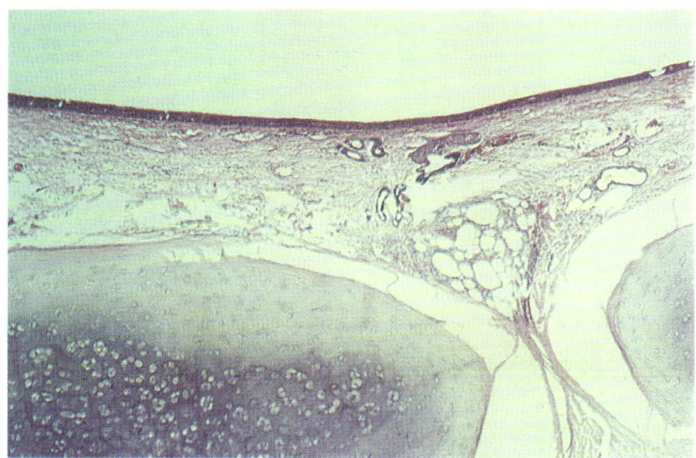

Fig. 19.2c. One week after cryosurgery. Regeneration of mucosa and degeneration of cartilage are seen

the whole experimental period, no perforation of the trachea occurred even in the membranous portion. This fact might be due to the time lag in degeneration and regeneration of the tracheal tissue components.

Recurrent Laryngeal Nerve: Six mongrel dogs (adult and a puppy) were used. Exposed recurrent laryngeal nerve was frozen at −60°C to −80°C for 1 + 1 minute or 30 + 30 seconds (2-cycle freezing), simulating the event when extensive cryosurgery would be done for thyroid cancer in man. The

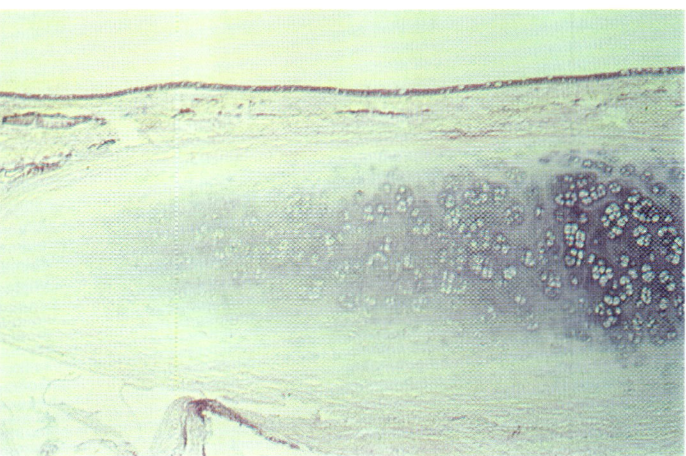

Fig. 19.2d. Three weeks later. Marked degeneration of cartilage is still obvious

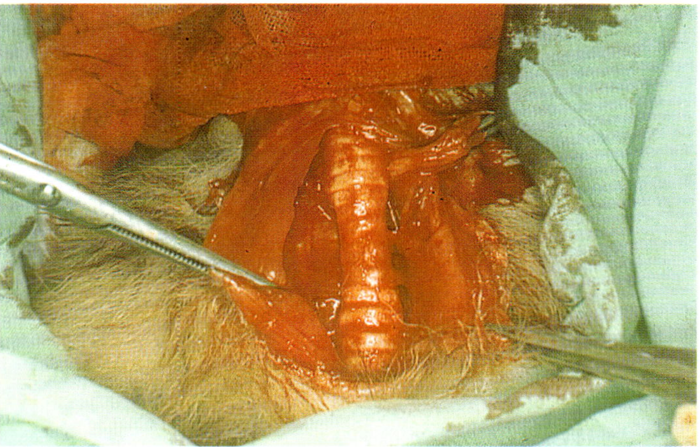

Fig. 19.3. Trachea of puppy 3 months after cryosurgery. Narrowing of the frozen site is observed

frozen area of the nerve extended for 1 to 3 cm in length. Movement of the vocal cord was observed every day during the first week, and then at one-week intervals with direct laryngoscopy. No movement of the vocal cord on the paralyzed side was noticed during the first 2 weeks. But 3 weeks later, a slight movement of the cord was observed, followed by complete recovery in 4 to 6 weeks.

19.2 Cryosurgery of Primary and Recurrent Thyroid Cancer in Man

Technique: Healthy skin covering the tumor was saved if possible, dissected from the tumor and retracted aside to expose the tumor, except in cases resulting in hazardous bleeding. Biopsy was taken prior to cryosurgery. The tumor was frozen using a heavy-duty cryogenic device, with LN_2 as the cryogen, with an appropriate cryoprobe and probe-tip adaptor to fit the size and shape of the tumor. Freezing was performed by the contact method, at a temperature of −100°C to −160°C for 5 to 10 minutes 2- or 3-cycle freezing, to the fractionated overlapping sites, if required. After cryosurgery, the wound was covered by the skin, with a drain. Necrotomy and freezing were repeated at 2- or 3-weeks' intervals. At necrotomy, usually no bleeding was observed. Radical surgery followed in some cases. In the cases in which the tumor was already necrotized in part and developing ulcers and bleeding when first seen, the cryoprobe was applied directly over the tumor and freezing procedures commenced. Wounds were covered later by a mesh skin graft, composite graft, or by a pedicled flap. During the healing process, the necrotized tissue was replaced by connective tissue, occasionally with calcification.

Clinical Results: Thirty-four patients with advanced thyroid cancer, 12 primary and 22 recurrent, received cryosurgery in our institution from July 1968 through January 2000. Cryosurgery was performed principally with intent of palliation but achieved even cure in some cases. Of 12 primary cases, 3 attained more than 10-year survival to date disease-free, and 2 died of geromarasmus after more than 4 years of disease-free interval. As regards recurrent cancer, 7 of 22 cases survived more than 10 years, all papillary adenocarcinoma, although some were lost to our follow-up. Six anaplastic cancer, including 4 primary cases, treated by cryosurgery, yielded poor results and died within 2 years.

A total of 42 patients with primary head-and-neck malignancies, including 12 thyroid cancer, had overall 1-, 3-, and 5-year survival rates of 66.7%, 59.6%, and 59.6%. When confined to primary advanced thyroid cancer, the number of cases is too small to evaluate, but those rates are 63.6%, 9.1%, and 27.3% respectively. As for recurrent cancer, the rates are 28.6%, 4.8%, and 66.7%, only for reference.

Case Reports

Case 1. A 71-year-old female, with a large recurrent tumor in the right neck, accompanied by intractable pain and paralysis of the right recurrent laryngeal nerve (Figs. 19.4a–c). Histology revealed papillary adenocarcinoma. The tumor was exposed to save healthy skin and frozen with a heavy-duty cryosurgical device using LN_2 as the cryogen, equipped with a special probe-tip adaptor, at −170°C for 10 minutes by the contact method, 4-cycle freezing (Fig. 19.4b). During the hospital stay, the same procedures followed by necrotomy were repeated at 2- to 3-week intervals for 5 times. Figure 19.4c shows the appearance at the time of discharge, 3 months after the first treatment. Although the tumor remnant was obvious, the initial bulky tumor was markedly reduced in size and the

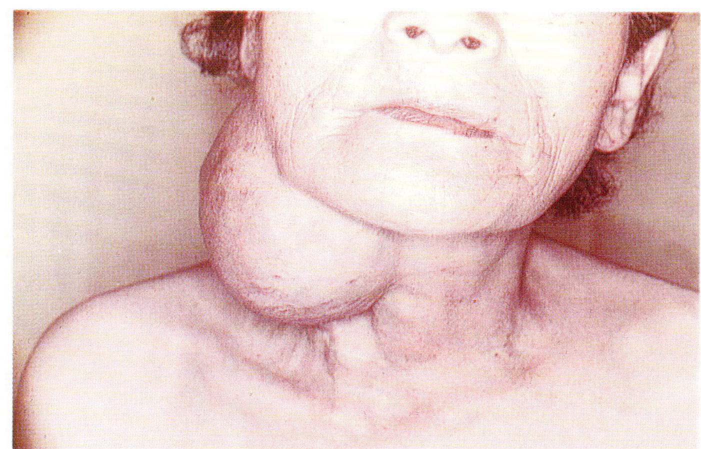

Fig.19.4a. A recurrent thyroid cancer, Case 1, female, 71 y, with intractable pain. Papillary adenocarcinoma, 11 × 8.5 cm

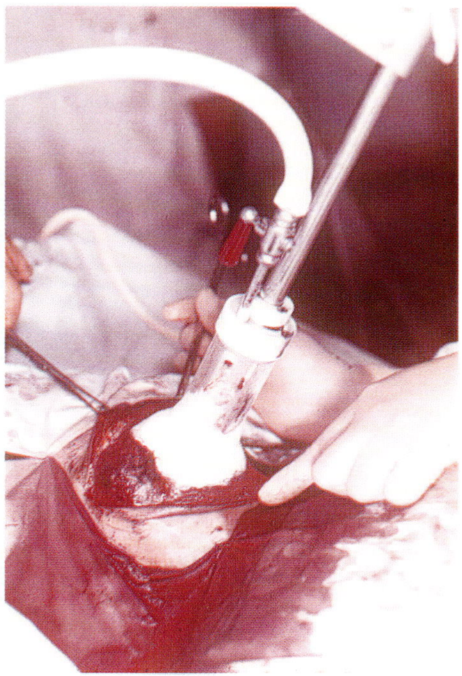

Fig. 19.4b. The tumor was exposed to save healthy skin and frozen with a 40 mm ø hemispherical probe-tip adaptor, −170°C, 4 cycles

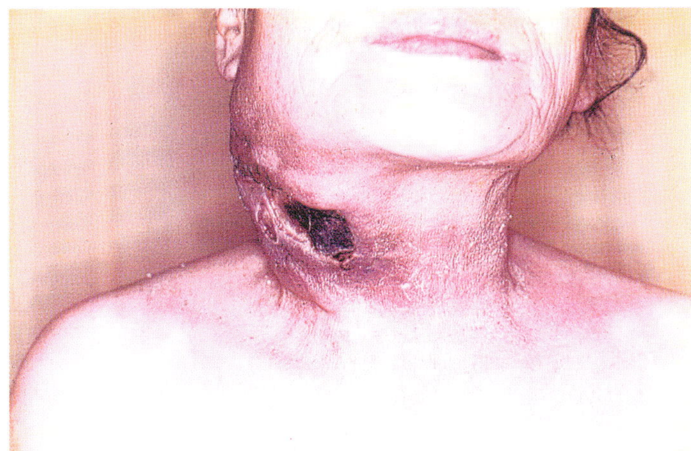

Fig. 19.4c. A photograph taken at the time of discharge, 3 months after the first cryosurgery

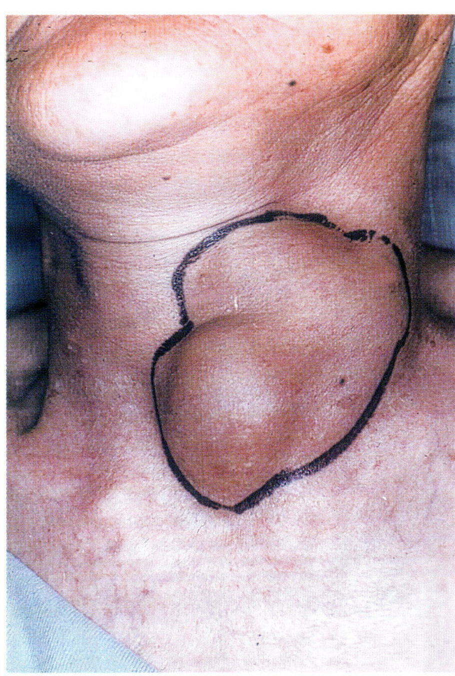

Fig. 19.5a. A recurrent thyroid cancer, Case 2, female, 65 y, with severe pain. Papillary adenocarcinoma, 8.5 × 7.5 cm. The common carotid artery was involved in the tumor

pain had disappeared. Sequential cryosurgery and necrotomy were able to reduce such a tumor with minimal blood loss.

Case 2. A 65-year-old female, with a painful recurrent tumor in the left neck, a papillary carcinoma (Figs. 19.5a–c). During cryosurgery, pulsation of the carotid artery was felt unchanged at the distal portion and the blood stream was maintained. Three weeks after the extensive cryotreatment of the tumor, the second ablative surgery was performed. The common carotid artery was

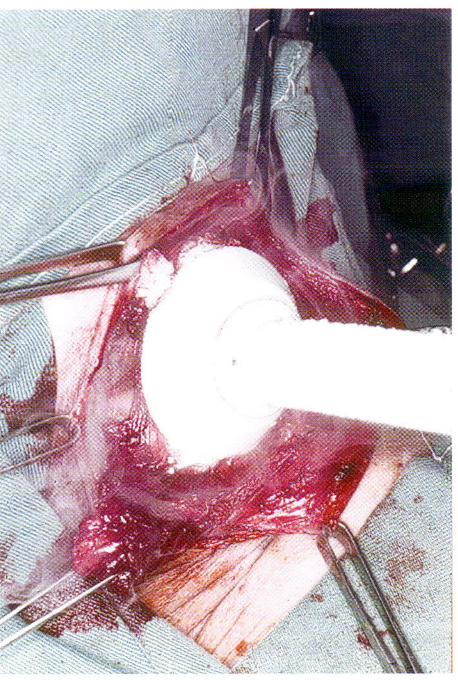

Fig. 19.5b. The tumor was exposed and frozen with a 40 mm ø hemispherical probe-tip adaptor at −170°C for 8 + 5 minutes (2 cycles)

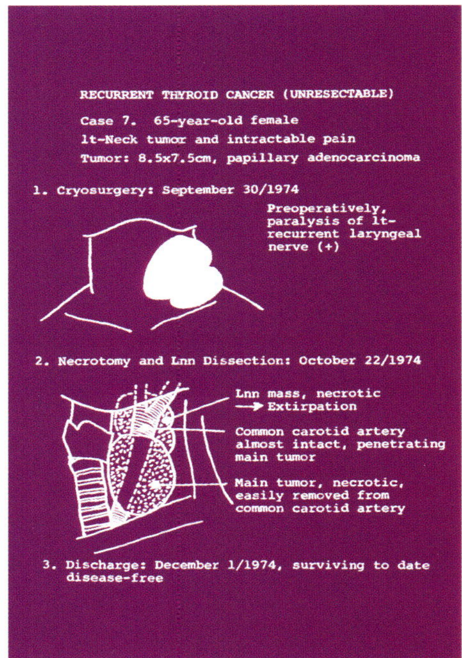

Fig. 19.5c. A schematic view of the tumor and explanation of Case 2

found almost intact, notwithstanding massive cryonecrosis of the surrounding tumor (Fig. 19.5c). Necrotized tumor was easily removed piece by piece with forceps from the artery. Total eradication of the tumor was achieved and a major artery

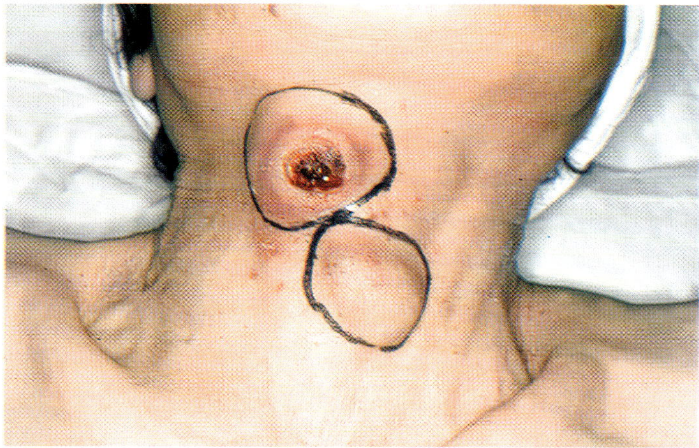

Fig. 19.6a. A recurrent thyroid cancer, Case 3, female, 62 y. Papillary adenocarcinoma. Bleeding, with intratracheal invasion, 6.6 × 3.5 cm

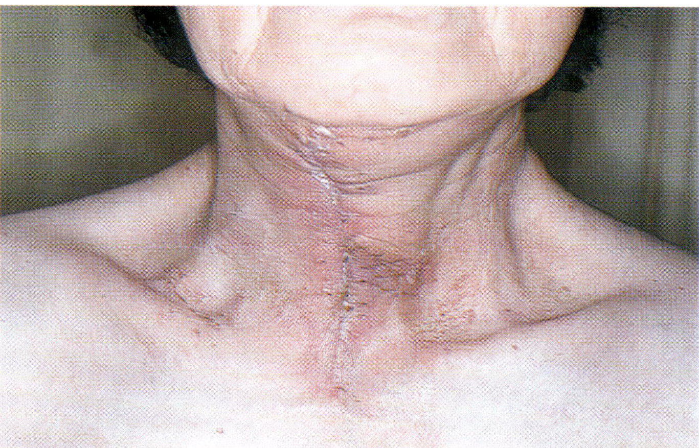

Fig. 19.6d. A photograph taken at discharge. The tracheostomy was closed

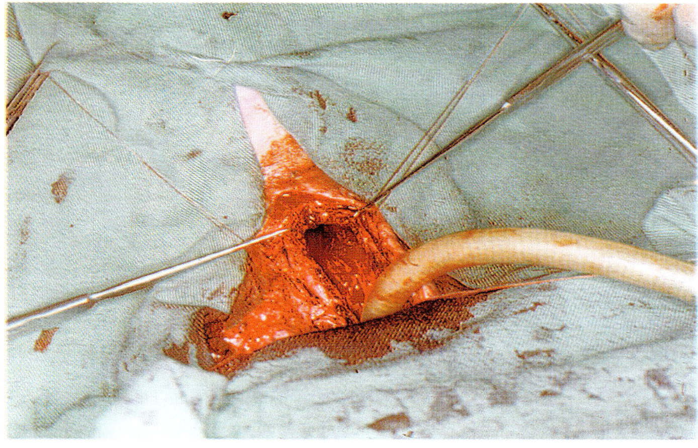

Fig. 19.6b. After extensive cryosurgery (upper part, −170°C for 5 + 7 min; lower part, −170°C for 5 + 7 min) and necrotomy, the tracheal wall was opened

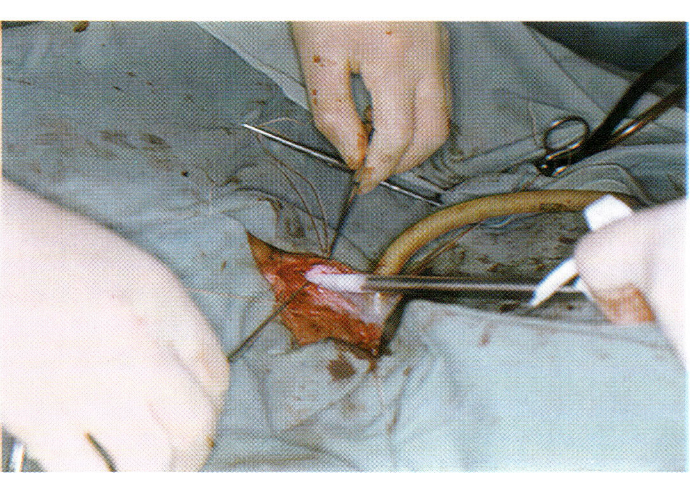

Fig. 19.6c. Intratracheal tumor (1), and left-paratracheal tumor (2) were frozen with 10 mm ø cylindrical probe-tip adaptor. (1): −120°C, 3 + 3 min; (2): −80°C, 3 + 3 min

was saved. The patient survived more than 10 years disease-free.

Case 3. A 62-year-old female, with a bleeding recurrent thyroid cancer with intratracheal invasion, and paralysis of the right recurrent laryngeal nerve. After extensive cryosurgery and necrotomy, the tracheal wall was opened. The intratracheal tumor and the left paratracheal tumor remnants were frozen (Fig. 19.6c). The tracheostomy was able to be closed and the patient survived since then more than 10 years disease-free.

19.3 Comments

Reports or comprehensive reviews of cryosurgery for the management of thyroid cancer are seldom seen in the literature. However, our experience has proved its advantage over conventional surgery in treating primary advanced, or recurrent unresectable thyroid cancer *safely*. Since most patients have large tumors with bleeding, a powerful LN_2 driven cryosurgical device is required. Freezing of the thyroid tumor may involve adjacent vital organs of the neck, such as trachea, recurrent laryngeal nerve, and common carotid artery.

Our experiments with dogs indicated that the recurrent laryngeal nerve restored its function after cryosurgery, although it was paralyzed temporarily. Clinically, in a 66-year-old female, with a recurrent papillary adenocarcinoma of the right thyroid, 5 × 6 cm, paralysis of the left recurrent laryngeal nerve due to the left primary lesion was observed when the patient was referred to us. Cryosurgery of the right bleeding tumor resulted in complete aphonia. However, it reversed 3 months later and the tracheostomy was closed. Freezing of the tracheal wall, not only the cartilagenous portion but also the membranous portion, resulted in no perforation, as also observed by Thomford et al. (13) and Neel et al. (9). As regards the common carotid artery, we have no experience with a blow-out of the artery thus far. Case 2 is an excellent example. Although numerous reports supported safety of the freezing of major blood vessels, some related freezing injury caused rupture of the artery (10). However, another clinical observation at radical neck dissection, direct freezing of the tumor-invading vascular wall, or normal external carotid artery and jugular vein, which had to be resected later, showed in no case any complication, i.e., no rupture, and no infection (4). Nevertheless, caution must be exercised on a patient who had been given irradiation in the past, and/or if the wound is seriously infected (1,2), which would create the danger of a blow-out of the artery, due to loss of regeneration activity of the tissue caused by irradiation or infection.

Clinically, cryosurgery is invaluable for the treatment of advanced thyroid cancer not only for reducing tumor bulk, arresting hemorrhage, and alleviating intractable pain, while not seriously damaging the juxtatumor vital organs of the neck, e.g., preserving major blood vessels. However, anaplastic thyroid cancer is contraindicated for cryosurgery: The outcome of all of the 6 cases (4 primary and 2 recurrent) was poor (11). A beneficial effect of a tumor-specific cryoimmunologic reaction elicited by cryosurgery would be expected (12), which will lead to reduction in size of the tumor bulk and improve quality of life of the patient, since the thyroid gland is known as one of the highly immunogeneic organs in man.

References

1. Chandler JR (1972) Cryosurgery of malignant neoplasms of the head and neck. JAMA 221: 387–390.
2. DeSanto LW (1972) The curative, palliative, and adjunctive uses of cryosurgery in the head and neck. Laryngoscope 82: 1282–1291.
3. Gage AA, Fazekas G, Riley EE Jr (1967) Freezing injury to large blood vessels in dogs with comments on the effect of experimental freezing of bile ducts. Surgery 61: 748–754.
4. Ganz H (1974) Experiments on cryosurgery of tumors at the great blood vessels in the neck. Minerva Medica 65: 3645–3647.
5. Klein H, Braess P, Ganz H (1973) Untersuchungen zur Kryotherapie an den grossen Halsgefässen beim Menschen. Arch Klin Exp Ohren Nasen Kehlkopf-Heilkd 205: 307–311.
6. Mandeville AF, McGabe BF (1967) Some observations on the cryobiology of blood vessels. Laryngoscope 77: 1328–1350.
7. Masui T, Tanaka S, Obata T, Toyoda K, Nagata H (1975) Experimental studies on the freezing of trachea and its adjacent organs and their response (1) J Jpn Soc Cryosurg 1: 50–56 (in Japanese).
8. Masui T, Watanabe S, Tanaka S, Nagata H (1976) Experimental studies on the freezing of head and neck organs (brain, trachea, and the adjacent organs) and their response (2) J Jpn Soc Cryosurg 2: 32–33 (in Japanese).
9. Neel HB III, Farrel KH, DeSanto LW, Payne WS, Sanderson DR (1973) Cryosurgery of respiratory structures. I. Cryonecrosis of trachea and bronchus. Laryngoscope 83: 1062–1071.
10. Schrott KM, Sigel A, Hermanek P (1971) Nebenwirkungen der Kryotherapie auf grosse Gefässe. Urologe 10: 73–80.
11. Tanaka S (1982) Cryosurgery of unresectable, advanced or recurrent thyroid cancer. In: Ui N, Torizuka K, Miyai K (eds.): Current problems in thyroid research, Excerpta Medica, Amsterdam, pp. 601–604 (International Congress Series No. 605).
12. Tanaka S (1982) Immunological aspects of cryosurgery in general surgery. Cryobiology 19: 247–262.
13. Thomford NR, Wilson WH, Blackburn ZD, Pace WG (1970) Morphological changes in canine trachea after freezing. Cryobiology 7: 19–26.
14. Unger RF, Feldman H, David E, Lehman R, Szdzuy D (1971) Über die Wirkung tiefer Temperaturen (Kryotechnik) an der Aorta abdominalis des Kaninchens. Z Exp Chir 4: 100–106.

20. Lymph Node Cryosurgery

Nikolai N. Korpan

20.1 Lymph Node Metastases

We have, world-wide, gathered the first clinical experience with patients with lymph node metastases, which have different etiologies. For the first time, new cryosurgical operations have been developed and used with clinical success in patients with lymph node metastases after breast cancer surgery, melanoma extirpation and hypernephroma extirpation performed with conventional methods.

We have also developed new subcutaneous (Figs. 20.1–20.2) cryosurgical operations and carried them out in numerous patients. The operation is normally carried out with local anesthesia. When an affected metastatic lymph node lies deep in soft tissue, the surgery should be carried out under general anesthesia, in order to be able to expose and dissect all the lymphnodes (Figs. 20.3–20.6). The operation is usually ended without a drain and the wound is closed by intracutaneous suture (Fig. 20.7).

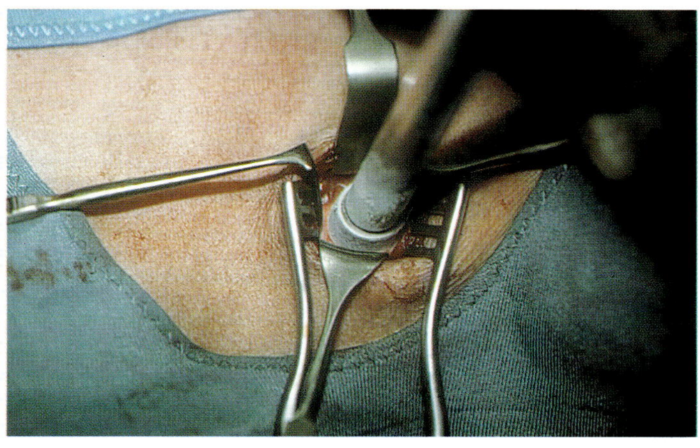

Fig. 20.1. Cervical node metastases from primary breast cancer, left-sided, 65-year-old woman. The technique of nodal subcutaneous cryosurgery (NSC), showing a disc probe 30 mm in diameter which is placed on the tumor mass at a temperature of −180°C for 3 minutes, with local anesthesia

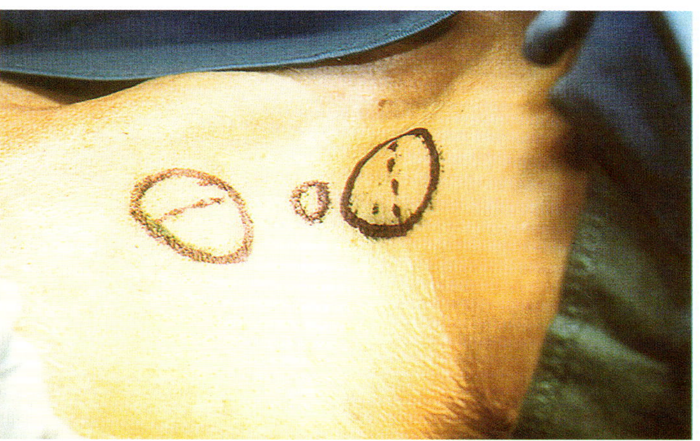

Fig. 20.3. Cervical node metastases from primary squamous cell carcinoma of the right shoulder, 72-year-old man. Preoperative view: Metastases to cervical lymph nodes are marked on the skin with the aid of ultrasound

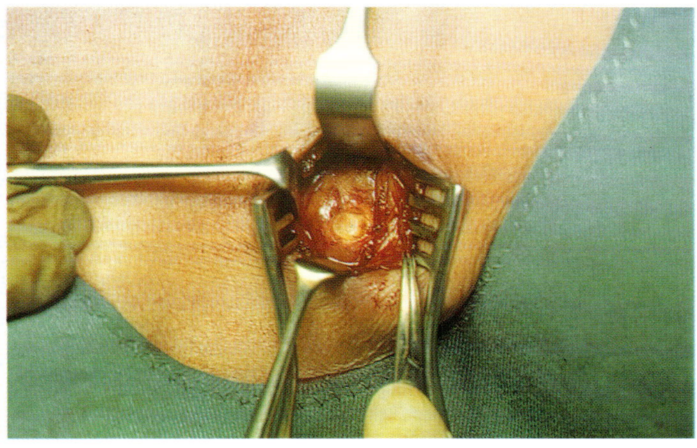

Fig. 20.2. NSC, same patient: Typical view of the post-cryosurgical zone, which measures 50 mm in diameter. Clearly demarcated post-cryosurgical zone

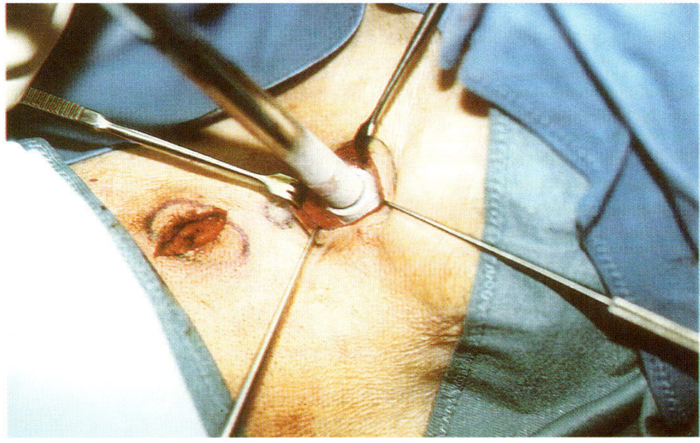

Fig. 20.4. The same patient. NSC: A cryoprobe with a diameter of 30 mm is applied on the one nodal metastasis at a temperature of −180°C for 3 minutes. A double freeze-thaw cycle is started using local anesthesia. Two treatment freeze-thaw cycles are usually needed

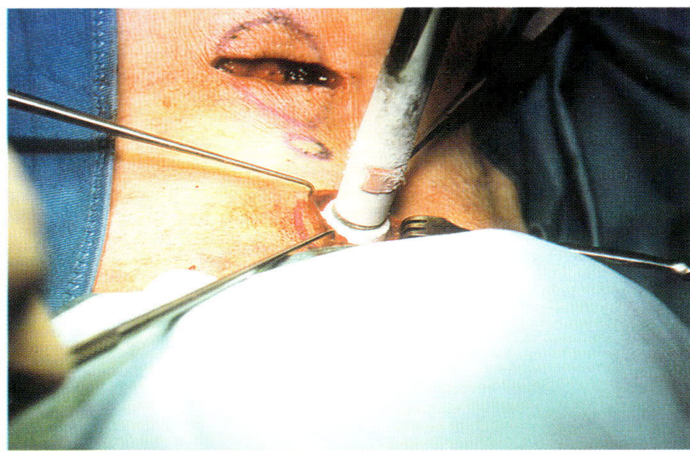

Fig. 20.5. NSC: A cryoprobe 40 mm in diameter is placed on the next cervical nodal metastasis at the same cryosurgical parameters

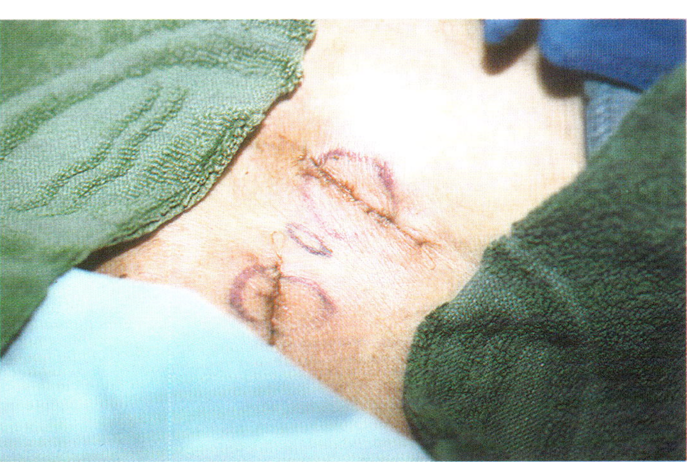

Fig. 20.7. NSC: Immediately after the cryosurgical treatment, final local appearance. View of the post-cryosurgical wound. No post-operative bleeding

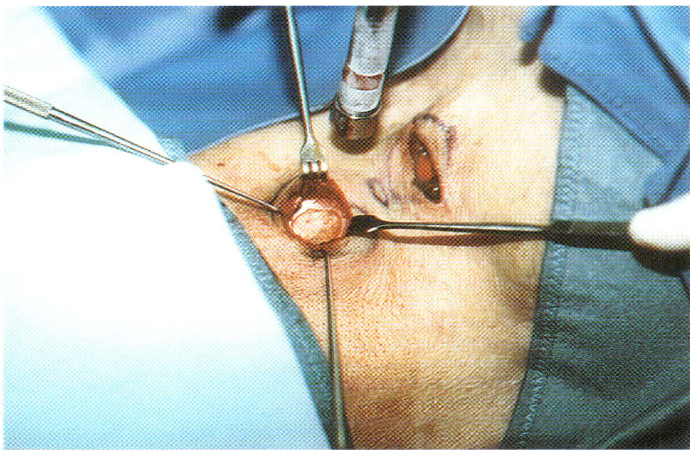

Fig. 20.6. NSC: Base view of the post-cryosurgical zone immediately after the thawing of the cryoprobe

21. Proctological Cryosurgery

Nikolai N. Korpan

21.1 Hemorrhoidal Nodules

Many new surgical and non-surgical approaches to the treatment of hemorrhoids have been described. Which is the most effective depends on the size and the grade of the hemorrhoid, but equally on the experience of the surgeon. Generally speaking, all the procedures give good results.

One of the modern treatment methods is the cryosurgical operation with all its advantages. These interventions are particularly indicated in patients with internal nodules and, as our 5-year experience shows, are highly promising (Fig. 21.1).

21.2 Rectal Cryosurgery

The treatment of a rectal carcinoma is essentially surgical. Many factors influence the choice of surgical management of the patient with rectal cancer: general condition of the patient, overweight, obstruction, location of tumor, presence of metastases, as well as the experience and preferences of the surgeon. What seems very promising for one patient may not necessarily be the best solution for another patient. Therefore, a variety of approaches can be developed.

According to the statistics palliative surgery is associated with morbidity of 20–40% and mortality of more than 10%. Endoscopic procedures can provide effective palliation with fewer complications. Many different local treatment strategies have been used to date.

Endoscopic cryosurgery is a simple, effective and safe treatment of resectable and nonresectable rectal carcinoma (Figs. 21.2–21.4).

21.3 Cancer of the Anal Region

The treatment of epidermoid cancer in the anal region has undergone important change. The use

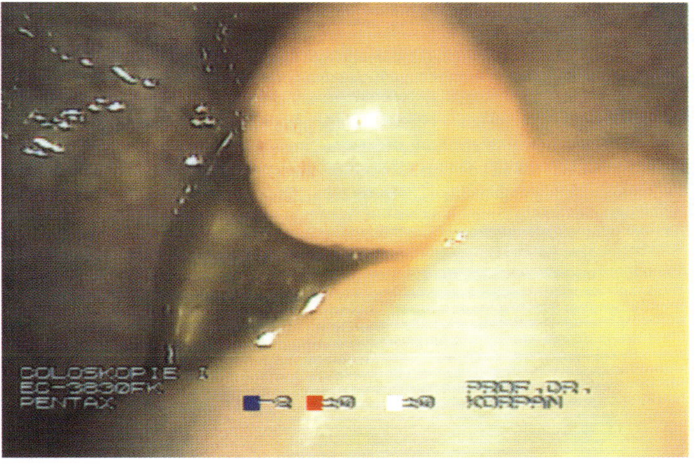

Fig. 21.2. Transrectal cryosurgery (TRC). Rectal adenocarcinoma in a 61-year-old man. Preoperative endoscopical view

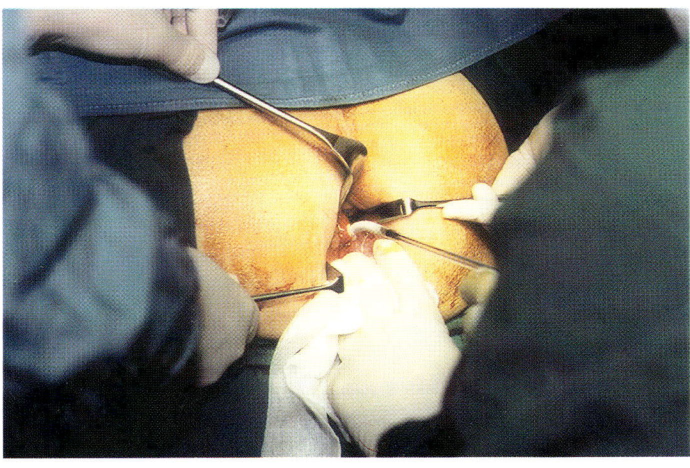

Fig. 21.1. Proctological cryosurgery (PC). Hemorrhoids, degree II, 37-year-old woman. The intraoperative view. The single cryosurgical freeze-thaw cycle is performed with the curved cryosurgical instrument for anorectal cryosurgery at a temperature of –80°C. The probe is placed against the pile for 20 seconds

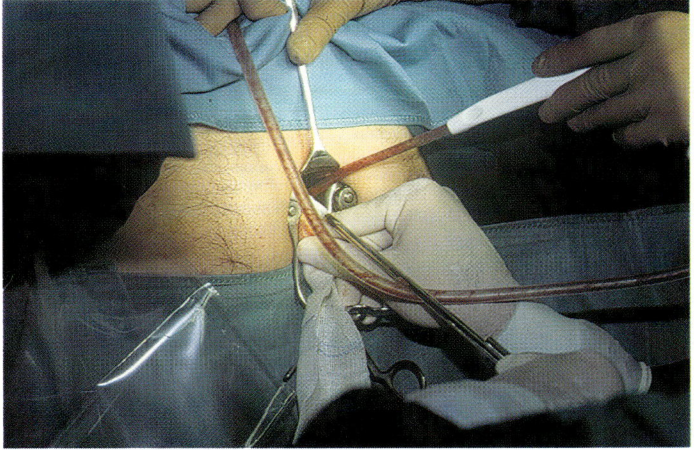

Fig. 21.3. The same patient. TRC: The tip of a curved cryosurgical instrument for anorectal cryosurgery is applied to the center of the tumor at a temperature of –180°C for 7 min. No bleeding after cryosurgery

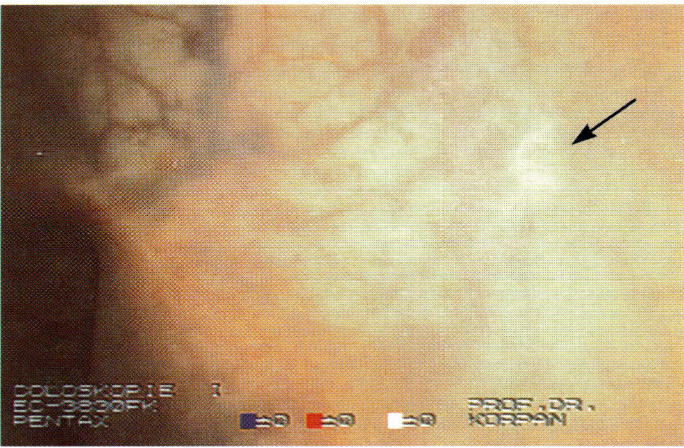

Fig. 21.4a. TRC: Coloscopical examination shows the excellent results 1 year after cryosurgery in the same patient. Only a post-cryosurgical "track" can be observed. No recurrence or metastases following a 14-month observation period

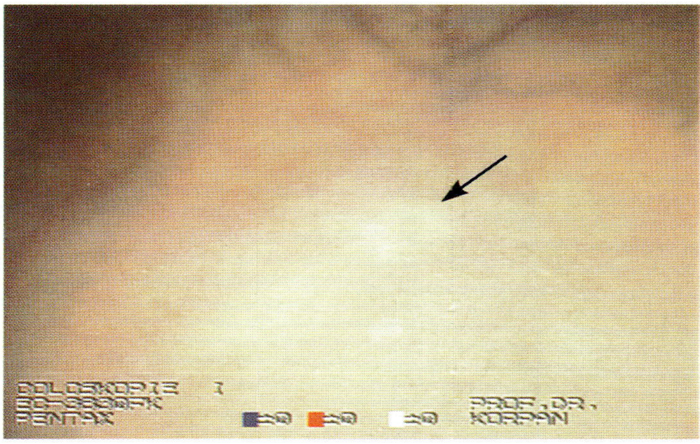

Fig. 21.4b. TRC: A post-cryosurgical "track" is clearly seen

of treatment modalities that include cryosurgery has led to increased survival as well as to the conservation of the sphincter muscle in most patients.

Superficial perianal skin cancer (e.g., squamous and basal cells) outside of the anal border can be effectively treated using the cryosurgical operating technique, so that the best results can be achieved in this patient group.

The treatment of Bowen's disease is a good indication for cryosurgery, with control of the margins. In the absence of the invasive tumor, Paget's disease can be treated with cryosurgery without skin grafting. Numerous biopsies of the edges are crucial. For malignant non-invasive tumors of the anal regions in the early stages a local cryosurgical procedure has been shown to be successful (Figs. 21.5–21.8).

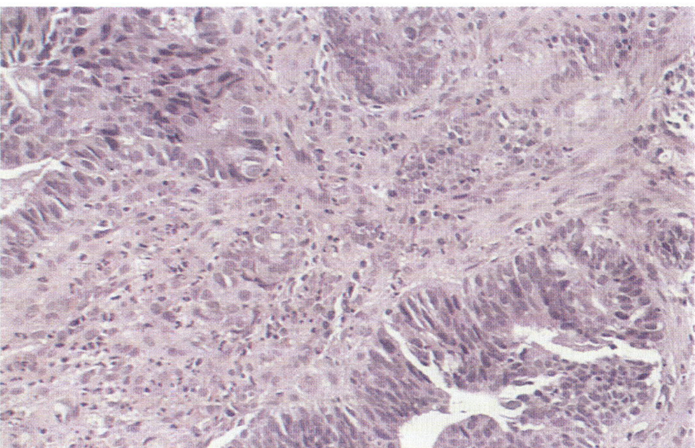

Fig. 21.5. Cancer of the anal region, 85-year-old woman. Histological section of a tubular adenocarcinoma of the colon, well to moderately well differentiated, infiltrating the muscularis mucosae between bundles of smooth muscle fibers. Hematoxylin and eosin staining. Magnification x600

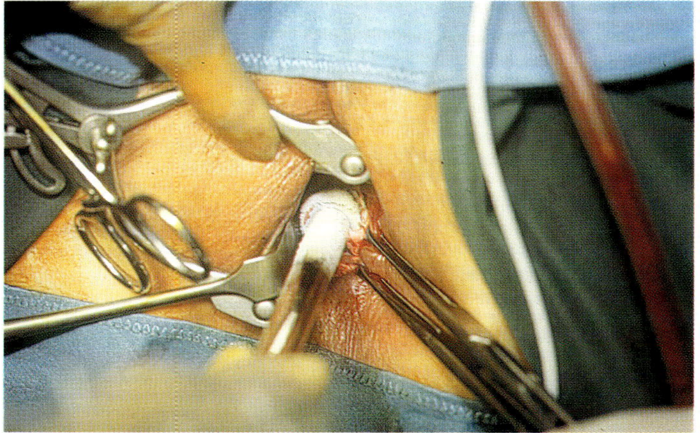

Fig. 21.6. Same patient. Base view of the technique of transanal cryosurgery (TAC), showing a disc probe 40 mm in diameter which is placed on the tumor mass at a temperature of −180°C for 3 min, with spinal anesthesia

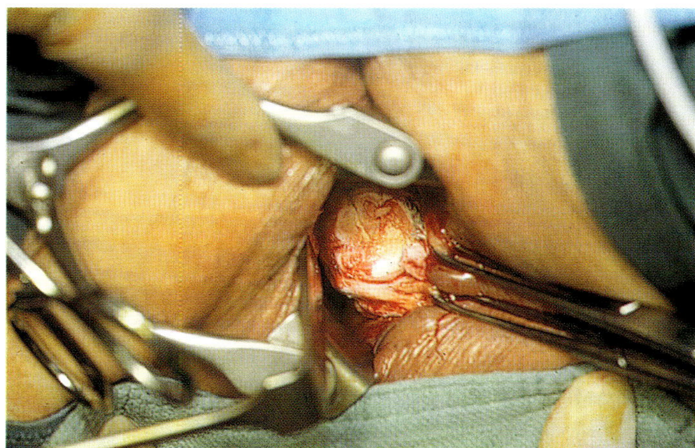

Fig. 21.7. Same patient. The post-cryosurgical zone immediately after the thawing of the cryoprobe measures 64 mm in diameter. The formed post-cryosurgical zone is clearly demarcated. A double freeze-thaw cycle was used

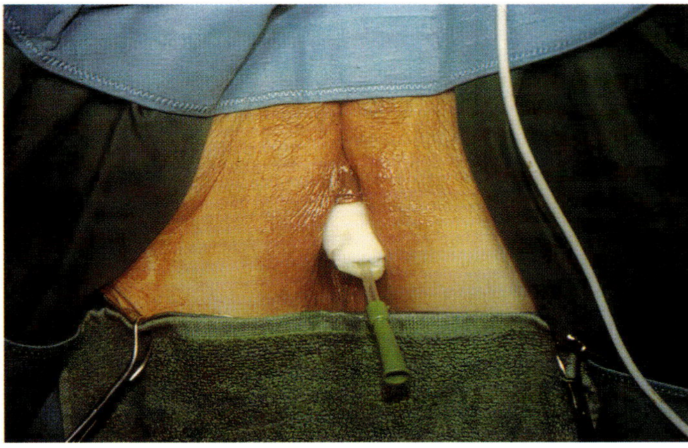

Fig. 21.8. TAC: Final local appearance, immediately after the cryosurgery in the same patient. View of the post-cryosurgical wound. No postoperative bleeding

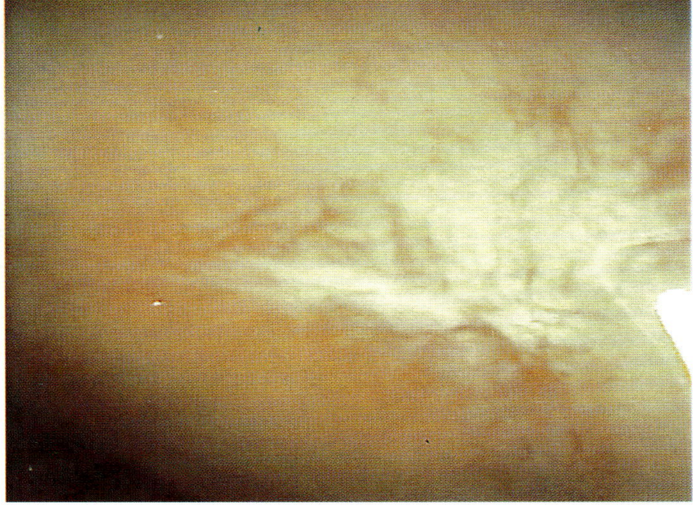

Fig. 21.9b. TAC: A post-cryosurgical "track" is clearly seen

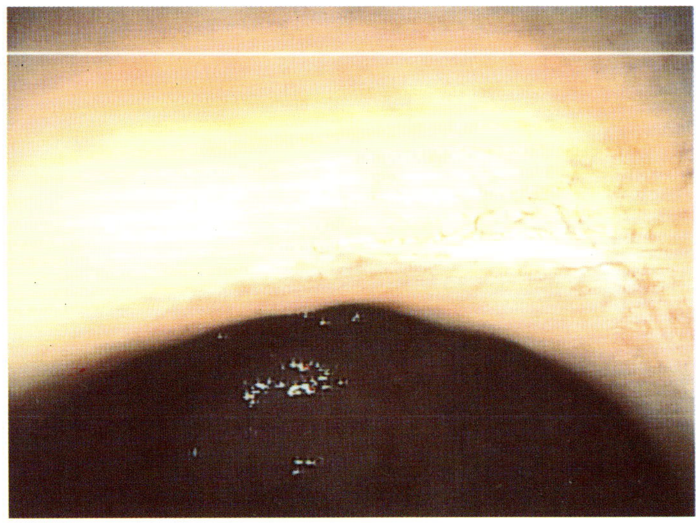

Fig. 21.9a. TAC: Coloscopic examination shows the excellent results 6 months after cryosurgery in the same patient. Only the post-cryosurgical "track" is visible. No recurrence or metastases following a 10-month observation period

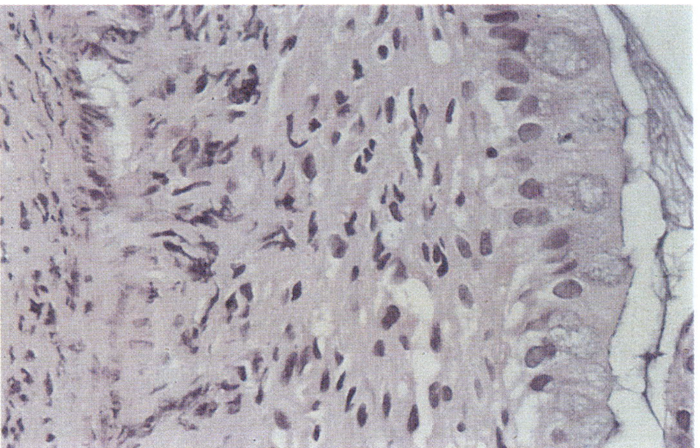

Fig. 21.10. Tumor-free mucosa of the colon, no inflammation worth mentioning 6 months after cryosurgery. Hematoxylin and eosin staining. Magnification ×200

Patients with recurring anal carcinoma after conventional surgery can be treated with cryosurgery in the framework of a multi-modality treatment. Such treatment including cryosurgery for locally advanced primary cancer of the anal canal can be a good palliative procedure, and in some cases even a curative method.

It may be expected that cryosurgery will already in the near future play a substantial role in patients with rectal and anal cancer.

22. Acute Total Body Hypothermia in Cryosurgery

Georgij G. Prokhorov with contributions by D. G. Prokhorov, A. P. Andreev, O. A. Litvinov, and A. V. Vlasova

22.0 Introduction

Cryosurgery as a method of malignant tumor destruction substantially expanded the opportunities for treatment of patients with incurable tumors and is successfully used in clinical practice. Cryosurgical methods are very effective in cases of extensive bilobar damage to the liver and spread of metastases into a portal fissure, where the possibilities for traditional surgical interventions are limited (Korpan 1998). The application of high-power cryosurgical equipment allows the successful solution of technical problems related to the destruction of large malignant tumors. When performing large-volume cryoablation, however, there is a real threat of severe complications due to acute total-body overcooling of the patient, which is clinically termed cryogenic shock (Morris 1998).

To understand the mechanisms of the occurrence and pathogenesis of cryogenic shock it is necessary to correctly understand the basics of cryosurgical intervention in terms of thermophysics as well as typical responses of the human body to acute total body hypothermia (ATBH).

22.1 Cryo-Treatment as General Cold Trauma

The thermophysical basis of cryosurgical operations is of practical interest. At present cryogenic destruction of tumors of large volume is carried out with equipment in which liquid nitrogen or argon are the cooling agents. The use of large amounts of the cooling agent may prove to be fatal to the patient. When six 4-mm cryoprobes are used simultaneously, an ice ball of 25–250 ml volume is formed, the temperature in its center being −186°C. The temperature on the surface of an ice ball is −4°C to −7°C, and the area of the surface which participates in the heat exchange between the cooled tissues and the whole body is 200 cm^2. An ice ball is surrounded by tissues of a local hypothermia zone, in which the microcirculation is maintained and there is an actual heat exchange between cryosystem and the patient.

The continuous work of the cryosystem at maximum power for 5–10 min is required for the complete formation of an ice ball. This time is reduced in case of close location of different probes and is increased with greater distance between them. The rate of ice ball formation is influenced by the local vascularization, especially the presence of large arteries in the area of ball formation. The process of ice spread ceases when the intensity of warming of an ice ball surface appears to be equal to the intensity of cooling from cryogenic probes.

Exposure of the tumor to low temperatures for a sufficient period of time is known to be necessary. Most researchers believe the minimal period of exposure to the lowest temperature to be not less than 10 min. During this period there is a continuous passage of liquid nitrogen to the cryoprobes.

The next stage of the operation is either active or passive thawing of the zone of cryoablation and repeated freezing, with the formation of an ice ball during a 10-min exposure. The formation of a ball at the second cycle occurs 3–5 min faster, the size of the ice ball is insignificantly larger, and the surface temperature is 5–7°C lower than during the first freezing cycle.

The size of a tumor is another major factor determining the total amount of cooling. For example, the destruction of a 15-cm tumor requires a change in position five times of 3.85 mm cryoneedles. There should be a double freeze-thaw cycle for each probe position.

It is obvious that cooling inevitably influences the total body temperature balance of the patient in the case of cryoablation of large-volume tumors. Severe complications following extensive cryoablation, resulting in lethal outcomes in the hours following the operation, are reported in the literature. A review of outcomes of cryosurgery on the liver (Morris 1998) has shown that the cause of lethal outcomes in 18% of cases is the development of cryoshock. Severe impairment of blood coagulation following cryogenic operations has been also described.

In spite of the fact that cryosurgery has been applied in oncology since 1961, the problem of postoperative total body hypothermia has became most important during the last decade, for the following reasons. First of all it is associated with the technical improvement of the cryoequipment as well as with advances in anesthesiology, that allowed the cryosurgical treatment of patients with large tumors. ATBH in cryosurgery is associated with underlying operational trauma, intravascular large volume infusions and anesthesia. It is difficult to study the pathogenesis of ATHB in cryosurgery because clinical evidence is lacking. At the same time there is a great deal of data on clinical experience with the treatment of ATBH. Not only clinical but also experimental studies deal with this problem.

22.2 Acute Cold Trauma in Medicine

ATBH has been known since the beginning of the 18th century from the descriptions of sea accidents in northern waters. Following the immersion of a person into cold water there is an intensive cooling of his body which can result in death within an hour (Carter 1995). In this situation the cooling rate of a human corresponds on a whole to that observed during extensive cryosurgical operations. For this reason, it is extremely important to acquire the necessary knowledge to manage ATBH.

Most researchers distinguish successive stages of hypothermia, which correspond to the mild, moderate, severe and most severe degree of cold injury. The decrease in rectal temperature serves as a criterion of the severity of hypothermia. In the literature, different researchers report various boundary values for rectal temperature. The severity of ATBH changes can be estimated by rectal temperature (see Table 22.1). These values are related to healthy individuals of young age as a rule. When performing large-volume cryosurgical operations, however, we usually deal with weak elderly patients. Taking this into account, we cannot consider the above data as absolute.

Blood circulation, lung ventilation, metabolism and other main vital factors in ATBH have been studied by Dubois (1937), Grosse-Brockhoff (1959), Eagan (1960), Joern et al. (1970), Akimov et al. (1977), Pokrovski et al. (1984), Burton (1995), Musacchia (1984).

The period during which adaptive mechanisms appear to be most effective has been referred to as a phase of compensation by Stark and Gollins. This phase corresponds to a mild degree of ATBH. The temperature of the "nucleus" of the body (rectal temperature at a depth of 10 cm) remains normal, but adaptive mechanisms become more pronounced. The reserves providing maintenance of thermal homeostasis are activated. This leads to stress response accompanied by discharge of catecholamines and glucocorticoids and increase in pulse and respiratory rate as well as in blood pressure. The activation of metabolic processes, hyperadrenalinemia, reflex spasm of skin vessels, physiologic tremor accompanied by contractile thermogenesis, and changes in diuresis are of compensatory character.

It is clear that for patients under anesthesia quick mobilization of the above protective responses is impossible. Here the action of thermoregulatory mechanisms appears to be possible only following a decrease in body temperature. The permissible fluctuations of the internal temperature of the brain are known to be 0.07–0.10°C (Lomber 1996). Hence, brain stem divisions responsible for the support of homeothermy possess a very high level of sensitivity to temperature fluctuations. The triggering of mechanisms of enhancing thermoproduction in response to blood temperature reduction takes some hours. As a result the patient in surgery seems to be physiologically unprotected against developing iatrogenic hypothermia.

The phase of decompensation (exhaustion) originally corresponds to a moderate degree of cold injury, the criterion of which is decrease of rectal temperature to 35–36°C. The human body is able to restore normal temperature within 18 hours after cooling ceases.

Hypothermia first alters calcium ion exchange between cells and interstitial space (Souilem 1995), and the synthesis of adenosine triphosphate is slowed down (Hochahka 1986). Disintegration of metabolic processes, activation of tissue enzymes and further calcium exchange disorders occur. Calcium transport directed against electric potential and concentration gradient are the most energy consuming and vulnerable processes when temperature is reduced.

The maintenance of temperature is important even from the point of view of simple maintenance of the rate of biochemical reactions. A reduction in body temperature of 1°C results in oxygen consumption reduction of 5–7% due to the suppression of basal metabolism (Rogers 1971). The slowing down of metabolic processes leads to even greater reduction of thermoproduction. To combat hypothermia the human body therefore must overcome a double barrier – restoration of metabolism with the subsequent restoration of tempera-

Table 22.1. The severity of ATBH (rectal temperature)

Severity/ Authors	E. Delorme (1956)	G. Klinzevich (1973)	A. Chudacov (1999)
Mild	30–35	32–34	N
Moderate	25–28	30–32	35–36
Severe	15–20	24–30	33–34
Most severe	–	< 24	< 33

ture. Nobles et al. (1990) described the mechanism of a "futile cycle". The term "futile" is considered from the point of view of synthesis of adenosine triphosphate, but it is due to metabolic thermoproduction that homeothermal organisms are capable of maintaining a constant temperature.

According to A. Chudakov (1999) there is consecutive triggering of a pathogenic chain of events, such as suppression of microcirculation (capillary stasis, venous and arterial spasm, sludge syndrome), impairment of the blood coagulation system (hypercoagulation, microthrombosis) and early cold hemolysis.

Increased oxygen consumption in the phase of "incomplete compensation" while the temperature is decreasing, aggravates hypoxia of tissues, with subsequent pericellular and perivasal edema. Hyperosmolar plasma has high viscosity that worsens its rheologic properties. The temperature reduction also considerably worsens the plastic properties of erythrocytes when passing along the capillaries. In this respect the results of clinical studies (Chudakov 1999) are of some interest. They demonstrated that high initial erythrocyte count in a patient is a negative factor predisposing to the most severe hypothermal traumas.

Vital system functions can be inhibited, with the development of multiple organ failure against a background of microcirculation disturbances. The direct action of cold on the permeability of capillary walls plays an important role in the formation of mechanisms of edema. Owing to loss of plasma volume, extracellular liquid is increased and there is an increase of viscosity of blood.

Hemolysis occurs in areas of local hypothermia. In cryosurgery this area can be a region surrounding an ice ball, where tissue temperature is within the range of −6°C to 37°C. The blood constituents in this region are exposed to intensive cooling and mechanical action by ice crystals. As a result an impairment occurs, which is associated with hemoglobinemia aggravating kidney, liver, heart and brain function disorders.

The phase of decompensation in cold trauma corresponds to the severity of cold injury. The rectal temperature falls to 33°C to 32°C. The restoration of normal body temperature is not possible until 24 hours after the exposure to cold has ended. The decompensation phase is accompanied by the suppression of basic vital functions, the inhibition of metabolism and the progression of general hypothermia (Cannon 1963; Milton 1967; Wainberg 1993). As a result there is an impairment of main adaptation mechanisms and homeostasis disorder (Ohkubo 1974; Mahood 1978), which result in the beginning of the process of morphological transformation (Carter 1995).

The clinical findings of hypothermal damage to the central nervous system manifest as general weakness, adynamia, speech confusion and dysarthria, movement disturbances, trismus, euphoria, depression, delirium, hallucinations, and loss of consciousness. The respiratory rate increases to 26–28 per min, there is rarely dry cough with scanty viscid sputum and bronchospasm. Rough respiration with dry rales is auscultated.

The patients show an accelerated pulse rate (up to 145 per min); the systolic pressure increases while diastolic pressure may be reduced.

The clinical laboratory findings show various changes. The number of erythrocytes appears to be increased up to $5.6 \times 10^{12}/l$, while hemoglobin rises up to 160 g/l. As hypothermia progresses, the tendency to augmentation of these findings remains, and hyperglycemia and glucosuria appear. Hyperglycemia is likely to be associated with stress response to cold and represents a compensatory response, which would encourage restoration of body temperature at the expense of enhanced metabolism. These compensatory mechanisms remain inactivated, however, because of the metabolism inhibition. Glucose not metabolized remains in the blood in high concentration, which is discharged with the urine. The hyperglucosemia is always manifest in patients during hypothermia. The initial rise in glucose level can be caused by stress. It is necessary, however, to take into account that tissues are not capable of utilizing glucose even at the usual rate owing to processes of metabolism inhibition. As a result extreme hyperglycemia and glucosuria occur.

The production of hyperosmolar components in the body contributes to survival under low temperature conditions. Hyperglycemia is the factor that increases cell resistance to freezing. Similarly, polyuria results in formation of hyperosmolar components capable of protecting tissues and cells from damage at cooling. At the same time the above shifts in the osmotic status of a body exert a negative action on the activity of the cardiovascular system and the microcirculation.

Under these conditions further metabolism inhibition and centralization of blood circulation occur, the microcirculation disturbances becoming more pronounced. The coagulogram shows typical changes, such as increase of recalcification time, rise of fibrinogen concentration up to 5.25 g/l, increase of tolerance to heparin. The thromboelastogram demonstrates a decrease of clot retraction time and clot formation time, and increase of maximum plasticity of thrombocytes. As disturbances progress, the disseminated intravascular coagulation syndrome develops with the accompanying micro- and macrothromboses. In addition to the electrolyte imbalance of calcium, there are severe balance disorders between potassium and sodium ions. Plasma concentration of free hemoglobin and iron ions increases, which encourages the development of a ferrite collapse.

Laboratory findings of hypothermia are as follows: hemoconcentration, hyperproteinemia, and rise of hematocrit. The blood test reveals an increase in erythrocytes and hemoglobin concentrations as well as a mild degree of leukopenia, hypokalemia in various degrees of severity, thrombocytopenia and disseminated intravascular coagulopathy developing later.

The gas composition values are difficult to estimate, since they are calculated for a temperature of 37°C. The hemoglobin dissociation curve is displaced to the left. Blood PO_2 is reduced.

There is a shift in the acid-base balance to decompensated metabolic acidosis.

The concentration of bilirubin (in general, of its direct fraction) and the activity of transferases rise moderately. A rise in creatinine and urea levels is observed. Proteinuria correlates with the gravity of cold injury.

ECG records repolarization phase disorder in 70% of the patients, in 7.7% of them right atrium arrhythmia is recorded. Judging from results of rheocardiography, the increase in the severity of cooling is accompanied by an increase in hemodynamic and cardiac rhythm impairment and increase of blood pressure.

The impairment of respiration frequently is manifest as a hyperventilation syndrome. Acute urine retention develops, a narcotic effect of cold on the central nervous system is evident.

In the phase of irreversible changes the patients are in coma, which corresponds to a severe degree of ATBH. In this state the body is not capable of restoring temperature balance by itself even after the discontinuation of cooling. Rectal temperature falls below 32°C. Respiration is slowed to 10 per min and becomes shallow. ECG records diffuse impairment of the repolarization phase in the myocardium. The arterial pressure reduces continuously. The rise of PO_2 and glucose concentration in the blood results from the deceleration of metabolic processes.

Hemorrhages in the vital organs, macrothrombosis of the aorta, heart and brain sinuses, and focal necrotic tissue changes are characteristic of the terminal phase. Acute cardiovascular, respiratory and cerebral disturbances, anuria, hepatic failure, pulmonary and brain edema, fibrillation and asystole precede the development of the terminal state and death of the patient.

Most scientists believe the cause of death due to ATBH to be vascular collapse following inhibition of vasomotoric center activity, and the cessation of cardiac and respiratory activity (Bullord and Rapp 1970; Simon and Iriki 1971). Death due to ATBH is inevitable when body temperature has fallen to +24°C. However, some unique cases of survival following a body temperature decrease to +18°C have been reported (Steele 1996).

Results of transitory hypothermia are mixed. When patients with ATBH are given aid in due time, the pathological processes associated with hypothermia regress.

Typical renal function disorders following mild cold injury are manifest as microhematuria and transitory short-term proteinuria. Proteinuria is characterized by a moderate degree of injury (up to 66 mg/l); while in case of a severe degree of injury the level of proteins in the urine is 165 mg/l, which is accompanied by cylindruria, hematuria, and leukocyturia.

In severe ATBH the disturbances persist for two weeks thereafter. A rise in blood levels of urea and creatinin in moderate injury is observed for 5–6 days, in severe injury for up to 14 days after ATBH. Effective renal blood flow and glomerular filtration are shown to be reduced.

Changes in ECG in the form of repolarization changes described above persist for 2 days after ATBH. The Makster exercise test taken by the patients caused tachycardia and discomfort in the heart even on the 6th day, which can be assessed as signs of myocardial dystrophy.

Severe ATBH was characterized by hemoglobin levels of 161 mg/l during 24 hours, leukopenia transforming into leukocytosis.

Biochemical data demonstrated hepatic and renal function disorders 33 hours after ATBH. Mean total bilirubin levels increased almost twice (up to 38.5 mcmol/l), whereas conjugated bilirubin increased 3 times (from 6.8 up to 21.5 mcmol/l).

The levels of serum liver function parameters increased. AST activity increased from 0.60 to 1.48 mmol/h/l, and ALT activity increased from 0.48 to 1.68 ± 0.10 mmol/h/l. There was an increase in urea from 7.64 to 11.22 ± 0.20 mmol/l and an increase in creatinine from 106.7 ± 1.2 to 194.1 ± 2.5 mmol/l. The calcium concentration level decreased from 3.23 to 2.86 ± 0.03 mmol/l. Serum amylase increased significantly in the warming period. The patients commonly present the signs of catarrhal disorders, temperature rise to subfebrile levels, and the exacerbation of chronic inflammatory diseases.

"Cryogenic shock" as defined by surgeons refers to acute hemodynamic disturbances and coagulopathy, developing during cryosurgical operations. It is evident that mechanisms of shock development differ from those described above. Surgeons consider blood temperature reduction of vital organs to play a major pathogenic role.

Blood loss accompanying ATBH is the most essential factor of loss of body resistance to cold. At the same time, a syndrome of mutual aggravation develops, i.e., cold trauma slows down the wound healing and the wound decreases the body's resistance to cold. The elderly, women and children tolerate ATBH poorly (Lushicky et al. 1985).

Some authors studying ATBH as a result of immersion into cold water, define the condition in which the patient dies some minutes after immersion as cold shock. In contrast to cryogenic shock, cold shock is assumed to develop as a result of acute CNS depression due to a powerful stream of afferent impulses from the skin surface (Kumanichkin 1954).

Cryosurgical hypothermia has much in common with ATBH in cold water. However, there are some differences.

First of all, anesthesia is an important factor in the patient's protection against triggering a number of negative reflex responses as well as functional overloading of the nervous and endocrine systems. When external irritation due to cold as described above is absent, reflex mechanisms of cutaneous and muscular vascular spasms are not triggered to the degree which occurs at cooling in cold water. Anesthesia should have a cryoprotective action on the patient, by switching off negative emotional and stress responses. On the other hand, it is stress response that allows the body to activate natural mechanisms to combat hypothermia.

We believe that a similar negative action of anesthesia should be taken into account. Moreover, hypothermia can be effectively prevented with certain measures, which can be implemented some days before the operation. Among these we would like to emphasize the administration of triiodothyronine for preliminary cryoprotection.

It is necessary to recognize that the mechanism of damage to internal organs is the same, as it results from contact of tissues with cooled blood. The carrier of cold is circulating blood both in ATBH from cold water immersion and from cryosurgery. The mechanisms of functional disturbances of heart, kidneys, liver and brain are thought to be quite similar.

Cryogenic injury inflicted in patients in extensive surgery can be compared with ATBH developing in weakened patients suffering from combined mechanical injury. A most negative factor in these patients is operational trauma. Thus, even routine median laparotomy can cause serious immunological damage in oncologic patients. The blood loss adds to this trauma.

22.3 Treatment of ATBH

Passive and active warming techniques are being employed in the treatment of ATBH. After exposure to cold is discontinued, wrapping the patients in blankets, or warming them with other means available makes it possible to restore body thermal balance.

Active internal warming is also used. This is drinking of hot beverages or irrigation of the stomach with warm water, inhalation of warm inhalants, intravenous administration of warm solutions.

Double blind studies demonstrated the effectiveness of oral intake of ephedrine (1 mg/kg) and caffeine (2.5 mg/kg) as inducers of thermogenesis, enhancing oxygen consumption. The results obtained showed a rectal temperature decrease in ATBH to occur more rarely (by 40%) than in the control group.

The thermostabilizing effect of sidnocarb taken orally at a dose of 30 mg increases the period during which a person may be safely immersed into cold water (without rectal temperature reduction).

Ketamine and nembutal are the preferred anesthetic drugs. Antioxidants, alpha receptor antagonists, metronidazol, cytochrome C, antiadrenergic medications, carbohydrate metabolites and substances improving their utilization (glucose, saccharose, insulin, arginine, phenamine) have been administered in the warming period.

It has been shown that polyethyleneoxide of molecular weight 400–1500 improves the rheologic properties of blood and diminishes the negative consequences of ATBH. The administration of hyperbaric oxygenation following warming of patients may also have a positive effect.

According to Klincevich (1973) the administration of cytitone, lobeline, caffeine and alcohol is contraindicated until complete body warming has been achieved.

Experimental data have shown that the prevention of ATBH and its complications is possible several days prior to cooling. In particular, pyrogenal in a 0.05 mg/kg dose given one day prior to exposure resulted in better survival (by 30%) of mice in cold water. Triiodothyronine in a 2 mg/kg dose for 3 days prior to cooling increased the rate of animal self warming by 40%.

Thermogenesis inducers and stimulators recommended for the treatment and prophylaxis of ATBH in cold water could not as a rule be used for hypothermia correction in oncologic patients during cryosurgery.

22.4 Clinical Experience in ATBH Studies

Our clinical evidence is based on 52 cryosurgical operations for prostate cancer (42 patients) and extensive metastatic involvement of liver (10 patients). The area involved amounted to as much as 1700 cm^3. The maximum amount of liver involvement was 2% of total body weight. Bilobar damage and metastases spreading either to the portal fissure or to the hepatic veins were considered to be indications for cryosurgery.

A liquid nitrogen based cryounit (Cryotech LCS 3000) was employed for cryosurgery. Five cryoprobes of 3.85-mm diameter as well as a cryoprobe of 40-mm diameter for the destruction of surface tumors were used.

The operations were performed under general anesthesia with nitrous oxide with additional epidural anesthesia. Body temperature was continuously monitored with an electrical thermometer placed on the chest or in the rectum.

As a prophylactic measure against hypothermal complications solutions warmed to +38°C were infused in all the patients during the operation. Body warming was carried out with electric blankets and thermal ventilators.

As a preventive measure against coagulopathy frozen plasma was administered to the patients intraoperatively, while heparin in the dose of 10–15000 IU daily was given immediately following the operation.

The maximum duration of surgery was 9 hours 25 min. Twelve freeze-thaw cycles with the help of five 3.85 mm cryoprobes were performed during this operation. The mass of metastatic involvement of the liver in this case was 1.5 l, which amounted to 2% of the total body mass. Reduction of rectal temperature by 1°C was noticed 45 min following the beginning of cryosurgery.

Body temperature decreased by 4°C, reaching 32°C by the end of the operation. There was intraoperative blood loss of 1200 ml. Blood pressure and pulse rate did not change.

Postoperatively the patients were treated in the intensive care unit. Two hours after the operation the dressings were soaked with blood, a mean of 500 ml of hemorrhagic fluid was discharged through drains from the abdominal cavity, there was a continuous decrease in blood pressure. The patients also received hemotransfusions.

Although intensive external warming and intravenous infusions of warm solutions continued and body temperature increased by 2°C to reach 34°C, one patient died 12 hours following the operation because of acute cardiovascular failure.

The analysis of body temperature changes made intraoperatively demonstrated that heat loss differs in different patients and does not bear a direct association with tumor size and cryoablation duration. When metastases spread in the proximity of the wall of the vena cava inferior and the formed ice ball partially involved the vein, compressing it, temperature fell more quickly. In fact, the continuous action of 5 cryoprobes for 15 min caused a temperature decrease of 0.5°C. At the same time, when cryoablation of a subcapsular metastasis of the same size in the liver was performed with the clamping of the hepatoduodenal ligament, body temperature did not change. These results show that anatomic characteristics of the operative area and, above all, the intensity of regional vascularization are significant for the consequences of cold trauma.

Hegenauer et al. (1988) recommend temporary clamping of the hepatoduodenal ligament in cases when liver metastases are large.

Specialists in thermophysics and cryobiology participated in the studies to determine the largest permissible volumes of cryosurgical intervention. It is obvious that there is a thermophysical barrier in cryosurgery. The theoretical background required clinical evidence. Special experiments were carried out with the aim of obtaining information on the temperature difference between an ice ball and the patient's body.

The experimental work included thermometric studies and monitoring of temperature in different areas inside an ice ball as well as in the tissues surrounding it, using 3.85-mm probes. Both single probe and multiple probes located at different distances from one another were used.

Control thermometry in the area of cryoablation with standard thermocouples of a cryosurgical system was performed. Body temperature of the patients was continuously monitored during surgery and postoperatively. The results of temperature control served as the basis for the subsequent calculations of thermal exchange parameters between the probes and the patient's body, according to thermophysical laws.

Calculations made by us showed that the amount of heat energy absorbed by the cryounit at the heat exchange zone around the ice ball, is equal to the amount of heat given off by the patient's body. Further mathematical calculations made it possible to set up formulas to determine body temperature changes depending upon the duration of cryosurgery and different numbers of cryoprobes.

Figure 22.1 shows the body temperature decrease in patients weighing 75 kg by the duration of operation, and by the number (one, three or five) 3.85 mm cryoprobes used.

The results of the study demonstrated that the duration and intensity of cryoablation has the greatest influence on the thermal balance of the patient. Thus the interrelationship of the parameters was complex. Continuous simultaneous use of five cryoprobes for 30 minutes resulted in a decrease in body temperature from 37.0°C to a potentially fatal level of 34.0°C. The simultaneous operation of three probes located at peaks of a triangle caused a fall in the patient's temperature by 3°C within four hours. The single cryoprobe did not have an appreciable influence on the thermal balance of the patient's body.

More powerful cryogenic equipment has advantages that allow the duration of exposure to cold to be reduced and to destroy tumors of large size. The interruption of blood circulation in the liver during cryosurgery by clamping the hepatic artery and portal vein also seems to contribute to reduction of the duration of hypothermia. The correlation between theoretical evidence and clinical findings made it possible to determine the maximum tumor volume that can be subjected to double freezing without the development of ATBH. This tumor volume has been found to be 0.7% of the total body mass of the patient. In case the total tumor mass exceeds this volume, it is necessary to apply effective cryoprotective methods.

The clinical consequences of ATBH were found to be various. They are always superimposed on the consequences of operational trauma and of inevitable damage to healthy liver tissue, and resorption of a cryodestroyed tumor mass.

The development of a moderate leukocytosis and an increase in activity of ALT and AST was observed. Anemia and a decrease in fibrinogen and platelets are influenced by volume of blood loss. Hemoglobinemia and hemoglobinuria were also typical for cryosurgical trauma and were due to the development of cold hemolysis at the

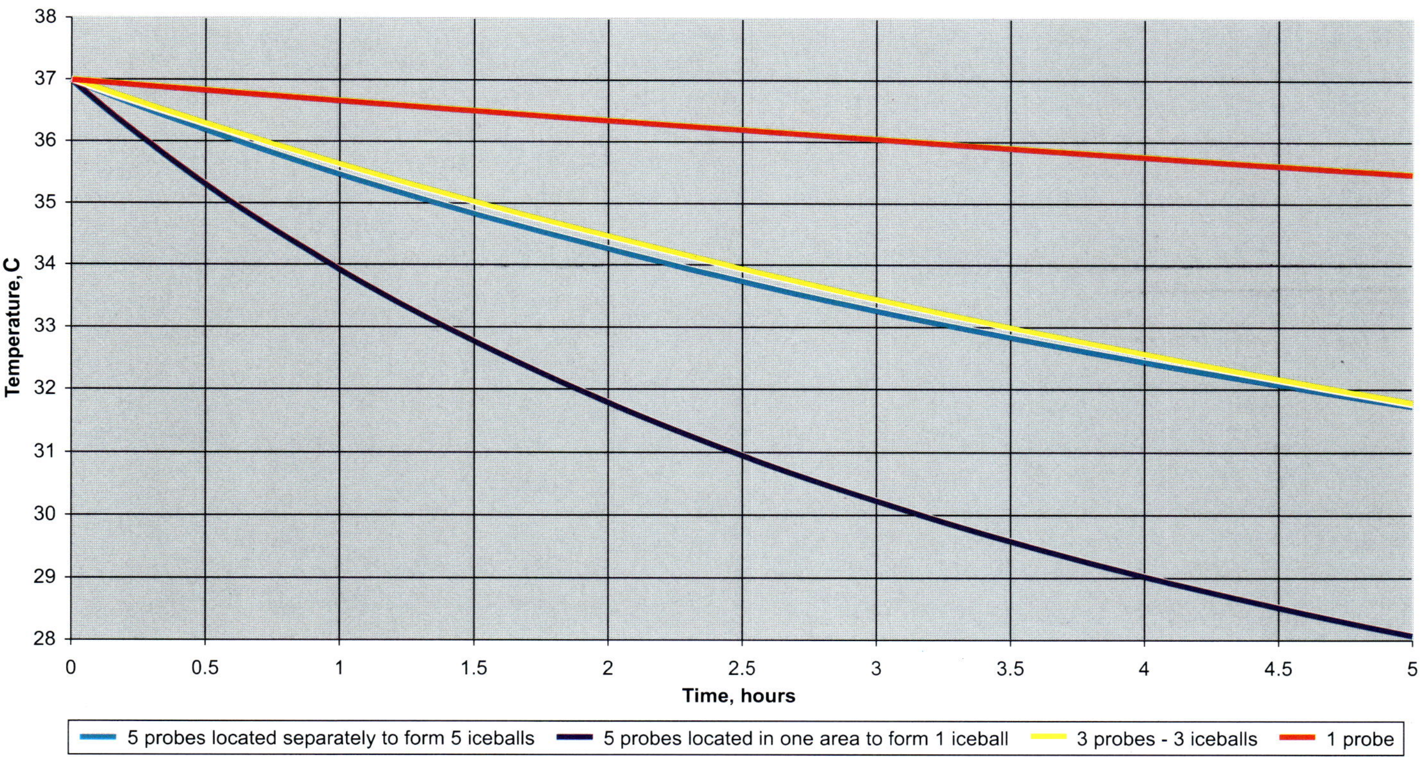

Fig. 22.1. Decrease of human body temperature during cryosurgical operation

cryodestruction area. This factor led to an increase in urea and creatinine levels in the blood.

The cryosurgical intervention aggravated renal function especially in long-standing cases.

All patients had subfebrile temperatures for up to 1 month postoperatively. The main feature of this hyperthermia was the absence of severe toxemia which is characteristic of severe infection complications. Antibiotic therapy did not influence significantly the temperature pattern. At the same time eosinophilia was seen that reflected complex changes in the immune status of the patients.

In considering the above data we arrived at the conclusion that cryogenic hypothermia has much in common with ATBH in cold water as far as clinical and laboratory findings are concerned.

The prevention of complications from cryo-ATBH should start with a preliminary estimation of the volume of the operation and assessment of its safety in terms of the probable development of cryogenic shock.

The indications for cryosurgery need to be thoroughly assessed in case tumor volume approaches 1% of body mass. If this volume is exceeded, radical tumor cryoablation (double freezing cycle) is not possible. Furthermore, cryosurgical shock may develop.

The use of active prophylaxis and preventive treatment of ATBH enables the above-mentioned limitations to be overcome and the indications for cryosurgery of large volume tumors to be extended.

The main prophylactic and treatment measures in ATBH occurring following cryosurgery are as follows: warming of the patient, prophylaxis for acute cardiovascular failure, correction of rheological blood properties, control of disseminated intravascular coagulation syndrome, and maintenance of forced diuresis.

The above measures are achieved by wrapping the patient in an electric blanket, application of heaters and thermal ventilation, aspiration of cold air from the cryodestruction area in the abdominal cavity, isolation of cooled area from surrounding organs with gauze pads, blood flow restriction at the site of cryoprobes by clamping the vessels, and application of the cryosurgical technique at maximum power when forming the ice ball.

Infusion fluids should be warmed to +37°C to +39°C. Protein solutions, native and frozen plasma are preferable. Dosage and rate of administration of anticoagulants and diuretics must be discussed with anesthesiologists.

The combination of cardiotonic medications, vasopressors, and diuretics for diuresis support should be set at levels not less than 100 ml per hour. This is of importance because the patients as a rule have severe accompanying abnormalities, anemia, hypoproteinemia and immunodeficiency.

Extracorporeal warming and high-frequency warming techniques allow full protection of the patient against ATBH during cryosurgery. Extracorporeal circulation apparatus allows control of the patient's body temperature with the purpose of creating controlled hypothermia, especially in cardiac operations.

Another way to solve the problem of prevention and treatment of cold injury is the application of general high-frequency hyperthermia in the treatment of oncologic patients (Balluzek et al. 1998).

At present, it is not difficult from the technical point of view to raise the body temperature to any given level. The problem is the necessity of cryosurgical interventions in patients with large tumors. Disseminated tumors seen by cryosurgeons as a rule represent the final stage of disease.

We believe that the problems encountered in ATBH in cryosurgery are closely connected with major problems in oncology, and will help oncologists find solutions in the future.

22.5 Conclusion

Acute total body cryohypothermia is a dangerous complication of cryoablation of large tumors. The indications for the cryosurgery are restricted if the volume of the tumor is more that 1% of the mass of the patient's body. The pathogenesis of acute total body cryohypothermia is characterized by homeostasis disorders, which are life threatening to patients, but do not have any specific clinical symptoms. Only the decrease of rectal temperature is a reliable test for cryohypothermia. The complications of hypothermia may be overlooked among clinical consequences of disease and operational trauma, and they demand special attention to be correctly diagnosed treated and prevented.

References

1. Akimov GA, Alishev V, Vershtein V, Bukov V (1977) General cooling of a body. Leningrad.
2. Balluzek FV, Morosova SI, Bolmusov JD et al. (1998) Hyperthermia in oncology - International congress "Hyperthermia in Clinical Oncology" 28–30 May 1998, Venice, Italy, 1998, p. 30.

3. Budd GM, Warhaft N (1966) Body temperature, shivering, blood pressure and heart rate during a standard cold stress in Australia and Antarctica. J Physiol 186: 216–232.
4. Bullord RW, Rapp GM (1970) Problems of body heat loss in water immersion. Aerosp Med 41. 1269–1277.
5. Burton AK, Edholm OG (1955) Man in a cold environment. London. p. 340.
6. Cannon RN (1963) Cold immersion J Roy Naval Med Serv 2: 88–92.
7. Carter N (1995) Terminal borrowing behavior a phenomenon of lethal hypothermia. Int J Legal Med 108(2): 116–119.
8. Chudakov A, Isakov V, Doronin Yu (1999) Acute Total Body Hypothermia in cold water. Saint-Petersburg, Russia.
9. Delorme E (1956) Hypothermia. Anasthesia 3: 11–14.
10. Dubois E (1951) Many different temperatures of human body and its parts West J Surg 59: 476–490.
11. Eagan CJ (1960) Unilateral cold adaptation to recurrent ice-water immersion. Physiologist 3: 51–56.
12. Grosse-Brockhoff F, Schoedel W (1942) The picture of acute super-cooling in animal experiments. Arch Exp Path Berlin 201: 417–422.
13. Hegenauer K et al. (1998) Optimization of cryosurgery of paracaval hepatic metastases by portal inflow occlusion. Abstract book of X World Congress of Cryosurgery 28 Oct –2 Nov. 1998. Orlando Florida 54–55.
14. Hochahka PW (1986) Defense strategies against hypoxia and hypothermia. Science 231 (4755): 234–241.
15. Joern AT, Shurlly JT, Brooks CA, Quenter CA, Pierce CM (1970) Short-term changes in sleep patterns on arrival at the South Polar plateau Arch Intern Med 125: 649–654.
16. Ivanov KP (1990) Basics of body energetic: theoretical and practical aspects. Science, Leningrad.
17. Klincevich GN (1973) Acute total body hypothermia. Leningrad.
18. Korpan N et al. (1998) Hepatic cryosurgery: long-term survival after palliative surgical cancer treatment, Part 2. Abstract book of X World Congress of Cryosurgery 28 Oct –2 Nov. 1998. Orlando, Florida 69–70.
19. Kumanichkin SD (1954) Acute total body hypothermia in cold water. Leningrad.
20. Lomber SG (1996) Learning and recall of form discrimination during reversible cooling deactivation of ventral-posterior suprasylvian cortex in the cat. Proc Natl Acad Sci USA 94(4): 1654–1658.
21. Lushicki MA, Myasnikov A, Zayceva K (1985) Clinical–histo-enzymological investigations of the wound process, combined with overcooling of a body in cold water. In: Cold Trauma, Leningrad, pp. 41–42.
22. Mahood JM, Evans A (1978) Accidental hypothermia, DIC and pancreatitis. NZ Med J 87: 283–284.
23. Milton C, Gee Gin K (1967) Human acclimatization to cold water immersion. Arch Environ Health 15: 568–579.
24. Morris D (1998) Hepatic cryotherapy – as well-established treatment for primary and secondary liver cancer. Abstract book X World Congress of Cryosurgery. 28 Oct – 2 Nov. 1998. Orlando Florida 58–59.
25. Musacchia XJ (1984) Hypothermia. Cryobiol 21(2): 583–599.
26. Nobles CD, Brown GC, Olive PN, Brand MD (1990) Futile cycle in mitochondria. J Biol Chem 265 (7): 12903–12909.
27. Ohkubo Y (1974) Basal metabolism and other physiological changes in the Antarctic. In: Edholm OG, Quenderson E (eds) Polar human biology. Year book Med Publishers (Chicago): 161–170.
28. Pokrovski VM, Sheih-Zade Yu, Vovereidt V (1984) Heart during hypothermia. Leningrad.
29. Rogers TA (1971) The clinical course of survival in the Arctic. Hawaii Med J 30: 31–34.
30. Simon E, Iriki M (1971) Ascending neurons highly sensitive to variations of spinal cord temperature. J Physiol 63(3): 415–417.
31. Souilem O (1995) Effects of moderate cooling on contractile responses in mouse vas deferens and it relations to calcium NS Arch Pharmacol 352(3): 337–345.
32. Stark IE, Gollins JV (1977) Methods in clinical trails in asthma. Dis Chest 71(4): 225–244.
33. Steele MT (1996) Forced air speeds rewarming in accidental hypothermia. Ann Emerg Med 27(4): 479–484.
34. Wainberg ED (1993) Hypothermia. Ann Energ Med 2(2): 370–377.

23. Cryomassage

Irina R. Khramova

23.0 Introduction

Cryomassage is the repeated short application of superficial cold on healthy body tissue with a cryoinstrument to accelerate the process of stimulation and biological regeneration in the case of an anemic or hyperemic skin surface.

23.1 Technique

A cryoinstrument driven by liquid nitrogen is used for the cryomassage. The cryoinstrument consists of a special lightweight bottle. The special cryoprobes are cylindrically formed. Cryoprobes varying in size with a diameter ranging from 5 to 30 mm can be used so that different parts of the body can be effectively massaged. A temperature ranging from −40°C to −50°C is applied. The cryomassage cycle lasts for 1 to 3 min. A complete treatment includes 3 to 6 cycles, once a month.

Cryomassage is especially indicated in the case of dry or 'aged and withered skin'. Why so? Because no injury to lipid- and protein-containing complexes and no vascular stasis in the skin occurs in the course of this effective cryosurgical treatment.

The effectiveness of cryomassage is enhanced when the skin is cleansed beforehand.

Metabolic processes and microcirculation is improved in the course of this cryogenic procedure, regenerating the patient's anemic or hyperemic skin surface. As a general rule, a stimulation and biological regeneration process can be observed in the skin.

Under the microscope, a regenerated new skin layer – epidermis – consisting of 10 to 20 layers of cells is observed. In the regenerated epithelium one can make out the basal, thorn and horny skin layers. These histological changes resulting from the cryomassage therapy could form the basis for the treatment of baldness. Future studies will provide clinical results in this regard.

Subject Index

SpringerMedicine

Mario Campanacci

Bone and Soft Tissue Tumors

Clinical Features, Imaging, Pathology and Treatment

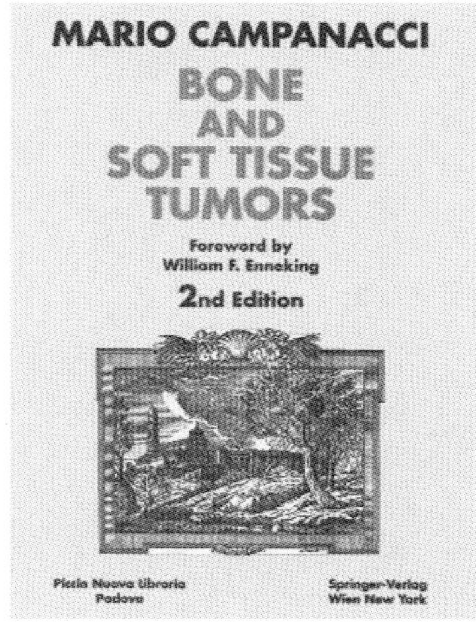

Foreword by William F. Enneking.
Second, completely revised edition.
1999. XX, 1319 pages. 1120 figures.
Hardcover DM 632,–, öS 4421,–, as of Jan. 2002 EUR 321,–
(Recommended retail prices)
All prices are net-prices subject to local VAT.
(Distribution rights: worldwide except Italy.
Jointly published with Piccin Nuova Libraria, Padova)
ISBN 3-211-83235-1

"This is an extraordinary book by an extraordinary author. Dr. Campanacci brings to the readers the vast experience in musculoskeletal oncology of the Rizzoli Orthopaedic Institute in Bologna. As such, he has had at his disposal the patient records, radiographs and pathologic material dating back to 1905. The wealth of clinical material that has been accumulated at the Rizzoli Institute, with exquisite documentation and maintenance is a unique resource and testimonial to not only the author but his predecessors. This book brings to the reader an almost unparalleled experience from one of the leading centers of musculoskeletal oncology in the world.
From the Foreword of William F. Enneking

This second english edition is an entirely new book. It has been thoroughly rewritten, from the first to the last word. About 30% of the pictures are new. The new book incorporates the accumulated personal experience of the author, covering over 20.000 inpatients and many more outpatients, the perusal of the literature of the last 10 years, the recent developments in imaging (particularly MRI), microscopic diagnosis (especially immunohistochemistry and electron microscopy) and the ultimate progress in surgical and non-surgical treatment modalities.
Mario Campanacci (1932–1999) was an orthopaedic surgeon and a pathologist with 40 years of experience (started in 1958 in the Laboratory of Pathology and Tumor Center of the Rizzoli Orthopaedic Institute) focused on musculoskeletal oncology. He was Professor of Orthopaedic Surgery and Pathology, University of Bologna, Director of the 1st Orthopaedic Clinic and of the Tumor Centre, Rizzoli Orthopaedic Institute, Bologna and Director of the Graduate School of Orthopaedics, University of Bologna.

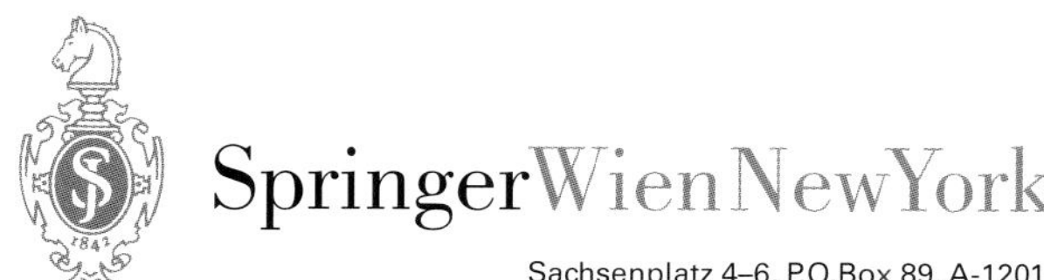

Springer-Verlag and the Environment